PRIDE VERSUS PREJUDICE

THE LITTMAN LIBRARY OF JEWISH CIVILIZATION

Dedicated to the memory of
LOUIS THOMAS SIDNEY LITTMAN
*who founded the Littman Library for the love of God
and as an act of charity in memory of his father*
JOSEPH AARON LITTMAN
and to the memory of
ROBERT JOSEPH LITTMAN
who continued what his father Louis had begun
יהא זכרם ברוך

'*Get wisdom, get understanding:
Forsake her not and she shall preserve thee*'
PROV. 4: 5

*The Littman Library of Jewish Civilization is a registered UK charity
Registered charity no.* 1000784

PRIDE VERSUS PREJUDICE

◆

Jewish Doctors and Lawyers in England, 1890–1990

◆

JOHN COOPER

London
The Littman Library of Jewish Civilization
in association with Liverpool University Press

The Littman Library of Jewish Civilization
Registered office: 4th floor, 7–10 Chandos Street, London WIG 9DQ

in association with Liverpool University Press
4 Cambridge Street, Liverpool L69 7ZU, UK
www.liverpooluniversitypress.co.uk/littman

Managing Editor: Connie Webber

Distributed in North America by
Oxford University Press Inc., 198 Madison Avenue,
New York, NY 10016, USA

First published 2003
First published in paperback 2012

Catalogue records for this book are available from the
British Library and the Library of Congress

ISBN 978–1–906764–42–5

Publishing co-ordinator: Janet Moth
Copy-editing: Gillian Bromley
Proof-reading: Cyril Cox
Index: John Cooper
Design: Pete Russell, Faringdon, Oxon.
Typeset by Footnote Graphics, Warminster, Wilts.

Printed and bound in Great Britain by
CPI Group (UK) Ltd., Croydon, CR0 4YY

*This publication has been supported
by a donation in memory of*

GEORGE J. WEBBER, LL.D.

*Barrister-at-law of the
Middle Temple and the Northern Circuit
sometime Reader in English Law,
University College London*

⚖

Author of *The Effect of War on Contracts* and
editor of the Fifth Edition of Batt's *Law of Master and Servant*;
he also wrote numerous articles, including:
'Natural Justice in English Case Law', 'The Reform of Legal Procedure',
'Safety of Tools and Employer's Liability', 'Trial by Newspaper',
'The Heritage of Jewish Law', and
'The Law and the Law Courts in the State of Israel'.

⚖

BORN IN MANCHESTER 1899
DIED IN LONDON 1982

⚖

Preface and Acknowledgements

I WOULD like to acknowledge the help of a number of archivists and librarians, in particular Esra Kahn and Aron Prys of the London School of Jewish Studies; Dalia Tracz of the Mocatta Library; and the staff at the British Library, the Law Society library, the Wellcome Library, and my local library in Swiss Cottage.

One discovery I made over the course of my researches was that the facilities for exploring the history of medicine are far superior to those existing for the study of the history of the legal profession; I would suggest, therefore, that there is a need for barristers and solicitors to set up a centre comparable to the Wellcome Library. I was fortunate, though, that my friend Graham Drucker allowed me to select books from his late brother Leon's collection; these provided many unexpected insights into the lives of Jewish lawyers.

Finally, I would like to thank all those who generously agreed to be interviewed and then tolerated what I had to say about them. The list of names is too long for them all to appear here, but everyone concerned is duly mentioned in the text and notes that follow. My thanks are also due to Mr David Freeman for allowing me to use material collected by his late wife Iris for her projected biography of Lord Goodman; to Dr Martin Sarner for making available data which he had compiled on London's Jewish doctors; to Dr Charles Daniels for giving me access to the pre-war records of the London Jewish Medical Society; to Dr Philip D'Arcy Hart for permitting me to look at records held by him; to Mrs Madeleine Gottlieb and her husband Craig for allowing me to inspect the papers of her late father Joseph Jackson; to Mrs Jessica Gillis for allowing me to see her husband's unpublished memoirs; and to Daniel Lightman, who gave me access to material on the career of his grandfather, Harold Lightman. My brother Rabbi Dr Martin Cooper has been a steady source of encouragement and help to me throughout the project. I have also benefited from the assistance of Judge Israel Finestein QC, Henry Grunwald QC, Dr Gerry Black, Dr Mervyn Goodman, Dr Joyce Bourne, Emma Klein, Aubrey Silverstone, Murray Freedman, and the late Monty Dobkin and Richard Sherrington.

I should like to record my deep gratitude to Connie Webber, managing editor of the Littman Library, for supporting this project and for her assistance throughout the development of the book, and to my editors Janet Moth and Gillian Bromley for ironing out infelicities in my original draft. If there are any errors of fact or judgement in the book, these faults are mine alone.

I want to thank my wife Judy for her sage counsel when I tried out some of my ideas on her, and for helping me to decipher Norman Bentwich's unintelligible diary entries. My daughter Flower and son Zaki and my brother-in-law Michael Teper sorted out problems with the word processor, and my nephew Jonathan Teper was a wizard with the software; for all this I am very grateful.

London JOHN COOPER
December 2001

Contents

Abbreviations

Medical Qualifications

BC, B.Ch., B.Chir.	Bachelor of Surgery
BM	Bachelor of Medicine
BS, Ch.B.	Bachelor of Surgery
DM	Doctor of Medicine
FRCP	Fellow of the Royal College of Physicians
FRCS	Fellow of the Royal College of Surgeons
FRS	Fellow of the Royal Society
LRCP	Licentiate of the Royal College of Physicians
LRCS	Licentiate of the Royal College of Surgeons
LSA	Licentiate of the Society of Apothecaries, London
MB	Bachelor of Medicine
MD	Doctor of Medicine
MRCP	Member of the Royal College of Physicians
MRCS	Member of the Royal College of Surgeons

Journals Cited in Footnotes

BMJ	*British Medical Journal*
JC	*Jewish Chronicle*

Introduction

M Y interest in Jews in the professions was awakened some years ago when I was browsing through an Australian rabbi's library which contained books on the history of Australian and New Zealand Jewry. From them I was astonished to learn of the difficulties placed in the way of refugee doctors from Germany and Austria wishing to requalify in these countries during the 1930s—difficulties so pronounced as almost to deny Jews any opportunity to follow a career as a lawyer or doctor in the glutted employment markets of the Western world during these years. Then there was my own family experience: one of my grandfathers was adamant in his opposition to my uncle's qualifying for a profession, seeing such a career as a well-trodden path to assimilation—a view that deterred many Jews from joining the professions. A third case that lodged in my memory was that of a high-flying Jewish surgeon in London after the Second World War, who—having grown up and qualified in England—was told that there was no place for him, as a Jew, in the most prestigious teaching hospitals. Over the years I have often wondered whether these were random facts or precious insights, and whether or not, with the requisite research, they could be woven into a coherent account. The answers are not straightforward, and therefore not easily summarized; indeed, the position has changed over time. Moreover, in surveying the history of the entry of Jews into the medical and legal professions there are many other factors to consider. Among them is the Jews' changing view of the prestige attached to each profession, the variations in their perception of the psychological and financial rewards to be gained from pursuing a career in medicine or the law, and the hierarchical structure of these professions. At the same time, just as England moved from being part of the British empire run by an elite contemptuous of immigrants, whom they viewed as inferior, so the Jews themselves imbibed new values. Furthermore, their class and status in today's multicultural society is no longer that of recent immigrants.

It would have been an impossible task to cover the history of Jews in all the principal professions. My choice to focus on medicine and the law was dictated in part by the factors mentioned above, in part for other practical and personal reasons. Medicine was the profession which Jews entered in the greatest numbers; moreover, it is well researched and the Wellcome Institute offers magnificent facilities for further research work. The law was of particular interest to me as the profession with which I was most closely acquainted in my own career as a solicitor.

So far there has been a paucity of books about Jews in the professions in England. A slim volume by Asher Tropp entitled *Jews in the Professions in Great Britain 1891–1991* covers all the professions, and as a consequence the author is unable to delineate in any detail the changing patterns of Jews' membership of the legal and medical professions. There is a magnificent book by Kenneth Collins, on Jews in the Scottish medical profession, *Go and Learn*; but this stops in 1945, and English conditions are sometimes depicted by other historians as differing widely from those pertaining in Scotland. Certain lacunae as far as English conditions are concerned are filled by Gerry Black's Ph.D. thesis, 'Health and Medical Care of the Jewish Poor in the East End of London 1880–1914' and his more recent *Lord Rothschild and the Barber* (2000). Apart from an important pioneering article by Phyllis Lachs on nineteenth-century Jewish barristers and Judge Finestein's in-depth survey of Sir George Jessel's career, little has been written about Anglo-Jewish lawyers. However, many of the trends in the professions in England are similar to those experienced in America, and more can be learned from the literature on the American legal profession, particularly Jerrold S. Auerbach's *Unequal Justice: Lawyers and Social Change in Modern America* and Erwin O. Smigel's *The Wall Street Lawyer*.[1]

This study also sets out to explain how an Anglo-Jewish immigrant population from eastern Europe, mainly proletarian in character, which arrived in England and Wales between 1880 and 1920 transformed itself socially and economically in the course of three generations. The founding fathers were principally tailors, cabinet-makers, street traders, and shopkeepers. Many of the children and grandchildren of these immigrants prospered in business enterprise, some of them founding companies with a national reputation; many others entered the professions of law and medicine. It is the latter with whom we are concerned.

Beginning with the Jewish doctors of the Victorian and Edwardian period, I seek to demonstrate why there were so few of them in England in comparison

---

[1] Asher Tropp, *Jews in the Professions in Great Britain 1891–1991* (London: Maccabeans, 1991); Kenneth Collins, *Go and Learn: The International Story of Jews and Medicine in Scotland* (Aberdeen: Aberdeen University Press, 1988); Gerry Black, 'Health and Medical Care of the Jewish Poor in the East End of London 1880–1914', Ph.D. diss. (Leicester University, 1987); id., *Lord Rothschild and the Barber* (London: Tymsder, 2000); Phyllis S. Lachs, 'A Study of a Professional Elite: Anglo-Jewish Barristers in the Nineteenth Century', *Jewish Social Studies*, 44 (1982), 125–34; Israel Finestein, 'Sir George Jessel, 1824–1883', *Transactions of the Jewish Historical Society of England*, 18 (1958), 243–83; Jerrold S. Auerbach, *Unequal Justice: Lawyers and Social Change in Modern America* (New York: Oxford University Press, 1972); id., 'From Rags to Robes: The Legal Profession, Social Mobility and the American Jewish Experience', *American Jewish Historical Quarterly*, 66/2 (Dec. 1976), 249–84; Erwin O. Smigel, *The Wall Street Lawyer: Professional Organization Man?* (Bloomington, Ind.: Indiana University Press, 1969).

with their numbers in Continental Europe. Notwithstanding some anti-semitism facing Jews trying to obtain hospital posts in the mid-nineteenth century, English and Welsh society was more open in the late Victorian and Edwardian years than it was to be between the two world wars, and a number of Jews rose to eminence in the medical profession, holding appointments as consultants in the London teaching hospitals and elsewhere. The next chapter is devoted to the entry of second-generation east European Jews—that is, the children of immigrants—into the medical profession. Having explained why medicine was so popular among young Jews from an immigrant background, and why it was more favoured as a career choice than the law, I show that the massive influx of Jews into the medical profession started during the First World War and continued into the 1920s and 1930s. Although there is a widespread belief among Anglo-Jewish historians that discrimination made entry into the medical profession difficult for Jews, finding a place in an English medical school was in fact—apart from a few isolated incidents—relatively straightforward for Jewish students during the inter-war period; however, problems arose when Jews from an immigrant background tried to obtain house appointments and staff positions in the leading London and provincial hospitals.

We next turn to the barristers of Victorian and Edwardian England. The Jewish giants of the Victorian Bar, men such as George Jessel, Judah Benjamin, and Arthur Cohen, devoted themselves to the practice of commercial and international law; they were followed by younger barristers, who likewise specialized in various aspects of commercial law or practised in the Chancery courts. Many of the prominent Jewish members of the Edwardian Bar were deeply involved in communal affairs and supplied much of the leadership of Anglo-Jewry. The number of Jews who held judicial office during the late Victorian and Edwardian eras was small, but between the world wars their number shrank still further, paralleling the dearth of consultant positions in teaching hospitals held by Jews with a positive Jewish identity. In Chapter 5 I explore the question whether the lack of Jews in the higher echelons of the legal profession had exclusively domestic causes or was connected with the rising tide of anti-semitism in Europe. If the number of Jews practising at the Bar increased in the years 1918 to 1939, very few of these new barristers came from east European Jewish families, and I attempt to explain why this was the case.

Between the chapters dealing with barristers and solicitors I pause to discuss Jews and the courts more generally between the early years of the century and the Second World War. Jews were keen litigants in the lower-level civil courts, particularly in the Whitechapel and Shoreditch county courts presided over from 1911 by Judge Cluer. Although an able judge, Cluer possessed many foibles and prejudices, and I try to ascertain whether Jewish litigants had their cases fairly tried and whether they were adequately represented by the Jewish barristers who regularly appeared there. I also consider the small minority of Jewish businessmen who were charged at the Old Bailey and quarter sessions with credit fraud, fraudulent claims against insurance companies, and illegal share-pushing schemes. The number of Jewish bankruptcies was also high, for Jewish businessmen tended to be risk-takers and entrepreneurs, always seeking new opportunities in the market—and sometimes, in the process, exposing themselves to prosecution. After the Second World War, many moved into the urban property market or took over sluggish public companies with hidden assets.

In the chapter on Jewish solicitors from 1890 to 1939, I show how the first Sir George Lewis (George Henry Lewis, 1833–1911) was a role model for later Jewish solicitors, both as a society lawyer and in his involvement with the arts world. I then examine the structure of Jewish law firms between the wars. Most were concentrated in the City, and were small; there were also a few firms connected with the Anglo-Jewish elite which represented banks and big business, certain others which acted for moneylenders or those in the world of the arts, and a few others associated with leading communal figures. In addition, a separate chapter is devoted to explaining why relatively few Jews from east European Jewish families joined the English legal profession before the Second World War and outlining when Jews from these immigrant families did move into the law. I also consider the problems faced by young Jewish lawyers and doctors setting up their own practices during the 1930s, and how seriously affected they were by antisemitism within the professions.

Even if antisemitism was sometimes common at the lower end of the professions in the 1930s, we need to ask whether this was a major factor influencing the entry of Jews into the professions or of relatively minor significance. With the rise of Nazism Jews were expelled from the professions in Germany, and because of the new agenda created by Hitler there was talk everywhere of the overcrowding of the professions by Jews. Anglo-Jewry was divided in its response to this crisis. On one side were the old Anglo-Jewish elite, supported by affluent businessmen and professionals from the most socially mobile east European Jewish families, who attempted to discourage young Jews from entering the professions of law and medicine through fear of inflaming antisemitic feeling; on the other side were the young Jewish students and successful professionals from immigrant families, who had faith in the future and held that there should be no self-imposed or other limits on the entry of Jews into the professions.

The sensitive position of Jews in the professions was aggravated by the influx of Jewish refugee doctors and lawyers after 1933. Some of these refugees from central Europe were brought up as Christians, or converted when they migrated to this country, as radical assimilation—either by converting to Christianity or by marrying a non-Jew—was an acute problem in Germany. During the Second World War approximately 4,000 doctors from central and eastern Europe, a large percentage of whom were Jewish or partially Jewish, practised in the United Kingdom or served with the Allied forces. After the war many were repatriated, but a considerable number stayed in Britain; most of them found work as general practitioners, although a few established themselves as consultants in Harley Street or continued with important scientific research. Jewish lawyers who had qualified in Germany found it much more difficult to join the English legal profession, but a small number were admitted as solicitors, a few qualified for the Bar or joined the restitution organizations, and a notable group became academic lawyers of distinction.

After the Second World War, under the twin influences of revulsion at the Holocaust and the cessation of attacks on British troops in Palestine after their withdrawal from the territory, antisemitism gradually subsided, and this together with a number of fresh developments transformed the position of Jews in the professions, particularly in respect of ease of entry into the professional elite. The enormous growth of work promoted by the Legal Aid and Advice Act 1949 improved the economic prospects for barristers and solicitors considerably; in addition, the post-war property boom, together with the increase of company work consequent on a spate of takeovers, hastened the expansion of the legal profession, enabling a much larger number of Jews to become solicitors and barristers. At the same time, the restrictions placed on the admission of Jewish partners by almost all the big City law firms until the 1970s (when the expansion of many law firms led to recruitment on a meritocratic basis) encouraged the growth of dynamic new Jewish firms, associated with businessmen of the same faith, participating in the property boom and the expansion of corporate activity. There was also a group of radical Jewish solicitors, who campaigned vigorously on social issues and took up contentious cases.

Before the Second World War none of the senior barristers in the criminal courts was Jewish; by the 1950s a number of distinguished Jewish silks were appearing in these courts. Through the skills of such as Morris Finer and Samuel Stamler, Jews from an east European immigrant background started to come to the fore in the commercial courts as well. Until the 1950s there had never been more than one Jewish judge sitting in the High Court, and until the 1960s never more than two. Thereafter, with the gradual decline of antisemitism and the concomitant expansion of the higher judiciary, opportunities for advancement became less scarce. After the Second World War, the first Jewish judges promoted to the High Court bench were from patrician families, but from 1968 onwards Jews from an east European immigrant background began to fill such vacancies. Similarly, with the inauguration of the National Health Service in 1948 Jews from an immigrant background began to be appointed as consultants in the chief London and provincial hospitals, instead of such appointments being regarded as exceptional.

Thus Jews moved from the periphery of the English legal and medical professions in the 1930s to their centre in the closing decades of the twentieth
century. The growing antisemitism in eastern and central Europe after the First
World War and the advent of Hitler in Germany in 1933 resulted in a backlash
against the acceptance of Jews in the higher ranks of the professions within the
western democracies, including England and the United States; and more generally there was concern about the overcrowding of the professions by Jews.
The sociologist Talcott Parsons believed that the professions possessed a basic-
ally liberal ethos, but new research on the professions in Germany and Hungary
has shown that there were many illiberal elements in the professions in the years
between the two world wars, so that conditions in England must be seen in this
wider context.[2]

The western democracies were reluctantly forced by the Nazis to confront
the issues of racism during the Second World War; in the course of that
struggle these issues became more sharply defined and were, at least in principle, resolved in favour of the Jews and the segregated black combatants in the
US forces. As the scale of the genocide perpetrated by the Germans became
clear, the democracies were forced to take a more robust stand on human rights
over the course of the war than they had assumed at the beginning. After the
war the remaining barriers against the acceptance of Jews in the professions in
Britain and the United States were slowly dismantled, as the democracies began
to implement the ideals for which they had been fighting. In addition, in 1948
President Truman issued an executive order desegregating the American army,
but the implementation of the reform proceeded at a slow pace.[3]

Some would view the advance of the Jews in the professions to the position
they occupied at the end of the twentieth century as an unalloyed triumph;
others, however, would regard it as a qualified success, for acculturation has
produced assimilation, and many of the Jews with notable achievements to their
credit had only tenuous links to their co-religionists.

A few words must be said about the terminology I have used in this book. A
group of wealthy Sephardi families from Spain and Portugal migrated into
Britain from the latter half of the seventeenth century onwards, intermarrying
with a smaller number of Ashkenazi Jews from central Europe, mainly from
Germany, who were international traders or stock or commodity brokers.
Together, the members of this group dominated the institutions of Anglo-
Jewry well into the nineteenth century and beyond. So frequent were marriages
within this group of families that they were known as the 'Cousinhood'. When

---

[2] Maria M. Kovacs, *Liberal Professions and Illiberal Politics: Hungary from the Hapsburgs to the Holocaust* (New York: Oxford University Press, 1994), p. xviii.

[3] Juan Williams, *Thurgood Marshall, American Revolutionary* (New York: Times Books, 1998), 169 and 170.

I refer to individuals from such families, I designate them as members of the 'Cousinhood' or the 'Anglo-Jewish elite' or as coming from 'patrician' families—these terms are used interchangeably. By the Edwardian era membership of this group of families had expanded considerably. Over time, members of these families, along with those of German Jewish merchants who had migrated to England before the large-scale settlement of Jews from eastern Europe in the 1880s, grew lax in their religious practices; many even left the Jewish community, either by converting to Christianity or by marrying non-Jews, a process known as 'radical assimilation'. This process of assimilation was not a matter purely of personal choice, but affected whole families stemming from eastern Europe, as well as later German migrants. At times I focus on members of such families who joined the elite of the legal or medical profession, because their story is also part of Anglo-Jewish history. Sometimes I refer to individuals who converted or married non-Jews, or who were the products of such marriages, as being of 'Jewish origin' or 'partially Jewish' or 'marginally Jewish'.

From here it is but a short step to defining what I mean, when I call an individual Jewish. Anyone whose mother is Jewish is accepted in Jewish law (halakhah) as being Jewish; I have gone beyond this, describing individuals with Jewish fathers and non-Jewish mothers as Jews, so long as they identified themselves as such. On this basis Gilbert Beyfus QC is defined as Jewish, but the consultant physician David Pyke is not. On the other hand, certain individuals, such as David Pyke and Nicholas Winton, because of their work with Jewish refugees in the 1930s and 1940s, had an 'unconscious identification' with Jews, and thus, I would argue, in this restricted sense had a form of Jewish identity.[4] It should also be remembered that individuals whose grandmothers and mothers were Jewish, even if the women had married non-Jews, are still recognized in halakhah as being Jewish. Among the doctors and lawyers considered in this book (leaving aside for the moment those who were refugees from Germany and Austria during the 1930s) there can be a dispute about the Jewish affiliation of no more than a mere handful.

Some British professionals on the left, while not denying they were Jewish, did not want to be affiliated or counted as such. Nevertheless, I have counted them in because their radicalism and permanent questioning are qualities that I would regard as being connected with Jewish values, albeit in a secular form.

With the refugees from central Europe there are greater problems in defining who was Jewish; and here I would use a looser definition. In central Europe a substantial number of Jewish parents raised their children as Christians in the hope that their offspring would escape opprobrium when they entered the professions. Thus the art historian Sir Ernst Gombrich (1909–2001), although

---

[4] *Evening Standard*, 14 Nov. 2001 (on Winton).

he was brought up as a Protestant pietist, insisted after his flight to England on describing himself as an Austrian Jew.[5] Similarly, Kurt Lipstein, though he was brought up as a Christian, wrote a paper on the contribution of German Jewish refugees to English law and included himself in the survey. I discuss in the following chapters a number of such refugee lawyers and doctors whose careers prospered in England and who in some way identified themselves as Jewish. Some refugees converted to Christianity, along with their young children, before they fled to England; but in many such cases the conversion was made out of opportunism and the adult refugee had no abiding interest in his new faith. An example of such a refugee would be the gynaecologist Emanuel Schleyer-Saunders. I have counted these individuals as Jewish. Refugees with one or more Jewish grandparents have also been included, where they sought employment by approaching Jewish charities or worked within a predominantly Jewish milieu. It would be churlish indeed not to consider these individuals as Jewish, when they had to escape from central Europe because of their Jewish ancestry, and when their flight and subsequent settlement in England compelled them to grapple with the problems of their identity. Even so, the overwhelming majority of the refugee doctors and lawyers I have discussed were fully Jewish.

This work chiefly deals with the careers of the children and grandchildren of immigrants from eastern Europe, who started arriving in Britain in large numbers from Russia, Russian Poland, Lithuania, Galicia, and Romania in the 1880s. After the Aliens Act of 1905 this migratory flood lessened somewhat. Vivian Lipman has estimated that an average of 4,000 or 5,000 Jews settled in Britain every year between 1906 and 1914—'about two-thirds of the annual average for the years 1891–1904'. By 1914, after which the First World War and the Aliens Act of 1919 brought Jewish migration from eastern Europe to a halt, the Jewish population of Britain had grown from 60,000 in 1880 to 300,000.[6]

When I refer to Jews from central Europe, I mean the geographical area which today embraces Germany and Austria, Slovakia, the Czech Republic and Hungary. Finally, when I discuss descendants of immigrants, I call the children of the original migrants second-generation immigrants and the grandchildren third-generation immigrants, according to a convention common in sociological literature.

*

Many times in the course of this introduction I have used the word 'antisemitism', and it is only reasonable to point out that there is an ongoing controversy among Anglo-Jewish historians as to the impact of antisemitism on the

---

[5] *Guardian*, 5 Nov. 2001 (obituary of Gombrich).
[6] Vivian Lipman, *Social History of the Jews in England 1850–1950* (London: Watts & Co., 1954), 143.

community's history. On one side of the debate is W. D. Rubinstein, who has argued that in modern Britain 'anti-semitism was minimal and almost always marginalised to the fringes of society, while Jewish life in Britain has almost always been a success story and has certainly lacked virtually any element of brutality and tragedy known on the continent'. According to Rubinstein, the view of his critics is flawed because it 'consists in a systematic exaggeration of both the volume and significance of modern British anti-semitism, hand-in-hand with an equally notable insensitivity to philo-semitism, mainstream hostility to extremists, and the explicit and implicit ways in which the British political and cultural system has invariably worked to marginalise extremists and anti-semites'.[7]

On the other side are Geoffrey Alderman and two historians from South-ampton University, David Cesarani and Tony Kushner. Cesarani has asserted that 'Jews were accepted not for who and what they were, but according to terms set by the English majority and cast in the liberal rhetoric of toleration and universalism', and Kushner noted that 'Such was the strength of anti-semitism that the state was put on the defensive by it and repeatedly capitulated to "anti-alien" panics, of which Jews were the prime victims. While antisemitism was considered acceptable, the Jews were deemed virtually unassimilable.' Kushner has further claimed that

'the antisemitism of exclusion' operated against all sections of Anglo-Jewry. To the elite it could be found in public schools, clubs and universities. To the new immigrants, dis-crimination—either at work or in the housing market—was common . . . it shaped the economic and social make-up of the [Anglo-]Jewish community. Jewish residential and employment patterns reflected both the reality and fear of non-Jewish hostility, as well as Jewish ethnic and religious solidarity.

Moreover, 'a case could be made that the most serious antisemitism was located amongst the lower middle classes', declared Kushner,

who felt threatened by the increasingly mobile Jewish population in the professions and in occupations such as shopkeeping, taxi driving and clerical positions . . . Indeed such discrimination was probably increasing during and after the [Second World] war. It would seem that this had a net effect of both slowing down the entry of the descendants of the East European Jews into the professions and of encouraging Jews to continue a tradition of economic independence.

British antisemitism also demanded that Jews conform to the habits and prac-tices of society at large, and 'that the price of toleration [and the emancipation contract] was to abandon any distinctiveness'.

[7] W. D. Rubinstein, *A History of the Jews in the English-Speaking World: Great Britain* (Basingstoke: Macmillan, 1996), 31-3.

Cesarani felt that 'The readiness [of Britain] to receive refugees from Germany in the 1930s was another casualty of anti-Jewish animosity and the resultant Jewish defensiveness.'[8] Moreover, Kushner asserted that

The children of immigrants attempting to enter the professions in the late 1930s and during World War II found that formal and informal barriers were placed in their way. Whilst not so pronounced as in the United States, there was a *numerus clausus* operating against Jews in the legal and medical schools. In 1945 for example, the Leeds School of Medicine was found to be blatantly discriminating against Jews.

Norman Cantor added that during the 1930s 'There were severe limitations on the entry of Jews to the better private schools, to Oxford and Cambridge, and to the learned professions. The Jews were alien and unwanted.'[9]

Whose hypothesis is the more attractive in this historical debate: Rubinstein's or that of the Cesarani–Kushner school? Can we draw any conclusions about this controversy from a study of the entry of Jews into the medical and legal professions in England and Wales in the period 1890–1990? It is my contention that such a study may provide some answers to these questions; but first it is necessary to clarify the issues, by examining whether or not there were any barriers obstructing the entry of Jews to the English medical and law schools, and by exploring whether or not there were any impediments to Jews setting up as medical practitioners or solicitors. Second, a distinction must be drawn between the careers of humdrum Jewish lawyers and doctors practising locally and those trying to gain entry into the elite of their profession, by becoming consultants in teaching hospitals or by joining the Bar and climbing to the top tiers of the judiciary. Even among solicitors there was a distinction between the high-street lawyers and the members of large City or West End law practices. Again, it needs to be asked: to what extent did those who reached the highest positions in their profession have to pay the price of conformity, surrendering their Jewish identity?

---

[8] David Cesarani, introduction to id. (ed.), *The Making of Anglo-Jewry* (Oxford: Blackwell, 1990), 1–11; Tony Kushner, *The Persistence of Prejudice: Antisemitism in British Society during the Second World War* (Manchester: Manchester University Press, 1989), 10; Geoffrey Alderman, *Modern British Jewry* (Oxford: Clarendon Press, 1998), *passim*.

[9] Tony Kushner, 'The Impact of British Anti-Semitism, 1918–1945', in Cesarani (ed.), *The Making of Anglo-Jewry*, 201; Norman F. Cantor, *The Sacred Chain: The History of the Jews* (New York: HarperPerennial, 1995), 360.

ONE

Victorian and Edwardian Jewish Doctors

ACCORDING to the historian Todd Endelman, 'With some exceptions, native English Jews were to be found in commerce and finance, not in the professions, the civil service, the universities, and the arts (although more Jews were entering these fields from year to year . . . In the absence of this [elsewhere prevalent] anticapitalist ethos, Anglo-Jewish sons tended to follow the occupational paths of their fathers and grandfathers [into commerce and finance].'[1] This analysis of the Anglo-Jewish occupational structure is supported by the pathologist and distinguished geneticist Redcliffe Salaman (1874–1955), who observed that in the late Victorian age fathers in upper-middle-class Anglo-Jewish households (such as his own) tried to place their sons in the family business, and only if this were not suitable would they urge them to go into the professions of law and medicine.[2] Addressing a dinner of the Maccabeans in October 1892, the great public health reformer Ernest Abraham Hart (1835–98) told this gathering of Jewish professionals:

It is interesting to me to consider the status of Jews in the Professions when I started and to compare it with the present. Such a Club as this would have been impossible. There were one or two barriers. I had the honour of being the first Jew in this Country who took a University scholarship and although I won several scholarships I did not go to Cambridge University because it would have been impossible for me, as a Jew, to obtain a degree. I was the first Jew who was ever a hospital surgeon attached to a public hospital in England. Now there are many. So you will see that I belong to a quite prehistoric period and yet I am only 63 years old.[3]

[1] Todd M. Endelman, 'The Social and Political Context of Conversion in Germany and England 1870–1914' in id. (ed.), *Jewish Apostasy in the Modern World* (New York: Holmes & Meier, 1987), 96, 97.

[2] Redcliffe Salaman, 'The Helmsman Takes Charge', unpublished memoirs (Royal London Hospital Archive, n.d.), 5. Salaman's life and career are discussed in more detail on pp. 34–6 below.

[3] Ronald A. Goodman, *The Maccabeans: The Founding Fathers and the Early Years* (London: Maccabeans, 1979), 14. A vigorous attempt was made to arouse Jewish sympathies among this new class of professionals and to stem assimilation by the foundation in 1891 by Herman Cohen, a barrister, of the Maccabeans, a social and dining club. It is still in existence and contains the foremost Jewish members of the professions. It established the Education Aid Society in 1897 to sponsor talented children from poor Jewish families who were seeking a higher education. For more about Hart, see pp. 17–22 below.

If Jews wanted a higher education in the early Victorian period, they had to go to the University of London, incorporated in 1837, which (unlike the two older universities of Oxford and Cambridge) was not affiliated to the established Church and allowed Jews to receive degrees. Elsewhere there were restrictions on the admission of Jews to the universities. An act of 1854 allowed Jews at Oxford to matriculate and to take the degree of bachelor without subscribing to religious tests, and two years later the Cambridge University Reform Act of 1856 abolished religious tests on graduation for all degrees, including medicine. The University Tests Act of 1871 not only brought the position at these two universities into alignment, but threw open fellowships and professorships to all suitable candidates irrespective of religious belief. Even so, before 1914 Jews from upper-class families availed themselves of the opportunities to study at the older universities to only a limited extent.[4]

Mindful, no doubt, of the potential obstacles, many parents from the Anglo-Jewish elite remained reluctant to allow their sons to study medicine. When Robert Waley Cohen (1877–1952) went up to Cambridge in 1896, he began by registering as a medical student and attended operations at Addenbrooke's Hospital. His father summoned the family doctor, the renowned Dr Sidney Phillips, 'to advise that Bob's grumbling appendix unfitted him for so arduous a life as that of a doctor'. Under this family pressure, after his first year at university Robert Waley Cohen switched to natural science; on graduating he joined the Shell Oil Company,[5] and went on to a notable career in industry.

Jewish parents in lower-middle-class families, such as shopkeepers in poor neighbourhoods, also attempted to thwart the ambitions of any of their children inclined to follow a career in medicine. For these families, it may well have been financial considerations that weighed most heavily; as a correspondent writing to the *Jewish Chronicle* in 1904 noted, 'No one expects a lawyer or a doctor to make a living before he is thirty.'[6] J. H. Levy (b. 1838), later a civil servant with the Board of Education, recounted how the eminent Jewish physician Dr Jonathan Pereira (1804–53) had made a house call on his mother when he was a schoolboy:

She likewise told him that the boy was anxious to be brought up to the medical profession, but she and his father [who were shopkeepers near London Docks] were opposed to it. 'Send him to me', said Dr Pereira. The boy went, and after being warned that he would have to work very hard if he wanted to practise medicine, received much valuable advice from the great man about his studies.

[4] Cecil Roth, 'The Jews in the English Universities', *Miscellanies of the Jewish Historical Society of England*, pt. iv (1942), 102–15; Todd M. Endelman, *Radical Assimilation in English Jewish History 1656–1945* (Bloomington, Ind.: Indiana University Press, 1990), 78–80.

[5] Robert Henriques, *Sir Robert Waley Cohen 1877–1952* (London: Secker & Warburg, 1966), 49. For more on Sidney Phillips, see pp. 32–3 below.   [6] *Jewish Chronicle*, 1 Apr. 1904, p. 19.

When Dr Pereira died suddenly, Levy's hopes of a medical career were shattered; in the absence of this source of moral and perhaps also financial support, 'His parents now insisted on putting him into business, for which he had not the slightest inclination'. Nevertheless, in the 1860s Levy became one of the first Jews to enter the Civil Service; 'and well I recollect', he declared, 'how astonished the head of my Department . . . was at a Jew . . . undertaking so unremunerative a post. He asked me whether I could not do better at my father's business.'[7]

Accordingly, the number of Jewish doctors remained small in Victorian England, both within and outside London. We should also remember that the Jewish population of London in 1882 was only 46,100, of whom 14.6 per cent were upper or upper-middle class and another 42.2 per cent were middle class, and that the total Jewish population of Britain was 60,000.[8] It was not always easy to establish oneself. A doctor writing to the *Jewish Chronicle* in 1883 claimed that English Jewry was prejudiced against going to a co-religionist for treatment, whereas Jewish general practitioners were plentiful in Germany because there the local Jewish communities patronized Jewish doctors. He nevertheless claimed that there were twenty-three registered Jewish medical practitioners in London, not twelve as suggested by Joseph Jacobs.[9] In Manchester in 1871 there were only two Jewish doctors, and it was not until 1894 that Dr Julius Friend became the first Jewish doctor to practise in Leeds.[10]

Speaking to the Maccabean Medical Dinner in 1907, some fifteen years after Hart had addressed the society, Dr Bertram Abrahams stated that

he felt bound to express his regret that so few Jewish young men had adopted the consulting branches of the profession. In Germany, where obvious and organised anti-Semitism prevailed, there were a large number of Jewish practitioners taking high honours. Here there was an increasing number of Jewish general practitioners doing good work, but in all the great teaching hospitals in London there were only three Jews upon the consulting staff, and it was a very great pity that the sons of the well-to-do Jews should take up the destructive professions such as the army and the law (laughter) instead of the more humane one of medicine.[11]

In 1909 there were eleven Jewish Royal Navy officers and fifty-one Jewish officers in the regular army—two of whom may have possessed medical qualifications, as they were serving in the Indian Medical Service—but there was also a considerable number of other officers of more remote Jewish origin.[12]

---

[7] *JC* 17 July 1908, p. 16. For more on Jonathan Pereira, see p. 16 below.

[8] Alderman, *Modern British Jewry*, 102–4; Endelman, *Radical Assimilation*, 74. Endelman took his class definitions, and the figures cited here, from the pioneering sociological study by Joseph Jacobs, *Studies in Jewish Statistics: Social, Vital and Anthropometric* (London: D. Nutt, 1891).

[9] *JC* 14 Sept. 1883.

[10] Bill Williams, *The Making of Manchester Jewry 1740–1875* (Manchester: Manchester University Press, 1985), 359.   [11] *JC* 24 May 1907, p. 25.

[12] Isidore Harris (ed.), *The Jewish Year Book 1909* (London: Greenberg & Co., 1909), 272–8.

Even if a young Jewish student enrolled for training in a medical school, it was not clear whether he would emerge as a general practitioner or stay on for a post-graduate course to become a consultant or a scientific researcher; sometimes, after a prolonged medical training had been completed, the newly qualified doctor decided for personal reasons to abandon medicine and to pursue some other career. Redcliffe Salaman, having obtained first-class honours in the natural science tripos at Cambridge University entered the London Hospital as a medical student in 1896, qualifying as a doctor in 1899. From his unpublished memoirs we can learn something of the stages by which high-flying students were earmarked for promotion within the hospital system, while their less able colleagues were encouraged to become general practitioners.

Salaman, because of his academic credentials, naturally gravitated to a select group of 'Oxford and Cambridge men, together with a few of the keenest men from elsewhere, [who] did quite unconsciously form a set . . . As my student years drew to a close I found myself one of a small group of men [at the London Hospital] who were marked out more or less definitely for the higher branches of the profession.' Nevertheless, few young members of the Anglo-Jewish elite attended Oxford and Cambridge in the late Victorian and Edwardian periods. While Salaman was an undergraduate at Trinity Hall in the 1890s a *minyan* (a quorum of ten men for prayers) could be raised by the Jewish students only by coercing one or two tradesmen to participate. In 1912, according to Basil Henriques, there was a total of thirty Jewish undergraduates in all the Oxford colleges, only a few of whom could have been studying medicine. At this time an Oxbridge degree was a prerequisite for progress to a top job in a London hospital (though by the Edwardian era provincial hospitals were awarding their own degrees); with so few Jews graduating from Oxford and Cambridge, there was inevitably only a very small number of Jewish physicians and surgeons in the top London hospitals. 'In those days', continued Salaman,

if one felt oneself destined to become a consultant in medicine or surgery one filled as many house appointments as possible at the hospital and held on till the opportunity arose of being created a Registrar; from that point of vantage the next step was to be elected by the governors an assistant physician or surgeon to the hospital. Up to that point the struggle . . . was how to maintain health and strength in the exhausting atmosphere of continuous hospital service; from then on it became in the main a problem of finance, moral courage and endurance, and not a little luck . . . The aspiring young man, now about 28 or 30 years of age, instead of thinking about getting married, had to muster every penny he could to acquire a brass plate and a footing, however slender, in Harley Street or its immediate neighbourhood.[13]

Immediately after their final examination, newly qualified doctors embarked on their first house appointment. Only the most favoured students secured posts in

13 Salaman, 'The Helmsman', 6, 23, 25; Endelman, *Radical Assimilation*, 79, 80.

the London teaching hospitals where they had been trained. Salaman came from an upper-middle-class family; his background was public school—St Paul's—and Cambridge; he was clever and very self-confident; and he was accepted by his teachers and the hospital authorities, never suffering from any antisemitic slights. Salaman was one of the fortunate ones, being selected as clinical assistant and house physician at the London Hospital; likewise, Albert Edward Mortimer Woolf (1884–1957), despite graduating from Cambridge with only third-class honours in the natural sciences tripos, part I, in 1905, secured appointments as house physician and house surgeon after finishing his training at the London Hospital. Other Jewish students belonging to Anglo-Jewish elite families also encountered few problems in obtaining suitable house appointments in leading hospitals and advancing up the career ladder in such institutions in mid-Victorian and Edwardian England.[14]

The evidence from early Victorian England seems to point in the opposite direction, but this, as we shall see, was a temporary phenomenon. The great London hospitals were controlled by boards of lay governors, who made all the appointments to the permanent senior medical staff, without bowing to the wishes of the existing consultants. Nepotism was rampant, family ties and friendship heavily influencing the selection of successful candidates. The governors tended to be establishment figures and to look askance at doctors with politically radical views or those who were not affiliated to the Anglican Church or one of the free churches. Hence Jewish candidates were sometimes rejected when they applied to become consultants. Joseph Gutteres Henriques (1795–1885) was trained at St Thomas's Hospital, where he was a favourite pupil of Sir Astley Cooper and Sir William Lawrence. He then went to Jamaica and

practised chiefly as an oculist, and was successful in performing many difficult operations, one of which was to remove two cataracts from his father's eyes . . . [Returning once again to England, he] began to practise in the Metropolis, but the dead weight of prejudice against Jews at that time was too great to admit of his being appointed a Consulting Physician at the Ophthalmic Hospital in Finsbury, for which position he was nominated.

He therefore retired from medical practice to devote himself to communal affairs. As senior warden of the Spanish and Portuguese Synagogue, he read the address to the Queen and Prince Albert on their marriage in 1842, and in the same year became one of the founders of the Reform Synagogue.[15]

[14] *JC* 25 Oct. 1901, p. 17; R. H. O. B. Robinson, W. R. LeFanu, and Cecil Wakeley (eds.), *Lives of the Fellows of the Royal College of Surgeons of England 1952–1964* (Edinburgh and London: Livingstone, 1970), 455, 456.

[15] M. Jeanne Paterson, *The Medical Profession in Mid-Victorian London* (Berkeley and Los Angeles: University of California Press, 1978), 138–71; *JC* 11 Sept. 1885, p. 14.

Again, the Cambridge-educated Daniel Whitaker Cohen MD, an assistant physician at St Thomas's Hospital, was three times nominated for the position of lecturer in forensic medicine at the school by the Committee of Lecturers, but was rejected because of antisemitic prejudice by the hospital's governing body. He engaged in a heated correspondence with the treasurer over this in 1852, but to no avail. In 1854 Cohen was forced to resign the post of assistant physician at the hospital, which he had held since 1846. The treasurer and governors of St Thomas's Hospital seem to have believed that in addition to providing medical care, it was a body imbued with Christian principles with which Dr Cohen's elevation was incompatible.[16]

A less clear-cut case of anti-Jewish prejudice was the difficulty encountered by Jonathan Pereira FRS (1804–53), when he sought an appointment to lecture at the medical school of St Bartholomew's Hospital in 1836. Dr Pereira became a member of the Royal College of Surgeons in 1825; in 1840 he gained his MD from Erlangen, Germany, and became a Licentiate of the Royal College of Physicians; and he was elected a Fellow of the Royal College of Physicians in 1845.[17] He was appointed Professor of Materia Medica at the Aldersgate Medical School in 1832 and also lectured in chemistry at the London Hospital, where he became an assistant physician in 1841 and a full consultant physician ten years later.[18] In 1839 he published *Materia Medica and Therapeutics*, a work which tried to set out the empirical principles of pharmacology and which earned him a European reputation, but which was criticized for showing a certain lack of originality. After studying the records of St Bartholomew's Hospital, Claire Hilton concluded that it was hard to ascertain whether the blocking of Jonathan Pereira's appointment by the governors of the hospital was motivated by rivalry between different London medical schools, leading to a disinclination on the part of the St Bartholomew's governors to appoint a candidate from Aldersgate and the London Hospital, or antisemitism.[19] In any case, Pereira's relationship with the Jewish community was somewhat equivocal: he married Louisa Ann Lucas at St Thomas's church, Winchester, in 1843. Nor was it only Jewish candidates who ruffled the sensibilities of the hospital governors. Thomas Hodgkin, a Quaker friend of the philanthropist Moses Montefiore, was active in the Aborigines' Protection Society and in 1837 clashed with the treasurer of Guy's Hospital, a leading light in the Hudson Bay Company which controlled

[16] Lindsay Patricia Granshaw, 'St Thomas's Hospital, London, 1850–1900', Ph.D. diss. (Bryn Mawr College, 1981), 331, 332.

[17] *Lancet*, 29 Jan. 1853, p. 124, 5 Feb. 1853, pp. 139–40 (obituaries of Pereira).

[18] Leslie G. Matthews, 'The Aldersgate Dispensary and the Aldersgate Medical School', *Pharmaceutical Historian*, 13/3 (Sept. 1983), 7–10; id., 'Will of Dr Jonathan Pereira', *Pharmaceutical Historian*, 14/1 (Mar. 1984), 5.

[19] Claire Hilton, 'St Bartholomew's Hospital, London, and its Jewish Connections', *Jewish Historical Studies*, 30 (1987–8), 26, 27.

the North American fur trade, thus destroying his chances of promotion to the position of assistant physician at the hospital.[20]

The eminent eye specialist John Zachariah Laurence (1829–70) was one of the first Jewish doctors to break through the barriers erected against the appointment of Jews as hospital surgeons. Educated at University College London, he went to Utrecht to study ophthalmology under Frans Cornelis Donders (1818–89), who formulated the modern concept of refraction and accommodation; there Laurence also benefited from the research undertaken during the 1850s by the pioneering German ophthalmologists Helmholtz and von Gräfe. He obtained his Fellowship of the Royal College of Surgeons in 1855 and in 1857 founded the South London Ophthalmic Hospital, the forerunner of the Royal Eye Hospital. He was first appointed as the surgeon of the Hospital for Epilepsy and Paralysis, later switching from general surgery to ophthalmology and becoming an ophthalmic surgeon at St Bartholomew's Hospital, Chatham (1866–9). He was not only highly skilled in his treatment of cataracts, but a brilliant diagnostician who identified a genetic condition known as the Laurence–Moon–Biedl syndrome. He was also the founder of the short-lived *Ophthalmic Review*, which conveyed the advances in research being made in Germany to a wider British audience. Yet although Laurence 'produced excellent work on ophthalmology, endocrinology, and genetics, [he] never achieved fame or financial success'.[21]

Another illustrious Anglo-Jewish figure of the Victorian period, not only in surgery but also in the area of public health, was Ernest Hart. Perhaps because his career in surgery was short-lived, while the major portion of his adult life was devoted to editing the *British Medical Journal* and using it as a platform to promote a series of important reforms in public health, he is a somewhat overlooked figure. Although contemporaries rated him highly, the changes which Hart, along with other reformers, helped to introduce were so widely accepted that they became essential elements of the Victorian public health infrastructure, and thus ceased to be regarded as noteworthy. In fact, Hart was probably the leading British public health reformer of the late nineteenth century, a worthy successor of Edwin Chadwick and John Simon.

On the debit side, it may be said that in some respects Hart did his own reputation few favours. His first wife died in suspicious circumstances in 1861, having drunk some tincture of aconite instead of a harmless laxative potion, an

[20] Louis Rosenfeld, *Thomas Hodgkin: Morbid Anatomist and Social Activist* (Lanham, Md.: Madison, 1993), 137–55, 179–82.

[21] Paterson, *The Medical Profession*, 266. See also *JC* 22 July 1870, p. 4; *Jewish Encyclopedia*, vol. vii (New York: Funk & Wagnalls, 1916), 648; Frederic Boase (ed.), *Modern English Biography*, vol. ii (London: Frank Cass, 1965), col. 317; Arnold Sorsby, 'John Zachariah Laurence: A Belated Tribute', *British Journal of Ophthalmology*, 16 (1932), 727–40.

event dramatized in Julia Frankau's novel of 1887, *Dr Phillips*. Although the inquest cleared Hart of any wrongdoing, the suspicion inevitably lingered that his attitude towards his wife was at best ambivalent and that unconsciously he contributed towards her death. A whiff of scandal clung to Hart as a consequence of this episode and some minor matters connected with his editorship of the *British Medical Journal*. In addition, he had an abrasive personality and relished provoking hostility in disputes over ideas—so much so that his enemies regarded him as a 'pushy' Jew.[22]

Hart's father was a dentist with a prosperous practice in west London. Ernest was educated at the City of London School, where the headmaster Dr Mortimer regarded him as 'the most capable lad whom he had ever educated', and gained the unusual distinction for a Jew of serving as school captain in the early 1850s, when he was two years younger than any previous appointee. He won a scholarship to Queens' College, Cambridge, but did not take it up because of the restrictions still affecting Jews at the older universities, and instead entered St George's Hospital, London, as a medical student. Here he had a brilliant career: at the end of his second year he gained prizes open to both second- and third-year students, and while still unqualified was appointed as demonstrator in anatomy.[23] 'He was always a favourite with his fellow students—bright, genial and witty,' recalled William Adams, a friend of Hart and one of his teachers, 'and he was also a favourite with the surgical staff, who appreciated his great abilities.'[24] While still undergoing his medical training during the Crimean War, Hart formed an association of medical students in London to press for better conditions for naval surgeons; the campaign, during which public meetings were staged and the support of a number of MPs gained, honed the political skills and reforming zeal that were to find their fullest expression in Hart's later endeavours in the public health cause. He had good connections with the Jewish community, and while serving as Mr Coulson's assistant in a busy City practice gained many patients—so many, indeed, that Hart admitted that his earnings for his first five years in practice in the late 1850s averaged £2,000 per annum, a not inconsiderable sum.[25] In 1856 he took the diploma of membership of the Royal College of Surgeons and became surgical registrar at St George's. He then attached himself to St Mary's; welcomed here, as at St George's, without prejudice, he became ophthalmic surgeon (1861–8), aural surgeon specializing in diseases of the ear (1865–8), and dean of the medical school (1863–9).

[22] W. J. Bartrip, *Mirror of Medicine: A History of the* British Medical Journal (Oxford: Clarendon Press, 1990), 64, 65, 78, 79; Frank Danby, *Dr Phillips: A Maida Vale Idyll* (London: Keynes, 1989), pp. v–xii; *JC* 30 June 1916, p. 20.
[23] *British Medical Journal*, 15 Jan. 1898, pp. 175–86; *Lancet*, 15 Jan. 1898, pp. 192, 193 (obituaries of Hart).   [24] *BMJ* 22 Jan. 1898, p. 237.   [25] *JC* 14 Jan. 1898, p. 12 (obituary of Hart).

He also devised a method of treating aneurism by flexion of the knee joint which attracted much attention in those pre-antiseptic days.[26]

Without doubt, Hart's talents and personal charm were such that, had he so wished, he could have advanced to the highest positions within the Victorian medical establishment. But, instead of staying in surgery, Hart plumped for an influential career in journalism and public health reform as editor of the *British Medical Journal*. He had shown a literary bent since his schooldays, when he outdistanced all competitors in essay writing. Indeed, it is said that the number of prizes he won was so great that he had to hire a cab to carry them home after each distribution.[27] Under Hart's editorship between 1866 and 1898, the circulation of the *British Medical Journal* rose from 2,500 in 1867 to 20,500 some thirty years later. He used his position on the journal to boost the membership of the British Medical Association, which was only 2,500 when he took over as editor; offering subscribers to the journal reduced-price subscription to the BMA, he saw the growth in the circulation of the journal accompanied by an increase in membership of the association to 17,000 by 1898. Hart also promoted the membership of the association by assisting in the formation of new branches during his holidays; in addition, for over twenty-five years he was chairman of its key Parliamentary Bills Committee. By the time of his death, Hart had built up the BMA from a small group with slender resources into a formidable force in medical and health politics.[28]

Hart's journalistic career had begun on the *Lancet*, where he worked from 1858 to 1866—when he was sacked after a falling-out with the editor, James Wakley. It was while employed by this journal that, in 1865, he took the initiative in founding a commission to inquire into the condition of the sick poor in London's workhouse infirmaries. Among the other members of the commission were Dr Francis Anstie, editor of the *Practitioner*, and the public health reformer Dr Carr. Dr Anstie carried out the bulk of the investigatory work, but it was Hart who established the general lines of the inquiry, as well as writing three of the reports on individual workhouses. It was also Hart who, in a journal article, coined the phrase 'state hospitals', when referring to what the poor law institutions could become. With fellow doctor Joseph Rogers and others, he formed the Association for the Improvement of the Infirmaries of Workhouses early in 1866, and in the words of one obituary writer 'led the crusade' which resulted in the passing of the Metropolitan Poor Act of 1867.[29] Although John Storr, a wealthy businessman and supporter of poor law reform, offered accommodation for the association, its office was located in Hart's home in Wimpole Street; from this, and from subsequent comments by contemporaries, it may be

[26] *BMJ* 15 Jan. 1898, p. 176.
[27] *JC* 14 Jan. 1898, p. 12.
[28] *BMJ* 15 Jan. 1898, pp. 175, 177; Bartrip, *Mirror of Medicine*, 71.
[29] *BMJ* 15 Jan. 1898, p. 177.

inferred that he seized day-to-day control of the operations of the association, as one of its honorary secretaries.

It was Hart who formulated the whole plan of reform. In April 1866, in an article in the *Fortnightly Review*, he outlined a scheme under which the sick poor were to be separated from the able-bodied, and consolidated infirmaries were to be established in place of the sick wards at present contained in each workhouse. As 'the sick poor of the metropolis are a charge upon' London, Hart argued that the cost of their care should fall on 'the whole area of London'. On 14 April 1867 a reform on these lines was presented by the association to Charles Villiers, then president of the Poor Law Board, who received the deputation sympathetically. Not to be outdone, Gathorne Hardy, who succeeded Villiers as president of the Poor Law Board in the new Conservative administration of 1867, introduced a Poor Law Amendment Bill that embodied the proposals of the reformers, providing for separate infirmaries to be set up for the sick poor of London, thereby removing them from contact with 'lunatics, imbeciles, persons with infectious diseases and the able-bodied'; and he agreed that the sick poor should to a limited degree be a common charge on the metropolis. In a tribute to Hart in June 1867 the secretary of the Metropolitan Workhouse Infirmaries Reform Association asserted that

Sir John Simeon MP . . . said that the success of the Association was due to 'the tact, earnestness, business power, and singular suggestiveness, displayed by Mr Hart: the gentleman had kept the whole thing together'. We propose to recognise Mr Hart's successful and unselfish labours in converting written words into political deeds, and public opinion into legislative action [by a testimonial].[30]

Athough many of the poor law administrators in the provincial towns followed the example of London, Hart noted that conditions were still deplorable in the remoter rural workhouses, where the sick were nursed by ignorant paupers instead of a trained nursing staff. He published a series of articles in the medical press exposing the situation in certain selected rural workhouses, aiming to rouse local opinion and to compel the Local Government Board to take action. As a result of Hart's efforts, as well as those of other agencies, in the last decade of the century the Local Government Board issued an order abolishing pauper nursing. In line with Hart's recommendations, it became government policy to provide the sick poor, the aged, and infants with the same standard of care as they would have received had they been treated in voluntary hospitals.[31]

In the 1880s, under the influence of his sister-in-law Henrietta Barnett, Hart turned his attention to the plight of pauper children. When a fire and an out-

[30] *Lancet*, 22 June 1867, 782; James E. O'Neill, 'Finding a Policy for the Sick Poor', *Victorian Studies*, 7/3 (Mar. 1964), 265–84. See also Joseph Rogers, *Reminiscences of a Workhouse Medical Officer* (London: Unwin, 1889), 48–61.   [31] *BMJ* 15 Jan. 1898, 177, 178.

break of food poisoning occurred at the Forest Gate School in south-east London, which housed such children, Hart organized a deputation which successfully pressed the government to appoint a departmental committee of inquiry in 1894. Hart was called as the first witness and 'marshalled his facts, arranged his arguments, and pressed his reforms on the Committee with a lucidity, comprehensiveness, and force which evidently carried great weight, for after hearing 75 witnesses the now famous Report embodied many of his suggestions, and in the main supported his conclusions'.[32] The report of the departmental committee in 1896 recommended that the large workhouse barrack schools should be abolished and that the children in them should be sent to scattered homes and cottages or boarded out with foster-parents, or that arrangements should be made for them to emigrate. The report concluded that housing children together in large numbers encouraged mental dullness; that the abundant use of machinery which was not found in ordinary households meant that girls could not learn simple household chores; and that the concentration of so many children caused the dissemination of illness, such as ophthalmia, ringworm, and skin diseases. To press for these reforms Mrs Barnett and her supporters, including Ernest Hart, established the State Children's Aid Association in November 1896 with the goal of removing children from any connection with the poor law. The biggest barrack school in the country, at Sutton, in Surrey, which housed 1,500 children, was broken up; the Metropolitan Asylums Board was given care of 'feeble-minded' children, and those suffering from ringworm and malnutrition. A new ophthalmic hospital school was built at Brentwood in small cottages each containing no more than ten children.[33]

Earlier in his career Hart had campaigned on a number of other issues, such as the attempt to curb baby-farming. John Brendon Curgenven, a fellow surgeon, had already tried to focus public attention on the issue, but without much success, because the charges against the women who ran the baby farms, chiefly providing homes for illegitimate infants for profit and ensuring they had a high mortality rate, were unsubstantiated. Hart devised a ruse to entrap these women, inserting newspaper advertisements for a nurse to look after such a child. A fellow reformer, Dr Wiltshire, posed as the father of an illegitimate child, thereby gaining entry into the homes of the women who replied to the advertisements—and, in the words of the *British Medical Journal*, 'exposing the details of the system of baby-farming and baby-murder . . . which . . . is now carried out in the metropolis and in the provinces, after a fashion destructive to life, utterly

[32] Ibid. 178.

[33] Henrietta Barnett, *Canon Barnett: His Life, Work and Friends* (London: Murray, 1921), 684–92; Alexander Michael Ross, 'The Care and Education of Pauper Children in England and Wales', Ph.D. diss. (London University, 1955), 109–16.

immoral, and not uncommonly felonious'.[34] According to George K. Behlmer, the historian of the campaign, 'More than anyone else the person responsible for making tangible these hazy suspicions was Ernest Hart.'[35] Yet despite the efforts of Hart and other reformers the movement against baby-farming 'went to sleep' for a time between the autumn of 1868 and the summer of 1870; not until the formation in October 1870 of the Infant Life Protection Society, in which Curgenven was the leading figure but in which Hart also played a part, was the campaign reactivated. The Infant Life Protection Act was passed in 1872. Outside London it was not vigorously enforced, while an important loophole remained in that private homes taking a single child could not be inspected—a gap in the law that was not filled until 1908. A by-product of the campaign was the passing of the Birth and Death Registration Act 1874, under which a failure to report a birth within forty-two days and a death within eight was followed by a 42*s*. fine. This reform was secured by the Infant Life Protection Society with the assistance of the Obstetrical Society and the BMA, whose Parliamentary Bills Committee was chaired by Hart.[36]

Hart was important and talented as a public health reformer capable of clearly grasping the big issues and devising bold strategies for improving the condition of the poor and defending the work of the medical profession. However, he 'possessed a most unscientific hatred of detail, and always referred to the microscopical work he did . . . as a rather pitiable waste of time. Hence the amount of original work to be accredited to him is entirely insignificant. His gift lay in generalisation, and in the clever application of scientific facts to matters of everyday life.'[37] Thus he concentrated on trying to dismantle the poor law system, by removing the sick and children from workhouses. Thus, through Hart's initiative, the British Medical Association defended compulsory vaccination, forcing the government in 1880 to abandon a bill which sought to relax the law. And, according to P. W. J. Bartrip, 'There are good grounds for viewing the outcome of the [*British Medical*] *Journal*'s campaign [orchestrated by Hart] to uphold animal experiments as one of its most notable successes.'[38]

When the governors of St Thomas's Hospital decided to appoint an ophthalmic surgeon in 1871 to head a new department, they chose Richard Liebreich (1830–1917), a German Jew who was regarded as one of 'the ablest Ophthalmic Surgeons in Europe'.[39] He studied medicine in Königsberg, Berlin, and Halle, then worked under Donders in Utrecht and was an assistant in von Gräfe's clinic in Berlin, thus serving under two of the founding fathers of ophthalmology.

[34] *BMJ* 25 Jan. 1868.
[35] George K. Behlmer, *Child Abuse and Moral Reform in England, 1870–1908* (Stanford, Calif.: Stanford University Press, 1982), 22–38, 150–7.
[36] Harry Hendrick, *Child Welfare in England 1872–1989* (London: Routledge, 1994), 47–9.
[37] *JC* 14 Jan. 1898, p. 13.   [38] Bartrip, *Mirror of Medicine*, 105–19.
[39] Granshaw, 'St Thomas's Hospital', 275–7.

Liebreich next established himself as an ophthalmologist in Paris from 1862 to 1870, when at the outbreak of the Franco-Prussian War he moved to London. He insisted that the general surgeons at St Thomas's should not treat ophthalmic cases, but left the actual running of his department to an assistant surgeon; owing to the commitments of a busy private practice, he was in attendance at the hospital on only two days a week. Liebreich designed and constructed two ophthalmoscopes which were widely adopted, one large and elaborate, the other portable. He gave special attention to ophthalmoscopy, publishing his first atlas on the subject in 1863. He also published a monograph on school life and its influence on sight in 1872. He was a talented painter and sculptor, and in 1878 resigned his hospital position and cut down on his hours of private practice to devote himself to art. As well as pursuing his own work, he also studied the works of such painters as Turner and Mulready to demonstrate that the developments in their use of colour were due to changes in their eyes. He retired to Paris, and died there in 1917.[40]

Felix Semon (1843–1921) was born in Danzig, Germany (now Gdańsk in Poland) of Jewish parentage. As a result of the business failure of his stockbroker father, Semon was not pressed to go into commerce like the great majority of educated young Jews, and was free to opt for a career in medicine, qualifying as an MD in Berlin in 1873 and pursuing his medical studies in Heidelberg, Berlin, Vienna, and Paris, and at St Thomas's in London. In Berlin, professionals, mingled only with one another; Semon remembered 'that the dislike of Jews was very general, and though, personally, I suffered from it much less than many of my co-religionists, yet I felt its existence on more than one occasion'. Because of the level of antisemitism in Germany Semon decided to move to London, where in 1875 he became a clinical assistant in the Throat Hospital in Golden Square under Britain's leading laryngologist Morell Mackenzie; he was much influenced in this choice of specialty by the advice received from Dr Liebreich, an old friend of his mother. He was admitted as a Member of the Royal College of Physicians in 1876 and became a Fellow in 1885. In 1882 he was appointed assistant physician in charge of the throat department at St Thomas's, and rose to the position of full physician in 1891; however, he resigned this post in 1897, partly owing to the increase of his private practice but also because he could not obtain permission from the hospital authorities to perform operations for cancer of the throat using surgical techniques of his own devising. He was one of the founders of the London Laryngological Society in 1893 and in 1884 of an international journal of laryngology, the *Internationales Centralblatt für Laryngologie*, of which he was editor for many years.[41] Knighted

[40] *BMJ* 10 Feb. 1917, 211 (obituary of Liebreich).

[41] Felix Semon, *The Autobiography of Sir Felix Semon* (London: Jarrold, 1926). On his family background see pp. 15–19, 31–4, and 60; on his medical education see pp. 63–5 and 79–85; on his decision to settle in England see pp. 88–103; on his work at St Thomas's Hospital see pp. 114–21 and 220–1; on his work for laryngology see pp. 222 and 223.

in 1897, in 1901 Semon was appointed physician extraordinary to King Edward VII and served the monarch until a dispute between them in 1908 (see page 29 below). Among his other illustrious patients were William Ewart Gladstone, Winston Churchill, and the opera star Nellie Melba.[42] He was awarded the KCVO in 1905.

Summing up his career, *The Times* stated that Semon found laryngology 'in its infancy'; he left it

an important and flourishing specialty. It was perhaps owing to his initiative that it long maintained a closer relationship with Berlin and Vienna than any other branch of medicine or surgery . . . His own work was chiefly in connection with cancer of the throat and with the functions and diseases of the motor nerves of the larynx.[43]

How are we to explain the prominence of Jewish doctors, particularly as surgeons, in the London teaching hospitals in late Victorian England? Part of the answer to this question lies in the increasing specialization of medicine and surgery. The Victorian hospitals were starting to open special departments for diseases of the eye, ear, and throat, for skin diseases, and for gynaecological problems. In 1850 Hermann Helmholtz (1821–93) invented the ophthalmoscope, which has been called 'the greatest discovery in the history of ophthalmology, not excepting the extraction of [a] cataract', while in Berlin Albrecht von Gräfe (1828–70) extended its application and became the greatest of eye surgeons.[44] By the 1870s Vienna was famous for its postgraduate instruction in laryngology and otology (diseases of the ear). However, Jews sometimes found promotion elusive within these hospital systems; hence the German Jewish doctors, such as Richard Liebreich, Felix Semon, and the eye surgeon Adolph Samelson, looked to England for advancement in their careers; for the chief London hospitals, eagerly seeking fresh talent to fill the positions in their newly burgeoning departments, whether the applicants were Jewish or not did not seem to matter. Once these departments became established, their selection procedures became more rigid and it was much harder for Jews to gain entry to them.

Moreover, most of these eminent Victorian Jewish doctors whether of German or English origin were only marginal Jews, born Jewish but with no affiliation to any Jewish organization or charity, and in many cases bringing their children up as Christians. Whereas Liebreich was steeped in the world of art, Semon toyed with the idea of becoming a concert pianist or composer, finally— wisely—coming to the conclusion that he did not possess sufficient talent;

[42] Semon, *Autobiography*, 217, 190–1, 236–43, 280–7.

[43] *The Times*, 3 Mar. 1921, p. 13 (obituary of Semon).

[44] Granshaw, 'St Thomas's Hospital', 273; Burton Chance, *Ophthalmology* (New York: Hafner, 1962), 65–8, 76–8.

neither man had strong ties to the Jewish community. Semon, according to the *Jewish Chronicle*, 'was entirely dissociated from the Jewish faith and the community to which he was born, and by his expressed wish the funeral tomorrow [Saturday] will take place privately at Golders Green'[45]—presumably, as it was a Saturday, in the crematorium rather than in any of the Jewish cemeteries. Semon himself confessed in his memoirs that 'The very fact that I do not believe in the exclusive truth of *any* religion, has prevented a change from the faith in which I was born'; yet he could not 'accustom himself to the rigid formalism of its [Judaism's] rites'. Even as a boy, Semon had decided to bring up any children he had 'in the State religion of their native land, and to leave it to themselves to form their own opinions later on', because 'he did not want to close many careers open to them'. As for Ernest Hart, it is true that he published a book entitled *The Mosaic Code of Sanitation* (1877), and that he said 'I was born a Jew, I am living as a Jew, and I shall die as a member of the great and glorious House of Israel'; yet his second wife, Alice Rowland (sister of Dame Henrietta Barnett) was non-Jewish. In fact, his brother-in-law Canon Barnett, the warden of the Toynbee Hall settlement in the East End, where university graduates lived while doing social work alongside their regular employment, conducted a memorial service for him on a Saturday in the St Marylebone church, after which he was cremated in Woking; but his ashes were nevertheless buried in the United Synagogue cemetery in Willesden.[46] (Although cremation is contrary to Jewish law, the United [Orthodox] Synagogue allowed burial of an urn, provided it was placed in a coffin.) Although John Zachariah Laurence and his wife were both adherents of the Jewish faith and were buried in the Balls Pond Road cemetery of the Reform Synagogue, their three young daughters, left without parental guidance, all intermarried; and this may indicate the loosening of the family's ties to Judaism.[47]

Outside London, particularly in Manchester, where a large German Jewish community had settled over the course of the nineteenth century—some having become assimilated, others founding the Manchester Reform Synagogue—there was a similar pattern of German Jewish doctors being recruited by hospitals because of their knowledge of the latest Continental advances in medicine. Adolph Samelson, who became surgeon to the Manchester Eye Hospital in the 1870s, had gained his MD in Berlin and had done some further training at von Gräfe's eye clinic.[48] Siegmund Moritz (1855–1932) had received his MD from the University of Würzburg in 1877 and became a Member of the Royal

[45] *JC* 4 Mar. 1921, p. 11.
[46] Semon, *Autobiography*, 32–4, 60; *BMJ* 15 Jan. 1898, 185–6; Bartrip, *Mirror of Medicine*, 91.
[47] Emma Klein, *Lost Jews* (Basingstoke: Macmillan, 1996), 25.
[48] For Samelson, see *The Medical Directory 1872* (London: J. & A. Churchill, 1872), 562.

College of Physicians in London in 1881. In addition to lecturing in laryngology and rhinology at Manchester University, he was senior physician to the Manchester Hospital for Consumption and Diseases of the Chest and Throat, and physician to the Victoria Memorial Jewish Hospital.[49]

Perhaps the most outstanding foreign-born Jewish doctor in Manchester at this time was Julius Dreschfeld (1845–1907). Born in Bavaria, he was educated partly at Owen's College in Manchester (the forerunner of Manchester University) and partly at the University of Würzburg, where Rudolf Virchow had established a school of pathology that used pioneering methods. After further study on the Continent, Dreschfeld qualified as a Licentiate of the Royal College of Physicians in London in 1869 and settled in Manchester. He was rapidly promoted, gaining the chair in pathology at Owen's College in 1881 and subsequently becoming professor of medicine. He organized one of the first pathological laboratories in Britain, specializing himself in the pathology of the nervous system. He was also extraordinarily gifted as a general physician, becoming one of the very few Jews to be appointed consultants at the Manchester Royal Infirmary before the 1960s, and acquired a huge consultancy practice in the north which left him with little leisure time.[50] After retiring from the Royal Infirmary, he became a consulting physician to the Manchester Jewish Hospital and the Home for Aged Jews.

Dr Dreschfeld was the most gifted man I ever had the good fortune to meet [one house physician declared]. He had a photographic memory and read the literature of the world. I well remember a neurologist bringing him a neurological case to see. Dreschfeld was taking a ward class and was followed by a trail of students. He examined the case carefully and gave his diagnosis which was quite different from that made by his colleague. He then continued with what Charcot had said about this disease and physicians in Berlin, St. Petersburg and other countries, leaving the neurologist thoroughly crestfallen . . . He was equally skilled with his treatment and had the highest sense of his duty to his patients, never sparing in thought or trouble.[51]

Dreschfeld's father Leopold, a dentist, was a member of the Manchester Reform Synagogue, and Julius for most of his life remained attached to the Jewish community. However, his second marriage was to a non-Jewish woman, and towards the end of his life he converted to Christianity. When he died he was interred in a Christian cemetery.[52] His drift from the Jewish community

[49] For obituaries of Moritz, see *JC* 19 Aug. 1932, p. 7, and *Lancet*, 20 Aug. 1932, 422.

[50] G. H. Brown (ed.), *Lives of the Fellows of the Royal College of Physicians of London 1826–1925* (London: Royal College of Physicians, 1955), 292; William Brockbank, *The Honorary Medical Staff of the Manchester Royal Infirmary 1830–1948* (Manchester: Manchester University Press, 1965), 73–4.

[51] Brockbank, *The Honorary Medical Staff*, 75.

[52] Williams, *The Making of Manchester Jewry*, 262, 311; Brockbank, *The Honorary Medical Staff*, 76; *JC* 21 June 1907, p. 32 (obituary of Dreschfeld).

resembled the life-pattern of many of the leading German Jewish doctors in London.

*

As the Jewish population in London increased from about 46,000 in 1880 to about 180,000 in 1914, so the number of Jewish medical practitioners also rose. From twenty-three in the early 1880s, by 1910 the number of clearly identifiable Jewish medical practitioners in the capital had climbed to ninety, but the true number may lie somewhere between this figure and 100, with a handful hidden behind names not easily recognizable as Jewish.[53] The majority of the doctors came from Ashkenazi and Sephardi families who had lived in London for many generations. Notable Sephardi names included David Aaron Belilios, David Henriques de Souza, Judah Moses Finzi,[54] and David Nunes Nabarro, while those stemming from old Ashkenazi families included Phineas Abraham, Alfred Eichholz, Charles Ralph Keyser, and Harold Albert Kisch. There was also another, smaller, group of medical practitioners who had been born abroad and had received their initial training in Germany and Austria—men such as Adam Augustus Breuer, Jacques Cohn, Ludwig Freyberger, and Heinrich Oppenheimer—and a further contingent who had attended medical college in Ireland before moving to England; these included Abraham Cohen, Myer Akiba Dutch, and Jacob Jaffé.

During the 1850s and 1860s the City synagogues employed Dr Asher Asher (1837–89), Dr Canstatt (1794–1874), and Dr Joseph Kisch (1806–90), who provided extensive medical relief for the Jewish poor until the system was phased out between 1873 and 1879.[55] In the 1890s a few Jewish doctors began practising in the East End, and by the Edwardian age there was a sizeable group of Jewish physicians catering for the medical needs of the Yiddish-speaking immigrants there, men such as Raphael Berman, George Chaikin, Marcus Woolf Cohen, William Moses Feldman, Joseph Klein, Solomon Krestin, Gustave Michael, Bernhard Morris, and Jacob Schumer. There were probably a few additional doctors of Jewish origin within the Christian medical missions in the East End, men such as Nathaniel Benoly, Bakhshi Isaac Rahim, George Hessenauer, and George William Sequeira.[56]

Gustave Michael (1863–1924) was practically the first Jewish medical man to

[53] *The Medical Directory 1910* (London: J. & A. Churchill, 1910), 59–370. I prefer to follow the figure of twenty-three doctors for the early 1880s, given by a London Jewish doctor who knew the identities of his colleagues, rather than that of twelve given by the pioneering sociologist Joseph Jacobs.

[54] *JC* 23 Jan. 1903 (obituary of Finzi).

[55] *JC* 6 Feb. 1874, p. 751, 7 Mar. 1890, p. 9 (obituaries of Canstatt and Kisch); Vivian Lipman, *A Century of Social Service 1859–1959: The History of the Jewish Board of Guardians* (London: Routledge & Kegan Paul, 1959), 17, 61–3; Cecil Roth, *The Great Synagogue 1690–1940* (London: Goldston, 1950), 200, 275.

[56] *The Medical Directory 1910*, 59–370; Wilfred S. Samuel, article on the Sequeira family, *JC* 3 Apr. 1953, p. 10.

settle in the East End of London, and was thus the pioneer of a large and increasing contingent:

He was a young Scotch graduate, was steeped in the culture of Edinburgh University, and except that he was endowed with a good Jewish education had no kind of affinity with the environment wherein he was to begin his life's work. But he had great ability, shrewdness, good judgment, and a most amicable disposition, qualities which secured for him, within a brief period, a success which was literally phenomenal. This imposed upon him a burden of unceasing work, by day and night, which became the habit of his life and which contributed to his breakdown when the emergencies of the war added to the burden of every medical man.[57]

Samuel Gordon, a novelist and friend of Dr Michael, 'doubted whether any of his many very able colleagues and rivals ever succeeded in displacing him in the affection and prestige he enjoyed in the district'.[58] He was also communally active, serving on the board of management of the Great Synagogue and on the council of the United Synagogue, and simultaneously as medical officer for the Home for Aged Jews, the Joel Emanuel Almshouses, and the Sara Pyke Home for Girls.[59]

One of the early Jewish physicians with a practice in the East End was Dr Phineas Gross (1868–1902). He too was severely overworked, and died at the age of 34, but he was praised for allaying his patients' 'pain with soothing and cheering words; and although strictness was enforced when necessity compelled, it was always mingled with gentleness and kindness'.[60] Another East End doctor, with a practice in the Commercial Road, was Bernhard Morris, who obtained his MD from Dorpat (Germany) in 1888 and requalified in Edinburgh in 1893. Described by one former patient as 'a socialist, a Jewish saint', he was a bachelor, slightly awkward in manner, of whom it used to be said that he did not take money from patients who could not afford to pay, but actually left them with some cash from his own pocket.[61]

Dr William Moses Feldman (1880–1939), later a consultant in paediatrics in Harley Street, started out as an assistant of Dr Morris. Anticipating many features of the strict regimen of baby-care promulgated by Dr Frederic Truby King (1858–1938)—a widely followed paediatrician who taught that 'regularity' in infant care 'was paramount'—Feldman published a manual in Yiddish for immigrant mothers in 1907; it is fortunate that his ideas were not rigidly followed, because he advised mothers to shorten the period of breast-feeding, which would have reduced the infants' protection against diseases.[62]

[57] *JC* 14 Mar. 1924, p. 10 (obituary of Michael).
[58] *JC* 21 Mar. 1924, p. 10 (additional obituary of Michael).
[59] *JC* 14 Mar. 1924, p. 10, 21 Mar. 1924, p. 10.   [60] *JC* 19 Dec. 1902 (obituary of Gross).
[61] Interview with Michael Cooper, 8 May 1997, on Bernhard Morris.
[62] John Cooper, *The Child in Jewish History* (Northvale, NJ: Aronson, 1996), 331, 332; on Feldman, see S. Levy (ed.), *The Jewish Year Book 1933* (London: Jewish Chronicle, 1933), 391. Research by Lara Marks and others has shown that immigrant mothers breast-fed for longer periods than others.

According to Bethel Solomons (1885–1965), 'not more than fifteen per cent [of newly qualified doctors] remained in Ireland. Many went into the Army, Navy, Indian and Colonial Medical Services, some went to Great Britain as assistants or partners; the remainder stayed in Ireland as general practitioners or specialists.'[63] Jewish medical graduates followed these trends. Selim M. Salaman and Asher Leventon joined the Indian Medical Service, but most moved to England, where employment opportunities were more numerous. Dr Henry Dutch (1862–1926) seems to have prospered. He lived at 8 Berkeley Street, off Piccadilly, served for twenty-five years on Westminster City Council, and was chief medical officer of the Jewish Lads' Brigade.[64] Dr Jacob Isaac Jaffé (1878–1918), like Gustave Michael, was a busy communal leader with a large practice whose own health succumbed to the added strain of voluntary medical war work. He was considered

a notable and energetic figure in the social and communal life of Stoke Newington, building up by professional ability, sheer personal charm, and untiring energy one of the largest practices in North London. In spite of the heavy demands of this practice, he found time to guide the destinies of the Stoke Newington Jewish Literary Society, to take part in the deliberations of the Board of Deputies (where he represented Limerick), and the Stoke Newington Borough Council.

He also participated fully in the work of the board of management of his local synagogue, besides sitting on the Council of the United Synagogue. He died at the age of 40.[65]

When King Edward VII ascended the throne in 1901 he surrounded himself with a coterie of assimilated Jewish bankers—the Rothschilds, the Sassoons, Baron Maurice de Hirsch, and Sir Ernest Cassel—with whom he socialized and shared his enthusiasm for horse-racing. Edward not only had a genuine affection for his wealthy Jewish friends, but also placed a high value on Jewish legal and medical advisers. Felix Semon had met him while he was Prince of Wales, after treating Lillie Langtry in 1888, and through his skill as a raconteur, his usefulness at bridge, and his prowess at shooting soon became a friend of the prince. Knighted by Queen Victoria, Semon was later appointed physician extraordinary to the king and treated Edward for recurring attacks of bronchial catarrh due to his heavy smoking—until in 1908 he fell out of royal favour by supplementing his successful treatment with a rebuke for the king's neglect of his own health. Thus the king was sending out signals to the medical world that Anglicized Jewish doctors were completely acceptable and that they could be promoted to the highest positions. Under the Liberal government elected in

[63] Bethel Solomons, *One Doctor in his Time* (London: Johnson, 1956), 34; Louis Hyman, *The Jews of Ireland* (London: Jewish Historical Society of England, 1972), 143–5.

[64] *JC* 21 May 1926, p. 14, *BMJ* 29 May 1926, 925, obituaries of Henry Dutch.

[65] *JC* 18 Oct. 1918, p. 12 (obituary of Jaffe).

1906, royal support for the social acceptance of Jews was reinforced by educational reforms facilitating their preparation for entry into the professions, as well as relaxation of the immigration rules and the gradual emergence of a more open society in the years before the First World War. Both the Jewish masses and some of the new members of the elite were identified with the Liberal Party, which welcomed Jewish parliamentary candidates: Isaacs, Samuel, and Montagu all became Cabinet ministers.[66]

Who were the outstanding Jewish medical men in London during the Edwardian era? Three names spring readily to mind: Dr Gustave Schorstein (1863–1906), Dr Bertram Abrahams (1870–1908), and Dr Sidney Philip Phillips (1851–1951). Both Schorstein and Abrahams suffered careers, and eventually lives, cut short by persistent ill-health. Schorstein was a brother-in-law of Claude Montefiore, the biblical scholar and founder in 1910 of the Liberal Synagogue (his sister Thérèse was Montefiore's first wife) and very much a member of the Anglo-Jewish establishment. Originally intended for the rabbinate, Schorstein was actively committed to the Anglo-Jewish community, participating in the work of the sanitary committee of the Jewish Board of Guardians, especially with regard to its attempts to eradicate tuberculosis, and criticizing the overwork caused by traditional teaching methods in the *cheder*, the Jewish religious school. 'Although he was no older than forty-three [at the time of his death] he had already attained the summit of his profession', proclaimed one obituary writer.

As physician of the London and Brompton Hospitals, as the possessor of a large private practice, and in many other capacities, he was widely known and held in the highest esteem by all classes, both within the community and without. His work at the London Hospital more particularly brought him into sympathetic relations with the East End poor, many of whom he had generously visited in their own homes, and who repaid his zealous devotion with the keenest appreciation.

For all his establishment connections, Schorstein had a genial manner and conversed with poor Jewish patients from the East End in Yiddish, besides making himself available to all and sundry, particularly underpaid teachers: a rare generosity of approach in so eminent a physician.[67]

Educated at the City of London School, Schorstein was a favourite pupil of its famous headmaster Dr Abbot. After studying classics at Oxford, he enrolled as a student in the London Hospital, where he qualified in 1889 and was appointed to the posts of house physician and house surgeon, positions which

[66] Alderman, *Modern British Jewry*, 210; Anthony Allfrey, *Edward VII and his Jewish Court* (London: Weidenfeld & Nicolson, 1991), 6–15, 203–5.

[67] *JC* 23 Nov. 1906, p. 10; *Lancet*, 24 Nov. 1906, 1481; *BMJ* 24 Nov. 1906, 1524 (obituaries of Schorstein).

were later withheld from the sons of east European Jewish immigrants. In 1894 he was appointed as assistant physician to Sir Stephen Mackenzie, and in 1897 he secured his fellowship of the Royal College of Physicians, adding an MD from Oxford in 1904. In 1905 he was promoted, being made a full physician at the London Hospital. At the same time, he devoted much attention to the study of tuberculosis and was a physician at the Brompton Hospital for Diseases of the Chest and Consumption; he also held lectureships in public health and medical pathology at the London Hospital.[68] One former student of his, paying tribute, remarked that

by the present generation of 'London' men he will be best remembered as a clinical teacher of rare merit. Those who had the privilege of working under him will ever cherish memories of the witty and instructive clinical talks to which they were entertained every Monday and Thursday. His large and enthusiastic following testified to his popularity as a bedside teacher. A polished and fluent speaker, his remarks were always closely followed not only by reason of their practical nature, but because of the wit and humour which invariably characterised them.[69]

According to the *Lancet*,

Dr Schorstein was not only a physician of singular acumen and sound knowledge but he had the rare faculty of infusing his own energy and capacity for organisation into others. He was devoted to the interests of both the Oxford Medical School and the London Hospital School and it was in great measure due to him that the former has become the centre of activity which it now is.[70]

'Apart from the teaching side of his duties Dr Schorstein was a favourite at the bedside,' declared a former pupil, 'especially in the children's wards . . . How well I remember his cheery greeting on entering a ward and his skilful but gentle examination of some little patient. On these occasions a coin of the realm would be observed to change hands to the intense satisfaction of the little one.' Redcliffe Salaman, another one of his students, described Schorstein as 'a man who was greatly respected and loved by everybody'. Suffering for some years from diabetes, Schorstein recuperated with annual visits to Carlsbad and Engadin in Switzerland, but eventually his exhausting labours took their toll and he died at the age of 43.[71]

Almost as brilliant was the career of Dr Bertram Abrahams, the son of L. B. Abrahams, the headmaster of the Jews' Free School. After attending the City of London and University College Schools he enrolled at University College medical school, from which he graduated in 1894, winning gold and silver

[68] *JC* 23 Nov. 1906, p. 10.   [69] *JC* 30 Nov. 1906, p. 11 (obituary of Schorstein).
[70] *Lancet*, 24 Nov. 1906, 1481 (obituary of Schorstein).
[71] *JC* 30 Nov. 1906, p. 11; Salaman, 'The Helmsman', 31.

medals for his outstanding academic achievements. He set up a consulting practice in Welbeck Street, where he rapidly acquired a reputation as an authority
on certain forms of disease. In 1898 he was appointed registrar and in 1903
assistant physician to the Westminster Hospital, where he lectured in physiology and medicine, and rose to become sub-dean of the medical school. In 1904 he
was elected a Fellow of the Royal College of Physicians. He was also one of the
first medical inspectors in the London County Council schools, and set up a
school for children suffering from favus, an infectious skin disease, where his
own methods of treatment were utilized.[72] Sir William Allchin, one of the consultants at the hospital, praised Abrahams as

a physician whose knowledge was based upon the soundest and most recent physiological and pathological principles, which his inborn ability and clinical acumen had
developed and applied . . . he had an exceptional power of imparting to others the
knowledge he possessed, and this in the clearest language, whether written or spoken . . .
and it is not going too far to say that for some years past a very considerable share of the
medical teaching at Westminster Hospital devolved upon him.[73]

So highly regarded was Abrahams that he was frequently consulted by colleagues, even by those senior to him in the medical profession. Had he lived
longer, instead of dying at 38 from a kidney disease, Abrahams would undoubt-
edly have achieved full consultant status.[74]

Abrahams was also deeply involved with the Jewish community. Before the
Jewish Athletic Association was formed in 1899, he took boys to Victoria Park
in Bethnal Green, where he gave them cricket coaching. He was closely connected with the Jewish Lads' Brigade, and 'When he was well enough to attend
camp he was the life and soul of the officers' mess, where his sparkling wit was
much appreciated.'[75] Abrahams also acted for five years as honorary secretary of
the Maccabeans, the body of the Jewish professionals.

The final member of this illustrious trio was Dr Sidney Philip Phillips, who,
in marked contrast to the sad fates of Schorstein and Abrahams, enjoyed a very
long as well as a highly distinguished career. The son of a City businessman, he
was educated at University College School, which at that time was housed in
the south wing of University College, and proceeded to the college itself and its
medical school. He qualified as a doctor in 1877, gaining the gold medal for
materia medica and therapy; he then served first as house physician and surgeon, and later as ophthalmic assistant and junior demonstrator in anatomy. He
briefly held the position of surgical registrar at the Middlesex Hospital before
moving to St Mary's Hospital, where he was appointed physician to the

[72] *JC* 26 June 1908, p. 10 (obituary of Abrahams).
[73] *Lancet*, 4 July 1908, 63–4 (obituary of Abrahams).
[74] *JC* 3 July 1908, p. 22, 10 July 1908, p. 14 (tributes to Abrahams).   [75] *JC* 26 June 1908, p. 10.

outpatients, becoming a full physician in 1896 on the retirement of Sir William Broadbent. He was also physician to the London Fever Hospital, the Paddington Green Hospital for Children, and the Lock Hospital, and published many papers on fevers and diseases of the heart and digestion.[76] 'Perhaps Phillips was best known at St. Mary's for his ward classes as medical tutor, which he carried on from 1890–1901', recalled Wilfred Harris, his colleague at St Mary's.

He had a good-natured, pawky humour, and was fond of teasing his students in class by laying simple traps, such as telling them to listen to the inaudible heart in a man with gross emphysema and then questioning them on what they had heard . . . In appearance he was tall and thin, with aquiline features, iron-grey hair, and a clipped moustache.[77]

Phillips belonged to one of the long-established Anglo-Jewish families—albeit one that went through difficult times financially (his father died before he had qualified)—and he established himself as a member of the Jewish elite with a bachelor residence at 3 Upper Brook Street, Grosvenor Square.

In contrast to Schorstein, Abrahams, and Phillips, Charles Joseph Singer (1876–1960) failed to prosper as a doctor, despite his many talents. He was the son of the Reverend Simeon Singer, a stalwart of the Orthodox United Synagogue (the majority grouping at this time) and the compiler of the daily prayer book authorized by the Chief Rabbi and affectionately known as Singer's *Siddur*. Charles studied zoology at Oxford and medicine at St Mary's, where he qualified in 1903. He then held some minor appointments at the Sussex County Hospital in Brighton and abroad, returning to London to become registrar at the Cancer Hospital in 1908.[78] When the post of registrar at St Mary's Hospital fell vacant, there were two candidates, Charles Singer and Charles Wilson (later Lord Moran). On the surface, Singer seemed by far the stronger candidate, having acquired the diploma for membership of the Royal College of Physicians by passing a tough postgraduate examination in internal medicine and by having served as a registrar elsewhere. By contrast, Wilson's student career, in his own words, 'had been quite devoid of distinction, I had not gone up for any of the annual prizes, I had not even a reputation for industry'. The non-Jewish Wilson, however, had been captain of the hospital rugby team, on the strength of which he had been appointed as Dr Sidney Phillips's house physician, from which he had progressed to the position of obstetric officer. It appears from Wilson's autobiographical notes that Singer was not 'altogether congenial to the physicians' at the hospital, Sidney Phillips and Wilfred Harris, who supported

[76] *JC* 2 Feb. 1951, p. 21.   [77] *BMJ* 3 Feb. 1951, 252 (obituary of Phillips).
[78] *JC* 17 June 1960, p. 30 (obituary of Singer). The Charles Joseph Singer Papers, Wellcome Library, London, include a curriculum vitae.

Wilson's candidature.[79] This may have been because of Singer's 'lowly' origins; many members of the established Anglo-Jewish elite were contemptuous of the children of immigrants, albeit their co-religionists. Singer later married Dorothea Waley Cohen, a member of the Anglo-Jewish upper class, and initially had not been welcomed by her family, as the son of a rabbi and a second-generation immigrant. Perhaps the doctors had a similar perception of him. Although Singer became a physician to the Dreadnought Hospital and established himself as a consultant in Brook Street, his career as a cancer specialist never progressed; following his election as FRCP in 1917, he decided on an academic career and a year later was appointed as lecturer in the history of biology at Oxford, eventually becoming professor of the history of medicine at the University of London in 1930 and a pioneer in this field in England. During the 1930s Singer was active on behalf of refugee Jewish doctors through the Society for the Protection of Science and Learning; but he abandoned the orthodoxy of his father and regarded the dietary laws and circumcision as 'piffle', sympathizing with Judaism solely as a prophetic faith.[80]

Jewish doctors not only had to overcome social barriers if they wished to reach the rank of consultant, they also had to survive a difficult apprenticeship as a houseman in a hospital, where a sudden bout of ill-health could demolish a career. 'As far as we were concerned, the first recognizable strain took place when, working in pairs, we did our maternity [stint prior to qualification]', wrote Salaman.

We were on duty for a fortnight; in that time each of us would deliver not less than 54 mothers, and after a preliminary visit each would leave about half the number to be dealt with by his partner. In addition, we visited each case every day for ten days . . . We were thus on for a month on end. The deliveries took place in the homes, many of which were the poorest imaginable and often totally unprepared for the event. Once I attended a woman in a naked garret, reached by a ladder. There was a broken down bed with a single blanket, a chair without a back, a tin basin without a towel, and the poor mother herself practically naked. Of food and drink there was none.

If the medical student encountered a difficult delivery, he could call on the assistance of the resident accoucheur, but the one Salaman encountered at the London Hospital was singularly 'incompetent', causing a baby to be lost through his negligence. 'The maternity fortnight was, as I look back on it now, a veritable nightmare', Salaman declared. 'I was no sooner in my bed at the hospital

[79] Richard Lovell, 'Choosing People: An Aspect of the Life of Lord Moran (1882–1977)', *Medical History*, 36 (1992), 444; id., *Churchill's Doctor: A Biography of Lord Moran* (London: Royal Society of Medicine, 1992), 13–17.

[80] Henriques, *Sir Robert Waley Cohen*, 165; see also a letter from Henry Curtis to Singer, 4 Nov. 1911 (PP/CJS/A3/1), and a copy letter from Singer to Redcliffe Salaman, 2 Nov. 1943 (PP/CJS/A16/1), both in the Singer Papers. Henry Curtis was a consultant to whom Singer sent a paper on cancer and whom he was trying to impress; the letter to Salaman contains Singer's views on Judaism.

than I was summoned to go to a case, I sat down to a meal and it was ten to one I never got beyond the first few mouthfuls, when I was off again . . . I lost all sense of time.'[81]

Some newly qualified doctors gained house appointments in the provinces; others passed straight into private practice; yet others, of the right social standing and educational attainments, having passed their final examinations filled the most junior positions in the leading London hospitals. 'Whether it was of a house physician or house surgeon, the work was equally exacting, the responsibility unmeasured', Salaman asserted.

Every twelve days one 'firm' on the medical and one on the surgical [ward] 'took in' having cleared as many as possible of the 70 odd beds which were under the particular physician or surgeon, in preparation for the reception of all the acute cases which might come in during the course of the next four days, as well as such reserved cases of serious illness which might be sent in by seniors in command of the 'firm'. During the taking-in period, the house physician, in addition to keeping an eye on his more acute cases in the evening, gave anaesthetics for his corresponding house-surgeon whilst he dealt with minor surgical cases. At half past eleven o'clock we . . . used to go to the Receiving-room for a cup of cocoa and a chat with sister, and then to bed, but rarely to sleep for we were alternately responsible for all the casualties which came in till midnight and on a Saturday night [with the hospital abutting the East End] . . . that was more or less a whole-time job for the house physician.

Moreover, Salaman contended,

So keen was our interest, so happy our mood, that we were blind to the dangers which threatened us, and what was worse, the governing body and [the hospital] authorities . . . never scented the danger when they worked us at top pressure without arranging for the break of even a day in a six months appointment.[82]

Hospitals at the turn of the century were infested with a lethal cocktail of germs, to which the grossly overworked young doctors frequently succumbed. There were as yet no antibiotics to combat the acute infections to which these doctors were prone to fall victim, nor were there any drugs to assist them if they contracted tuberculosis; streptomycin was not discovered until 1943. 'The trouble began during my first year of office', Salaman remembered.

The casualties all occurred within the 'set'. One of the house-men developed a septic throat, carried on for a few days, collapsed, was put to bed, and in about a week, was dead. We were saddened but regarded it as a passing misfortune. Before two years had passed, apart from those who fell sick, and recovered to a greater or less degree, four more died in exactly the same way, including my very dear friend, R. W. Payne. In addition, one other went down with Pthisis [tuberculosis] but recovered sufficiently after some years to go back to work.[83]

---

[81] Salaman, 'The Helmsman', 27, 28, 40.   [82] Ibid. 27, 40, 41.   [83] Ibid. 26, 41, 42, 44.

In 1901 Salaman took up the position of director of the enlarged Pathological Institute at the London Hospital, as he had scruples about competing with his less well-off colleagues for the hospital appointments in clinical medicine. Unfortunately, soon afterwards in 1903 he suffered a serious breakdown in his health when he contracted tuberculosis, and his medical career was brought to a premature end; he became a plant geneticist and director of the Potato Virus Research Station at Cambridge.[84] Salaman's close friend Charles Samuel Myers (1873–1946), after graduating with an MB from St Bartholomew's Hospital, suffered a similar setback to his health. After travelling to Egypt to recuperate, he taught physiology at Cambridge, then switched to psychology and opened the first English experimental psychology laboratory at Cambridge in 1912.[85] Other potential high-flyers, such as Charles Gabriel Seligman (1873–1940), the superintendent of the Clinical Laboratory at St Thomas's Hospital from 1901 to 1904, also felt unable to continue with a career in medicine; Seligman seems simply to have lost interest, subsequently enjoying a distinguished career as an anthropologist.[86]

Reviewing the evidence, it appears that in the late Victorian age assimilated German-born Jews and English Jews from well-connected families could secure positions as surgeons in the leading London teaching hospitals. During the Edwardian age, although it was difficult for Jews to enter the new specialties in surgery, Jews from upper-middle-class or from old Ashkenazi families were appointed as consultant physicians in the principal teaching hospitals in London and elsewhere, such as the Manchester Royal Infirmary. In Leeds, Albert Sidney Frankau Leyton (1869–1921), the professor of pathology, who concentrated on cancer research and later became dean of the medical school, was of Jewish origin, though he had married a non-Jew and severed his links with the Jewish community.[87] The situation was much more fluid as far as prestigious jobs were concerned than it became for the children of east European immigrants between the two world wars. It is possible that the failure of Charles Singer, despite a brilliant academic record, to secure a hospital appointment commensurate with his talent may be a harbinger of the fraught situation that was to obtain between the wars; for Singer was not a member of the Anglo-Jewish patrician class and many doors remained closed to him. It is possible that had Charles Keyser FRCS (1874–1910), a surgeon at the London Cancer

[84] Redcliffe Salaman, *The History and Social Influence of the Potato* (Cambridge: Cambridge University Press, 1985), pp. xxix, xxx, xxxi.

[85] 'Charles Samuel Myers', in L. G. Wickham Legg and E. T. Williams (eds.), *Dictionary of National Biography 1941–1950* (London: Oxford University Press, 1959), 613, 614.

[86] 'Charles Gabriel Seligman', in L. G. Wickham Legg (ed.), *Dictionary of National Biography 1931–1940* (London: Oxford University Press, 1949), 802.

[87] *Lives of the Fellows of the Royal College of Physicians of London*, 438, on A. S. F. Leyton.

Hospital, not died at the age of 36 he might have obtained an appointment at a teaching hospital. However, it is significant that Dr Maro Tuchmann, an expert on bladder and kidney diseases, who died in 1902 in his early sixties and was a member of the Hampstead United Synagogue, resigned as assistant surgeon to the German Hospital in London because of religious difficulties.[88]

Compared with the late Victorian group of consultants, their Edwardian successors Gustave Schorstein and Bertram Abrahams were much more closely involved with the Anglo-Jewish community. Even Sidney Phillips was associated with the Maccabeans, the organization of Jewish professionals, and I have already noted the depth of Schorstein's commitment to East End Jewry.

Outside the hospital system, there were a couple of outstanding Jewish medical experts who deserve mention: Dr Alfred Eichholz (1869–1933) and Dr Montague David Eder (1866–1936). Eichholz was awarded a first-class degree in both parts of the natural science tripos at Cambridge, and in 1893 was elected a fellow of his college—one of the first two Jewish fellows at the university. He was later made university demonstrator in physiology. After qualifying as a doctor, Eichholz served as the medical inspector of schools in Lambeth. When he appeared before the Inter-Departmental Committee on Physical Deterioration which reported in 1904 he became a star witness, exposing the conditions in the Johanna Street School, where 90 per cent of the children had so little to eat they were unable to study properly. Dr Eichholz testified that 'if the medical officer went round the schools and certified a child as obviously ill he ought to be excluded from further employment out of school', agreeing that his proposal would result in a medical man being engaged by every local authority. Never close to more politically minded public health experts like George Newman or Arthur Newsholme, Eichholz was passed over when a new post of chief medical officer to the Board of Education was created in 1907. He did, however, join the Board of Education as assistant medical officer, and rose to the position of chief medical inspector in 1919. Here he became even better acquainted with the medical, sanitary, and hygienic aspects of schools, and worked with schools for blind, deaf, and dumb children.[89]

While at Cambridge, Eichholz fell under the spell of Solomon Schechter, from whom 'he caught an overmastering belief in the vitality and growth of Judaism and an intense admiration for its literature'. In 1895 he married Ruth, the second daughter of Chief Rabbi Adler, and when the Union of Hebrew and Religion Classes was formed around 1910 Eichholz became a moving spirit in the organization. After the First World War, Jewish education was co-ordinated not only in London but in the provinces as well, and Eichholz was chosen to head

---

[88] *JC* 1 July 1910, p. 9 (obituary of Keyser), 31 Oct. 1902, p. 3 (obituary of Tuchmann).

[89] *JC* 10 Feb. 1933, pp. 12–13 (obituary of Eichholz); Bentley B. Gilbert, *The Evolution of National Insurance in Great Britain* (London: Joseph, 1966), 89 and 133.

the new Central Committee for Jewish Education. He was also vice-president of the Jewish Health Organization and chairman of the New West End Synagogue League of Social Service.[90]

Montague David Eder, better known as David Eder, seems to have embodied what was best in the spirit of openness in Edwardian England. After attending St Bartholomew's medical school, Eder qualified as a doctor in 1895 and obtained an MD from Bogotá in Colombia; in 1905 he practised briefly at 55 Commercial Road in the East End before moving to Charlotte Street in the West End, where he tended to the needs of working-class and immigrant patients.[91] A member of the Fabian Society and of the Independent Labour Party from its early days, he became an enthusiastic supporter of Margaret McMillan's campaign for child health, helping at the school clinic in Bow which was set up in 1908 and then moving to the larger clinic which was opened in Deptford in 1910. As one of the three directors, he attended regularly and wrote many of the annual reports for Miss McMillan.

At Deptford an eye-witness records Eder's unfailing cheerfulness and ingenuity when eye-testing had to be done in a little black-cupboard of a room, tonsils operated on when beds must be improvised on the spot, extra money collected here, there and everywhere, when it was found that the open-air life inaugurated by Miss McMillan so increased these slum children's appetites that the . . . usual 'institution diet' became totally impossible.

With Dr James Kerr, the medical officer of the London County Council, he established the journal *School Hygiene* in 1910; he became its editor and used its pages to campaign for an expansion of the network of school clinics.[92]

Until recently it was believed that a national system of school clinics was established by a far-seeing civil servant, Sir Robert Morant; but N. D. Daglish has questioned this and shown that Morant was not so much concerned with Margaret McMillan's emphasis on the 'Therapeutic Remedial side' of the project. Instead, Daglish credited Morant's appointee George Newman, the chief medical officer of the Board of Education, 'with the creation and development of the school medical service'.[93] However, this is to ignore the fact that Newman wanted to proceed slowly with the development of school clinics, and that it was pressure from Margaret McMillan and more especially David Eder that forced him to move more quickly. In an editorial by Eder in *School Hygiene* in

[90] *JC* 10 Feb. 1933, pp. 12–13. *The Jewish Year Book 1933*, 386.

[91] *David Eder: Memoirs of a Modern Pioneer*, ed. J. B. Hobman (London: Gollancz, 1945), 41, 48, 73–7; *JC* 3 Apr. 1936, p. 12 (obituary of Eder).

[92] M. D. Eder and R. Tribe, 'Report on the Deptford School Clinic', *School Hygiene* (Mar. 1911); M. D. Eder, 'Report on the Deptford School Clinic', *School Hygiene* (Oct. 1911).

[93] N. D. Daglish, 'Robert Morant's Hidden Agenda? The Origins of the Medical Treatment of Schoolchildren', *History of Education*, 19/2 (1990), 139–48.

August 1910 it was suggested that 'Just as a recalcitrant Board had, a short time ago, to be driven to some pronouncement upon medical inspection, it will have to be driven by parents, teachers, and doctors, rightly indignant at the present chaos, to make up its mind about treatment.' Elsewhere in the journal he pointed out that 'The diseases for which there is no proper provision are dental decay, defects of vision, simple eye diseases, "running ears", adenoids, and enlarged tonsils, skin diseases such as ringworm and pediculosis.' Again, in February 1911, in an examination of Newman's report for 1909, Eder asserted that any criticism of it should be based 'upon a failure to take advantage to the full of "spade work" already done, not only in actual medical inspection in this country and abroad, but also in the fields of medical and surgical therapeutics . . . the probable or suitable lines for further development are not suggested'. Discussing Newman's report for 1910, *School Hygiene* declared that 'This year the report goes further; an entire section is devoted to school clinics . . . it is even laid down that whether a centre termed a "school clinic" be or not be used in any scheme of treatment, the method and spirit of the school clinic should be adopted . . . a clear line of advance is indicated much more strongly than has been the case in the previous years.'[94] Newman, under pressure from *School Hygiene* and the school doctors, broached the question of a grant at meetings with Lloyd George, the Chancellor of the Exchequer, on 3 August and 25 October 1911; in 1912 Newman and Christopher Addison, after several years of determined persuasion, secured a grant of £60,000 per annum from the government to assist the running of school clinics.[95]

Eder was also an early practitioner of psychoanalysis in England. In 1912 he opened a consulting room in Welbeck Street; here he saw surplus patients sent to him by Ernest Jones, who had coached him for his medical examinations. The following year, together with Jones, who was the senior partner in this venture, he formed the London Psycho-Analytic Society. Freud hailed Eder 'as the first, and for a time the only doctor to practise the new therapy [psychoanalysis] in England', but this was not strictly true; credit for this pioneering role must be given to Jones. However, the latter served briefly as professor of psychiatry in Canada prior to the First World War, and at that time Eder was the only psychoanalytic practitioner in England.

In 1916 Eder was placed in charge of a hospital in Malta for troops traumatized by the war, and a year later he published a notable study, *War Shock*. Encountering opposition to psychoanalysis within the army, he returned to London to resume his medical practice and also to work as a physician to the

---

[94] *School Hygiene* (May 1910, Aug. 1910, Feb. 1911, Dec. 1911).

[95] John M. Eyler, *Sir Arthur Newsholme and State Medicine 1885–1935* (Cambridge: Cambridge University Press, 1997), 322–4; George Newman, Diary, 3 Aug. 1911, Oct. 1911, MH139/1, National Archives.

Ministry of Pensions neurological clinic. Having drifted into Jungian circles before the First World War, which led to a cooling in his relationship with Ernest Jones, he rejoined the British Psycho-Analytical Society in 1923 and in the same year went to Budapest for eight months for analysis with Sandor Ferenczi, who developed a more interactional model of psychoanalysis rather than concentrating solely on the patient's internal world. On his return, Eder was appointed physician to the London Clinic of Psycho-Analysis; also, renewing his earlier interest in children and young people, he established the Institute for the Treatment of Delinquency.[96]

'Following long days at his Welbeck Street consulting-rooms', wrote W. F. Purves,

he [Eder] used to put in several hours every evening in a little room at the junction of Charlotte Street and Percy Street, as a real 'poor man's doctor'. Whether patients had money or not did not seem to matter at all to Eder: the poorest got the same sympathetic attention as his richest patients further west. And, after these hectic hours of work among the cosmopolitan poor—including unlucky artists, writers, waiters, working women, and women of the streets—for whose medicine and other requirements he often paid—off he would rush to some East End political or educational meeting that lasted well on towards midnight . . . civilians and soldiers . . . [received] the same devoted service . . . as . . . the richest officer or captain of industry who went to him for psycho-analytical treatment after a nervous breakdown.[97]

Influenced by his cousin Israel Zangwill, Eder became a member of the council of the Jewish Territorial Organization (the ITO) in 1906, and two years later went on an expedition to Cyrenaica in North Africa to investigate whether a Jewish colony could be established there. In 1917 he declared that 'We studied other territories in Australia, Canada, Africa and America, but without any fruitful results . . . And so having completed the circle, I came back to the original scheme of the Zionists, viz., Palestine, including Mesopotamia.'[98] Having been persuaded by Chaim Weizmann to join the Zionist Commission in Palestine in 1918 as a medical expert and representative of the ITO to advise the British authorities, Eder did not finally return to Britain until August 1922. Disease spread rapidly through the population of Palestine during the war, and 5,000 Jewish children were left as orphans. Under Eder's direction new orphanages were opened in Jerusalem and Jaffa, while the bulk of the orphans were boarded out among suitable families, and unsatisfactory institutions were closed. 'Drawing upon his experience in London, where he had been a pioneer of school clinics, he [Eder] arranged for every child to be regularly examined for trachoma, thus saving many from blindness.'[99] Workshops and land colonies (a form of smallholding) were also started, to occupy the unemployed.

[96] Eder, *Memoirs*, 89–116; Vincent Brome, *Ernest Jones* (London: Caliban, 1982), 105, 121, 210, 211.
[97] Cited in Eder, *Memoirs*, 129.   [98] *JC* 13 Apr. 1917, p. 10.   [99] *JC* 21 Mar. 1919, p. 21.

Eder took on the responsibility of acting as the principal spokesman for the Zionist movement in talks with the British authorities. On his return to London, he devoted himself to Zionist activities, and in particular to the preparatory work necessary before the Hebrew University could be opened. He was chairman of the Advisory Committee which devised the first schemes for the science departments, he established the organization of the Friends of the Hebrew University in Britain, and he conceived and organized the official ceremony marking the opening of the university in 1925. From 1933 until his untimely death in 1936, Eder assumed the leadership of the campaign for the entry of refugee doctors into Britain.[100]

Jewish doctors in the 1890s and the Edwardian age were more intimately concerned with the daily tribulations of the poorer sections of the population than their colleagues as a whole. For doctors from upper-middle-class Anglo-Jewish families, there was a communal tradition of public service. Redcliffe Salaman deliberately chose to study at the London Hospital, which was situated in the East End, so that he could gain an intimate knowledge of the Jewish immigrant population. Schorstein, Bertram Abrahams, and Dr Alfred Eichholz all in their different ways were imbued with the same notions of communal service. Dr David Eder was a transitional figure, a socialist and Zionist who shared Jewish concerns while reaching out to a wider public. From the 1890s, Jewish general practitioners able to speak Yiddish opened surgeries in the East End, where the bulk of the Anglo-Jewish immigrant population was located. Here they competed with the charitable dispensaries and doctors from the Christian missions; their income remained precarious until a system of panel practices was inaugurated under the provisions of Part 1 of the National Insurance Act 1911.

Edwardian England was in many respects an open society, yet paradoxically the number of Jewish consultants in teaching hospitals remained small. This can be explained by the numerical insignificance of upper-class Jewish families in late Victorian Britain, by their preference for sending their sons into commerce rather than into the professions, and by the paucity of Jews studying biology and natural science at Oxford and Cambridge, the departments from which the elite of the medical profession was recruited. It must also be remembered that working in a hospital in the Edwardian age was a hazardous occupation. Many medical students and doctors were incapacitated by disease, resulting in death or such serious invalidity that they had to embark on new careers. Thus Salaman and Myers moved out of medicine. Even if doctors started climbing the ranks of the hospital hierarchy, there was no guarantee that their careers would be long; as we have seen, Schorstein and Abrahams died prematurely.

[100] Eder, *Memoirs*, 134–96.

Medicine in that era was a dismal science. Jewish doctors who did not belong to the patrician class or were not socially assimilated usually drifted into the ranks of the general practitioners. Because so few Jews were trying to reach consultant status, such appointments as were made raised little apprehension.

TWO

The Entry of East European Jews into Medicine, 1914–1939

THIS chapter seeks to establish why so many young Jews from east European immigrant backgrounds in England set out to become doctors, when this trend began, and how it gathered momentum. It considers the rate of recruitment of Jewish medical students in London and the leading provincial centres with large immigrant populations—Manchester, Leeds, and Liverpool; and I discuss whether or not there was antisemitism in the admissions policy of the medical schools, and how important antipathy towards Jews was among English medical students.

According to Calvin Goldscheider and Alan Zuckerman (writing about America),

Working in more skilled and stable occupations, Jews earned more money than did other immigrant groups. Their relative income and occupational security made it easier for Jews to invest in the schooling of their children. This combined with the permanency of their immigration, urban residence, and the availability and access to public education. Together, these structural factors explain why Jewish children were in school longer than other immigrant groups and why Jews accounted for relatively high percentages of those who attended schools and universities in the large cities of the Northeast [United States]. As in Western Europe, occupation, residence, and access account for educational attainment levels.[1]

However, this is not the whole story, at least not for England, where many Jewish medical students, although not the majority, came from poor households. An additional important factor is the strong tradition of Bible and Talmud study among Jews. Joel Perlmann, after examining a sample of 12,000 individuals from different ethnic backgrounds in Providence, Rhode Island, asserted that certain shared cultural values and the love of learning were as important in explaining the high levels of Jewish educational attainment as the

---

[1] Calvin Goldscheider and Alan S. Zuckerman, *The Transformation of the Jews* (Chicago: University of Chicago Press, 1984), 168.

structural factors emphasized by Goldscheider and Zuckerman.[2] 'Western-isation did not affect this instinct [for learning]', noted D. B. Stanhill in 1932. 'It merely secularised the character of the learning. The thirst for knowledge in the emancipated continental Jew at the University today is no less keen than that of his grandfather at the *Yeshibah* fifty years ago.'[3] As Perlmann put it, 'The point is not so much the level of learning achieved, but rather the honorable place learning enjoyed in the traditional culture.'[4] Again, it was argued by 'Watchman' in the *Jewish Chronicle* in 1932 that 'in the case of the Jewish father [in England] respect for scholarship plays its part, quite as much as the desire to do his best for the child. As a trader himself, too, he feels several inches added to his social stature, when he hears his own son addressed as "Doctor".'[5] The secretary of the Glasgow Jewish students' society corroborated this when he referred to 'the great respect, almost veneration, in which the profession is held by the community . . . and the consequent desire of parents to see their sons reap the benefits of such a position'. It is noteworthy that the sons of rabbis and cantors, precisely those with a tradition of learning in their families, were often among the first to enrol as medical students in England, and that they provided role models for their peers, encouraging other Jewish students to emulate them, thus quickening the pace of Jewish attendance at medical schools.[6]

The concentration of the immigrant generation in England in the tailoring, cabinet-making, and shopkeeping businesses meant that Jewish families favoured self-employment—an inclination further encouraged by the difficulty of maintaining strict sabbath observance when working for non-Jewish or public authority employers. The professions of medicine and law were more prestigious and generated higher incomes than the manual occupations or shopkeeping, but nevertheless were based on the same model of self-employment, and this attracted upwardly mobile Jewish men and women into them. Moreover, employment prospects in the medical profession were believed to be reasonably good.[7]

During the 1930s in England Jewish parents worried about past pogroms in their countries of origin and about the present gloomy situation in central and eastern Europe. 'In the case especially of Jewish doctors,' Arnold Goodman declared,

[2] Joel Perlmann, *Ethnic Differences: Schooling and Social Structure Among the Irish, Italians, Jews and Blacks in an American City 1880–1935* (Cambridge: Cambridge University Press, 1988), 122–60; Cooper, *The Child in Jewish History*, 305–7, 349–53.   [3] *JC* 18 Mar. 1932, p. 17 (Stanhill).
[4] Perlmann, *Ethnic Differences*, pp. 160–2.   [5] 'Watchman', *JC* 5 Feb. 1932, p. 11.
[6] Geoffrey D. M. Blok, 'Jewish Students at the Universities of Great Britain and Ireland Excluding London, 1936–1939: A Survey', *Sociological Review*, 34/3, 34/4 (1942), 189, 190.
[7] Seymour Wakov, *Lawyers in the Making* (Chicago: Aldine, 1965), ch. 3 by Joseph Zelan ('The Role of Occupational Inheritance'), esp. p. 50; Blok, 'Jewish Students', 190.

it is the parents who are inclined to advise their sons to become doctors out of a desire for their security. Most Jews . . . have their bags packed, metaphorically speaking, and a medical degree is a highly portable qualification . . . There are no realistic Jewish mothers who are unaware that medicine is one of the few professions—the law is another— where their sons can compete on equal terms with non-Jews.[8]

Surveys showed that Jewish children, because of their upbringing, had high levels of self-esteem, but that this was combined with a feeling of insecurity bred by their minority group status; the combination of the two gave them a competitive edge in examinations and in the marketplace.[9]

On the Continent, where the same social trends had occurred among Jews a generation or two earlier than in England, a considerable proportion of doctors were Jewish by the 1920s and 1930s. As early as 1890 Jews comprised 47.8 per cent of the medical students in the University of Vienna. In the Austrian capital, a city a quarter of the size of London but with about the same Jewish population level of 200,000, there were between 3,000 and 4,000 Jewish doctors in 1932. By the end of the nineteenth century, Jews constituted 16 per cent of the German medical profession. In 1930 there were 2,138 Jewish doctors in the region of Berlin, 1,965 men and 173 women: about a third of the total number of doctors, a proportion which they had already reached by the beginning of the century. In Prussia as a whole, in 1925 approximately 18 per cent of doctors were Jewish.[10]

The social factors responsible for the vast expansion in the number of Anglo-Jewish medical students were to be found throughout Jewish immigrant communities from eastern Europe across the English-speaking world. The Jewish achievement was all the more spectacular in that it started from such a low level. A survey of immigrants to the United States during the period 1899–1910 ascertained that, whereas 617 Italians had medical qualifications, only 290 Jewish arrivals were similarly trained to practise medicine.[11] In ten major cities surveyed in the United States, the number of Jewish doctors graduating increased from seven in 1875–80 to 277 in 1896–1900, 977 in 1911–15 and 2,313 in 1931–5. By 1934, of the 33,000 applications for admission to medical school, 60

[8] David Selbourne, *Not An Englishman: Conversations with Lord Goodman* (London: Sinclair-Stevenson, 1993), 57; Arnold Goodman, *Tell Them I'm On My Way: Memoirs* (London: Chapman, 1993), 22.   [9] Cooper, *The Child in Jewish History*, 354, 352.

[10] For Austria see Marsha L. Rozenblit, *The Jews of Vienna 1867–1914: Assimilation and Identity* (Albany, NY: State University Press of New York, 1983), 221; *JC* 27 Jan. 1928, 12 Feb. 1932, p. 23. For Germany see Robert N. Proctor, *Racial Hygiene: Medicine Under the Nazis* (Cambridge, Mass.: Harvard University Press, 1988), 142; *JC* 11 Apr. 1930, p. 29; Arthur Ruppin, *The Jews in the Modern World* (London: Macmillan, 1934), 218, 219.

[11] Thomas Kessner, *The Golden Door: Italian and Jewish Immigrant Mobility in New York City 1880–1915* (New York: Oxford University Press, 1977), 33.

per cent came from Jews.[12] In 1920, 7 per cent of entrants to the medical school attached to the University of Toronto in Canada were Jewish; this figure rose to 17 per cent in 1925 and 27 per cent in 1932. While the bulk of the fathers of these aspiring doctors were businessmen, between a third and a quarter were artisans.[13] Similarly, when Kenneth Collins investigated the occupational background of the fathers of Jewish medical students in Glasgow between 1924 and 1945, he found that almost one quarter (23.8 per cent) were artisans, mostly employed in the tailoring trade or as cabinet-makers; the majority of the fathers, as in Canada, were businessmen.[14]

Why did so many Anglo-Jewish students opt for a career in medicine rather than the law until after the Second World War? Several factors contributed to this preference. For one thing, the prestige of medicine was higher among the Jewish community than that of the law; for another, the community as a whole had not advanced far enough, economically and socially, by the inter-war period to forge the right connections to ensure a steady flow of work in the legal profession. Also, it was probably less expensive to train as a doctor in England than to become articled to a solicitor or wait to build up a practice as a barrister. For instance, the fees for a five-year course in the Leeds Medical School in 1915–16 were £27. 11s. od., inclusive of library and union fees, for the course leading up to the first examination at the end of year one, together with an additional payment of £115. 2s. 6d. for completing the rest of the course; the payment of the latter sum could, if necessary, be spread over four years.[15] When N. M. Jacoby enrolled as a student at Guy's Hospital medical school in 1928, he paid fees of £34. 13s. od. for a year's tuition, plus a £5 subscription to the Clubs Union; and he stayed there for six years.[16] Just as important as the general level of fees was the availability of numerous scholarships for financially impoverished medical students, as well as the assistance from the Education Aid Society that was targeted at bright but impecunious Jewish medical students. In contrast, the usual premium paid for articles to a solicitor before 1939 was £300 for five years (three years if the trainee had passed his Higher School Certificate), although higher and lower sums could be charged; scholarships in this field were scarce, and the Education Aid Society was reluctant to give grants to budding lawyers that would encourage poor boys to join already overcrowded professions.

[12] Jacob A. Goldberg, 'Jews in the Medical Profession: A National Survey', *Jewish Social Studies*, 1 (July 1939), 329; Leon Sokoloff, 'The Rise and Decline of the Jewish Quota in Medical School Admissions', *Bulletin of the New York Academy of Medicine*, 68 (1992), 498.

[13] R. D. Gidney and W. J. Millar, 'Medical Students at the University of Toronto 1910–1940: A Profile', *Canadian Bulletin of Medical History*, 13/1 (1996), 29–52.

[14] Collins, *Go and Learn*, 89–92.

[15] *The University of Leeds Calendar 1915–1916* (Leeds: Jowett & Sewry, 1915), 480–3.

[16] N. M. Jacoby, *A Journey through Medicine* (Sussex: Book Guild, 1991), 18, 19.

The Education Aid Society, which had been set up at the end of the nineteenth century, was led by members of the Anglo-Jewish establishment such as Robert Waley Cohen and Royalton Kisch (on whom see p. 180 below). It assisted Jewish students of all kinds—musicians, artists, those taking various degrees— but the main emphasis was on helping students of science, which included medicine. By 1930, it claimed, '42 students trained with the Society's help have qualified in medicine and are doing well, one or two having specialised in certain branches of the profession'.[17] The society's resources appear to have been minuscule: its income from subscriptions and donations was just £565 in 1937, and though this amount was supplemented by successful professionals repaying their student loans,[18] difficulties commonly arose in connection with repayment by students who, after qualifying, 'entered into financial negotiations in order to buy a practice which resulted in their incurring a debt the repayment of which took priority over their debt to the Society'.[19] To qualify for a grant, applicants had to show exceptional qualities of mind and personality and not be merely of average ability. Sometimes the society successfully picked out a future high-flyer; on other occasions they made an unimaginative choice, telling a future permanent secretary to the Treasury that in view of his poor family circumstances he should make a career in commerce, and rejecting an application for financial assistance from a future professor of psychiatry at Cambridge.[20]

It is worth examining a few examples of the Education Aid Society's work with students of medicine. Eli Velinsky of Leeds, who had won one of the two medical scholarships awarded by the city in 1928, applied for a grant of about £50. He was deemed to be a worthy applicant and it was decided 'to lend one of the Society's microscopes, to buy in London the books required from time to time and to make grants for apparatus, instruments, examination fees etc. as they were needed'. Simon Yudkin (later a consultant paediatrician at the Whittington Hospital in Highgate, north London), who had completed the final conjoint examinations, in anticipation of a grant from the society, 'borrowed £26-1s-od from a friend to pay his diploma and registration fees'. In April 1937 he was voted the money for the diploma and a sum to cover the final MB fee.[21] His brother John Yudkin became professor of physiology at London University. Their mother, after the premature death of her husband, had raised five sons by taking in six lodgers and by knitting sweaters. Another young man experienced the death of his father, a repairing tailor, soon after he had gained a state scholarship to study medicine. His mother earned £80 per annum as a

---

[17] Education Aid Society, *Objects, Methods and Progress* (London, 1930), 3–5, 8.
[18] Education Aid Society, *Annual Report 1937*, 12. [19] Ibid. 7.
[20] Education Aid Society, Minute Book, General Committee, 27 Sept. 1934, 14 Apr., 9 June, 19 July 1937, Southampton University, Parkes Library, MS 135 AJ/35/5.
[21] Education Aid Society, Minute Book, General Committee, 19 Sept. 1928, 1 Mar., 14 Apr., 9 June, 19 July 1937, Southampton University, Parkes Library, MS 135 AJ/35/5.

repairing tailoress, and the young man used his scholarship money to help maintain the family, including a brother who was still at school. 'In spite of this extreme poverty the lad did exceptionally well in his medical studies and it was only in his fifth year, when his scholarships came to an end, that he received a loan from the Society.'[22] Thus many of the doctors aided by the charity came from the poorer strata of the Jewish immigrant community.

Nearly all the recipients of this aid who were bent on becoming doctors were male. Yet increasing numbers of women were seeking to enter the medical profession. On the eve of the First World War, 30 per cent of the first generation of female students enrolled in Prussian medical schools and 60 per cent of the female medical students in the University of Vienna were Jewish.[23] In 1916 the *Jewish Chronicle* proclaimed that 'Miss FRANKLIN is by no means the first Jewess in this country to take a medical degree—quite a number are to be found in the East End of London, while another Jewess, Miss UMANSKI of Leeds, even holds a public medical appointment.'[24] A perusal of the pass lists at London medical schools, excluding the first year's examination, revealed that there were at least twenty-four female Jewish medical students enrolled in them between 1914 and 1924. In England as a whole the proportion of Jewish women students studying medicine in the years 1936–9 was higher than among non-Jewish women students: 20 per cent as opposed to 15 per cent. Many of these pioneering women doctors, such as Elsie Landau and Sybil Grace Mocatta, specialized in gynaecology, or in problems of birth control and the nurture of infants and children.[25] Vera Weizmann, the wife of the first president of Israel, who requalified as a doctor in Manchester in 1913 after studying in Geneva, was appointed medical officer to the local infant clinics, where she introduced 'improved methods of diet-and-weight control for the babies under . . . [her] care'.[26] Dr Amy Herbert pioneered the development of the Manchester Child Guidance Clinic during the 1930s. Dr Eveline Cohen, who was born in Tasmania, was one of the first Jewish women to practise medicine in England, taking up infant welfare work in Jewish centres in the East End before the First World War and continuing after the war until 1920; she died prematurely in 1922. Dr Deborah David (1900–94) moved from the Jewish Maternity (Bearsted Memorial) Hospital in Stoke Newington, east London, to become senior resident medical officer at the Birkenhead and Wirral Children's Hospital, where she stayed until the outbreak of the Second World War.[27]

[22] Kalman Jacob Mann, *Reflections on a Life in Health Care* (Jerusalem: Rubin Mass, 1994), 22.

[23] Aletta Jacobs, *Memories: My Life as an International Leader in Health, Suffrage, and Peace* (New York: Feminist Press at the City University of New York, 1996), 228 n. 8.

[24] *JC* 10 Nov. 1916, p. 6. [25] Blok, 'Jewish Students', 192.

[26] Vera Weizmann, *The Impossible Takes Longer* (London: Hamilton, 1967), 41.

[27] *JC* 9 Feb. 1940, 20 (obituary of Herbert), 20 Jan. 1922, p. 12 (obituary of Cohen), and 26 Feb. 1994 (obituary of David).

The growth in the number of Jewish doctors of both sexes, in both London and the provinces, accelerated markedly in the 1920s and 1930s. From a total of between 90 and 100 in 1910, their number in the capital had soared to about 500 in 1932, according to an estimate by Dr Maurice Sorsby, who, as the founder of the London Jewish Hospital Medical Society in 1928, was in a position to know. By 1938, Sorsby claimed, there were some 750 Jewish doctors and 150 Jewish dentists working in London. He suggested that 'in fairness to English Jews it must be pointed out that their numbers in medicine were insignificant until recently, their influx into medicine being largely a post-[First World] War phenomenon'.[28] In fact, this movement of the second generation of east European Jewish immigrants into the medical profession on a large scale began during the First World War, when many potential medical students from the upper and middle classes were serving in the armed forces, thereby creating a surplus of places in the medical schools. For the same reason, the London Hospital began to accept women applicants, who were duly given house appointments when they qualified. As a result of these anomalous wartime circumstances, there were about thirty Jewish medical students in the London Hospital by the spring of 1918, a marked increase over pre-war numbers.[29]

The incomers were by no means universally welcomed. In 1918 Lord Knutsford, the chairman of the London Hospital, admitted that

What had happened . . . was that, in view of the drain caused by the War the Hospital had been accepting for some time past students of various nationalities and creeds of a different type and of a different social standing to those formerly received and the experiment had not been successful. The Authorities therefore had been obliged to decide not to take Students in future, whatever their religion, who came below a certain standard.

Certain of the medical students at the London Hospital had always been prone to antisemitic outbursts, and while these were not on anything like the scale of the Continental hatred of Jews, they were none the less disturbing and irritating to the Jewish students against whom the hostility was directed. When Redcliffe Salaman was a student at the London Hospital in the 1890s, one of these unpleasant students directed abuse against 'a shy, cultured, somewhat gauche but peculiarly inoffensive young man', calling him 'that disgusting b——y Jew, etc.'. Salaman took strong exception to these remarks, forcing

[28] *JC* 12 Feb. 1932, p. 23, 29 Apr. 1938, p. 13. Previously, in 1928, Maurice Sorsby had formed the opinion that there were 450 Jewish doctors in the whole of the United Kingdom and Eire, perhaps an underestimate: *JC* 27 Jan. 1928.

[29] A. E. Clark-Kennedy, *The London. A Study of the Voluntary Hospital System: The Second Hundred Years*, 2 vols. (London: Pitman Medical, 1962–3), ii. 178; memorandum of C. H. L. Emanuel, 24 June 1918, containing Knutsford's remarks, Board of Deputies Archive, Greater London Record Office, Acc. 3121 C/13/3/8; Israel Zangwill to Lucien Wolf, 6 May 1918, ibid., Acc. 3121 C/13/3/8.

the accuser to utter 'some excuse'. Nevertheless, such incidents involving members of old Anglo-Jewish families were relatively trivial, hardly warranting depiction as the 'antisemitism of exclusion' which 'operated against all sections of Anglo-Jewry' including the elite at university.[30]

What was new was a pernicious anti-aliens campaign unleashed against the east European immigrants, most of them Jewish, who had come to Britain at the end of the nineteenth century and into the twentieth, which hardened still further during the First World War into xenophobic hysteria against all foreigners. Jewish immigrants were accused of taking homes and jobs away from the local population, and later of refusing to enlist in the British army, for which a number were deported. In the face of the Bolshevik Revolution in Russia in October 1917 and the perceived threat of world revolution, particular suspicion was directed against Russian immigrants, resulting in a number of campaigns to curtail their rights. In 1918 a measure was introduced stipulating that, in order to be eligible for London County Council scholarships to school or higher education institutions, students would have to British and to have been born in Britain; in 1923 preference was given to British citizens in the allocation of council housing.[31] According to Sharman Kadish, there was

a significant increase in the incidence and extent of domestic antisemitism . . . The belief that the October Revolution was a 'Jewish plot' gained currency even in sections of the 'respectable' press. Anti-Bolshevism became entangled with antisemitism in the public mind. It also got mixed up with anti-alienism. Immigrants were treated as suspect . . . And, immediately after the war, rumours of impending revolution took hold in Britain.[32]

In this climate, the influx of Russian Jewish students into the London Hospital during the war years of 1914–18 on a much larger scale than hitherto exacerbated existing ethnic and class tensions. On 6 May 1918 Israel Zangwill, an important Anglo-Jewish novelist and public figure, wrote to Lucien Wolf, a journalist, foreign policy expert, and active participant in the work of the League of Nations, suggesting that complaints made to him by some of the students were so serious that they should be taken up by the Board of Deputies, the representative body of British Jewry. He explained how two leaders representing the Jewish medical students at the London Hospital had approached him, telling him that

the general atmosphere from the behaviour of nurses, doctors and officials is almost intolerable, but that the matter is now reaching a more serious stage in the refusal of

[30] Salaman, 'The Helmsman', 24; Kushner, *The Persistence of Prejudice*, 10.

[31] Alderman, *Modern British Jewry*, 235–41, 251, 256–7.

[32] Sharman Kadish, *Bolsheviks and British Jews: The Anglo-Jewish Community, Britain and the Russian Revolution* (London: Frank Cass, 1992), 226–30, 243.

traditional appointments. Thus, [Emanuel] Miller, a brilliant student [of Russian Jewish origin] and Member of the Officers' Training Corps (as everyone is) did not get the usual appointment at the Hospital, the three months practice preparatory to going to War. Forshaw, the surgical Registrar, is very anti-Semitic. Morris, the House Governor, said to Sennett: 'I would rather not give jobs to Jews'. Even a great surgeon has played to a sneering gallery of Christian students and nurses, and said: 'When I operate on a Jew or German my knife is always liable to slip.'[33]

As a result of this complaint, a somewhat acrimonious correspondence developed between members of the Jewish community and Lord Knutsford, the hospital chairman, during May and June 1918. As more and more Jewish communal figures were drawn into this dispute, a series of misunderstandings occurred, as letters were disclosed to third parties without the knowledge or approval of the original authors. Irked by the sight of a letter from Zangwill which suggested that Jews should curtail their charitable contributions to the London Hospital unless the Jewish students were better treated, Knutsford exclaimed to Wolf, 'That letter from Zangwill is enough to make me Anti-Semitic . . . We have done our best for the Jews in every way more so than for any other race and of late we have been shamefully treated by them . . . I will propose that we never do take another student.' But in another fuller and more candid letter sent by Knutsford to Zangwill on the same date he went much further, adding:

Lately we have had some very bad dirty students whom we have had to sit on, and they said it was because they were Jews. I hoped that such a statement would not be believed by anyone who knew the reputation of the London Hospital . . . A Jew student the other day was found drunk. He was taken to the Residents' Sick Room, and when there found to have Syphilis and Gonorrhoea. The Nurses who attended him actually 'retched' from the smell of him, he was so filthy. The House Governor saw him and said we could not keep him as a student—and he at once said 'Because I am a Jew I suppose', and I presume he is the one from whom you have heard.[34]

An attempt was made by the Board of Deputies to arrange a meeting between Alfred Salmon and some of the Jewish medical students to allow them to air their grievances in front of him. Salmon, the chairman of J. H. Lyons, was a long-standing Jewish member of the London Hospital Committee, who had made available fourteen company vans to collect wounded soldiers from France at Waterloo Station as well as for transporting hospital supplies. However, both Salmon and H. S. Q. Henriques, a barrister and chairman of the Board of Deputies' Law and Parliamentary Committee who attended the meeting as a spokesman for Anglo-Jewry, were upper-middle-class members of the Anglo-

[33] Israel Zangwill to Lucien Wolf, 6 May 1918, Board of Deputies Archive, Acc. 3121 C/13/3/8.
[34] Lord Knutsford to Lucien Wolf, 25 May 1918, ibid., Acc. 3121 C/13/3/8; Lord Knutsford to Israel Zangwill, 25 May 1918, Royal London Hospital Archive, LH/A/25/13.

Jewish establishment; they were extremely sympathetic to the hospital administration, whose class viewpoint they shared, and sceptical of the claims of Jewish medical students from a poor east European background. Too wide a gulf
separated them from the culture of these students; their Anglicized Judaism
was a pale reflection of the warm-blooded piety characteristic of many of the
households of their Russian brethren from which these students came. Ignoring
the students' charges against the teaching staff and nurses, Salmon denied that
the management of the hospital was prejudiced against Jews. 'I might mention
too', he wrote to Charles Emanuel, the secretary of the Board of Deputies, 'that
the late Mr Nathaniel Cohen, who was also on the [London Hospital] Committee, frequently pointed [out] to me the fact that this institution was peculiarly
free from any such taint [of antisemitism], with which view I am in complete
accord.' In a sharp exchange with Emanuel on 4 June 1918, Salmon adamantly
refused to take any further action in the matter.[35]

On 6 June 1918 the leaders of the London Hospital Jewish medical students,
having called a meeting to discuss the issue of antisemitism at the hospital,
wrote to Emanuel. They told him that while their student body were all of the
same opinion 'that anti-Semitism is indeed rife at the Hospital', they were
divided as to whether they should press for action to be taken: some wanted to
proceed with the complaint, but others believed 'that any steps taken would
only prejudice adversely the position of the Jews'. At a meeting between Henriques and Emanuel on the one side, and Lord Knutsford on the other,
Henriques seized on the divisions of opinion among the Jewish students and
minimized their grievances, emphasizing that 'the Students themselves had
suggested that the complaints should not be proceeded with'. It was in reply
to Henriques that Knutsford made his comment, quoted above, that 'The
Authorities . . . had been obliged to decide not to take Students in future, who
came below a certain standard.' Choosing just one of the charges made against
the hospital, he demonstrated that is was unfounded, and went on to say that 'no
objection would be raised against any student on account of his religion nor on
account of the fact that he was descended from Foreign parents'. As we shall
see, this assertion was disingenuous; lower-class students from a Russian
Jewish background would continue to be discriminated against at the London
Hospital.[36]

Any considered analysis of Lord Knutsford's remarks must conclude that he
was perpetuating a number of anti-Jewish stereotypes, by making allegations
that lapsed into myth. First of all he repeated the canard that all east European

[35] Clark-Kennedy, *The London*, ii. 175; Alfred Salmon to C. H. L. Emanuel, 27 May 1918, 4 June
1918, Board of Deputies Archive, Acc. 3121 C/13/3/8.

[36] S. Jeger and J. Maurice Winnett to C. H. L. Emanuel, 6 May 1918, memorandum of C. H. L.
Emanuel, 24 June 1918, Board of Deputies Archive, Acc. 3121 C/13/3/8.

Jews were dirty and unhygienic. New European notions of hygiene and cleanliness evolved in the nineteenth century, and were adopted by the Jews as much as other groups; indeed, many observers agreed that working-class east European Jewish homes and countenances were cleaner than those of their non-Jewish neighbours from the same class.[37] Second, Knutsford was perpetuating the antisemitic view that Jews were a source of infection and disease, particularly venereal disease. Maybe there was a maverick east European immigrant student at the London Hospital who had a drinking problem and suffered from syphilis and gonorrhoea, although Knutsford's account seems to be highly coloured and somewhat exaggerated, yet the historical evidence points, if anything, in the opposite direction to Knutsford's implication: Dr Jacob Snowman admitted in 1920 that 'Syphilis was almost absent among Jewish mothers till recently, but I fear that we cannot boast that happy state of things now.' The war had generally resulted in a loosening of morals, and Knutsford was at fault by trying to present his case as typical for someone of a Jewish immigrant background. According to Sander Gilman,

The literature on syphilis . . . contains a substantial discussion of the special relationship of Jews to the transmission and meaning of syphilis. For it is not only in the act of circumcision that this association is made—it is in the general risk of the Jews as carriers of syphilis and the generalized fear that such disease would undermine the strength of the body politic.

By dwelling on a possible case of syphilis among the Jewish medical students, Knutsford lent credence to racist stereotypes, thus fostering attitudes that continued to limit the number of Russian Jewish students allowed to enter the London Hospital medical school.[38]

In the autumn of 1918 there were fresh complaints to the Board of Deputies from Russian Jewish applicants to the London Hospital, which sent each of them an identical letter of rejection. It stated 'that only students of British Nationality are for the present eligible for admission'.[39] The London University Jewish Students' Union was concerned 'that the primary reason of the rejection of all four students in question was not their nationality but the fact that they were Jews'. Emanuel, having tired of the students' complaints, now took a position more in sympathy with the views of the hospital authorities, writing to Henriques that 'I do not see that we can possibly question this, particularly in view of the Hospital's experience of certain of their foreign students as explained to us by Lord Knutsford.'[40] Once again, the social and

[37] Cooper, *The Child in Jewish History*, 327–30.
[38] Sander Gilman, *The Jew's Body* (Routledge: London, 1991), 96–102; *JC* 28 May 1920.
[39] Copy rejection letter, 6 Sept. 1918, from William Wright, Dean of the London Hospital.
[40] Charles Landau to C. H. L. Emanuel, 14 Oct. 1918, C. H. L. Emanuel to H. S. Q. Henriques, 18 Nov. 1918, Board of Deputies Archive, Acc. 3121 C13/3/8.

cultural outlook of the Anglo-Jewish establishment was more in harmony with that of the hospital authorities than either was with the views of the Jewish student groups. Not all the capital's medical schools, however, adopted the hostile attitude of the London Hospital, and at least three of the rejected students, Philip Inwald, Jack Shulman, and A. G. Silver—all of whom had in any case already passed their first MB elsewhere—later qualified at the Middlesex Hospital.

Students often commenced their medical training with a year at the East London College or another similar establishment, such as King's College or Chelsea College, before applying for admission to a medical school. Here they received a basic grounding in chemistry, physics, biology, and zoology in a single course that prepared them for medical school. Because of its location, the East London College was important for poor Jewish students living in the East End. Many of the young Jewish men who studied there were scholarship winners who had attended one of the grammar schools supported by the London County Council, such as the Central Foundation School, Raine's Foundation, the Davenant Foundation, Parmiters, and the Grocers' School.[41] Alex Sakula, later a consultant physician in Dorking, praised his teachers at the Davenant Foundation for transforming 'Jewish boys into English gentlemen'.[42] However, useful though the East London College was for Jewish students, here too they faced anti-Jewish prejudice. One of the lecturers at the college, Mr Mudge, was an antisemite, who not only allocated back seats in the lecture hall to Jewish students, but gave a talk to the college Officer Training Corps entitled 'Revolution, how it is caused and how to stamp it out', to which Jewish students were ostentatiously not invited and about which their non-Jewish colleagues were too embarrassed to speak to them. Such incidents reflected the 'Red Scare', the fear of revolution spreading from Russia, which lingered in post-war Britain. On a more personal, less political level, Jewish students at the college in the 1920s were sometimes harassed by petty antisemitic pranks, such as having a pin stuck in them, or the writing on the college notice board of cheap jibe: 'Of all the Jews in this abode the Halperinians are most *à la mode*.'[43]

In 1927 M. S. Holzman, a young Jewish student with a Palestinian and Australian background, who had studied at the East London College for his first MB, was refused admission into the London Hospital; Redcliffe Salaman, as an ex-member of its staff enjoying a certain clout with the hospital authori-

---

[41] W. Victor Sefton, 'Growing up Jewish in London 1920–1950: A Perspective from 1973', in Dov Noy and Issachar Ben-Ami (eds.), *Studies in the Cultural Life of the Jews in England* (Jerusalem: Magnes, 1975), 321.   [42] Interview with Alex Sakula, 10 Apr. 2000.

[43] London Hospital Medical College Minute Book, 14 Feb. 1919, Royal London Hospital Archive, MC/A/2/12; ibid. 16 Jan. 1922, MC/A/2/13; M. S. Holzman to Redcliffe Salaman, 7 Mar. and 12 Mar. 1927, Redcliffe Nathan Salaman Papers, Cambridge University Library, Add. MS 8171, Box 1.

ties, particularly with its governor, E. W. Morris, successfully intervened to secure a place for him. Salaman informed Holzman on 5 March 1927 that

In the event of your getting into the London . . . I feel sure that you will not find any anti-Semitism among the authorities. Their reasons for excluding persons of whom the majority are Jews, is not because they are Jews, but very largely because they are foreigners, and they have to make a choice . . . The choice however, may not always be wisely or even carefully made.

One reason why Holzman had been rejected in the first instance was that the hospital authorities found his manners too curt. 'I must remind you,' wrote Salaman to Holzman on 28 March 1927,

that much weight is placed in this country on good, not to say, facile manners . . . little things [are disliked], such as: sitting down in a room before you are asked to; not getting up when the owner of the room or the responsible person comes in; answering questions curtly, and without an occasional 'Yes, sir', which is often much resented.[44]

In 1927, of the six Jewish students taking the first-year preparatory course at the London College that usually served to qualify students for entry to the London Hospital, four were refused admission by the hospital to complete their training as doctors. Yet, despite the difficulties which Jewish students of east European origin encountered at the London Hospital, they continued to find places available in the capital's other medical schools, such as those at University College Hospital, Guy's, King's College Hospital, St Bartholomew's, the Middlesex, and the London School of Medicine for Women—though few Jewish students attended St Mary's and hardly any were admitted by St Thomas's. Thus the discriminatory admissions policy practised by the London Hospital medical school in the 1920s was not an insuperable barrier for foreign-born Jews determined on a medical career; and eventually, around the same time that the restrictions on the eligibility of Jews for scholarships were lifted by the London County Council (LCC) in 1928 (until that time they were still classed as aliens), the complaints against the bias of the London Hospital in its selection of medical students faded away.[45]

During the 1930s the antisemitism of a small group of students in the London teaching hospitals became more vehement, as Mosley's British Union of Fascists and Arnold Leese's Imperial Fascist League took to the streets of

[44] Redcliffe Salaman to M. S. Holzman, 5 Mar., 28 Mar. 1927, Redcliffe Salaman to E. W. Morris, 22 Mar. 1927, E. W. Morris to Redcliffe Salaman, 27 Mar. 1927, Redcliffe Salaman to E. W. Morris, 28 Mar., 6 May 1927, Redcliffe Nathan Salaman Papers, Cambridge University Library, Add. MS 8171, Box 1.

[45] M. S. Holzman to Redcliffe Salaman, 6 Feb. 1927, Redcliffe Salaman Papers, Cambridge University Library, Add. MS 8171, Box 1; Alderman, *Modern British Jewry*, 258, 259.

London. The fascists' activities and influence, however, peaked in the summer of 1936 and went into decline after the 'Battle of Cable Street'.[46] Kalman Jacob Mann, who attended University College Hospital medical school from 1931 to 1937, reported that

> most of the Jewish students I met were poor people and like me, they did not go to the cafeteria to buy lunch. They too brought sandwiches from home and we all met in the locker room to eat our lunch. About this time the . . . Officers Training Corps . . . was active and many of these people leaned towards fascism. On one occasion as we entered the room we found written on the lockers: 'No Jews are allowed to eat here!' We decided this had to be reported and we informed the Dean, Dr Kirk, who . . . was quite upset when he heard about the incident. He then allocated a room where we Jewish students could go to eat our sandwiches.

On another occasion, one of the more thuggish students kept on putting his feet on Mann's shoulders during a lecture until Mann stood up and interrupted the lecture, to warn his tormentor to stop.[47]

In March 1935 the University College Hospital magazine carried a blatantly offensive article. 'We get the dregs of the world's students because we can get nothing else . . . Are there no medical schools in Palestine, in Poland, in India, Africa or Baluchistan? . . . The only tolerable foreigners are the unselfish ones and they are few!' It went on: 'It [the silence room] was filled with polychromatic faces, broken English and strange odours. We could not get near the ping-pong table except on a Saturday when the synagogues are open.' After a meeting of the college medical society the offending issue of the magazine was withdrawn from circulation, and an apology was printed in the next number.[48] Kalman Mann also recalled a fight over the use of the table-tennis table, which was brought to an end only when he almost throttled one of the antisemitic louts who was trying to interrupt his game.[49]

Writing in 1939, G. R. Young noted that 'The students of this country, especially in the medical faculties have at times made themselves notorious by their attitude towards their fellow Jewish students. Students in a London Hospital two or three years ago chalked up slogans on the walls to the effect, "Throw out the Jews . . .".'[50] At St Bartholomew's there was a group of fascist students who published a short-lived magazine called *Argent and Sable*. The October 1939 issue ran a 'Hymn to Hitler' which contained the lines:

> Fear not to attack the Jews;
> They have but their life to lose.
> And if thou shouldst need their money
> They still have their milk and honey.

[46] Kushner, *The Persistence of Prejudice*, 15–47; Morris Beckman, *The Hackney Crucible* (London: Vallentine Mitchell, 1996), 155–73.   [47] Mann, *Reflections*, 26, 27.   [48] *JC* 22 Mar. 1935.
[49] Mann, *Reflections*, 27.   [50] Quoted in Rubinstein, *History of the Jews*, 291.

Claire Hilton has argued that there was a quota for Jewish students entering Bart's during the 1930s, as the intake of Jewish students was consistently small;[51] but if such a quota existed it was not always rigidly enforced, because twelve Jewish students were admitted in 1937. The conclusion must be that the many and various openings in the London medical schools meant that most English Jewish applicants could in the end find a place to study medicine. Indeed, the Middlesex Hospital's philosemitic policy on admissions earned it the affectionate nickname of 'the Yiddlesex'. Refugee doctors who were requalifying, and medical students from Germany and other parts of central and eastern Europe, however, encountered great difficulties in finding suitable places in England during the 1930s.[52]

Antisemitic attitudes were not confined to the London medical schools. At Manchester University some of the more Anglicized Jewish students shunned those of their co-religionists who were of a more pronounced east European origin and shabbily dressed, mixing instead with the English students, some of whom were very antisemitic, particularly the rugger crowd. Dr Louis Rich, who qualified in 1933, recalled one of them shouting, 'Come on, let's have a pogrom!' On another occasion, a Jewish dental student had his sideburns shaved off. Most of the Jewish students here ate their sandwiches in an area of the locker room which they called 'the Ritz', where they discussed such issues as Zionism and internationalism. At the Leeds University School of Medicine, too, there were occasional lapses of good taste. A facetious letter appeared in the Medical Society magazine inviting subscriptions to a society whose headquarters were located in 'Raby Street, Sheenyville'. The point to note is the repeated association of Jews with disease.[53]

*

The *Medical Directory* entries for Leeds in 1910 show the names of at least three Jewish doctors: Dr Julius Friend, Dr Moses Umanski, and Professor A. S. F. Grunbaum (1869–1921), who later changed his surname to Leyton because of the anti-German feeling during the First World War.[54] Of the two general practitioners, Julius Friend (1867–1949) was the most Anglicized and the most well established in the city, his parents having migrated to Leeds from Poland in 1847. He was a bitter opponent of the unhygienic methods of some of the *mohelim* (ritual circumcisers); nevertheless, he thought that Jewish children were better fed than those of their non-Jewish neighbours, and endowed with a

---

[51] Hilton, 'St Bartholomew's Hospital', 33–4, 49–50.   [52] Blok, 'Jewish Students', 190.
[53] Dr Louis Rich, interview transcript deposited at the Manchester Jewish Museum; *JC* 18 Mar. 1932, p. 8.
[54] *The Medical Directory 1910*, 747; *Lives of the Fellows of the Royal College of Physicians of London*, iv. 438 (obituary of Leyton [Grunbaum]).

superior physique as a result. 'I do not consider size and weight of so much importance as superior bone formation', he declared, 'evident in the straight limbs and better teeth of our children.' He encouraged athletics and physical culture among Jewish young men, and was a robust supporter of the Jewish Lads' Brigade. He was also active in attempting to raise funds for the Jewish branch of the Leeds Association for the Prevention and Care of Consumptives—the incidence of the disease was rising among adults in the early years of the twentieth century, and in 1910 Jews occupied 20 per cent of the beds in one sanatorium—and for more than forty years he was chairman of the parent body of the association in Leeds. He was honorary physician to the St Faith's Rescue Home, the Leeds Jewish Board of Guardians and—despite his initial opposition—to the Herzl–Moser Hospital, the new Jewish hospital in Leeds founded in 1905. He sat on the Leeds City Council as a Conservative, serving on the health and improvement committees in the 1920s.[55]

Dr Moses Umanski (1862–1936) presents a marked contrast to the Anglicized Julius Friend. A native of Ekaterinoslav in south Russia, he graduated from Kharkov and Berlin universities as well as studying in London before settling in Leeds. As a student in Kharkov he had been a vigorous supporter of Hovevei Zion movement—the first fully fledged Zionist movement which wanted to see the Jews restored to their ancient homeland—led by Dr Leon Pinsker (1831–91), author of *Auto-emancipation* (1882). After moving to Britain, he helped to found the Leeds Hebrew Literary Society in 1893 and the English Zionist Federation in 1899. According to his obituarist, he 'introduced the Zionist movement into Leeds and was rewarded by bitter opposition which affected his professional income. Beloved by the poor, for whom he always had a smile and an encouraging word, he had his eventual reward in seeing the various societies and institutions which he and his remarkable wife established, grow from strength to strength.' As honorary medical officer to the Leeds Talmud Torah, Dr Umanski noted that there were underfed and starving children in the city's Jewish community, and was instrumental in founding the Jewish Soup Kitchen and Children's Free Dinners' Association in October 1903 with the financial assistance of Alderman Moser of Bradford. By 1905, 200 children were sitting down to daily dinners in Leeds of bread, soup, and meat. Above all, at a meeting of the local Zionist societies Dr Umanski persuaded Alderman Moser, a wealthy businessman and Zionist supporter, to put up the funds for the setting up of the Herzl–Moser Hospital. At the outset the scheme for a Jewish hospital in Leeds was bitterly opposed by the local Jewish establishment, including Dr Friend (although, as noted above, he subsequently served the hospital as an honorary physician); they thought it would encourage a ghetto mentality and

[55] *JC* 7 Feb. 1902, p. 8, 26 Aug. 1904, p. 19, 21 Dec. 1906, p. 32, 29 July 1910, p. 11, 18 Feb. 1949, p. 18 (obituary of Friend).

wanted, on the contrary, to see more mixing of Jews with their non-Jewish neighbours. When the nursing home was opened in 1905 in a private house, it comprised two wards and a small surgery with accommodation for ten patients. By 1907 some twenty-seven operations had been performed in the Herzl–Moser Hospital and 130 out-patients had been seen.[56]

Julius Friend was not only the first Jewish doctor to be trained in Leeds, where he qualified in 1894 by becoming a Licentiate of the Society of Apothecaries (London), but was also the first Jewish general practitioner in the town. Leeds's next Jewish medical student, Julian Landman, also trained in Manchester, where he was awarded his MB and Ch.B. in 1905. He was followed by Isaac Barnett Bernstein, who trained in Leeds before qualifying as a doctor on passing the London conjoint examination in 1911. Two more Jewish doctors, Julius Barnet Sinson and Henry Caplan, graduated from Leeds University in the same year; Harry Angel and Samuel Samuel followed suit in 1912; another two, Herman Louis Taylor and Harry Sinson, graduated in 1913; and Harry Shokett and Sam Nathaniel Cohen qualified in the following year. Graduating in the same year as her male colleague Jacob Rosencwige, Augusta Landman, the daughter of Dr Moses Umanski, became the first woman to qualify as a doctor in Leeds in 1915. The pattern in Leeds remained the same until 1920, with one or two Jews graduating as doctors, apart from 1917 when three students qualified: Saul Adler, Israel Liberman, and Isaac Silverstein. Many of these early graduates left Leeds once they had qualified; Taylor and Shokett moved to Newcastle and Augusta Landman to London, where she specialized in child psychology and acted as a consultant to the Marriage Guidance Council and the Family Planning Association.[57]

As in London, the situation changed dramatically during the First World War, which saw an influx of women students and Jews into the Leeds School of Medicine, as large numbers of public schoolboys who would normally have constituted the intake of new students flocked to join the armed forces. The result of these changes in the selection of trainees was that in 1920 five Jewish doctors graduated from Leeds University: Louis Gordon, Reuben Sacks, Jack Science, Harry Sienblum, and Morris Shernovitch. An equal number graduated in the following year, including two women, Bessie Goodson and Osra Muriel Phillips; and in 1922 the full effect of the wartime changes in the composition of the student body at the school became fully apparent, when no fewer than eleven Jewish doctors graduated. The number of Jewish doctors trained by the

[56] *JC* 21 Sept. 1900, p. 8, 18 Nov. 1904, p. 20, 2 Dec. 1904, p. 24 (correspondence about the proposed hospital), 29 June 1906, Leeds Supplement, 9 Nov. 1906, p. 35, 3 Jan. 1908, p. 30, 15 May 1936, p. 12 (obituary of Umanski), 4 Mar. 1938, p. 24 (tribute to Umanski).
[57] University of Leeds Graduation List 1915–1922, Faculty of Medicine Students' Record, vols. i and ii, *University of Leeds Calendar 1904–1905* to *1921–1922*, all in University of Leeds Archive; *JC* 24 Dec. 1916, 21 Jan. 1966, p. 21 (obituary of Landman).

Leeds School of Medicine remained high throughout the inter-war period.[58] In addition to these graduates of the Leeds medical school, a number of other Jewish students trained in Leeds, but obtained their final qualifications as MRCS or LRCP from the Conjoint Board of the Royal Colleges of Physicians and Surgeons in London in the early 1920s. Among those who took this route were Max Rosencwige, Jack Bernstein, Abraham Isaac Solberg, and George Klionsky; a couple of others completed their training in Edinburgh. Archibald Sinson, who left the Leeds School of Medicine in unhappy circumstances, after accusations of and subsequent conviction for theft, graduated as MD from Columbia University in 1924, announcing that he intended to specialize in the diseases of children.[59]

By 1931 the *Jewish Chronicle* could declare that

For the past quarter of a century and more, the number of Jewish students who have studied medicine at the [Leeds] School and who have taken their Medical Degrees there is exceptionally large, and the Jews of Leeds naturally harbour no small gratitude to the University and Medical Associations for these privileges granted unstintedly and without any bias whatsoever. At the present time the Jewish students form at least twenty-five per cent of the total students of the Medical School.[60]

Some tensions did, however, develop within the medical school because of the multitude of Jewish students, and Joseph Robson (1906–90) 'studied medicine at Leeds University but chose, because of antisemitism he encountered from one of the academic staff, to take his finals in London [in 1931]. "Foreigners" like him, he was told, were not entitled to any advancement in their profession.'[61] On the other hand, so grateful were the bulk of the Jewish medical graduates from Leeds that a committee of them raised £550 in 1933 to endow a Jewish community fellowship at the medical school; and when an antisemitic letter appeared in the Leeds University medical society magazine in February 1932, there was an abject apology on behalf of the editorial staff and the principals of the school of medicine for this unintentional editorial oversight.[62]

It may be deduced from the increase of Jewish students in the medical faculty at Leeds University that as a result of the scholarship ladders introduced in the early years of the twentieth century by local authorities with Liberal and Fabian members, bright Jewish pupils from poor households were advancing in limited numbers through the school system by means of scholarships and then going on

[58] S. T. Anning and W. K. J. Walls, *A History of the Leeds School of Medicine: One and a Half Centuries 1831–1981* (Leeds: Leeds University Press, 1982), 96, 97; University of Leeds Graduation List 1915–1922, Leeds Faculty of Medicine Students' Record, vols. i and ii, University of Leeds Archive.

[59] *JC* 6 June 1924, p. 15 (on Sinson); Leeds University Faculty of Medicine Students' Record, vol. iii, no. 604 (Archibald Sinson). [60] *JC* 8 May 1931, p. 26.

[61] *JC* 14 Sept. 1990, p. 32 (obituary of Robson). [62] *JC* 4 Aug. 1933, p. 25, 1 Apr. 1932, p. 29.

to medical college. 'There is a veritable colony of the most promising Jewish students at the University,' wrote M. J. Landa in 1906, 'all sons of poor men, I believe, who have gained scholarships.'[63] In 1910 the *Jewish Chronicle* reported that

As usual, Leeds had its yearly quantum of University successes. The large number of Jews in secondary schools and at the University, is, no doubt, due to a certain extent to the local scholarship scheme, but also in a large measure to the aptitude of the children, and the zeal and self-sacrifice of the parents. Nearly all those who have succeeded in attaining the higher reaches of education are almost entirely dependent on scholarships and other external support. Nevertheless, the number of these is yearly increasing.[64]

In 1909 over 50 per cent of the candidates who passed the Northern Universities Matriculation exam for entry into university were Jewish, while in the following year six out of the twenty scholarships awarded by this matriculation board were gained by Jews.[65]

Take the career of Herman Louis Taylor, who started his education at the Leylands Council School, 'which has produced in recent years so unique a list of Jewish talent'. He went by scholarship to the Central High School, matriculating in 1908 and obtaining a senior city scholarship to the Leeds medical school, from which he graduated in 1913. He was appointed prosecutor in anatomy at the medical school and distinguished himself in surgery there. He was also a good Hebrew scholar, teaching the subject for many years. He married a sister of his partner, Dr Shokett; their son was the late Peter Murray Taylor, Baron Taylor of Gosforth, Lord Chief Justice from 1992 to 1997.[66]

Hyman Goodman, too, held a city scholarship in 1913 to study medicine in Leeds; but it was not renewed a year later, and he found himself 'in such straits that he is unable to find the money to get instruments and books & to pay his college fees'. According to information supplied to the dean of the medical faculty of Leeds University, Goodman 'has no visible means of subsistence & relies . . . on the help of two sisters who are able to gain a livelihood'. Dr Myer Coplans, a Jewish member of the faculty and an agent of the Education Aid Society, recommended that Goodman abandon his medical studies for a science course; but Goodman, who was a bright student able to absorb information easily, persisted with his medical studies and qualified by passing the conjoint examination in 1919.[67]

[63] *JC* 28 Dec. 1906, p. 26.   [64] *JC* 8 July 1910, p. 13.
[65] *JC* 6 Aug. 1909, p. 10, 12 Aug. 1910, p. 11.   [66] *JC* 2 Jan. 1914, p. 34.
[67] Alfred Makower to de Burgh Birch, 12 Nov. 1914, de Burgh Birch to Alfred Makower, 13 Nov. 1914, correspondence attached to Leeds Faculty of Medicine Students' Record, vol. ii, no. 544. Birch was the dean of the medical faculty; Makower was on the committee of the Education Aid Society.

For all the difficulties faced by students such as Goodman in their struggle to continue with medical training, the discipline was attractive to many, not least because scholarships and grants were more readily available and employment prospects better than in many other fields. During the late 1930s, 'Two Jewish students . . . changed their course from Science to Medicine', claimed the secretary of the Leeds Jewish Students' Association, 'because of the bogey of unemployment among Leeds teachers (naturally more acute among Jews) . . . Two Jewish students, after spending three years at school trying to get Arts scholarships finally came to the University as Medical students.'[68]

In 1919 there were nine Jewish doctors in the *Medical Directory* for Leeds, out of a total of 285; or, to put it another way, 3.16 per cent of the doctors in Leeds were Jewish. The next decade showed the greatest increase in the percentage of Jewish doctors in Leeds. In 1929 thirty-seven (9.48 per cent) of the 390 doctors in Leeds were Jewish. By 1939 fifty out of the 430 doctors in Leeds were Jewish—nearly 12 per cent.[69]

Although Liverpool had a Jewish population of only 7,500 in 1906, a third of the size of the community in Leeds, it was, in contrast to Leeds, an old-established Jewish centre, with 2,500 members as far back as 1850. While the main occupations of most first-generation east European Jewish immigrants in London and the provincial towns were cabinet-making, tailoring, and market trading or peddling, there was a stratum of Jewish inhabitants in Liverpool who were more prosperous. There were at least four Jewish doctors in Liverpool in 1910—Abraham Ellenbogen, Julius Ellenbogen, Isaac Harris, and Max Loewenthal; possibly five, if Karl August Grossman was Jewish. In 1919 there were still, somewhat surprisingly, only four Jewish doctors—Julius Ellenbogen, Loewenthal, M. B. Strock, and V. I. Levy—out of a total of 458 practitioners in the city: less than 1 per cent of the total.[70]

Liverpool, being an international seaport, was more open and welcoming to immigrants than inland towns such as Leeds. Both Harris, who was an MD from Königsberg (1904), and Loewenthal, who had obtained an MD from Würzburg (1892), were examples of such German-trained immigrants. Strock, who had studied at the universities of St Petersburg and Paris, was awarded an MD from Liverpool in 1920. With its key position in international trade and its old-established, prosperous Jewish elite, Liverpool attracted many Jewish

[68] Blok, 'Jewish Students', 190.

[69] The names of all the Jewish doctors practising in Leeds in 1919, 1929, and 1939 were compiled from the reports of the pass lists of the School of Medicine of the University of Leeds which appeared in the *Jewish Chronicle* and the School of Medicine records preserved in the University of Leeds Archive. *The Medical Directory 1919* (London: J. & A. Churchill, 1919), 1162, *Medical Directory 1929* (London: J. & A. Churchill, 1929), 1244, 1245, *Medical Directory 1939* (London: J. &. A. Churchill, 1939), 1376, 1377.

[70] *Medical Directory 1910*, 1122, 1123; *Medical Directory 1919*, 1163, 1164.

doctors from abroad who served as role models for the younger generation of immigrants and their children. This encouraged the move of second-generation Jewish immigrants into the professions in the 1920s and 1930s, when the number of Jewish doctors in Liverpool increased rapidly. In 1929 there were twenty-nine (thirty if Theodore Lasker was Jewish) out of a total of 650, or 4.62 per cent; by 1939 sixty-five out of 693 doctors were Jewish: 9.38 per cent.

Among the reasons for the increase in Jewish doctors in Liverpool in the 1930s was the prominent position in the Liverpool medical school of Professor Henry Cohen (1900–77), who himself came from an east European immigrant family and was appointed professor of medicine at the university in 1934. At the town's Royal Infirmary, where he was senior physician, he assisted in the promotion of a number of Jews, such as Maurice Pappworth and Isaac Ansell, to the level of registrar.[71] According to Dr Mervyn Goodman, 'There were [also] a number of Jewish doctors in the neighbouring areas such as Wallesey, Birkenhead and one, Dr Fox, in Chester', who were 'traditionally part of the Merseyside Jewish Community and most of them were Liverpool Graduates'.[72] The total of sixty-five Jewish doctors practising in Liverpool in 1939 far outstripped the fifty located in Leeds in a Jewish community three times the size of Liverpool's—a discrepancy attributable to the reluctance of the Leeds medical school to employ Jews and the hostility Jewish practitioners encountered in that city. Because of these adverse conditions before the Second World War, a few Leeds-trained doctors practised in the Liverpool area.

Of all the provincial cities in England, Manchester and Salford had the largest Jewish population before the First World War, rising from 2,000 in 1850 to 30,000 in 1910, thus exceeding the Jewish population of Leeds which had risen to 25,000 during the Edwardian era.[73] Within this well-established Jewish community there were already thirteen Jewish medical practitioners in 1910: Harry Louis Becker, Meyer Joseph Bernstein, Joseph Dulberg, Nathan Charles Haring, Henry Graff, Solomon Levy, Sidney Messulam, Siegmund Moritz, Bendit Saul, Helen G. Saul, Victor S. Saul, Walter O. Steinthal, and Wilfred M. Steinthal.[74] The number rose to seventeen in 1919.

At this period there was already a flourishing and somewhat secularized German Jewish mercantile community in Manchester which made it an attractive venue for physicians trained on the Continent. Among these were Dr Julius Dreschfeld and Dr Siegmund Moritz, discussed in Chapter 1 above, and Dr

[71] N. Kokosalakis, *Ethnic Identity and Religion: Tradition and Change in Liverpool Jewry* (Washington: University Press of America, 1982), 167, 170, 179; *Medical Directory 1910*, 1122, 1123; *Medical Directory 1929*, 1246, 1247; *Medical Directory 1929*, 1378–80. I have also consulted the pass lists of the Liverpool Medical School which appeared in the *JC*.

[72] Letter from Dr Mervyn Goodman to the author, 21 Sept. 1996.

[73] Lipman, *Social History of the Jews in England*, 160, 171.

[74] *Medical Directory 1910*, 1125, 1126; *Medical Directory 1919*, 1166, 1167.

Adolph Wahltuch (1837–1907); another was Dr Simon Finkelstein (1865–1906), an assistant physician to one of the principal hospitals in Vienna and a founder, with the wealthy industrial chemist Dr Charles Dreyfus and Dr Nathan Charles Haring, of the Manchester Jewish Hospital in 1903. Like Moses Umanski, his counterpart in Leeds, Dreyfus, the chief protagonist in Manchester of the movement for a Jewish hospital, was a leading Zionist; and, like Umanski in Leeds, he had to overcome opposition to his project from the local communal establishment. Haring, the only outstanding Anglo-Jewish doctor in Manchester, was a physician at the Hospital for Consumption and Diseases of the Throat and chairman of the medical board of the Manchester Jewish Hospital from its inception. Another important physician at the Manchester Jewish Hospital was Dr Joseph Dulberg, who had obtained his LL D from the University of Leipzig in 1884 and his MD from the University of Würzburg in 1891, and during the First World War was neurologist to the Western Command Discharge Centre.

The extent of these individuals' engagement in Jewish communal affairs varied. Although Wahltuch was not Orthodox, he was well versed in Hebrew, a supporter of Jewish education, and a founder of the South Manchester Synagogue; Dulberg served on the committee of the Manchester Old Hebrew Congregation. Other doctors had a more secular Jewish orientation. Dr Solomon Herbert (1875–1940) was a member of Poale Zion, the left-wing Zionist party, and the founder of the local Fabian Society, whereas Haring was not only chairman of the Jerusalem University Society but a sponsor of a B'nai B'rith lodge.[75]

In 1919 there were seventeen Jewish doctors in Manchester and Salford, out of a total of 555: 3.06 per cent. By 1929 the number had increased to fifty-one out of a total of 728, or 7 per cent; by 1939 it had almost doubled to ninety-three out of 771 doctors, or 12.06 per cent: the highest total figure, and the highest percentage, in all the provincial English towns. Even so, there are grounds for believing that this is still a serious underestimate.[76] An investigation by the Jewish Health Organization revealed that in 1937 there were 108 Jewish doctors in Manchester out of 760: 14.21 per cent of the total.[77]

[75] Williams, *The Making of Manchester Jewry*, 81–4, 127, 128, 169, 260; *JC* 8 June 1906, p. 36 (obituary of Finkelstein), 6 Dec. 1907, p. 23 (obituary of Wahltuch), 17 Apr. 1925, p. 8 (obituary of Dulberg), 1 Feb. 1929, p. 8 (obituary of Haring), 9 Feb. 1940, p. 20 (obituary of Herbert); on Dulberg, see Isidore Harris (ed.), *The Jewish Year Book 1922* (London: Jewish Chronicle, 1922), 184. The B'nai B'rith was an organization of the Jewish middle class established to pursue charitable and cultural purposes and to defend Jewish interests around the world.

[76] *Medical Directory 1919*, 1166, 1167; *Medical Directory 1929*, 1249, 1250; *Medical Directory 1939*, 1381–3. I have also consulted the pass lists of the Manchester University Medical School published in the *JC*.

[77] Memorandum on the Statistical Investigations conducted by the Jewish Health Organisation, 23 Apr. 1937, Acc. 3121 B4/JHO, Board of Deputies Archive.

Apart from their scholarship route to success, another common theme in the careers of Jewish doctors in the provinces at this period was that many of them were the sons of rabbis or other officials in the Jewish community, men with regular work and steady incomes. With no clear-cut employment prospects, their children were frequently attracted by a career in medicine, as it combined learning with public service: a more secular version of the communal service undertaken by the older generation. Examples are J. B. Sinson, Harry Sinson, and Archibald Sinson, the sons of Rabbi N. Sinson of Leeds; Professor Saul Adler, also from Leeds, whose father was a rabbi but preferred to earn his living by keeping a shop; and the four Shlosberg brothers in Manchester, all of them the sons and grandsons of a rabbi. Dr Shokett, the grandson of Rabbi Palterovitch, won scholarships to the Central High School in Leeds and a senior city scholarship to the city's medical school; he also had a good talmudic training and was a proficient Hebraist. Some trainee doctors had abandoned a rabbinical career. William Moses Feldman (1880–1939) came to Britain from Pinsk in Russia (now Belarus) at the age of 8 and studied rabbinics at Jews' College in London before embarking on a medical career. Both Dr Bendit Saul (d. 1933) and his brother Dr Victor Saul (1868–1936) were intended by their father for the ministry and also studied at Jews' College before they decided to become doctors. Henry Graff (1873–1916) studied in yeshivas in Russia and migrated to Ireland in the 1890s, when 'by dint of hard work and study in his spare time he took the triple qualifications of the Royal Colleges of Physicians and Surgeons of Ireland in 1900, obtaining numerous prizes and distinctions'; he then settled in Manchester as a doctor.[78]

Among the Jews of eastern Europe a broad educated elite studied the Talmud, and many of the Jewish doctors of the inter-war years in England were the direct descendants of this educated minority. David Perk, writing in 1924 from the school of medicine in Leeds, explained that a Talmudical Society had been started by the students which could boast twenty-two members.[79] As noted above, the sons of the rabbis served as role models for their contemporaries, encouraging an influx of Jewish students into the medical profession. By the 1920s and 1930s, however, a wider section of the English Jewish community was prospering economically, and it was from among the children of these businessmen, as well as the bright scholarship holders from more humble origins, that the new generation of Jewish medical students was being recruited.

[78] Daniel Gavron, *Saul Adler: Pioneer of Tropical Medicine* (Rehovot: Balaban, 1997), 8, 9, 12; *JC* 14 Oct. 1910; 10 July 1914, p. 24. *JC* 7 July 1939, p. 15 (obituary of Feldman), 14 Aug. 1936, p. 8 (obituary of Saul), 8 Sept. 1916, p. 18 (obituary of Graff). Other examples are Dr Hyman Franklin and Dr Samuel Samuel, *JC* 29 Dec. 1916 and 26 Dec. 1919, p. 22.

[79] *JC* 8 Feb. 1924, p. 19 (letter of David Perk). Professor Israel Doniach (1911–2001), a leading expert on thyroid cancer, was the son of a scholar in Hebrew and Aramaic: *The Times*, 2 Mar. 2001; *JC* 9 Mar. 2001 (obituary of Doniach).

All three cities discussed above, Leeds, Liverpool, and Manchester, had seen the number of Jewish physicians practising in their area substantially increase in the 1920s, from nine to thirty-seven in Leeds, from four to thirty in Liverpool, and from seventeen to fifty-one in Manchester; but while the growth in numbers continued in the 1930s, in the great trading cities of Liverpool and Manchester the rate was much faster (116 per cent and 82 per cent respectively) than in Leeds (35 per cent), where the labour market was less elastic. Nevertheless, by the end of the 1930s both Leeds and Manchester had a similar proportion of Jewish doctors among their medical practitioners, a figure approaching 12 per cent. Liverpool lagged slightly behind; here just under 10 per cent of the doctors were Jewish. However, these figures for 1939 may represent a 2 per cent underestimate of the actual proportion of Jewish doctors practising in these towns, if the 1937 survey of Manchester by the Jewish Health Organization was valid. Adding an additional 2 per cent on to my own estimates for 1939 would give us fifty-nine Jewish doctors in Leeds, seventy-nine in Liverpool, and 108 in Manchester.

To understand the admissions policy of the English medical schools during the 1920s and 1930s, it is necessary to place it in a wider context. In Germany after 1933, Jewish students were brusquely ejected from the medical faculties. In Poland in 1935, Jewish students had to sit apart from other students in the lecture halls, on a separate 'ghetto bench'; at Warsaw University the Jewish medical students were regularly and violently assaulted by antisemitic ruffians from other faculties, and in one especially nasty incident two Jewish girls were thrown out of the windows on to the pavement below.[80]

Even in the United States the majority of the medical schools placed tight restrictions on the admission of Jewish applicants during the inter-war period. There was a sharp discrepancy between the proportion of Jewish applicants to these schools and the percentage actually admitted. Over 60 per cent of the 33,000 applications for admission to these medical schools in 1934 were from Jews, but it was estimated that at this time just 17 per cent of the medical students in America were Jewish. As a result of this policy, in 1936–7 there were 550 non-university Jewish medical students from America studying in Scotland, together with a smaller number enrolled in British university medical schools.[81] Whereas the population of Scotland was only one-ninth that of England, its medical schools produced two-thirds as many medical graduates; as a result, a large number of Scottish-trained Jewish doctors sought employment in England. Conditions in Ireland were similar, with the majority of

[80] Moshe Prywes, *Prisoner of Hope* (Hanover, NE: Brandeis University Press, 1996), 66–71.

[81] Leon Sokoloff, 'The Rise and Decline of the Jewish Quota in Medical School Admissions', *Bulletin of the New York Academy of Medicine*, 68 (1992), 497–517; Goldberg, 'Jews in the Medical Profession'; Blok, 'Jewish Students', 192, 193; Collins, *Go and Learn*, 98–132.

Jewish medical graduates coming across to England for work. By 1939 they had helped to push the number of Jewish doctors in London up to around 800.

By comparison, England was a markedly less hostile environment for Jews wishing to enter the medical profession between the wars. There were difficulties placed in the way of foreign-born east European Jewish students, for example by the London Hospital in the 1920s, and from time to time antisemitic incidents occurred there and at other hospitals, but they were perpetrated by fringe elements. The authorities in charge of the medical faculty at University College took determined action against unruly behaviour by fascist students during the 1930s, and in any case fascism as a political force in England was on the wane by the end of 1936. Few Jews ventured into St Thomas's Hospital medical school or that associated with the Charing Cross Hospital, and only a slightly larger number entered St Mary's; but there were many other medical schools in London to which Jews could gain admission, and the provincial medical schools had a large intake of Jewish students and do not appear to have placed any restrictions on their admission between the wars. It was probably more difficult during these years for black or female students to find a place in a medical school than for Jews; of the seven London medical schools which agreed to accept women students during the First World War, six reversed their decision between 1919 and 1928, giving as their excuse the lack of rugby players or the reluctance of Oxbridge men to apply for admission.[82] Yet there was a higher proportion of Jewish girls studying medicine than among their non-Jewish counterparts. Nor do any of the antisemitic incidents that took place in England during the 1930s bear any comparison, either in scale or in the depth of the hatred shown, with the anti-Jewish measures and activities spreading across central and eastern Europe in these years.

[82] James Stuart Garner, 'The Great Experiment: The Admission of Women Students to St Mary's Hospital Medical School, 1916–1925', *Medical History*, 42 (1998), 68–88; London Hospital Medical College Minute Book, 24 Oct. 1921, 21 Nov. 1921, Royal London Hospital Archive, MC/A/2/13.

THREE

Jewish General Practitioners and Consultants between the World Wars

NEWLY qualified doctors of the 1920s and 1930s sought practical experience as housemen in hospitals. A position of this kind, which usually lasted for six months or a year, was the standard first step in a doctor's career, although as yet it was not compulsory. However, even the top students, if they were the children of east European Jewish immigrants, sometimes found it difficult to obtain these positions in the London teaching hospitals or such institutions as the Manchester Royal Infirmary during the 1920s, though it became slightly easier in the following decade. The general practitioner and communal leader Dr Bernard Homa claimed that in order to fill one of these positions at Bart's, it was necessary to have passed the primary FRCS exam—or to be a member of the hospital rugby team. He ended up in 1923 as house physician at the Royal Berkshire Hospital in Reading;[1] Solomon Wand, despite graduating in 1921 with distinction in medicine, could find no vacancy for a houseman in the Manchester teaching hospitals because of the prejudice against Jews and instead became house surgeon to Dr Robinson at the local infirmary in Warrington.[2] On the other hand, Dr Louise Aronovich (b. 1885), whose father had been a prosperous cotton merchant, was in 1926 made a clinical assistant at the Manchester Royal Infirmary, where she was treated 'as one of themselves'.[3]

In 1937 the Education Aid Society reported that 'All medical students [assisted by the society] recently qualified have obtained positions and four of them secured House Appointments in London Hospitals.'[4] One of these students, who filled the position of house physician at University College Hospital,

[1] Bernard Homa, *Footprints in the Sands of Time* (Charfield, Glos.: Charfield, 1990), 65, 66.

[2] Zoe Josephs (ed.), *Birmingham Jewry*, vol. ii: *More Aspects 1740–1930* (Birmingham: Birmingham Jewish History Research Group, 1984), 75.

[3] Dr Louise Aronovich, transcript of interview (Oct. 1976) deposited at the Manchester Jewish Museum.

[4] Education Aid Society, *Annual Report 1937*, 6, Southampton University, Parkes Library; Education Aid Society, Minute Book, General Committee, 9 June 1937, Southampton University, Parkes Library.

was Simon Yudkin; others who secured such appointments at the same hospital were Moss Albert and Kalman Mann.[5] Yet Jewish students completing their medical training in Leeds and other provincial towns found difficulties in obtaining employment. In Leeds in 1922 the local board of guardians chose a Catholic doctor as medical officer for a certain district, although the Jewish contender Dr Morris Shernovitch was better qualified and had satisfactorily performed his duties as deputy, on grounds that non-Jewish women would not want to be examined by a Jewish doctor.[6] In spite of being the top student of his year in the Leeds school of medicine Dr Harry Edelston (born Edelstein), when he qualified as a doctor in 1924, could not find employment until he discovered an opening in psychiatry, 'then the Cinderella of the medical profession'.[7]

On 21 June 1930 an advertisement appeared in the *British Medical Journal* in the following terms: 'Wanted, Midlands, Assistant [doctor] . . . male. Panel 1,950 and private. Receipts £2,700. Good House and garden available. No Jews or men of colour.' When a protest was made by the *Jewish Chronicle*, the deputy medical secretary of the BMA expressed his regret and stated, 'It is not the custom of the British Medical Association to allow any invidious stipulations to appear in such advertisements.'[8] There were further complaints in 1937 and 1938 from Dr J. L. Blonstein about similar antisemitic advertisements in the *British Medical Journal*; again they elicited an apology from the BMA.[9] Such prejudice as did exist bears no comparison with the Nazi animus against all Jewish doctors, and by and large a more tolerant tradition prevailed in Britain. Nevertheless, during the 1920s and 1930s many newly qualified doctors Anglicized their surnames, and sometimes their first names as well, in order to conceal their Jewish origin. Hence in Leeds, for example, Israel Liberman changed his name to John Morrison Lever, Harry Sienblum became Harry Shaw, Jacob Rosencwige became Jack Rose, and Morris Shernovitch was transformed into Morris Sherwin. Solomon Gordon changed only his first name, becoming John Gordon; Alec Katz, Leon Cohen, and Jack Cohen changed their surnames, becoming Jackson, Collins, and Coleman respectively.[10]

Some doctors going into general practice started their careers by the route of becoming assistant to a well-established practitioner, with a view to entering into partnership later, if the parties suited each other. Many, however, purchased their practices, usually beginning in a working-class neighbourhood. Bernard Homa commenced his career by renting two rooms from a friend in Hackney early in 1924. As progress was slow, he was pleased when an elderly

[5] Mann, *Reflections*, 35, 36. [6] *JC* 24 Feb. 1922, p. 34, 24 Mar. 1922, p. 30.

[7] *JC* 8 Apr. 1994, p. 15 (obituary of Edelston). [8] *JC* 27 June 1930, p. 10, 4 July 1930, p. 8.

[9] Copy letter assistant secretary of BMA to Dr J. L. Blonstein, 14 Nov. 1938, Dr J. L. Blonstein to A. G. Brotman, 15 Nov. 1938, Acc. 3121/B4/B25.

[10] Faculty of Medicine Students' Record, vol. ii, Leeds University Archive.

local practitioner invited him to buy his practice, which was situated near Dalston Junction. This was a dispensing practice with private patients, but Homa also began to take on panel patients, besides purchasing a panel practice in Shoreditch. Under the system of panel practices, which had been set up under the provisions of the National Insurance Act 1911, workers contributing to the state national insurance scheme had a right to treatment by a doctor on the local list or 'panel'; the doctors on these panels were paid from the national insurance fund. The panel practices were more stable than practices with a large percentage of private patients, who could quickly melt away, especially when a new young doctor took over the practice. 'The residents of the district, especially to the South of Dalston Lane were mainly drawn from the upper working classes. Most of the patients were non-Jewish but about twenty percent were co-religionists', Homa remembered.[11] Similarly, Dr Myer Cohen (b. 1895), another Leeds-trained physician, bought a practice in Walthamstow from an Irish doctor with both panel and private patients in 1927. It was a big midwifery practice, again with few Jewish patients.[12] In London at this time there were agencies which, for a commission, found practices for doctors to purchase; one of these was run by a Jew, Dr Eustace Chesser, and was said to favour co-religionists.[13] All the Jewish doctors interviewed by Zoe Josephs in Birmingham purchased panel practices, often in run-down neighbourhoods, later enrolling private patients and moving to more fashionable houses in areas like Edgbaston. There was a limited range of medicines: 'Kaolin for indigestion, a diarrhoea mixture and cough linctus', recalled Dr Hyman Hamilton; 'I made them up myself.'[14]

Practices usually changed hands for a sum equivalent to the income generated over a two-year period. When Dr Lionel Stoll started as a general practitioner during the mid-1930s, he could not afford to buy a large practice, so he purchased a smaller one in Adelaide Road, Hampstead, for under £2,000 with the aid of a loan from the Midland Bank which was repaid over seven years. Because the opportunity for the purchase had arisen on the death of the previous practitioner, Dr Stoll was able to buy it for a sum equivalent to only one and a half times the annual income.[15]

A number of Jewish women established practices in the working-class neighbourhoods of London. One such was Dr Liba Zarchi (1882–1929), who specialized in infant care and in gynaecological problems. Zarchi, a descendant of the hasidic master Rabbi Levi Itzhok of Berditchev (1740–1809), was born in Russia in affluent and cultured surroundings; educated at the University of Freiburg, she later requalified in London. 'She became one of the medical officers of the

[11] Homa, *Footprints*, 66–9.
[12] Dr Myer Cohen and Dr Cecilia Cohen, transcript of interview recording deposited at the Jewish Museum, Finchley.
[13] Interview with Dr Lionel Stoll, 28 Sept. 2000.
[14] Josephs, *Birmingham Jewry*, ii. 77–9.
[15] Interview with Dr Lionel Stoll, 28 Sept. 2000.

infant welfare centres established in connection with the Jewish Maternity Home and St. George's Infant Welfare Centre, besides practising privately in the East End and North London.' According to Dr Maurice Sorsby, 'She blended professional activity with those little acts of charity that made one who received them cherish her memory, not only as a skilful healer, but as a sympathetic helper of all those who were in need of help.'[16]

Another in a similar mould was Dr Hannah Billig (1901–87). Although there were books everywhere in her parents' home, she came from a poor family; her father acted as a beadle in one of the East End synagogues and rolled cigarettes for a living. Nevertheless, two of her brothers and a sister also became medical practitioners. With the aid of scholarships, Hannah trained at the Royal Free Hospital in London, and qualified in 1925. She wanted to go into medical research, but was hampered by lack of money; so for a time she was an assistant pathologist at the Elizabeth Garrett Anderson Hospital for women, and then a medical officer at the Jewish Maternity Hospital. 'To my knowledge,' stated Bertha Venitt, a schoolfriend,

Hannah was not interested in private patients. She mostly cared for the poor, and whether they paid her or not, she still visited them . . . The front room of a house in Cable Street [in the East End] was the waiting room (which was always packed) and behind that room was the surgery . . . The majority of her patients were Jewish but she treated everybody irrespectively. Gynaecology was her speciality—especially babies, and I would say also the elderly.

Like many doctors, she would often be called out at night to deliver babies, particularly when the East London Nursing Society was short of staff. During the Second World War she was awarded the George Medal for tending dockers injured in bombed warehouses, despite having broken her leg; later she served in the Indian Army Medical Service, as a result of which she was awarded the MBE for her work in Calcutta during the famine of 1944 and 1945. Utterly dedicated to her patients and used to working long hours, she never married.[17]

John Efron has pointed out that one of the distinguishing features of Jewish physicians in the modern period, as distinct from their predecessors, has been their concern not only for individual patients but for the health of the Jewish community as a whole. With this wider concern in mind, Russian Jewish doctors established the OSE (Society for the Preservation of the Health of Jews) in St Petersburg in 1912, and in 1923 a branch of this body was set up in London as the Jewish Health Organization of Great Britain, with Dr Redcliffe Salaman

---

[16] *JC* 8 Feb. 1929, p. 10 (obituary of Zarchi); ibid., tribute by Maurice Sorsby.

[17] Melvyn H. Brooks, *Dr Hannah Billig 1901–1987. The Angel of Cable Street: Memories* (Israel: Karkur, 1993), 8, 9, 14–19, 26–35 (Bertha Venitt cited on p. 28); Pamela Melnikoff, 'An Apple-Eating Angel', *JC* 1 Aug. 1997.

as its leading light.[18] This was a society composed partly of consultants from the London Jewish Hospital, notably Dr Hugh Gainsborough, and partly of general practitioners and communal workers. Among its Jewish doctors was a prominent Russian contingent, namely Dr M. Schwarzman (originally from Odessa), a physician in charge of the radiological department of the London Jewish Hospital, Dr Noah Pines, and Dr Yankel Krupenia; its first secretary was the historian Michael Postan. Its annual income reached £1,669. 18s. 2d. in 1927, but by 1932 it was able to raise only £381 in subscriptions and £241 in donations, thereby causing financial problems for its pioneering child guidance and dental clinics.

The Jewish Health Organization sponsored regular lectures in the Whitechapel Art Gallery on public health concerns, drawing audiences of 700, as well as arranging for speakers to address Jewish societies, trade union branches, and clubs, and distributing pamphlets in Yiddish and English.[19] It also carried out a series of investigations into the defective vision of Jewish schoolchildren (concluding that it was a genetic predisposition rather than induced by excessive hours of study in Hebrew classes after school) and into the intelligence of these children, demolishing research by Professor Pearson that purported to show that they were mentally inferior, and indeed proving the contrary. This was important, as it meant that Jewish candidates for hospital places (as well as those seeking to enter the law) were not burdened by such canards. While its long-serving secretary David Cheyney (1893–1962) remained at its helm until 1943, the Jewish Health Organization weathered the acute shortage of funds precipitated by the Second World War; but once he was forced out of office by Redcliffe Salaman after he alleged that irregularities had been committed by Dr Schwarzman, the society went into terminal decline.[20]

For those aiming at a hospital career, to become a consultant it was necessary to hold the basic qualification to practise as a doctor, the MRCS or LRCP of the Conjoint Board, or an MB, BS from a recognized university, plus either the FRCS or MRCP. The steps that had to be taken to progress from house physician or house surgeon to registrar in the late Victorian period have been described in Chapter 1 above; twenty or thirty years later little had changed. Moreover, anyone applying for the post of consultant in a London teaching hospital before the Second World War had to get between fifty and one hundred copies of the application specially printed and distributed to all members

---

[18] John M. Efron, *Medicine and the German Jews* (New Haven: Yale University Press, 2001), 64; W. B. Lowbury, 'The Jewish Health Organization: Its Origin and its Work', *JC Supplement*, 25 Mar. 1927, pp. vi, vii.

[19] Jewish Health Organization of Great Britain, *Annual Reports* 1923–5; *JC* 29 Apr. 1932, p. 13.

[20] Jewish Health Organization of Great Britain, *Annual Reports* 1927, pp. 10–16, 1940; *JC* 30 Mar. 1962 (obituary of Cheyney); David Cheyney papers in the possession of the author.

of the staff, and to call personally on every existing consultant, unless they declined the offer. Many of these visits were inevitably perfunctory, as some of the consultants would already have their own favoured candidates for the position.[21]

Before the establishment of the National Health Service in 1948, consultants were appointed only in teaching and specialized hospitals, all of which were located in London and other major cities. Many of the consultants served both the teaching and the specialized hospitals, thereby reducing the number of vacancies for newcomers wishing to embark on a career as a consultant. Consultant physicians diagnosed and advised on treatment; consultant surgeons conducted the more difficult operations. Outside the local authority hospitals, consultancy positions were part-time and unpaid, the consultants being expected to earn their living from the fees paid by their private patients.[22] Rose Hacker wrote that

You had to work for nothing in a hospital with a successful consultant who would gradually send you patients . . . You either had to have money or marry money. If Harold [her former boyfriend] had intended to be a general practitioner my father could have helped to put up the money to buy him a practice, but not to keep him in the hope of getting into Harley Street.[23]

However, in local authority hospitals with specialist units, including those run by the London County Council, the consultants were paid employees and worked full-time; and the staff were of varied origin, including Englishmen, Jews, and those from Commonwealth countries such as Australia and South Africa. The only realistic path open to sons and daughters of east European Jewish immigrants wanting to become specialists in the 1920s and 1930s was to apply for posts in these local authority hospitals or in a specifically Jewish institution. The financial pressure involved often meant postponing marriage, sometimes into their forties—a constraint not experienced to the same degree by those going into general practice.

'In contrast to the varied origins of those in local authority hospitals,' claimed Dr N. M. Jacoby,

parochialism and a modicum of nepotism were *de rigueur* in teaching hospitals and their associated medical schools [between the two world wars]. When I entered the wards in 1931, almost the entire staff of Guy's were home bred, and several were the sons and sons-in-law of previous consultants. It was many years later before the appointment of an outsider was anything but a remote possibility. This position continued with very

---

[21] Jacoby, *Journey*, 34, 35, 45.   [22] Ibid. 44, 45.
[23] Rose Hacker, *Abraham's Daughter: The Autobiography of Rose Hacker* (London: Deptford Forum, 1996), 38.

few exceptions until the establishment of the NHS. There was also a disinclination to appoint a consultant who had trained in some other part of England, and the aversion was even more marked across the national boundaries.

Moreover, it was the period when Hitlerism was in the ascendant: there was no conspicuous lack of antisemitism in the UK, and a few consultants felt in no way obliged to restrain themselves.[24]

How did Jews fare in the teaching hospitals? One Harley Street physician complained in 1926 that Jews were excluded from the plum hospital jobs, and Claire Hilton has argued that during the inter-war period Jews were barred from occupying the commanding heights of medicine: posts in the teaching hospitals in general surgery, as physicians, and in gynaecology.[25] However, while this may be largely true, there were a number of exceptions to the rule. Harold Albert Kisch (1880–1959), a member of an old Anglo-Jewish family, was a consulting surgeon to the Royal National Throat, Nose and Ear Hospital, University College Hospital, and the London Jewish Hospital. The surgeon Edward Gustave Slesinger (1888–1975) was not only head of the fracture department at Guy's Hospital and chairman of its board of governors, but also an honorary consultant to the London Jewish Hospital in the 1930s. Sir Stanford Cade (1895–1973), born in St Petersburg as the son of a diamond merchant called Kadinsky, underwent a process of Anglicization as a young man; having severed most of his ties with the Jewish community, he emerged as a leading figure in the British medical establishment. He was consulting surgeon to the Westminster Hospital from 1924 until his retirement in 1960, an expert in the field of cancer surgery and radiotherapy, and director of surgical studies at the Royal College of Surgeons; his outstanding surgical skills brought him promotion to the rank of air vice-marshal of the RAF during the Second World War. Lionel Richard Fifield was a brilliant consulting surgeon at the London Hospital, who converted to Judaism prior to his marriage at the Orthodox Shackwell Lane Synagogue, but unfortunately died young in a road accident.[26]

More typical of the career pattern of Anglo-Jewish surgeons in these years was that of David Levi (1901–94), who despite being hailed by his fellow surgeons as 'perhaps the last of the great general surgeons in London', was nevertheless unable to gain promotion to a consultancy at a teaching hospital. His family was well established in England: an ancestor born in London in 1742

[24] Jacoby, *Journey*, 44, 45.

[25] Endelman, *Radical Assimilation*, 195; Hilton, 'St Bartholomew's Hospital', 33, 34.

[26] *JC* 14 Aug. 1959, p. 9 (obituary of Kisch); *Lives of the Fellows of the Royal College of Surgeons 1952–1964*, 230; *Lives of the Fellows of the Royal College of Surgeons 1974–1982* (1988), 366, 367 (on Slesinger); *Lives of the Fellows of the Royal College of Surgeons 1965–1973* (1981), 53, 54; Gordon Wolstenholme (ed.), *Lives of the Fellows of the Royal College of Physicians of London Continued to 1975* (Oxford: IRL, 1982), 79 (on Cade); *JC* 23 Mar. 1928, p. 12 and *BMJ* 31 Mar. 1928 (obituary of Fifield).

worked making shoes and hats while translating the prayer books for the Ash-kenazi and Sephardi communities. David attended St Mary's Hospital for his training, relying on scholarships to see him through medical school; but though he won a succession of prizes, and became an FRCS at the early age of 23, he was never offered the posts at the hospital that would have set him on the ladder to a consultancy position. Yet, according to *The Times* obituarist, 'He was equally proficient with abdominal, orthopaedic, urological, gynaecological and thoracic operations, but he excelled as a paediatric surgeon, where his delicacy of touch (resulting in minimal scarring) and speed were recognised by other practition-ers as outstanding.' He secured an international reputation for the surgical treatment of babies with a constricted pylorus (the opening from the stomach into the duodenum). He 'tackled operations with great finesse and speed in the pre-War era of still rudimentary anaesthesia'. Among the hospitals where he served as a consultant were the Westminster Children's Hospital, Luton and Dunstable Hospital, Harefield Hospital, Southall Hospital, Hanwell Cottage Hospital, and the London Jewish Hospital. From 1928 to 1966 he lectured in anatomy at St Mary's medical school; a unique feature of his lectures was that he drew the anatomical diagrams on the blackboard with both hands. Blessed with indefatigable energy as a surgeon, he yet found time for many years to serve as the warden of the West London Synagogue.[27]

For the east European immigrant community, the breakthrough came with the appointment of Arnold Sorsby (born Ahron Sourasky, 1900–80) as surgeon to the Royal Eye Hospital in 1931. Born in Bialystok, Arnold was educated partly in Antwerp, where his father worked in the diamond industry, and partly at the Central High School and University in Leeds, where he moved with his family at the age of 14. Within seven years he had qualified as a doctor in Leeds, racing ahead for a short while of his elder brother Maurice, who subsequently also became a consultant surgeon. Arnold gained his FRCS in London in 1928, having been awarded the equivalent qualification from Edin-burgh a year earlier, and received his MD from Leeds in 1929. He was ophthal-mic surgeon to the Hampstead General Hospital, the London Jewish Hospital, and the West End Hospital for Nervous Diseases.[28] From 1931 to 1966 he served as a surgeon to the Royal Eye Hospital; from 1934 to 1938 he was dean of its medical school, and from 1943 to 1966 held the position of research professor at the Royal College of Surgeons under the aegis of the Royal Eye Hospital, a position that was specially created for him. When working at the London Jewish Hospital, he had noticed an unusual number of cases of trachoma; this kindled an interest in the treatment of this condition, on which he became a leading

[27] *The Times*, 28 July 1994; *JC* 5 Aug. 1994, p. 17 (obituaries of Levi).
[28] Interview with the late Mrs Sophie Phillips, 5 Dec. 1996; *Medical Directory 1930*, 308.

authority.[29] He sat on the World Health Organization advisory panel on the disease, and was a member of several other international organizations in a similar capacity. He was also director of the Medical Research Council unit on ophthalmic genetics and editor of the *Journal of Medical Genetics*.[30] Quieter and less ebullient than his brother Maurice, he was an intellectually intimidating figure.[31] Despite his Orthodox background, he changed his surname after qualifying professionally and married out of the faith, distancing himself from his family's Zionism as he moved up the career ladder. He became a strong British supporter of the Freeland League, which tried in vain to settle large numbers of Jews in north-west Australia rather than Palestine during the Second World War, a scheme akin to that proposed by Zangwill's Jewish Territorial Organization.[32]

Another somewhat unusual figure was the eminent gynaecologist Muriel Elsie Landau (Mrs Muriel Sacks, 1895–1972). Her staunchly Orthodox family had come to Britain in the mid-nineteenth century but had not assimilated (her sister Annie Landau went on to become headmistress of the Evelina de Rothschild School in Jerusalem). Brought up in London, where her father was a successful businessman, Elsie Landau entered the London School of Medicine for Women in October 1913, qualifying with the MRCS, LRCP, and MB, BS in 1918; two years later she became a Fellow of the Royal College of Surgeons, the first Jewish woman to achieve this. At the early age of 26 she was appointed to the consulting staff at the Elizabeth Garrett Anderson Hospital, where she specialized in gynaecology and obstetrics—at a time when there were very few Jewish gynaecologists in England—but she also practised in general surgery, and eventually became the senior consulting surgeon there.[33] According to her son, the psychiatrist Oliver Sacks, 'There was nothing she loved more than a challenging delivery—an arm presentation, a breech—brought off successfully.' She occasionally brought home a foetus: 'she dissected several of these for me, and then she insisted, though I was only eleven, that I dissect them myself.' In addition, she was a gynaecologist at the London Jewish Hospital and a surgeon at the Marie Curie Hospital, where she personally treated cancer patients with radium, a task later left to radiotherapists. She was an outstanding figure, 'one of that small band of second generation medical women who showed that

[29] *JC* 23 Mar. 1980, p. 14; *Lives of the Fellows of the Royal College of Surgeons 1974–1982*, 372 (obituaries of Arnold Sorsby). Trachoma was another of the alleged 'Jewish diseases'.

[30] *Lives of the Fellows of the Royal College of Surgeons 1974–1982*, 372; *JC* 24 Dec. 1026, p. 22 (lecture by Dr A. Sourasky).

[31] *Lives of the Fellows of the Royal College of Surgeons 1974–1982*, 372; interview with the late Mrs Sophie Phillips and Mrs Daniels, 5 Dec. 1996.

[32] Michael Blakeney, *Australia and the Jewish Refugees* (Sydney: Croom Helm, 1985), 253–80. Interview with the late Mrs Sophie Phillips and Mrs Daniels, 5 Dec. 1996.

[33] *Lancet*, 2 Dec. 1972; *BMJ* 2 Dec. 1972 (obituaries of Muriel Elsie Landau).

surgical skill is by no means an exclusively male accomplishment . . . She was also that somewhat *rara avis* among surgeons, a good medical doctor, and this quality, combined with a rare humanity, attracted a large and varied practice'— and, it might be added, countless numbers of students. As an early feminist, she had no qualms about suckling her own infant in front of the class when lecturing on breastfeeding.[34] She also wrote a pioneering work on the menopause, *Women of Forty* (1956), which had a wide circulation. With her husband, Dr Samuel Sacks, she fostered Jewish culture in her home, where they ran a Hebrew-speaking circle. Three of their four sons became doctors—including the afore-mentioned Oliver, author of several books, including *The Man Who Mistook his Wife for a Hat*. Mrs Sacks was a regular worshipper at the Cricklewood United Synagogue, and for over seventeen years chaired the doctors' and dentists' group of the Joint Palestine Appeal, the principal Zionist charity of the 1930s and 1940s.[35]

As far as physicians in the big London hospitals were concerned, the trends established in late Victorian and Edwardian England continued and a few Jews were to be found on the staff of these institutions. Otto Fritz Leyton (1874–1938), who changed his name from Grunbaum during the First World War, was a consulting physician at the London Hospital during the 1920s and 1930s as well as being an able scientist. He started the manufacture of insulin for the treatment of diabetic patients, when it was not readily available in Britain, and he was the first in the hospital to employ modern methods of blood trans-fusion.[36] Sir Adolphe Abrahams (1883–1967), the brother of the Olympic cham-pion athlete Harold Abrahams, was appointed as a consultant physician at the Westminster Hospital in 1920, rising to become dean of its medical school—the most senior position in the profession to be held by a Jew since Ernest Hart served as dean of St Mary's medical school in the 1860s. He specialized in gastroenterological subjects and 'was a physician of the old school to whom a detailed history and clinical examination were of basic importance, and of more importance and interest than the results of laboratory investigations, which came last to confirm or refute the clinical diagnosis'.[37] Lord Goodman, how-ever, gives a withering account of Abrahams in his memoirs, describing him as looking 'like a plucked hen; he was very tiny—I reckon about 5 ft 4 in', and castigating him for misdiagnosing a gall bladder that urgently needed removal

[34] Oliver Sacks, *Uncle Tungsten: Memories of a Chemical Boyhood* (London: Picador, 2001), 237, 240–1; interview with Elliot Elias Philipp, 16 Nov. 1998; *Lancet*, 2 Dec. 1972.

[35] *JC* 28 May 1920, p. 22, 1 Dec. 1972, p. 34 (obituary of Elsie Sacks).

[36] *Lives of the Fellows of the Royal College of Physicians*, vol. v, ed. Richard Trail (1968), 502; *Lancet*, 29 Jan. 1938, *BMJ* 29 Jan. 1938 (obituary of Leyton).

[37] *Lives of the Fellows of the Royal College of Physicians*, vol. vi, ed. Gordon Wolstenholme (1982), 1–3 (obituary of Abrahams).

as an inflamed appendix.[38] Philip Montagu D'Arcy Hart (b. 1900), a grandson of the banker and leader of Orthodox Jewry the first Lord Swaythling (1832–1911), held the positions of assistant physician and lecturer in clinical medicine at University College Hospital from 1934 to 1937; he was offered a full consultancy at the hospital, but this would have left him with no time to pursue an interest in medical research, so rather than accept it he resigned his post as assistant physician.[39]

The outstanding physician of Jewish origin in England between the world wars was Sir Arthur Frederick Hurst (1879–1944), who became the senior consulting physician to Guy's Hospital. He was the son of a German Jewish wool merchant from Bradford, William Martin Hertz, and the daughter of Baruch Halle, a London merchant. Two members of his father's side of the family were distinguished scientists: Heinrich Hertz, who gave his name to the measurement of electromagnetic frequency, and Gustav Hertz, who shared (with James Franck) the Nobel Prize for physics in 1925. Arthur Hurst graduated with a first-class degree in physiology from Oxford, going on to win gold medals for medicine and surgery in exams at Guy's Hospital in 1904. After studying in Munich, Paris, and the United States, he was appointed assistant physician at Guy's in charge of the neurology department in 1906, becoming a full physician in 1918 and retiring in 1939. With Sir James Mackenzie and Sir Thomas Lewis, he inaugurated the scientific investigation of physiological phenomena in Britain, as opposed to the established technique of reliance on the correlation of 'clinical findings with morbid anatomy' through dissection and observation. In 1908 Hurst adopted the use of X-rays to explore digestive disorders, feeding his students 'bismuth meals', later replaced by barium. According to Alex Sakula, he was able 'to throw further light on diseases of the oesophagus (such as achalasia), duodenal ulcer and disorders of the bowel (such as ulcerative colitis and dyschezia). His *Constipation and Allied Intestinal Disorders* (1909) and his Goulstonian Lectures (1911) . . . entitled *Sensibility of the Alimentary Canal* remain classics of their kind.' During the First World War, as a pupil of the French psychologist and neurologist Pierre Janet, he successfully treated shell-shocked soldiers by suggestion, without devising any new methods of treatment. After the war he continued with his researches on the alimentary tract and established the basis for the treatment of peptic ulcer and constipation. His work on achlorhydria, the absence of hydrochloric acid in the stomach, was a landmark, as he identified the possible association with pernicious anaemia and gastric carcinoma. In 1936 Hurst formed a gastroenterology club which was the precursor of the British Society of Gastroenterology, and he is now recognized as the

[38] Goodman, *Tell Them I'm On My Way*, 82–3.

[39] *Medical Directory 1953*, i. 141 (on Philip Montagu D'Arcy Hart); interview with Philip Montagu D'Arcy Hart, 8 Sept. 1997.

father of British gastroenterology. Almost too fluent in speaking and writing, Hurst was sometimes inclined to erect theories hastily which he had later to retract.[40]

It remained almost impossible for doctors from east European Jewish families to secure positions as consultant physicians at the chief London hospitals. Although William Moses Feldman (1880–1939) had published *Ante-Natal and Post-Natal Child Physiology* in 1920 and *Ante-Natal and Post-Natal Child Hygiene* in 1927, he did not add FRCP to his other qualifications until 1935, and though he was ambitious and would have liked a job at a teaching hospital, the best he could do was to open a Harley Street practice in the mid-1920s. This was itself a considerable achievement, setting the seal on his advance from general practice in the East End to specialist status. He also held non-resident appointments at the London Hospital, and was later physician to St Mary's Hospital for Women and Children and the East End Dispensary.[41]

The exception to the rule was Hugh Gainsborough (Hyman Hirsh Ginsberg, 1893–1980), who became consulting physician to St George's Hospital. Born in Leeds of Russian and Dutch Jewish parentage—his father was a grocer and later a confectioner—Gainsborough was Cambridge-educated and became a distinguished scientist. In 1926, at the age of 32, he was appointed consultant at St George's; he married in the same year, by which time he had Anglicized his name. Gainsborough was one of the first in Europe to use insulin to manage diabetes, setting up clinics for this purpose at St George's and the London Jewish Hospital. Certain diseases, of which diabetes was one, were widely thought of as affecting Jews more than the bulk of the population, and it is noteworthy that this sometimes influenced the direction of clinical practice of Jewish doctors; both Gainsborough and Otto Fritz Leyton pioneered the insulin treatment for diabetes. By patient laboratory analysis, Gainsborough also 'established many basic observations on cholesterol metabolism', which is so important a factor in heart disease.[42]

Gainsborough was also exceptional in his closeness to the Jewish community. Nearly all the other surgeons and physicians mentioned here were from the older Anglo-Jewish families and had the most tenuous connections with the Jewish community; with the exception of Abrahams, who had arrived from

[40] Alex Sakula, 'Sir Arthur Hurst (1879–1944), Master of Medicine', *Journal of Medical Biography*, 7 (1999), 125–9; Arthur Hurst, *A Twentieth Century Physician* (London: Arnold, 1949), 6, 58, 65–72; L. G. Wickham Legg and E. T. Williams (eds.), *Dictionary of National Biography 1941–1950* (Oxford: Oxford University Press, 1959), 417, 418; *BMJ* 26 Aug. 1944, pp. 292, 293 (obituary of Arthur Hurst).

[41] *Lives of the Fellows of the Royal College of Physicians*, vol. v (1970), 127; *JC* 7 July 1939, p. 15, 14 July 1939, p. 10 (obituary of William Moses Feldman); London Hospital Medical College Minute Book 19, Feb. 1920, Royal London Hospital Archive, MC/A/2/13; *Medical Directory 1925*, 103.

[42] *BMJ* 7 Feb. 1981, p. 487 (obituary of Gainsborough); birth and marriage certificates for Hugh Gainsborough.

South Africa as a boy, these families were Ashkenazi Jews who had lived in England at least since the nineteenth century. Many of them, for example, Otto Leyton, Adolphe Abrahams, and Arthur Hurst, married non-Jewish women. Gainsborough, by contrast, was associated with Jewish institutions and was married in the United Orthodox St John's Wood Synagogue to the daughter of Leopold Pilichowski, a well-known Jewish artist. For a time Gainsborough served as chairman of the executive of the Jewish Health Organization of Great Britain, and before that presided over a sub-committee of the Jewish Medical and Dental Emergency Association which drew up an alternative list of drugs and spas with a view to imposing a medical boycott of Germany. Possibly the price Gainsborough paid for being catapulted out of his social class in his youth was a stutter.[43]

Most Jews in medical practice between the wars filled hospital positions in dermatology, anatomy, pathology, psychiatry, and radiography. One particularly outstanding individual whose name springs to mind is Professor Samson Wright (1899–1956), who was promoted to the chair of physiology at the Middlesex Hospital medical school at the unusually young age of 31. Awarded the gold medal when he took his MB examination in 1922, he was immediately appointed as a demonstrator in the physiology department, succeeding his mentor Professor Swale Vincent as head of the department in 1930. 'Samson Wright was the greatest teacher of physiology of his generation,' declared Professor A. C. Keele.

He was supreme in knowledge of his subject, in critical analysis, and in power of exposition. He could make the most difficult topic seem simple, and no one could more effectively stimulate the student to think for himself. His lectures were lively, provocative, and memorable, and in his later years were frequently punctuated by apt illustrations from history, literature, politics, and religion.[44]

His *Applied Physiology* went through nine editions, securing his international reputation; and as editor he established *Physiological Abstracts* as the premier journal in its field. He also made notable contributions to physiological research, particularly by being, with Selladurai, the first to show that 'oxygen lack directly depressed the respiratory centre' and delineating chemical transmission in the central nervous system. Alongside this glittering professional career, Samson Wright yet found the time to be vice-president of the Board of Deputies and an enthusiastic Zionist; he was president of the Jewish National Fund and the driving force in the Friends of the Anti-Tuberculosis League of Palestine,

[43] Annual report of the Jewish Health Organisation of Great Britain for 1940, University College London Library; Laurance Phillips, *London Jewish Hospital Medical Society* (London, 1964), 8; copy letter Mrs Celia Cheyney to Redcliffe Salaman, 24 Aug. 1924, in the possession of the author.

[44] J. J. Astor *et al.*, *Professor Samson Wright (1899–1956) in Memoriam* (London: Favil, 1956), 1–38.

which helped eradicate the disease among the immigrants who had fled to Israel in the early years of the state. On David Eder's death in 1936, he took over the leadership of the campaign to secure admission to England for refugee doctors from central Europe.[45]

In the 1920s and 1930s any Jewish doctor in the northern cities who wished to become a consultant had to head for London. Whereas the London Jewish Hospital provided good opportunities for Jews to gain experience in surgery and as physicians to advance their careers, the provincial Jewish hospitals in Manchester and Leeds were smaller and relied on the whole on local non-Jewish consultants to fill their more senior positions. Hence Maurice Sorsby (1899–1949), like his younger brother Arnold, left Leeds for the capital in the 1920s. There was friendly rivalry between the two brothers, each spurring the other on to greater academic success. Although Arnold was the first to qualify as a doctor, Maurice obtained an Edinburgh FRCS in 1925, two years before his brother, and an MD from Leeds in 1925, four years before him. He was the first locally trained Jewish doctor to be appointed a house surgeon in the Leeds General Infirmary since Julian Landman at the beginning of the century. Maurice Sorsby held staff appointments at the London Jewish Hospital and the Plaistow Children's Hospital, and was consulting ear, nose, and throat surgeon to the London County Council hospitals. He was mainly interested in inter-cranial complications of ear disease and general aspects of the cancer problem, such as its distribution across the population. In *Cancer and Race* (1931) he concluded that the incidence of cancer 'in different parts of the world showed that the total cancer rate in Jews was everywhere approximately the same as that of the general population, though the distribution according to the organs affected varied considerably. The latter differences could in most cases be explained by environmental factors.'

Maurice, a keen Zionist and socialist brought up in an Orthodox east European household, nevertheless had the energy and charm to win the friendship of Lord Moynihan, his medical tutor at Leeds, and of Arnold Goodman Levy and David Eder from the older generation of Anglo-Jewish doctors, despite their divergent backgrounds.[46] Maurice not only founded the London Jewish Hospital Medical Society, now the London Jewish Medical Society, but with Eder formed the Jewish Medical and Dental Emergency Association to deal with the crisis affecting Jewish doctors in Germany and central Europe after 1933.[47] Unfortunately, Maurice's career came to a premature end on the

[45] *JC* 16 Mar. 1956, p. 11 (obituary of Wright); Alex Sakula, 'Samson Wright (1899–1956): Physiologist Extraordinary', *Journal of the Royal Society of Medicine*, 92 (Sept. 1999), 484–6.
[46] *JC* 8 Jan. 1926, p. 14, 15 Apr. 1949, p. 15, *BMJ* 23 Apr. 1949 (obituary of Maurice Sorsby).
[47] Phillips, *London Jewish Hospital Medical Society*, 10.

eve of the Second World War, when he was forced to retire because of a serious illness; he moved to Los Angeles for his health, and died there in 1949.

Among the newly qualified doctors who quit Manchester for London in the 1930s were Eli Davis and Albert Davis (not related). Albert Davis was one of eight children, but the only one to have student potential. Because family finances were tight, Davis had to establish himself in a career as quickly as possible. He left school at 16 to attend Manchester medical school, where he encountered 'little overt antisemitism'. However, despite coming third in the final MB, Ch.B. exams in 1925, he failed to secure a house surgeon job at the university hospital. 'I missed out again at the next round,' he recalled,

and went to see the medical committee chairman who said there had been some injustice and took me on his team. I subsequently went on to [become] house surgeon and registrar in the Royal Infirmary, St Mary's and Christie Hospitals and took postgraduates in Vienna and Lyons and got a Dickenson scholarship to work on the pelvic neuroanatomy at the University. I took the MD and the FRCS in 1931 and the Ch.M. the same year, with the Hunterian Professorship at the Royal College of Surgeons in 1933. I waited for the Registrar post at St Mary's, the stepping stone up to the future consultancy, in confidence but didn't get it. It was given to an Australian of lesser experience and qualifications on the grounds of preference for the Commonwealth, but I soon learned the truth of many previous warnings that there was no question of appointing a Jew to any senior post in any specialty in Manchester.[48]

In the mid-1930s Albert Davis obtained an appointment as a gynaecologist at the Jewish Maternity Hospital in London—though he almost missed out here too, as according to the hospital minutes one of the consultants, Mr O'Sullivan, tried to veto the appointment on the grounds that Davis was Jewish. However, he secured subsequent appointments as a gynaecologist and obstetrician, to the French Hospital and two big London County Council hospitals in St Giles and Dulwich, without difficulty.[49]

A few years before Davis's appointment, in 1930, there had been considerable disquiet in the Jewish press over the failure of the Jewish Maternity Hospital to appoint a Jew to its medical staff when a vacancy occurred; for Jews were excluded from positions in similar but non-Jewish organizations. 'This is the second occasion within the last two years that distinguished Jewish consultants have been turned down in favour of non-Jewish candidates', claimed Dr A. D. Woolf. 'I am also told that the same state of affairs exists in the appointment of the Junior Medical Staff, non-Jews are selected where there are equally good Jewish candidates.' Two of the medical staff of the London Jewish Hospital, Dr Mandel and Dr A. H. Levy, who were also on the honorary staff of the Maternity Hospital, resigned their positions at the latter institution in protest at

[48] Albert Davis, letter to the author, 18 Apr. 1997.   [49] *JC* 30 Oct. 1931, p. 26.

this policy.[50] This public controversy in the Jewish press probably eased Albert Davis's appointment.

Eli Davis (1908–97) was born in Lithuania, arriving in Manchester when he was 12 months old. On leaving school he won the only medical scholarship of his year, and went on to Manchester University. Choosing to take his scientific degrees before his medical finals, he was awarded a B.Sc. in physiology in 1929 with first-class honours and an M.Sc. in 1930, all of which delayed his qualification as a doctor by two years. He was a houseman at the Manchester Royal Infirmary, where he studied with the consultant neurologist and physician Mr Oliver, a non-Jew, who was friendly towards him and invited him to his home. Eli Davis gained his MB, Ch.B. in 1933 and his MD in 1935, followed by his MRCP London in 1937. Moving to London, he held several posts in London County Council hospitals: physician at St Stephen's Hospital, senior resident physician at St Alfege's Hospital, and later, in 1943, deputy medical superintendent and senior resident physician at St Andrew's Hospital in Bow.[51]

Unusually for someone of Jewish origin, Norman Kletts (1895–1955) held the position of consultant physician to the Manchester Royal Infirmary between 1934 and 1955. As the son of Louis Kletz, a manufacturer and local Jewish communal leader, he fitted into the pattern of successful scions from the older Anglo-Jewish families established in England since the nineteenth century; but he had few ties to the Jewish community and had married a non-Jewish woman. His 'awkward prejudices, expressed forcibly' incurred the ire of his colleagues[52]—although it has been suggested that Klett's brilliance as a lecturer aroused the jealousy of those around him, provoking unfair comments. He has also been praised for encouraging able trainee Jewish consultants.[53]

In contrast to the medical schools and hospitals in Leeds and Manchester, which with a few exceptions such as Kletts and Dr John Gordon, lecturer in bacteriology at Leeds, were virtually closed to Jews, Liverpool was a much more open environment, where a number of Jews held important medical appointments between the wars.[54] Henry Cohen (1900–77), later Lord Cohen of Birkenhead, was the youngest of five children of Isaac Cohen, a Jewish scholar who came to England with his wife Dora and established himself in Liverpool as a draper. The family, which was of east European origin, was so poor that

[50] *JC* 28 Feb. 1930, p. 6, 7 Mar. 1930, p. 12, 14 Mar. 1930, p. 11, 4 July 1930, p. 7.

[51] Interview with the late Professor Eli Davis, 22 Aug. 1996; *Medical Directory 1939*, 79; *Medical Directory 1942*, 73; *Medical Directory 1943*, 73.

[52] *Lives of the Fellows of the Royal College of Physicians*, vol. v (1970), 233 (obituary of Kletts).

[53] Private information.

[54] Julius Silman, *Signifying Nothing* (London: Minerva, 1997), 67; *Jewish Chronicle*, 8 Jan. 1926 (on Dr John Gordon); Brockbank, *The Honorary Medical Staff*, 229, 230. Even so, there was believed to be an unwritten rule in Liverpool as late as the mid-1950s that only one Jew could be appointed at consultant level in each specialty in teaching hospitals (private information).

during his student years, to save the tram fare, Henry used to walk all the way to the university from Merseyside. He graduated from Liverpool University as MB, Ch.B. in 1922, with first-class honours and a distinction in every subject of the curriculum—an unprecedented achievement. In 1924 he was awarded his MD with special merit. After further study in London and Paris he was appointed assistant physician at the Liverpool Royal Infirmary, and at the age of 34 he was made professor of medicine at Liverpool University and promoted to senior physician at the Infirmary.

Cohen had a remarkable memory. 'Thus, he remembered the details of nearly every patient he had ever seen and of nearly every paper he had ever read; he had "total recall"', wrote a colleague in a tribute in the *Lancet*. 'As a result, he was a marvellous diagnostician whose reputation was legendary. But he also had that ability to discriminate and foresee accurately the immediate and remote consequences of any action or inaction, a quality we term judgment . . . But Henry . . . was a warm, understanding and compassionate man . . . Small wonder that he had an enormous reputation as a physician and a vast practice.' Widely read, Cohen was also a brilliant platform orator; his addresses, delivered in a beautiful speaking voice, sparkled with wit and erudition, and his services as a lecturer were called upon on many occasions.[55]

From 1934 until the end of the Second World War, Cohen rose rapidly in eminence within the medical profession to become a figure of national importance. Among his published works were *New Pathways in Medicine* (1935), *Nature, Method and Purpose of Diagnosis* (1943), and *The Evolution of Modern Medicine* (1958). Although he had marvellous clarity of mind and was held in awe by his colleagues, he was not an original thinker, nor did he make any outstanding scientific discovery, despite being provided with a research team by the university because of his interest in neurology. For these reasons his reputation has declined somewhat since his death.[56]

In addition to his clinical skills, Cohen will be remembered for his great administrative talents. As a young professor in Liverpool he had to amalgamate three teaching hospitals and four general ones into a single administrative unit. In his attempt to overcome their rivalries he encountered much hostility and jealousy, which in turn fuelled his own insecurity; although he promoted a number of talented young Jewish doctors to the position of registrar, his own sense of rivalry forced them to leave and seek positions elsewhere. According

    [55] Lord Blake and C. S. Nicholls (eds.), *Dictionary of National Biography 1971–1980* (Oxford: Oxford University Press, 1986), 161, 162; *Lancet*, 20 Aug. 1977, pp. 413–14, *BMJ* 20 Aug. 1977, p. 525 (obituary of Cohen).
    [56] *Dictionary of National Biography 1971–1980*, 161; *Lancet*, 20 Aug. 1977; interviews with Dr Mervyn Goodman, 2 Oct. 1996; private information; Thomas Kelly, *For the Advancement of Learning: The University of Liverpool 1881–1981* (Liverpool: Liverpool University Press, 1981), 250.

to a colleague, 'There have been other leaders in clinical medicine who have given great public service in promoting the health and welfare of the nation, including the NHS. In this century, and perhaps in all our history, there has certainly been no-one who has done more than Henry Cohen, and if there is one who has done as much I could not name him.'[57] He was the first vice-chairman of the Standing Medical Advisory Committee of the Ministry of Health, and its chairman from 1947 until he retired from the position in 1963. Presiding over numerous committees, Cohen devised the categories under which drugs were classified for use in the National Health Service, organized the national scheme of poliomyelitis vaccination, and helped prepare reports on the medical care of epileptics and on staphylococcal infections in hospital. A British Medical Association committee chaired by Cohen in 1950 stipulated that all doctors should be residents in a hospital for one year before enrolling with the General Medical Council, and furthermore that they should undergo three years of postgraduate vocational training. While the first point was incorporated in the Medical Act 1950, postgraduate training was not introduced until the 1970s, and Cohen has been criticized for being opposed to health centres until his last years. Cohen was president of the BMA from 1950 to 1952 and of the GMC from 1961 to 1973; in the latter capacity he presided over the disciplinary hearings for doctors, thereby partially fulfilling a youthful ambition to practise law.[58]

Although in later life he was not so Orthodox as in his youth, Henry Cohen continued to feel intensely Jewish. When he was sworn in as a peer, he took the oath with his head covered, following Jewish tradition. For many years he was president of the King David Schools in Liverpool, upbraiding members of his community who preferred to send their children to non-Jewish schools and watching proudly as the number of pupils enrolled grew from 160 to 680. He was also president of the Liverpool Home for Aged Jews. He defended shechitah (the ritual slaughter of animals) in the House of Lords when a bill was introduced opposing the practice. 'The speech was a tour de force, combining great eloquence with cogent argument, detailed scientific knowledge and a warm appreciation of the cardinal concepts of Judaism.' Deeply attached to his mother, he had a long-standing relationship with his secretary, whom he did not marry because she was not Jewish.[59]

Other Jews succeeded in the middle ranks of the medical profession in Liverpool; these included Morris Datnow, Maurice Silverstone, and Emanuel Lourie, while Reuben Lipman (1901–56), a Leeds-trained practitioner, was a

[57] *Lancet*, 20 Aug. 1977; *Dictionary of National Biography 1971–1980*, 162.

[58] Charles Webster (ed.), *General Practice under the National Health Service 1948–1997* (Oxford: Clarendon Press, 1998), 7, 25.

[59] *JC* 20 Feb. 1970, p. 19, 12 Aug. 1977, p. 11 (obituary of Cohen).

consultant at the Liverpool Psychiatric Clinic. Maurice Silverstone (1905–56) was appointed to the consultant staff of the Liverpool Royal Infirmary as assistant surgeon, and at the time of his death was a consulting surgeon at four local hospitals as well as a lecturer in clinical surgery at Liverpool University. Despite poor health, he worked to the last, 'operating in the morning on the day of his death'.[60] Morris Myer Datnow (1901–62), who was born in South Africa, completed his medical training at Liverpool University, qualifying as an FRCS at Edinburgh in 1932 and gaining his fellowship of the Royal College of Gynaecologists in 1939. He joined the Liverpool University staff in 1925, eventually being promoted to lecturer in clinical obstetrics and gynaecology. He held gynaecological positions on the staff of the Women's Hospital Liverpool, the Liverpool Maternity Hospital, and the Royal Southern Hospital. Datnow was also part of the research team under William Blair Bell at Liverpool which investigated the place of chemotherapy in the treatment of cancer.[61] Dr Emanuel Lourie (1904–56), who was also born in South Africa, was for a time director of the department of chemotherapy at the Liverpool School of Tropical Medicine before he joined the World Health Organization as head of the biological standardization section.[62]

Other Jewish consultants in Liverpool teaching hospitals at this time were Jack Bernstien; Alex Tumarkin, an ENT surgeon; and Jack Berkson, an ophthalmologist. Dr Isaac Jackson-Lipkin (1895–1975) was a descendant of Rabbi Israel Salanter (1810–83), who founded the Musar movement, a Jewish ethical grouping whose members engaged in self-examination and expressed a contempt for worldly vanities. Jackson-Lipkin was a brilliant student, winning gold and silver medals; but his relations with Henry Cohen were frosty, possibly because he was not given a teaching hospital appointment.[63] Dr Jackson-Lipkin was one of the leaders of Liverpool Jewry; Datnow was junior warden of the Liverpool Old Hebrew Congregation; Maurice Silverstone 'took a keen interest in the affairs of the local congregation'; and Dr Reuben Lipman not only played a valuable role in the Liverpool Jewish Medical Society, but participated in many aspects of local Jewish life.[64]

Saul Adler FRS (1895–1966) was born in Karelitz in Byelorussia and brought at the age of 5 to Leeds, where he was educated and graduated as a doctor in 1917. He came from a family which was imbued with the ideals of the Haskalah,

[60] *JC* 5 Oct. 1956, p. 27 (obituary of Silverstone); R. H. O. B. Robinson and W. R. Le Fanu (eds.), *Lives of the Fellows of the Royal College of Surgeons of England 1905–1956* (London: E. & S. Livingstone, 1970) (obituary of Silverstone).

[61] *JC* 6 July 1962 (obituary of Datnow); John Peel (ed.), *Lives of the Fellows of the Royal College of Obstetricians and Gynaecologists* (London: Heinemann, 1976), 124, 125 (obituary of Datnow).

[62] *JC* 17 Aug. 1956, p. 13 (obituary of Lourie).

[63] *JC JC* 20 June 1975, p. 12 (obituary of Jackson-Lipkin); Dr Mervyn Goodman, letters to the author, 8, 20 Aug. 1999.   [64] *JC* 3 Aug. 1965, p. 20 (obituary of Lipman).

the Jewish Enlightenment, and Zionism, as a result of which he had learned to speak Hebrew. After gaining a diploma in tropical medicine in Liverpool, Adler joined the Liverpool School of Tropical Medicine as a clinical assistant in 1921. For three years he was based in Freetown, Sierra Leone, where he carried out research into malaria and other tropical diseases. While on holiday in Britain, Chaim Weizmann, the future first president of Israel, offered him a position as an assistant in the Microbiological Department of the Hebrew University, Jerusalem, an offer which Adler accepted with alacrity; he took up the post in 1924. Here he headed a commission of the Royal Society on Kala Azar (leishmaniasis), showing how the disease was transmitted from sandflies to humans in the Mediterranean area. He also did important work on theileriosis as a cause of the death of cows and devised an effective form of vaccination. He was appointed professor of parasitology in Jerusalem in 1929, and in 1944 became chairman of the Pre-Faculty of Medicine at the Hebrew University, while in 1957 he was elected Fellow of the Royal Society for his outstanding contribution to medical research. His 1960 translation of Darwin's *Origin of Species* into Hebrew has become a classic, showing that scientific literature could be translated into that language;[65] today such translations are a commonplace of academic life.

In the past, the Jewish community has made arrangements with, among others, the London Hospital, the German Hospital, and the Metropolitan Hospital for the provision of Jewish wards and kosher food; but the immigrant population in the East End did not feel that this was sufficient. Many of them were religious Jews, who wanted to feel able to perform all the practices of their faith in friendly surroundings when in a hospital at a time of physical and mental stress; they also wanted to communicate easily with Yiddish-speaking doctors and nurses to secure the maximum benefit from their treatment. Unable to reach agreement with the London Hospital for a Yiddish-speaking doctor, the East End Jews, under the leadership of Isador Berliner, a barber, collected funds to purchase a site in Stepney for a Jewish hospital. Thus it came about that the London Jewish Hospital opened the doors of its outpatient department in July 1919 and an inpatient department some two years later.[66] Almost all the nursing staff and porters at the hospital were Jewish, as were most of the honorary medical staff by 1933.[67] While the percentage of non-Jewish patients at the hospital varied between 20 and 35 per cent during the 1920s and 1930s, it increased considerably after the Second World War. A student nurse who joined the hospital in 1969 'described the [London Jewish] Hospital as unique, with its own special homely ambience, particularly on Friday evenings and

[65] Gavron, *Saul Adler*, 1–196; Rivka Ashbel, *As Much As We Could Do* (Jerusalem: Magnes, 1989), 56–63.　　　　[66] Black, *Lord Rothschild and the Barber*, 29–34, 47–8, 52–8, 65.
[67] *Jewish Year Book 1933*, ed. S. Levy (London: Jewish Chronicle, 1933), 125–6.

Saturdays when the nurses lit candles in every ward, *cholas* [sabbath loaves] were served, and there were services in the synagogue. [Dr] Elsie Landau invariably brought a home made cheesecake to each session she attended.' However, by the 1960s the facilities and equipment at a small hospital were no longer sufficient to cope with the changing pattern of medical practice and the bulk of the Jewish population of London had moved away from the East End. The hospital could not secure state funding for a major renovation and it was forced to close in September 1979.[68]

In the 1930s and 1940s the London Jewish Hospital was a safe haven for competent and clever Jewish physicians and surgeons who wished to avoid some of the tribulations of the very competitive employment market of those years. As a trainee surgeon Israel Preiskel (1907–85) did not bother to try very hard to apply for appointments in the 1930s at institutions other than the London Jewish Hospital because he 'realised it was so difficult'. Ian (Isaac) Gordon (1906–94), a prizewinning student at St Bartholomew's who went on to become senior consultant physician at the London Jewish Hospital, explained the general situation judiciously, remarking that

there was a certain amount of resistance [to appointing Jews to senior positions]. It was one thing to have appointed a junior person, another thing is to appoint someone who is your colleague and if you appoint a colleague you want someone who is your peer rather than someone who is a different species. And I think we regarded ourselves as a somewhat different species, as they did . . . I wasn't conscious of any anti-Semitism, but I was conscious of the fact that if a Jew and a non-Jew applied, there was an element which would favour, other things being equal, the non-Jew rather than the Jew, because the Jew was an unknown quantity in many respects.

He then related how a teacher with whom he was friendly advised him that he would be wasting his time to apply for a vacancy in one of the major London teaching hospitals, as 'they won't have another Jew there'. By this time Gordon had already applied for the job, and he believed that the person who was appointed did not match up to the requirements of the position. 'But there were already two Jews there and asking to appoint a third Jew was asking them to swallow too many Jews in one go . . . There were one or two other people I know, certainly very well up, brilliant in many respects, who should have been appointed to senior posts who were not appointed, and the only reason I can think of was because they were Jewish.' Since the Second World War, he added, Jews no longer lived in a small area and the 'non-Jewish community will be able to mix more intimately with Jews and be able to assess them differently'.[69]

[68] Black, *Lord Rothschild and the Barber*, 90, 127, 129–35.
[69] National Sound Archive, British Library, London, C525/77 (Israel Preiskel), C525/78 (Isaac [Ian] Gordon). Ian Gordon was Louis Littman's cardiologist.

Gordon's views were underscored by Robert Henriques, whose family were members of the Cousinhood.

The 'new Englishman' had found a way of earning a living; many were established in business progressing steadily through boom and slump; already the younger generation had started to enter the professions . . . But they were not yet Englishmen . . . They lived in densely settled 'Jewish areas' where their social life was restricted to the company of other Jews of similar origins. Even those who had been born and educated in England spoke an identifiably Jewish variety of English rather than a local dialect; and Yiddish remained the language of the home, the market and the street. Their taste in food, the way they dressed, walked, moved their hands, eyes and mouths, no less than the way their minds worked, all reflected the cultural heritage of the distinctively Jewish life in the 'Pale of Settlement' whence they or their parents had fled.[70]

His description recalls the debate that had occurred in Vienna in 1876, when the professor of medicine Theodor Billroth had objected to the influx of Jewish medical students from Galicia and Hungary, exclaiming that 'no Jew, like no Iranian, Frenchman, or New Zealander, or an African can ever become a German . . . even if they write literature and think in the German language more beautifully and better than many a genuine German native'.[71]

Who were the senior Jewish staff at the London Jewish Hospital? Simon Isaac Levy (1900–59) was senior consulting surgeon to both the London Jewish Hospital and the All Saints' Hospital for Genito-Urinary Diseases. 'Good looks, a commanding presence, keen intelligence, professional integrity, charm of manner, an engaging personality, outstanding skill and ability, all these he possessed in abundant measure', noted his colleague Israel Preiskel. 'His interest in general surgery and in urology was essentially practical rather than academic, and he practised it like a master. History, examination, diagnosis, all were models of painstaking accuracy. His clinical judgment was superb and his operative technique beautiful to watch.' He was brilliant with patients, worrying about them more than anyone else and achieving superior results. A matron, however, reported that the staff were frightened of him and that he was inclined to be bad-tempered.[72] Israel Preiskel passed his fellowship examination for the Royal College of Surgeons at the age of 23 and was appointed a consultant surgeon at the London Jewish Hospital in 1947; he remained there until it closed in 1978, specializing in genito-urinary diseases.[73] Another remarkable general surgeon who practised at the hospital was David Levi, whose career has been discussed earlier in this chapter. When Harold Chapple (1881–1945), the non-Jew who

---

[70] Henriques, *Sir Robert Waley Cohen*, 264, 265.

[71] Brigitte Hamann, *Hitler's Vienna: A Dictator's Apprenticeship* (New York: Oxford University Press, 1999), 329, 330.   [72] *JC* 16 Jan. 1959, p. 12; *Lancet*, 24 Jan. 1959 (obituary of Levy).

[73] *JC* 2 Aug. 1985, p. 12 (obituary of Preiskel); *Lives of the Fellows of the Royal College of Surgeons 1983–1990*, ed. Ian Lyle and Selwyn Taylor (1995), 302.

was also senior obstetric surgeon and gynaecologist at Guy's, retired from the staff, he was replaced by two Jewish gynaecologists, Elsie Landau and Albert Davis (also discussed individually above). Among the other senior Jewish staff at the London Jewish Hospital were Julius Burnford (1878–1972), a physician at the West London Hospital; Hugh Gainsborough, a physician at St George's; Geoffrey Konstam (1900–62), a consultant cardiologist who set up a cardiographic unit at the West London Hospital; Harold Avery, an East End boy who became senior physician to the Italian Hospital; and Ian Gordon, who, along with Preiskel could converse easily with Yiddish-speaking patients. Gordon reckoned that the consultant staff at the hospital were of 'tip top' quality.[74]

Prior to the First World War, the few Jews from the Anglo-Jewish elite who opted for a career in medicine rather than in commerce either consciously followed an assimilationist ideology or were in any event sophisticated and not markedly Jewish in manner; they were regarded as acceptable colleagues by consultants in the leading hospitals. At this time the career horizons of the east European Jewish immigrants were limited and as yet hardly any of their children studied medicine, let alone applied for positions in hospitals. Whereas upper-class Jews were beyond the reach of petty antisemitism, the immigrant families escaped unscathed from the prevalent rancour against aliens as far as entry to the professions was concerned because such careers were beyond the scope of their ambitions.

By the inter-war period the position of Jews trying to become consultants had changed somewhat. It was now at least possible for both members of the older Anglo-Jewish families and a few doctors from immigrant families to obtain positions as physicians and surgeons in the teaching hospitals of London; of the two groups, the surgeons tended to have a slightly more varied background, two being Russian-born and one a convert to Judaism. However, to reach this rank it was almost invariably necessary for Jewish doctors to camouflage themselves, by mingling with their colleagues, often by marrying non-Jewish women, and, above all, by not openly avowing their Jewish identity. Leyton, Abrahams, Slesinger, and Cade had all married out of the faith, as had Norman Kletts in Manchester. Stanford Cade passed as a Pole, while Adolphe Abrahams would not admit to being of the same faith as a voluble and demanding Jewish patient, despite having been an inveterate letter-writer to the *Jewish Chronicle* in his youth. Whereas Maurice Sorsby did not attempt to mask his Jewish identity, and indeed espoused Zionism, his more successful younger brother Arnold not only married out but was prepared to obscure his Jewish identity by disavowing Zionism and by supporting an organization which

<hr />

[74] *Lancet*, 10 Mar. 1962, p. 546 (obituary of Konstam); *JC* 17 Feb. 1961, p. 6 (on Harold Avery), 7 Oct. 1964, p. 21 (obituary of Gordon); Black, *Lord Rothschild and the Barber*, 96–107; National Sound Archive C525/78 (Isaac Gordon).

pressed for the settlement of Jewish refugees in Australia. Despite having Jewish forebears on both sides of the family, Sir Arthur Hurst's parents had married in church and he was a nominal Christian; but he was sympathetic to Jewish students and his daughter married a Jew. As dean of the Westminster Medical School, Adolphe Abrahams advised one Jewish student to Anglicize his surname, and assisted him in gaining a place to study medicine. Thus, even when they had personally espoused an assimilationist ideology, many of these doctors were still helpful to aspirant Jewish students. Other families from the Anglo-Jewish upper class had already chosen the path of radical assimilation. Sir Claude Howard Stanley Frankau (1883–1967), a consultant surgeon at St George's, was a member of such a family: his father, Frederick Joseph Frankau, a barrister, had married in church and severed all connections with the Jewish community.

During the 1930s, as the fascist threat grew at home and abroad, antisemitism in Britain reached a new level of intensity which did not begin to subside until the middle of the Second World War. At the same time a large number of bright young Jewish doctors who had begun as scholarship boys from an east European immigrant background were clamouring for admission into the higher staff levels of the top hospitals. These young men and women were widely regarded as low-class foreigners, imbued with strange and dangerous ideologies and odd manners, who could not be absorbed into the system; indeed, in the view of their opponents they mustered in such numbers that, if admitted, they threatened to overwhelm these institutions. The answer was to accept the small number of qualified Jews with public school and Oxbridge backgrounds as colleagues, and to make room for a token number of Jews from immigrant families, provided they were willing to accommodate themselves to the expectations and ideas of the leaders of the profession. Otherwise, the only openings for the children of east European immigrants at consultant level in London were in the London Jewish Hospital and the London County Council hospitals; outside London, with the exception of Liverpool, they were confined to the smaller provincial hospitals. In much the same way, Jewish hospitals in the United States 'furnished opportunities for internships and residencies that Jewish, Catholic and black doctors were denied elsewhere and staff appointments so that they could attend patients needing hospitalization'.[75]

Nevertheless, there were some outstanding figures among the children of east European immigrants who refused to conform to such an assimilationist lifestyle. The names that spring to mind are those of Professor Samson Wright, a brilliant physiologist, who did not practise as a physician; Professor Henry Cohen, a physician of genius in Liverpool, later to become an illustrious figure in national medical politics; and Professor Saul Adler of the Hebrew Univer-

[75] Paul Starr, *The Social Transformation of American Medicine* (New York: Basic Books, 1982), 173, 174.

sity, a scientific expert in tropical medicine, who was elected an FRS after the Second World War, becoming part of the English scientific establishment. In a sense all three were anomalies, as none gained a national reputation as a physician or surgeon in the top London hospitals. Too much voluntary work in Jewish causes fell on to the few who were prepared to help, and David Eder, Maurice Sorsby, and Samson Wright burned themselves out campaigning for refugee doctors and Zionist projects. Apart from these names, only one scholarship boy from an immigrant family reached the top of the profession in London without denying his Jewish identity: the physician Hugh Gainsborough (although even he Anglicized his name).

As far as the general practitioners were concerned, there were occasional problems when Jews applied for public appointments; and sometimes antisemitism was encountered in applying for the post of doctor's assistant, though the *British Medical Journal* banned discriminatory advertisements. But there were no such impediments when newly qualified doctors purchased practices, and here Jews could compete freely in the open market with everyone else.

FOUR

Jewish Barristers in the Victorian and Edwardian Era 1890–1914

THE first Anglo-Jewish barrister was Sir Francis Goldsmid (1808–78), who was called to the Bar in Lincoln's Inn in January 1833 and was elevated to the rank of Queen's Counsel in 1858; he practised for over twenty-five years, retiring after succeeding to his father's title and estates in 1859. To avoid breaking the sabbath, Goldsmid practised in the Court of Chancery, which dealt with property disputes and where it was always much easier to avoid inconveniently timed appearances than in the common law courts.[1] In 1860 he was elected to Parliament, becoming only the fourth Jewish MP. Sitting as a Liberal, he was dubbed 'the Member for Jewry' and made powerful speeches in defence of the Jews of the Danubian provinces, Russia, and Poland. The first Jew to appear regularly in the common law courts was Sir John Simon (1818–97); born in Jamaica, he was called to the Bar in the Middle Temple in 1842 and rose to the rank of serjeant-at-law in 1864 and QC in 1868. Earlier, in 1858, he acted as assistant to judges in county courts, becoming the first Jew to hold judicial office in England. As a serjeant, Simon later acted as a commissioner of assize in the Manchester and Liverpool criminal courts and presided over the City of London Court. Among his notable achievements as a barrister, Simon assisted Edwin James QC, MP in the defence of Dr Bernard, a radical French physician and political refugee in Britain, when in 1858 he was charged with complicity in the attempted assassination of Napoleon III by Orsini and the murder of others in Paris. Simon, who at one point had thought of becoming a rabbi, was one of the first English Jews to deny the authenticity of the Oral Law and was an early stalwart of the religious reform movement, which perhaps explains his ability to bridge the worlds of Judaism and the law. In 1868 he was elected MP for Dewsbury, becoming known as 'the Member for Jewry' on Goldsmid's death,

---

[1] D. W. Marks and A. Lowy, *Memoir of Sir Francis Goldsmid* (London: Kegan Paul, Trench & Co., 1882), 15–17, 72, 73, 156, 157. Nathaniel Basevi, Benjamin Disraeli's cousin, was called to the Bar before Goldsmid but he had converted to Christianity.

but his sharp criticism of Gladstone for failing adequately to condemn the anti-Jewish measures enacted by the Romanian government—which in 1866 declared Jews members of a 'vagabond race', subject to expulsion—kept him out of office. An advanced Liberal, he was a supporter of home rule for Ireland and the abolition of capital punishment.[2]

George Jessel (1824–83) was the son of a prosperous diamond merchant and railway company director who was also a considerable Jewish communal figure. Jessel studied philosophy, mathematics, and botany at University College London, and was called to the Bar in 1847. Starting his career as a conveyancer, he switched to advocacy and gained a reputation by appearing in a number of railway cases in the Court of Chancery, especially for the company of which his father was a director. 'No Jewish solicitor ever employed him', his son wrote, 'till he had an extensive practice at the Bar, and in fact, in the early years of his professional career no Jewish solicitor could have kept a Chancery barrister in wig powder.' By 1871 it was estimated that Jessel was enjoying an income of £29,000, earnings higher than anyone else had hitherto achieved at the Bar.[3]

In 1868, three years after becoming a QC, Jessel was elected Liberal MP for Dover, and in 1871 Gladstone appointed him Solicitor-General. The first Jew to become a High Court judge, he was Master of the Rolls from 1873 until 1881, after which he was promoted to sit in the Court of Appeal. *The Times* said that 'it was his unique distinction that he was one of the most erudite of case lawyers and also the most courageous of Judges in handling authorities . . . Unlike the ordinary authority-monger, he was the master, not the slave of precedents.' He was perhaps the greatest of equity judges, confident enough to refashion the law to make it consonant with the needs of Victorian industrial society. 'Whether it was a question of real property, or charter-parties, or the custom of the Stock Exchange, or brokerage in Mincing Lane,' asserted the president of the Law Society, 'he knew them all as if his life had been spent in the City instead of at Lincoln's Inn.' His scientific training allied to a prodigious memory enabled him to make judgments rapidly; and in the famous case of *Commissioners of Sewers* v. *Glasse* (1874), dealing with rights of common over Epping Forest, which occupied twenty-three days and the testimony of over 100 witnesses, he delivered his sixteen-page oral judgment immediately at the conclusion of counsels' speeches. In *Pooley* v. *Driver* (1876) Jessel established the principles underlying the modern law of partnership; and in *Emma Silver Mining Company* v. *Grant*

    [2] *Jewish Encyclopedia* (New York: Funk & Wagnalls, 1916), xi. 369 (on Sir John Simon); Israel Finestein, 'Serjeant Sir John Simon M.', *JC* 26 Oct. 1956, pp. 17, 25; Jasper Ridley, *Napoleon III and Eugénie* (London: Constable, 1979), 430–2.
    [3] Arthur L. Goodhart, *Five Jewish Lawyers of the Common Law* (London: Oxford University Press, 1949), 16–23; Finestein, 'Sir George Jessel'; Daniel Dunman, *The English and Colonial Bars in the Nineteenth Century* (London: Croom Helm, 1983), 145.

(1879) he defined the nature of the fiduciary relationship between a promoter and the company which he set up.[4]

Judah Philip Benjamin (1811–84), of Sephardi origin, was a leader of the Federal Bar in America and later Secretary of State of the Southern Confederate States during the Civil War; in 1865, when the Southern cause was lost, he fled to England. Here, at the age of 54, he began his legal career all over again. He became a pupil of Charles Pollock, whose father, the Chief Baron of the Exchequer Sir Frederick Pollack, persuaded his son to take on the distinguished American lawyer in his large mercantile practice, and was called to the Bar in 1866. His task, as an outsider, was not easy. Benjamin complained to a relative, Mrs Kruttschnitt, that 'The growth of business here is so very slow and the competition so severe that the attorneys give their briefs, whenever they possibly can, to barristers who are connected or related with them or their families.' To eke out a living while slowly building up his practice, Benjamin wrote a treatise on the sale of personal property; known as *Benjamin on Sales* (1868), it was one of the first English law texts to be grounded on basic principles, instead of being a collection of cases with notes. It became a legal classic, and served the additional purpose of making his name known to a wider circle of lawyers.[5]

Notwithstanding his initial difficulties, Benjamin's American legal experience gave him certain advantages which rapidly propelled him to the pinnacle of the English Bar. 'His clients [in New Orleans] were numerous, their business being principally of a mercantile character, and few men had a sounder or wider range of knowledge and experience of the law-merchant, including shipping, insurance and foreign trading than Benjamin', claimed Pollock. He was also a brilliant orator, excelling at presenting long, technical legal arguments to judges and equally persuasive with juries. In 1872 he was made a QC, just six years after being called. Increasingly he restricted his appearances to the highest tribunals in the land—the Court of Appeal, the House of Lords, and the Judicial Committee of the Privy Council—where his knowledge of constitutional, commercial, and maritime law was almost unrivalled. From an income of £495 in 1867, Benjamin's earnings increased dramatically after he took silk, peaking in 1880 at £15,792. In 1876 Benjamin's name made headlines in *The Times*, when he successfully represented Keyn, the captain of a German ship, in his appeal against the manslaughter conviction resulting from the death of a passenger after his vessel had collided with an English steamer. Benjamin enhanced his reputation in the appeal of Keyn against the Crown which is known in international law as the *Franconia* case. By stating an abstract proposition which he

[4] Finestein, 'Sir George Jessel', 245, 271, 273.

[5] Goodhart, *Five Jewish Lawyers*, 10–15; Eli N. Evans, *Judah P. Benjamin: The Jewish Confederate* (New York: Free Press, 1988), 326–48.

gradually developed in the course of presenting his client's case, Benjamin played an important role in persuading judges to recast commercial law to make it more adaptable to the exigencies of modern trading conditions and to prevent it from ossifying.[6]

A barrister who frequently clashed with Benjamin in the highest courts was Arthur Cohen QC (1829–1914), a grandson of the illustrious Levi Barent Cohen (1740–1808), from whom most of the leading Anglo-Jewish families were descended, and closely linked to several of these families. He was a nephew of Sir Moses Montefiore and his wife Judith. Through the good offices of his uncle, who wrote to Albert, the Prince Consort and Chancellor of Cambridge University, and secured his intervention on the young man's behalf, Arthur was able to go up to Magadalene College, Cambridge, despite the general prohibition on Jews being admitted to membership of Cambridge colleges at this time. In 1853 he was placed as fifth wrangler in the mathematics tripos. Four years later he was called to the Bar, where he soon acquired a great reputation as a pre-eminent authority because of his 'knowledge of international law and commercial law—in particular insurance and banking cases'. He frequently acted for the Alliance Insurance Company, with which his uncle Sir Moses Montefiore was connected, claiming to have been concerned in every significant insurance case of his time. In one year 'his income as a junior counsel was £8,000—figures which imply an immense amount of writing, revising, arguing and attending'. One distinguished lawyer recollected: 'It was the commonest thing in those days for solicitors in the City who could not agree on the legal rights of their respective clients to submit the matter in dispute upon an agreed case to Cohen, and agree to be bound by his decision.' According to *The Times*, 'He was a scientific lawyer . . . He had a large knowledge and a firm grasp of principles, and he followed them out slowly but tenaciously and logically', in a beautifully modulated voice.

Cohen was appointed junior counsel to Sir Roundell Palmer in the famous Geneva arbitration in 1872, resolving the case of the *Alabama*, a Southern privateer that preyed on shipping of the Northern American states without much hindrance from the British navy. After taking silk in 1874, he appeared in a number of other international arbitrations and in 1875 was appointed a judge of the Cinque Courts because of his profound knowledge of marine and insurance law. In *Ashbury* v. *Riche* (1875) he argued 'important issues as to the powers of statutory companies [and in] *The British S. African Company* v. *The Mozambique Company* [he] raised a question as to the right to sue in England for trespass to land abroad'. He was an important Jewish communal office-holder, serving as vice-president of Jews' College and as president of the Board of

---

[6] Evans, *Judah P. Benjamin*, 345, 372–99.

Deputies, a position from which he resigned when his daughter married outside the faith.[7]

Joseph Jacobs, who examined the professional directories, estimated that in the early 1880s there were twenty-seven Jewish barristers out of a total of 2,640, or 1.02 per cent. But Phyllis Lachs has suggested that this figure is too low; she found that as many as seventy-five Jewish men gained admission to the Bar between 1833, when Goldsmid was called, and 1870, and that between 1870 and 1900 they were joined by another 106 co-religionists. Thus at least fifty or sixty Jewish men, possibly more, may have been practising at the Bar during the 1880s, which would mean that over 2 per cent of barristers could have been Jewish. Moreover, if we follow Daniel Dunman and reduce the total number of practising barristers to a maximum of 1,450 in 1885, it is possible that as many as 3 per cent of the late Victorian Bar were Jewish.[8] At this time (around 1880) the Jewish population of Britain was just 60,000, or 0.2 per cent of the total population of about 30 million.

It is illuminating to focus on the careers of some of the late Victorian and Edwardian Jewish barristers. Sidney Woolf QC (1844–92) died at the age of 47 from tuberculosis, a death hastened by 'his excessive devotion to the interests of his clients'. His father was an extremely prosperous West End tailor and outfitter, who in his grandson Leonard Woolf's words 'educated his [seven] sons out of their class'. Sidney Woolf's elder brother David was already in practice in King Street in the City as a solicitor, and after qualifying Sidney initially joined him as a partner; but he was determined to change direction and was called to the Bar in 1873. Because of his experience as a solicitor in a small City office, 'He stepped at once into practice in mercantile cases: and was not even without some experience of criminal law' and bankruptcy matters. He was distinguished more by qualities of industry and enterprise 'and by his fairness and amiability than by the most commanding qualities of eloquence'. He wrote books on adulteration, compensation, and the *Winding-Up of Companies by the Court* (1891), but *The Times* remarked that 'his practice lay chiefly in the Bankruptcy Court', where at the time of his death he was the leading figure. According to Mr Registrar Linklater, Woolf was admired in the Bankruptcy Court for 'that subtlety in legal argument, and that appreciation of fine points, which are proper to the race who produced the Ethics of the Fathers'. He was appointed a QC in 1890. 'My father worked so hard and continually', recalled Leonard Woolf, 'that we saw less of him than we and, I think, he would have liked'; but

---

[7] *JC* 10 Nov. 1905, p. 10, 6 Nov. 1914, pp. 14 and 15 (obituary of Cohen); Israel Finestein, 'Arthur Cohen, QC (1829–1914)', in John M. Shaftesley, *Remember the Days* (London: Jewish Historical Society of England, 1966), 279–302; Lucy Cohen, *Arthur Cohen* (London: Bickers & Son, 1919), 47, 134–41.

[8] Jacobs, *Studies in Jewish Statistics*, 41, 42; Lachs, 'A Study of a Professional Elite'; Dunman, *The English and Colonial Bars*, 8.

as a QC Woolf was earning an income in excess of £5,000 per annum in the early 1890s.[9]

Like Woolf, Lionel Edward Pyke QC (1854–99) was also struck down prematurely by tuberculosis and died aged 44. Although his father compelled him to go into the family business of dealing in diamonds and precious metals, he was determined to pursue a career at the Bar, and graduated from University College London with a first-class degree in law in 1873. He was called to the Bar in 1877. 'Mr Pyke took up for his recreation the pursuit of yachting, owned a yacht and gained as a young man experience which stood him in good stead in his distinguished career in the Admiralty Court . . . He practised in commercial law generally with a leaning towards maritime cases.' A firm of solicitors, Messrs Irvine and Hodges, were asked by a friend to brief him on an important case, 'But with due regard to their client's interest, they provided the young barrister with two leaders. It chanced that both these learned gentlemen had engagements elsewhere. Mr Pyke was left to fight the battle by himself, and so impressed the solicitors that they henceforth gave him all the work they had to bestow on his branch of the profession.' Pyke came from an upper-middle-class Anglo-Jewish family and was thus able to indulge his taste for yachting; unusually for a Jew, he mastered the intricacies of seamanship, and after he took silk in 1892 immediately gained for himself a leading position in the Admiralty Court.

Both Woolf and Pyke had close links with the business world and were able to establish themselves as leading players at the commercial Bar, following the example of George Jessel, Judah Benjamin, and Arthur Cohen, who had shown earlier how this could be accomplished. Both Woolf and Pyke were also extremely hard-working, with an infinite capacity to master small details; and, like some of the overworked hospital doctors of the time, they succumbed to disease and died young.[10]

David Lindo Alexander KC (1842–1922) was the son of Joshua Alexander, a solicitor and communal worker, and grew to surpass his father as a communal leader. 'Educated at Cambridge he was permitted to dine with a Jewish family instead of in hall. His father was anxious that his son should observe the laws of *kasher* food.' Alexander read conveyancing law with Professor Jacob Waley (1818–73), a leading figure in Anglo-Jewry whose practice covered some of the largest settled landed estates in the country, and Judge Ellis. Called to the Bar in 1886, he took silk in 1892 and became a bencher of Lincoln's Inn in 1895, participating in the administration of the Inn to which he belonged. He was

[9] *JC* 18 Mar. 1892, p. 11, *The Times*, 15 Mar. 1892 (obituary of Woolf); Leonard Woolf, *Sowing an Autobiography of the Years 1880 to 1904* (London: Hogarth, 1960), 25, 27; Sidney Woolf, *The Winding-Up of Companies by the Court* (London: Reeves & Turner, 1891).

[10] *JC* 31 Mar. 1899, pp. 15, 18; 7 Apr. 1899.

exact and precise in his legal work and opinions. When he first started to practise, he was one of a very small number of Jews at the Bar, and his work lay chiefly among Jewish solicitors. But, as he became better known, his *clientele* grew extensively. Having become related through the marriages of his sisters to the [Jewish] Beddington family, who were largely interested in land, his connections supplied a valuable nucleus of practice for a real-property lawyer. He was a hard worker, but it is surprising that he should have accomplished so much in face of the distractions he suffered throughout his married life, in consequence of the ill-health of his wife, over whom he watched with the tenderest solicitude.[11]

Whereas the Jewish communal activities of Sidney Woolf and Lionel Pyke diminished as their legal practices increasingly dominated their lives, D. L. Alexander managed to be active in both spheres; and there were a number of other wealthy Jewish barristers who gave priority to their Jewish communal concerns over the demands of their legal careers, to the detriment of the latter. The busier his legal practice grew, the less time Woolf had to devote to communal work, but he had served as warden of the West London Reform Synagogue in Upper Berkeley Street and was on its council at the time of his death. Earlier on in his career, Woolf was an energetic supporter of the Westminster Jews' Free School and was also a council member of the Anglo-Jewish Association (AJA) as well as a committee member of the Aged Needy Society. So too, at the start of his career, Lionel Pyke was an active member of the AJA council and wrote letters to the *Jewish Chronicle* about the deteriorating position of the Jews in Romania and other parts of eastern Europe. Unfortunately, because of his professional commitments, Pyke was later left with 'little time for communal pursuits'.[12]

In contrast D. L. Alexander, despite a busy legal career, was immersed in communal life. As well as serving on the Council of Jews' College and the AJA, he devoted much energy to the National Vigilance Association (a non-Jewish pressure group advocating 'social purity'). When the health of Sir Joseph Sebag Montefiore, the president of the Board of Deputies, began to fade at the turn of the century, the government of the Board rapidly devolved on Alexander, who was vice-president. 'He became permanent Chairman of the Law and Parliamentary Committee, the most important department of the Deputies' work. This Committee which held its meetings at Mr Alexander's Chambers in Old Square [Lincoln's Inn]—and afterwards, at his house, 11, York Gate—watches and initiates all legislation affecting English Jews.'[13] He was elected president of the Board in 1903, but as its principal committee was completely under his control already, this merely gave official effect to the existing situation. As an editorial in the *Jewish Chronicle* put it, 'Mr Alexander was zealous and hard-

---

[11] *JC* 20 Feb. 1903, p. 9, 11 Jan. 1907, p. 22, 5 May, 1922, pp. 7, 13.
[12] *JC* 18 Mar. 1892, p. 11, 31 Mar. 1899, p. 15.   [13] *JC* 20 Feb. 1903, p. 9.

working, but he was also arbitrary and unyielding, self-centred and utterly in-
capable of adjusting himself to the new times and conditions which arose in the
community during his Presidentship. In opinion, he was frequently palpably
prejudiced.' Unwilling to respond to the growing forces of democracy in the
Board, he was forced to resign in 1917 owing to an ill-timed anti-Zionist mani-
festo sent to *The Times* without proper prior consultation with his colleagues.[14]

Another barrister who was able to combine a successful legal career with an
active role in Jewish communal life was Albert Henry Jessel QC (1864–1917).
His father Henry Jessel, a brother of Sir George Jessel, 'dealt with some important drafts and cases' and sat as a deputy county court judge for Paddington.
Albert was educated at Clifton and Balliol College, Oxford, and was called to
the Bar in 1889. He devoted himself to Chancery work, 'and thus in pursuit of
his profession did not frequently come under public notice. His legal knowledge was considerable, and he rapidly acquired a large practice.' He contributed
to several textbooks on company law. He was made a KC in 1906 and a bencher
of Lincoln's Inn in 1911, 'and acted in a judicial capacity on more than one occasion'. He came to prominence in the United Synagogue Council as a 'trenchant
debater' and was vice-president from 1899 until 1917. Jessel 'was always worth
hearing, his speeches being distinguished for their practical common sense and
lively wit'. However,

essentially occidental in his upbringing and sympathies, Mr Jessel was not in accord
with the administrators of Jews' College in their desire to produce a high standard of
rabbinical learning at the expense, as Mr Jessel thought, of English culture. He resisted
many attempts to obtain an increased grant to the College from the United Synagogue
and brought into these discussions a warmth and acrimony that often surprised his
friends.[15]

Yet another upper-middle-class Jewish barrister was Henry Hyman Haldin KC
(1863–1931). Haldin was educated at Balliol College, Oxford, where he read
classics and history, and was called to the Bar in 1886. He acquired a large legal
practice, 'being frequently retained in important Stock Exchange and City
actions, having specialized and become an authority in Commercial Law'. He
sat as a justice of the peace for Buckinghamshire and as a young man was a keen
athlete, captaining the Norfolk County Rugby Club. He was also an important
Jewish communal figure, helping to found the Maccabeans, the organization of
Jewish professionals, in 1891; and he served for a time as chairman of the Law
and Parliamentary Committee of the Board of Deputies.[16]

Among those wealthy barristers who neglected their legal practice in order to
devote their time to communal and philanthropic endeavours were Henry

[14] *JC* 11 Jan. 1907, p. 22, 3 Mar. 1922, p. 31, 5 May 1922, p. 13.
[15] *JC* 10 Feb. 1905, p. 14, 5 Jan. 1917, p. 14 (obituary of Jessel).   [16] *JC* 4 Dec. 1931, p. 11.

Lucas, Benjamin Kisch, and Felix Davis. Henry Lucas (1842–1910) was called to the Bar at Lincoln's Inn in 1869, but 'His legal work did not bring him under prominent public notice; he practised till his retirement in 1891 as an equity draughtsman and conveyancer.' He was left with ample time to assist in the running of the Jews' Orphan Asylum and the Westminster Jews' Free School; later he became treasurer and, in 1887, vice-president of the United Synagogue; he helped steer the newly formed Jewish Religious Education Board (formerly the Jewish Association for the Diffusion of Religious Knowledge, founded 1860) through many financial crises. His colleague Albert Henry Jessel 'always regarded him as an admirable type of a Jewish gentleman and an English gentleman. He combined the best Jewish qualities and the best English qualities.' In his country home at Bramblehurst, East Grinstead, Sussex, where he lived in some style, he acted as lord of the manor, devising many charitable schemes for the locality; he also raised substantial funds for University College Hospital.[17]

Benjamin Kisch (1842–1919), having studied mathematics and science at University College London, decided to embark upon law as a profession, studying conveyancing with Professor Waley and Chancery law with a Mr Eddis. He was called to the Bar in 1866 and retired in 1912. He never married and had inherited a sufficient fortune to gratify both his philanthropic inclinations and his taste for the good life, eventually making his home at 52 Gloucester Terrace, Hyde Park. 'Mr Kisch had early in his legal career good briefs, including a participation in the Acerdeckne litigation, but his intense interest in the fate of his less fortunate coreligionists induced him to devote a constantly increasing proportion of his time to communal affairs.' He was chairman of the executive of the AJA for thirty-six years and also served the organization as a vice-president. He was intensely interested in educational matters, serving on the management committees of the Jews' Free School, the Stepney Jewish School, and the Evelina de Rothschild School for Girls in Jerusalem. 'Although [Kisch was] a hesitating speaker, he invariably spoke to good effect and was listened to with much deference.'[18]

Felix Davis (1863–1916) was educated at Harrow and Cambridge, where he secured a first-class degree in law in 1886 and was called to the Bar in the same year. A man of considerable means, he lived in London at 12 Upper Hamilton Terrace, St John's Wood. He practised for a time on the Western Circuit, after which he attended the London and Middlesex Sessions which dealt with criminal cases. However,

he never occupied himself seriously with the law as a practising barrister, and even the meagre work he undertook in this direction was frequently associated with a desire to be helpful to the unfortunate men who found themselves in the dock . . . His friends

[17] *JC* 11 Nov. 1910, p. 7, 18 Nov. 1910, pp. 10, 11.   [18] *JC* 7 Mar. 1913, pp. 13, 14.

frequently wondered why he never 'went far' at the Bar, seeing how well fitted he appeared to be for a successful legal career. Quite unconsciously he, on one occasion, provided the explanation. 'My trouble has always been that I have been able to see the other man's point of view.'

Davis was a splendid example of the old type of Anglo-Jewish communal worker. He was active in various committees of the Norwood Jewish Orphanage (formerly the Jews' Orphan Asylum); he was treasurer and later, in 1911, vice-president of the United Synagogue; and, as chairman of the synagogue's visitation committee, he provided assistance to discharged prisoners.

Instinctively they felt that they stood before a real friend whose sole desire it was to help them, and . . . they responded to his fine and manly treatment of them, and left him strengthened and hopeful in their outlook on life. The care with which he watched their progress, the ready ear he always gave them, and the pride he took in their regeneration—and his successes were many—proved how near his heart this work lay.[19]

Many of the leading Jewish barristers in the Victorian and Edwardian era came from families belonging to the established Anglo-Jewish plutocracy, whether of Ashkenazi or Sephardi origin; those who did not generally had fathers who were dynamic businessmen, or some close relative or connection had opened a solicitor's office. George Jessel's father was one of the most substantial diamond merchants in London, as well as a successful investor in the Oxford–Worcester–Wolverhampton railway; Lionel Edward Pyke's father was an equally wealthy diamond and metal dealer. Benjamin Woolf, the father of Sidney Woolf, carried on a flourishing high-class tailoring business in Regent Street and Piccadilly. Even grander in scale was the Alliance Insurance Company, to which Arthur Cohen had family ties. When the sons of the Victorian Anglo-Jewish elite became barristers, they naturally gravitated into the commercial Bar because their families' business links meant that a steady flow of such cases came their way—and sometimes their early training suited them for this type of legal work. Adolph Max Langdon, for example, later KC, 'as a junior . . . enjoyed a good practice, particularly in commercial cases'; his father, H. N. Lazarus, was a member of the firm of S. L. Behrens, merchant bankers and textile manufacturers.[20]

To this list of barristers practising in the various branches of commercial law we should add the names of Israel Davis (1847–1927) and Sir Benjamin Arthur Cohen KC (1862–1942), the son of Arthur Cohen.[21] If the family aspired to joining the ranks of the landed gentry, its scions would become members of the Chancery Bar, where they specialized in land law and drafting conveyancing

---

[19] *JC* 27 Oct. 1916, p. 10.   [20] *JC* 12 Feb. 1904, p. 7 (on Langdon).

[21] *JC* 28 Jan. 1927, p. 20 (obituary of Davis, who 'did a considerable amount of work in Patent and Trade mark cases' before becoming a newspaper proprietor).

deeds. Yet because the Jewish business families had been steeped in commerce for generations, they were often reluctant to allow their sons to go into a profession. Only after a few years in the family business was Pyke allowed to become a barrister; and Rufus Isaacs's father and relatives did not approve of his studying for the Bar.

Among the smaller group of Jewish barristers practising in the criminal courts were Charles Zeffertt, Israel Alexander Symmons, and Edward Abinger. Zeffertt, who qualified as a barrister in 1908, became a 'well-known member of the Common Law Bar' and had an extensive criminal practice; he died in 1921. Symmons, born in the early 1860s, was called to the Bar in 1885 and in 1911 was the first Jew to be appointed a stipendiary magistrate; he died in 1923.[22] Abinger (1859–1929) was called to the Bar in 1887 and appeared frequently in the North and South London Sessions and the Old Bailey. Like so many of his fellow Jewish barristers, he was considerably aided by the fact that both his father and his uncle, Michael Abrahams, were well-known solicitors. Within six months of being called to the Bar he was already successfully defending a client, Franz Schultz, on a charge of murder. Abinger was a doughty fighter, 'and I don't mind confessing', he declared in his memoirs, 'that my pugnacious proclivities very often involved me in a wordy warfare with the Judge before whom I was appearing'. Because of his reputation as a skilful cross-examiner, he secured a certain amount of work in the Chancery Division. He also prosecuted the owners of financial journals who blackmailed the promoters of companies by hinting that they would publish articles alleging that particular companies were insolvent, when they were in possession of other information showing that this was palpable falsehood.[23]

But Abinger was best known for his tenacious defence in 1911 of Stinie Morrison, a Jewish thief from the East End charged with murder, who had never been convicted of any crimes of violence. According to a figure from the underworld, Morrison 'was handicapped by lack of funds to brief a good criminal lawyer, he had to be satisfied with a good trier and that is all that could be said of the lawyer, Mr Edward Abinger'. Nevertheless, Winston Churchill, the then Home Secretary, reprieved Morrison from hanging on Abinger's insistence, as the prosecution had suppressed evidence about a forged cheque. It is probable that Morrison was used by members of an anarchist gang as a decoy to lure the victim of the murder into a trap because they feared he was about to inform on them to the police, a prostitute later confessed to Abinger and to a Home Office official that her husband, who had fled to America, came home on the night of

[22] *JC* 6 May 1921 (obituary of Zeffert), 3 Aug. 1923, p. 8 (obituary of Symmons), 31 May 1929, p. 10 (obituary of Abinger).
[23] Edward Abinger, *Forty Years at the Bar* (London: Hutchinson, 1930), 21, 22, 26–69, 165, 166, 211–17, 253–6.

the murder with his clothing covered in blood, threatening her life if she spoke out.[24]

Perhaps the most outstanding achiever among the Jewish barristers of this period was Rufus Isaacs (1860–1935), first marquess of Reading, who in turn was successively Solicitor-General, Attorney-General, Lord Chief Justice, British ambassador to the United States, Viceroy of India, and Foreign Secretary— positions most of which had never before been filled by a Jew. His climb to the upper reaches of the judiciary was based on the solid foundation of his career at the English Bar, where he and Sir Edward Carson were the dominant figures during the Edwardian age.[25]

Rufus Daniel Isaacs, like so many of his predecessors among Jewish members of the Bar, came from a successful commercial family. His father, Joseph Isaacs, was a wholesale fruit merchant who imported citrus fruit from Italy and Spain; his uncle Sir Henry Isaacs had at one time been Lord Mayor of London. Seemingly destined for a mercantile career in the family business, Rufus was partly educated at Kahn's School in Brussels to acquire fluency in French, and also spent some time in Germany to learn the language. When at home in London the young Isaacs lived in Finsbury Square in the City, mixing within an exclusively Jewish circle and attending synagogue and Hebrew classes regularly. In fact, Isaacs's family was then a typically Victorian Orthodox Jewish one: his uncle Henry Isaacs sat on the interim executive of the United Synagogue; and at the beginning of the twentieth century, Rufus Isaacs was himself busy presiding over the distribution of prizes at Hebrew classes. However, his was a wild and unruly youth; he served as a ship's boy on a cargo ship for a couple of years, at which point he seems to have discarded the remaining remnants of Jewish practice to which he had hitherto adhered, and he also enjoyed a short career on the Stock Exchange before being declared a defaulter. Eventually, in 1887, after a period of study, he was called to the Bar; he married in the same year at the West London Reform Synagogue, a shift from the Orthodox United Synagogue of his youth.[26]

Because his father's extensive fruit business led to litigation from time to time, Isaacs received briefs relating to these disputes from Lowless & Company, a prominent firm of commercial lawyers in the City. During his first year at the Bar, 1887/8, Isaacs earned fees of £519, rising to £750 during his second

[24] Raphael Samuel, *East End Underworld: Chapters in the Life of Arthur Harding* (London: Routledge & Kegan Paul, 1981), 143–5; F. G. Clarke, *Will-O-Wisp: Peter the Painter and the Anti-Tsarist Terrorists in Britain and Australia* (Melbourne: Oxford University Press, 1983), 71, 86, 119. Sir Harry Bodkin Poland (1829–1928), who was half-Jewish, was the Crown prosecutor at the Central Criminal Court from 1865 to 1888.

[25] Gerald Rufus Isaacs, *Rufus Isaacs, First Marquess of Reading*, vol. ii: *1914–1935* (London: Hutchinson, 1945).

[26] Isaacs, *Rufus Isaacs*, vol. i: *1860–1914* (London: Hutchinson, 1942), 1–43.

year—quite considerable sums. He was also instructed by Algernon Sydney, his family's solicitor and a well-known Jewish communal lawyer, to assist a leader, Sir Henry James QC, in the famous case of *Chetwynd* v. *Durham*, a libel action involving Lord Durham arising out of a case of chicanery among the horse-racing fraternity. Gradually he began appearing more regularly in county and magistrates' courts, and receiving instructions to draft pleadings in High Court actions. In 1895 a special Commercial Court was opened at the behest of business leaders, offering clients a more rapid procedure. From his brief forays into the commercial world and his experience of the Stock Exchange, Isaacs had a sure grasp of financial instruments and business contracts allied to an aptitude for figures and the intricacies of business accounts. Thus armed, he rose rapidly to become one of the leading juniors in the commercial Bar. He also enhanced his reputation in the trade union case of *Allen* v. *Flood*, which ended in the House of Lords in 1896. Soon Isaacs was earning £7,000 a year, mostly from lucrative commercial cases, and when in 1898 he successfully applied for silk he became the youngest QC at the English Bar.[27]

Although Rufus Isaacs appeared to have found his niche, in the mould of his Jewish predecessors, as a celebrity at the commercial Bar, he soon stepped outside these limits—a process facilitated by his friendship with the eminent solicitor Sir George Lewis and, after his own election as Liberal MP for Reading in 1904, with the leading Liberal and future Prime Minister Lloyd George. At the beginning of the twentieth century Isaacs began to appear in a wider range of actions, particularly libel and high society cases which attracted considerable attention in the national press. In *Arthur Chamberlain* v. *The Star* (1901) Isaacs represented the newspaper; by telling the jury that his client's remarks were directed against Joseph and Austen Chamberlain, both of whom were ministers of the Crown, for favouritism in the award of government contracts to a family firm, and not against Arthur Chamberlain, he limited the award of damages against the newspaper to £200. For *The Star* this was a triumph. In 1908 he appeared for Lloyd George in an action against another newspaper, *The People*, for repeating gross calumnies about the statesman's private life, winning for the newly appointed Chancellor of the Exchequer a large sum in damages which was paid to charity. He continued to put his financial acumen to good use: in 1904 his technical mastery of share and other financial manipulations between companies enabled Isaacs to persuade a jury that the financier Whittaker Wright was guilty of fraud. Among the high society cases in which Isaacs was involved were the Gordon custody case (1902), the 'Gaiety Divorce' case, *Bryce* v. *Bryce and Pape* (1907), and *R.* v.

[27] Derek Walker-Smith, *Lord Reading and his Cases* (London: Chapman & Hall, 1934), 33–5, 59, 60; Isaacs, *Rufus Isaacs*, i. 47–54, 60–5.

Siever, an Old Bailey trial connected with a dispute among the horse-racing fraternity.[28]

Isaacs was possessed of remarkable gifts as an advocate. Blessed with a photographic memory, he would rise at four or five o'clock in the morning to master his brief before appearing in court.

A solicitor who had instructed him in a certain case once remarked that, although it was the most complicated case in his experience Mr. Isaacs . . . came into court, after one night's study of the facts, and conducted the case for two days almost without a note. 'He knew more about that case and the intricacies of it than either of the principals, and could tell each of them more about their own doings than they knew themselves.'[29]

By the early years of the century Isaacs had acquired a reputation as a most formidable cross-examiner of witnesses.

He never bullied a witness or dictated to a jury, and rarely argued with a judge. His methods were the more deadly ones of sweet reasonableness. He was always good tempered, and the height of courtesy. 'When . . . you hear him unravel some difficult case and deal with some slippery witness (and his cross-examination is a marvel of penetrating serenity) you see at once the secret of his success—a perfect grasp of his subject, and, perhaps chiefly, an invariable courtesy and charm of manner' . . . It was said that . . . [he] never troubled about the cheap device of making a flurried witness contradict himself; but convinced the witness before long that his safest plan was to make a clean breast of the matter. His deadliest suggestions were, as often as not, taken in all seriousness by the witness, so blandly and innocently were they expressed.

Isaacs did not desire to sweep a jury off its feet by a torrent of eloquence, but preferred to guide it quietly through the complexities of a difficult case. This was a style of speaking also eminently suited to judges sitting alone without juries, as was the practice in commercial cases.[30]

In 1910 Rufus Isaacs was appointed Solicitor-General and knighted at the same time. Immediately he was involved in the controversy surrounding the Archer–Shee case, concerning a naval cadet at Dartmouth who was falsely accused of theft—a case later famously dramatized by Terence Rattigan in *The Winslow Boy*. Towards the end of the year, Sir Rufus was promoted to become Attorney-General. On 2 February 1912 he prosecuted Mr and Mrs Seddon at the Old Bailey for the murder of their lodger, a Miss Barrow, his first and only murder trial, while Sir Edward Marshall Hall defended Frederick Henry Seddon and more junior counsel appeared for his wife. Once the Crown's scientific expert demonstrated that Miss Barrow could have died from arsenic poisoning, it was left to Rufus Isaacs to undermine Frederick Seddon's credi-

[28] Isaacs, *Rufus Isaacs*, i. 76–81, 119–54, 178–9, 190–219; Walker-Smith, *Lord Reading*, 119–54, 190–219.   [29] *JC* 3 Jan. 1936, p. 26 (obituary of Isaacs).   [30] Ibid.

bility in a day-long cross-examination. According to Mr Justice Humphreys, who was in the Treasury team,

In such a case the explanation of the accused, if given in the witness box, is of the first importance, and this trial was distinguished by the most deadly cross-examination of an accused person which I can recall—all the more deadly because it was perfectly fair . . . During that time the Attorney-General never raised his voice, never argued with the witness, never interrupted an answer, and scarcely put a leading question. The questions and the manner of putting them were pre-eminently fair. Seddon was taken through the history of the case and invited to give his own explanation of every material matter. The result was to turn what was always a strongish case into a conclusive one.

Influenced by her demeanour in the witness box and the judge's summing up, the jury found Mrs Seddon not guilty, while her husband was convicted of murder.[31]

In going on from advocacy to a prestigious judicial career, Isaacs was unusual among Jewish lawyers of the period. During the nineteenth century and the Edwardian era several ambitious Jewish barristers, including George Jessel and Arthur Cohen as well as Rufus himself, stood for election to Parliament as Liberal MPs as a route to judicial office. A few were successful: Sir George Jessel was appointed Solicitor-General in 1871 and Master of the Rolls, the third highest judicial office in the country, in 1873. However, when Arthur Cohen QC, MP was offered a High Court judgeship in 1881, he refused it on Gladstone's insistence because the relinquishment of his parliamentary seat consequent on his acceptance would have given rise to a risky by-election. When Lord Herschell, the new Lord Chancellor, who although a Conservative was partly of Jewish origin and thus had ambivalent feelings in the matter, refused to renew Gladstone's offer of a place on the High Court bench to Cohen, a quip went the rounds: 'What can Cohen expect of Herschell but a Passover?' The eminent jurist Albert Dicey asked: 'Why . . . was [Cohen,] a man whose presence would certainly have added strength and dignity to the Court of Appeal, to the Judicial Committee of the Privy Council, or to the House of Lords, as a final Court of Appeal, never placed in a position to which such a consummate master of English law had a moral claim?' The answer, he suggested, lay in 'the weaknesses of party government'; 'if judicial appointments were made by judges' and he had himself been more 'pushing', Dicey averred, Cohen would have long been on the bench.[32] Woolf, too, had unfulfilled parliamentary ambitions, and Pyke stood unsuccessfully as the Liberal candidate for a Wiltshire constituency in 1895; both hankered after judicial office.[33]

---

[31] Isaacs, *Rufus Isaacs*, i. 185, 188–91, 199, 211–20.   [32] Cohen, *Arthur Cohen*, 72–6, 86, 212.
[33] *JC* 18 Mar. 1892, p. 11, 31 Mar. 1899, p. 18.

Apart from Jessel and Isaacs, there was one Jewish Judge of the Admiralty Court and another in the Queen's Bench Division of the High Court; a half-Jew, Sir Archibald Levin Smith—a great cricket player—was briefly Master of the Rolls from 1900 until his premature death in 1901. Sir Harry Poland (1829–1928), a brilliant prosecuting counsel, 'might have been a High Court Judge had he chosen; but his work at the Bar had been largely criminal; he was wealthy, he had no ties and preferred to remain at the Bar'.[34] When the Maccabeans gave a dinner in honour of Adolph Langdon in 1904 there were some optimistic predictions about his soon adorning the High Court bench; but the highest appointment he achieved was that of recorder—of Burnley in 1909, and later of Salford.[35] Samuel Henry Emanuel KC (1866–1925), a treasurer of the United Synagogue and an influential chairman of Jews' College, held office as recorder of Winchester in 1915; as such, like Langdon in the north-west, he presided over important local criminal courts. Religiously observant himself, Emanuel was so deeply concerned about Jewish education that he took the initiative to ensure that the United Synagogue's religion classes (or 'Hebrew classes', as they were known) were placed on a sound financial basis by levying a charge on seatholders of the synagogue for this purpose.[36] Despite his background in an illustrious family and his considerable academic achievements at Oxford and thereafter, Henry Straus Quixano Henriques KC (1866–1925) never advanced further than assistant county court judge.[37] Phyllis Lachs concluded that the number of Jewish judicial appointments was 'disproportionately small for [the] sixty-seven years' following Goldsmid's call to the Bar in 1833, a sentiment with which it is hard to disagree; but this may be due to the fact that Jews were not sufficiently entrenched within the patronage system of the Liberal party until the Edwardian era and to the long periods of Conservative party rule.[38]

In October 1913 Sir Rufus Isaacs was sworn in as Lord Chief Justice despite the adverse publicity caused by the Marconi affair the previous year, in which his profiting from the sale of shares exposed him to allegations of impropriety if not actual wrongdoing. At the same time he was made a baron, taking the title of Lord Reading. As Attorney-General he was entitled to this preferment, and had been irritated when he was not appointed by Asquith to fill the vacant office

[34] Paul H. Emden, *Jews of Britain* (London: Sampson Low, Marston, 1943), 187; J. R. H. Weaver (ed.), *Dictionary of National Biography* (London: Oxford University Press, 1937), 683, 684 (on 'Sir Harry Bodkin Poland'); *The Recollections of Sir Henry Dickens KC* (London: Heinemann, 1934), 185.

[35] *JC* 4 Nov. 1904, p. 7, 19 Mar. 1909, p. 14 (on Langdon).

[36] *JC* 22 May 1925, p. 25 (obituary of Emanuel).

[37] *JC* 20 Nov. 1925, p. 19 (obituary of Henriques); *Transactions of the Jewish Historical Society of England 1924–1927*, vol. xi (1928), 247–51 (obituary of Henriques).

[38] Lachs, 'A Study of a Professional Elite', 131, 132.

of Lord Chancellor in June 1912, it being considered at the time questionable whether a Jew was qualified to hold this office.[39]

The Times in 1921 was of the opinion that Lord Reading 'was never a lawyer in the sense in which Benjamin and Jessel were lawyers, and though he had many of the qualities of a good judge, it may be doubted whether legal history will put him among the great Lord Chief Justices. He made no law, [and] few of his judgments will be remembered.' According to Derek Walker-Smith, 'he had neither the monumental legal erudition nor the literary ability to make judgments of the very first rank . . . in being rather less good on the Bench than he had been in practice in the Courts, Lord Reading was not widely different from the mass of very successful advocates, who became judges'.[40] One of his few notable judgments was in the case of *R.* v. *Christie* (1914), which dealt with the admissibility of evidence. Here he decided that statements made in the presence of an accused and denied by him at the time are not made admissible in evidence because the person who made the statements is called at the trial. Reading concluded that 'the test was, would the jury have come to the same conclusion if the evidence had been rejected? It was not enough to say that they might have come to the same conclusion; the Court must feel certain that they would.' He also reiterated the important principle that the onus of establishing the guilt of the accused beyond reasonable doubt always lay on the prosecution, not the defence, in *R.* v. *Schama* and *R.* v. *Abramovitch* (1914).[41]

Rufus Isaacs's attitude to Judaism was curiously ambivalent. His mother, Sarah (*née* Davis) was opposed to Orthodoxy and had encouraged him not to follow the traditional Jewish religious practices followed by his father's family without putting anything in their place. As his son recorded,

Though he never severed connection with Judaism and left in his will instructions that at his funeral there was to be 'a simple Jewish service', he never made any pretence of observing even the most solemn occasions of the Jewish year, and never entered a

---

[39] *Halsbury's Laws of England* suggested that it was unconstitutional for anyone but a Protestant to hold the office of Lord Chancellor, which involved being 'keeper of the King's conscience', because a Jew, for example, would not be able to join the monarch at worship. This was disputed by H. S. Q. Henriques, who showed in an article that there was no legal reason why a Jew could not be Lord Chancellor (H. S. Q. Henriques, 'The Question Whether a Jew Can Be Lord Chancellor of England', *Transactions of the Jewish Historical Society 1915–1917*, viii (1918), 55–62). However, the 4th edn. of *Halsbury's Laws of England*, vol. viii (2), (London: Butterworths, 1996), edited by Lord Hailsham, suggests that, despite the passing of the Lord Chancellor (Tenure of Office and Discharge of Ecclesiastical Function) Act 1974 and the repeal of various other statutes, 'it is still unclear whether a person professing the Jewish religion would be appointed Lord Chancellor without clarifying legislation' (p. 332). This is not universally agreed: one Jewish lawyer to whom I spoke about this still thought that the 1974 Act, which allows Roman Catholics to occupy the office of Lord Chancellor, also makes it possible for Jews to do so.

[40] Isaacs, *Rufus Isaacs*, i. 224, 275–9; Walker-Smith, *Lord Reading*, 389.

[41] *R.* v. *Christie* (1913), *The Times Law Reports*, vol. xxx, 1913–14, pp. 41, 42; *R.* v. *Schama*, *R.* v. *Abramovitch* (1914), *The Times Law Reports*, vol. xli, pp. 88, 89.

synagogue save for a wedding or memorial service. Yet he was far from either atheist or agnostic; he clung to the simple and central article of his faith, the belief in One God, but he felt that obedience to so simple a creed required neither church nor synagogue.[42]

Nevertheless, this was the man who, as Lord Chief Justice, rebuked Sir Ernest Wild in 1920 in the Court of Criminal Appeal for saying, ' "A Jew I suppose?" It produces, I confess, an unpleasant impression on me when I read it [because of its prejudicial undertones]. It is not in the prisoner's favour that it is put.' Yet despite a certain robust combativeness when confronting an antisemitic remark hurled at him at the hustings or aired in court, Isaacs did not feel deep pride in being Jewish—unlike his friend and fellow Liberal MP Alfred Mond (Lord Mond), whose daughter Eva married Isaacs's son. Had he been granted his life over again, Isaacs admitted, he would have preferred to have been born as a Unitarian, considering even Liberal Judaism no better than the Orthodox creed. His son, the second Lord Reading, would have been quite happy to marry his half-Jewish wife in church, but the vicar would not permit this. When this lady, Eva, marchioness of Reading, decided to convert to Judaism during the 1930s, Rufus Isaacs made her promise not to disturb the children's Christian beliefs. Not surprisingly, their son Michael brought up his children as Christians. While one daughter retained her allegiance to Christianity, another, Joan, identified with her mother and entered the Jewish faith.[43]

'A few days before the re-opening of the Law Courts,' wrote Benjamin Grad in 1914,

I asked a Jewish barrister 'Why should not Lord Reading [now Lord Chief Justice] have a procession of lawyers to the Synagogue, just like the Roman Catholic judges have theirs to Westminster Cathedral?' The reply I received was, 'Why, if you suggest such a thing to Lord Reading he will simply laugh at you' . . . I believe that any thoughtful reader will agree with the statement that in England a considerable number of Jews of the 'upper classes' remain professing Jews because their English friends attend Church Services.

While the Bar was very much intertwined with the Church of England, particularly in the memorial services for benchers from the various Inns of Court, Jewish barristers were encouraged to form a parallel attachment to Judaism, without risking making waves as far as their non-Jewish colleagues were concerned. Moreover, the *Jewish Chronicle* declared in 1892:

While it [the Jewish public] brands as a profanation the public-spirited behaviour of the obscure individual who courageously does his duty by attending an inquest or trial on the Sabbath, it reads of Jewish Queen's Counsel pleading and of Jewish Judges sitting

---

[42] Isaacs, *Rufus Isaacs*, i. 37, 38.
[43] Eva Reading, *For the Record: Memoirs of Eva, Marchioness of Reading* (London: Hutchinson, 1973), 37, 38, 147–51.

on the bench on that day, and displays no emotion save pride at the honour thus conferred on the race and faith.

On the other hand, D. L. Alexander, as leader of the Bar in the High Court during the latter part of his career, was instrumental in securing from the Vacation Judge a holiday for Jewish practitioners on the Day of Atonement.[44]

In so far as public service to the Jewish community was concerned, Isaacs, who held no office in communal institutions, remained the exception rather than the rule, and even he in his younger days had distributed prizes at Hebrew classes. Many of the barristers mentioned here, such as D. L. Alexander, Albert Henry Jessel, Arthur Cohen, Samuel Henry Emanuel, Adolph Max Langdon, and Henry Henriques, were guided by the principle of *noblesse oblige*, and gave considerable amounts of time and energy to directing the affairs of the Board of Deputies and the United Synagogue, and, to a lesser degree, the Jewish Board of Guardians—Alexander was the Board's honorary secretary from 1883 until 1893, and Langdon filled a similar position in the Board at Manchester. There was also a group of wealthy Jewish barristers who gave priority to their communal and philanthropic endeavours at the expense of their careers; and it is possible that H. S. Q. Henriques's high-profile advocacy in a number of cases involving Jews may have blighted the progress of his career at the Bar.[45]

Promotion to the highest judicial offices in the late Victorian and Edwardian era depended on party patronage, and so long as a candidate had such support, antisemitic outbursts against individuals seeking such office counted for little. This can best be seen in Rufus Isaacs's triumphant later career, despite the antisemitic clouds which threatened to engulf his career at the time of the Marconi scandal. Nor did the waves of anti-alien feeling in the country touch the Anglicized Jewish elite who were so prominent at the commercial Bar.

[44] *JC* 27 Nov. 1914, p. 11; 9 Sept. 1892, p. 11, 5 May 1922, p. 13.
[45] Lipman, *A Century of Social Service*, 260; *JC* 4 Nov. 1904, p. 7 (on Langdon).

FIVE

Jews at the Bar from 1918 Until the End of the Second World War

ACCORDING to Harry Sacher (1881–1971), himself a barrister and journal-ist, there were three different routes to success for members of the Bar. One was to be a member of a busy set of chambers, where surplus work would be passed on to its most junior members. The second was to have a close connec-tion with a solicitor. 'To know solicitors who are prepared to nurse the aspirant is the easiest road to success,' Sacher claimed,

but it must be accompanied by adeptness in law or advocacy. There are so many seeking briefs, and, like patients, clients are so impatient of being practised on, that a solicitor, however benevolent, cannot take many risks. Good chambers are chambers in which there is a barrister with a first-class practice, for whom you devil. They bring you into contact with solicitors, some crumbs may fall to you from the big man's table, and should he rise to higher things—take silk for instance, you may inherit something of his practice.

The third way of succeeding was to write an authoritative legal text, so that one became recognized as the leading expert in the field; again, this would attract the attention of solicitors and, one hoped, their instructions.[1]

In 1934 it was estimated that 5 per cent of practising barristers were Jewish, which meant that there were approximately 100 Jewish members of the Bar.[2] In 1924 there were seven Jewish King's Counsel out of a total of about 300—namely, D. L. Alexander, B. A. Cohen, S. H. Emanuel, H. H. Haldin, H. S. Q. Hen-riques, A. M. Langdon, and S. Mayer. During the 1920s and 1930s the bulk of these barristers continued to come from the most affluent Anglo-Jewish fami-lies or from families which were closely linked to the legal profession; very few originated from an east European Jewish immigrant background. A young man (or woman: Helena Normanton became the first female barrister to practise in England in 1922) who wished to become a barrister had to pay entrance fees of £200 to the Inn of Court which he had decided to join. In the Middle Temple,

[1] Harry Sacher, *Zionist Portraits and Other Essays* (London: Blond, 1959), 327.
[2] Board of Deputies Archive, Acc. 3121 B4/PM/42, Report of the Vocational Advisory Committee of the B'nai B'rith First Lodge of England [Sept. 1934], 1.

one of the Inns, students dined in messes of four, each of which was allotted a couple of bottles of wine; some students chose to dine with Muslims so as to have more wine to drink. Having passed his Bar final examinations, the student paid another £150 to receive the licence to practise, plus a fee of either 100 guineas for the right to read in a barrister's chambers for a year or 50 guineas for a shorter period of six months. Harry Sacher chose to be a pupil in the chambers of Hugh Fraser, who 'was the recognised authority on the law of defamation, and also on election law, and many cases in these branches came to him. He was a very sound lawyer, and as a pupil you had the privilege of looking at his papers and discussing them with him.'[3]

In England between the world wars the legal professions were 'the exclusive spheres of the aristocracy and plutocracy'. Among those Jews called to the Bar in 1923 and 1924 were Henry Cecil Leon BA, LLB (Cantab.), of 4 Cleveland Gardens, Bayswater, better known as the novelist Henry Cecil; Paul Henry Maurice Oppenheimer BA (Oxon.), of 9 Kensington Palace Gardens; and Harold Maurice Abrahams BA (Cantab.), of Hodford Road, Golders Green, whose parents lived in Rodney Court, Maida Vale. Both the Oxbridge education of these young men and the addresses of their families in London indicate something of their wealth and their privileged background, although Henry Cecil claimed in his memoirs that 'My parents were not at all well off' and 'had to be exceptionally economical' to send him to public school and Cambridge. There was a reluctance among solicitors and their clients to entrust their private and confidential business to a Jew, especially one from an east European immigrant background, who was regarded as a foreigner. Even if the client was willing to entrust his affairs to a Jew, 'The lawyer will be unknown to the client unless both move in the same social sphere, and the most important legal work necessarily comes from clients in the higher walks of life.' Thus, unless the aspiring barrister was a member of the Anglo–Jewish elite and sufficiently Anglicized, he would not have the manners or the social skills to win the confidence of instructing solicitors and their clients.[4]

Describing the situation between the wars, Sydney Aylett stated that

Duncan was the odd man out in an otherwise Jewish chambers [at 4 Elm Court]. There was at that time in the Temple, and indeed in some chambers there still is, a kind of Masonry. There was Catholic, Jewish, Irish and English Protestant chambers and most of the work came from solicitors of a similar persuasion. This did not of course apply to the more brilliant barristers whose Opinions and Pleadings were sought when it was considered necessary, and if the clients could afford them. There were also those cham-

---

[3] Sacher, *Zionist Portraits*, 326; W. Summerfield, 'Anglo-Jewry and the Law: (1) The Legal Profession', *JC Supplement*, 28 Apr. 1922, p. vi.

[4] *JC* 28 Nov. 1923, p. 9, 21 Nov. 1924, p. 6. Summerfield, 'Anglo-Jewry and the Law', p. vi; Henry Cecil [Leon], *Memories and Reminiscences* (London: Hutchinson, 1975).

bers where it was possible for the chief clerk to pick and choose, taking in only those barristers whom he considered were likely quickly to succeed, and whom he thought would eventually rise to the top of their profession. Packer was one of these, he didn't particularly like having a predominantly Jewish chambers, he wanted men on their merits and that was why he fostered Duncan.[5]

On the other hand, when William Frankel, a future editor of the *Jewish Chronicle* who was called to the Bar in 1944, applied to Cyril Salmon to become a member of his chambers, he was refused on the grounds that he did not wish to turn his chambers into a Jewish set, by having too many co-religionists. Certain solicitors' firms in the inter-war years, particularly those in the City, would not send instructions to Jewish barristers. Addressing the Jessel Society as late as 1979, the High Court judge Sir Sebag Shaw commented that there were still 'two or three sets of chambers in the Temple where a Jew has never been a member'.[6]

As yet, there were a few rich pickings to be had from legal aid for ambitious young barristers. Under the Poor Prisoners' Defence Act (1930), which provided for the representation of defendants with 'insufficient means' to hire their own barristers, advocates received the sum of 3 guineas for representing a client in a case. 'Before a case began an accused was invited to choose any barrister who happened to be sitting robed in court,' David Napley recalled, 'so that at the beginning of each case the court would miraculously fill with masses of white-wigged briefless barristers, while contemporaneously all the barristers who had already established themselves would just as mysteriously disappear into thin air.'[7] In the higher criminal courts, representation was similarly arranged by means of 'dock briefs' which were inadequately paid. From the 1920s onwards there was a Poor Persons Scheme for divorce, available to clients whose income was no more than £2 a week. Henry Cecil candidly admitted that when he was called to the Bar in 1923 'there was not then enough work to go round'.[8]

As in the Victorian age, many Jewish barristers of the inter-war period had fathers or other close relatives who were solicitors. Norman Bentwich's father Herbert was a solicitor, who became a barrister himself, while his uncle Albert Solomon was also a solicitor; both Fredman Ashe Lincoln and Frederick Landau's fathers were solicitors deeply involved in communal work; Alan King-Hamilton's father had a family law practice and arranged for his son, when he was about to become a trainee barrister, to have prior litigation experience with

[5] Sydney Aylett, *Under the Wigs* (London: Eyre Methuen, 1978), 29.

[6] Interview with William Frankel, 23 July 1998; interview with the late Fredman Ashe Lincoln, 19 Mar. 1996; *JC* 30 Mar. 1979, p. 29.

[7] David Napley, *Not Without Prejudice: The Memoirs of Sir David Napley* (London: Harrap, 1982), 30.   [8] Cecil, *Memories*, 23.

Joynson-Hicks & Company. Seymour Karminski (1902–72), who built up a successful divorce practice at the Bar, was married to the granddaughter of the society solicitor Sir George Lewis.[9]

Even if the young barrister had good connections, there was no guarantee that he would build up a flourishing practice at the Bar. The diary of Norman Bentwich (1883–1971) for 1910 makes dismal reading. On 3 February he wrote: 'Chambers are as usual lethargic'; ten days later he exclaimed: 'No legal excitements this week: and dull plodding on the Privy Council Book.' A month later, he stated that 'Monday began another year but no change in the outlook.' On 13 March he confided, 'Another Brief and another settlement before it fructified.'[10] Looking back in his memoirs, Bentwich remembered that having been 'called to the Bar in 1908, I practised in the Chancery Courts for four years; but I was not very busy with briefs, and I did not appear in any *cause célèbre*'. When he was asked to defend two youths from Whitechapel on a charge of murder, Bentwich did not have any more luck. 'Lord Swaythling, who had been asked to provide the money for the defence, wrote to me that he had done so,' Bentwich recalled, 'and had directed the solicitors to brief me'; but unknown to him the solicitors had chosen another counsel to represent the youths.[11] After compiling a volume entitled *Bentwich's Privy Council Practice*, he decided to leave the English Bar and in 1912 successfully applied for the post of inspector in the Egyptian Native Courts. At the last moment Sir Rufus Isaacs, who was then Attorney-General, on the strength of Bentwich's expertise invited him 'to "devil" for him in two appeal cases in which he was appearing before the Privy Council', but Bentwich never wavered in his determination to leave. He was the Attorney-General in Palestine between 1921 and 1931, and during his years in this office laid the foundations of a new legal system which, with modifications, was adopted by the State of Israel.[12]

His contemporary Harry Sacher was born in the East End, attended Jews' Free School and Cowper Street School, and after graduating from Oxford with a first-class degree in history decided to make a career at the Bar. Sacher claimed that 'The chambers I entered were not very fruitful. The leading man was a Welsh M.P. and Silk, the others needed for themselves all the work they could get . . . it was fortunate I could earn my living as a journalist. Very few cases, and those ill-paid, came my way.' Motivated by his strong Zionist inclinations and paucity of work, Sacher was drawn like Bentwich to Palestine; emigrating in 1920, he engaged a clerk fluent in both Hebrew and Arabic and

[9] Alan King-Hamilton, *And Nothing but the Truth* (London: Weidenfeld & Nicolson, 1982), 2, 15–16.

[10] Norman Bentwich's diary, 3 Feb., 13 Feb., 9 Mar., 13 Mar. 1910, Central Zionist Archive, Jerusalem, A255/881.

[11] Norman Bentwich, *My Seventy Seven Years* (London: Routledge & Kegan Paul, 1962), 20–8.

[12] *JC* 16 Apr. 1971, p. 35 (obituary of Norman Bentwich).

opened an office. He stayed for some ten years, 'becoming the foremost practitioner at the Palestinian Bar'. In Palestine, he wrote, an 'advocate had to be prepared to take and do any kind of legal work, defend a murderer [from an Arab village trying to uphold his family honour], register a company, conduct a civil action, fight a land claim, and persuade or dissuade an official'. Not only did Sacher, along with other colleagues, feel obliged to defend Jews arrested after the riots of 1920 and do other mundane Zionist work, he also took over the administration of Jewish Palestine when the land of Israel was in the throes of a financial crisis. Either side of his stint at the Palestinian Bar, Sacher worked as a journalist, rising to become one of the chief correspondents of the *Manchester Guardian*. He was described by Redcliffe Salaman in 1931 as 'a gentlemanly man, quiet but very capable of holding his own when put to it . . . He married Simon Marks' sister and has recently become in consequence very well-to-do.'[13]

Sara Moshkowitz, who migrated to Britain after the Russian Revolution, was the first Jewish woman to be called to the Bar in England, in November 1925. She was followed by a number of others, including Dorothy Stone (1908–95), a sister of Harold Lever, the barrister and Labour Cabinet minister, and Leslie Lever, a solicitor and communal worker. 'At the age of 20 she [Stone] passed the Bar Finals but could not be called for another year, when she became, as a member of Neville Laski's chambers, the youngest practising barrister on the Northern Circuit.' Having studied international law in Russia, Moshkowitz joined a chambers in Lincoln's Inn. Speaking in 1928, she pointed out that there was 'a tremendous prejudice to be overcome from every sphere with which we come into contact. Some look upon us as intruders, and there is that supercilious condescending attitude.' Moreover, she asserted that 'Individual solicitors find that some women are extremely good, but they are afraid that the lay public does not want a woman counsel and do not trust women with legal work. Therefore they are afraid of losing their practices or alienating their clients and so they do not brief women.' Like Bentwich and Sacher, Sara Moshkowitz decided to further her career in Palestine, where she qualified for the local Bar and specialized in commercial law; but she encountered problems later when she found that she was unable to master Hebrew.[14]

Bertram Benjamin Benas (1880–1968) was born in Liverpool, the son of Baron Louis Benas, a banker and communal worker. Educated at the universi-

[13] Sacher, *Zionist Portraits*, 328–40; R. N. Salaman to Fred [unidentified correspondent], 24 Jan. 1931, Redcliffe Nathan Salaman Papers, Cambridge University Library, Add. MS 8171, Box I (Simon Marks was the founder of Marks & Spencer); *JC* 1 Sept. 1961, p. 13 (eightieth birthday tribute to Sacher).
[14] *JC* 2 Mar. 1928, p. 25, 11 Aug. 1939, p. 24 (for Sara Moshkowitz); *The Times*, 21 Mar. 1995 (obituary of Stone); see also *JC* 2 Dec. 1994, p. 23 (obituary of Edith Cohen, who was called to the Bar in 1930).

ties of Manchester and Liverpool, he was called to the Bar in 1906, after which he practised as an equity draughtsman and conveyancing counsel for sixty years. According to his biographer Sefton Temkin, Benas 'cannot be said to have built up a practice of any great significance', while another source has remarked that he died in 'genteel poverty'. He wrote a book on Zionism in 1919 and a few years later two legal volumes, one with Judge Essenhigh called *Common Law and Chancery Pleadings* (1919) and the other with Lord Justice Scott, a work entitled *The New Law of Property Explained* (1925). A very busy literary and communal figure in Liverpool, he never quite fulfilled the promise of his youth.[15]

The difficulties facing Jews from immigrant families attempting to start out at the Bar are illustrated by the career of Eli Cashdan (1905–98). His prospective father-in-law stipulated before his marriage that he did not want him to become a rabbi with a congregation and urged him instead to qualify for the Bar, which he did in 1933. Unfortunately his father-in-law, who dabbled in property and had connections with solicitors, died a year after the marriage; and with his death all Cashdan's hope of becoming established as a barrister vanished: during his first year at the Bar, Cashdan earned between £8 and £10. Perturbed by this setback, he renewed his career in Jewish education, eventually becoming a tutor at Jews' College.[16]

The paucity of work available at the Bar for new entrants continued throughout the inter-war years and into the 1950s, and until that decade few young Jewish men and women from modest east European backgrounds attempted to enter the Bar. Salmond Levin (b. 1905) studied law at Leeds and was called to the Bar in Lincoln's Inn; but, unable to find adequate work as a lawyer, he opted for a career in commerce.[17] When Sefton Temkin (1917–96) resigned as secretary of the AJA in 1951 to read for the Bar, he incorrectly believed that he had made sufficient contacts to guarantee his success; handicapped by a stammer, by 1959 he was disillusioned enough to leave for the United States to take up a career as a Jewish historian.[18]

There were, notwithstanding the formidable potential obstacles, several Jewish barristers who achieved a measure of success in the English courts in the 1920s and 1930s. Neville Laski KC (1890–1969), whose father Nathan Laski was a wealthy cotton merchant and communal leader in Manchester who had emigrated from Russian Poland, was called to the Bar in 1913. Writing somewhat less than twenty years later, a correspondent in the *Jewish Chronicle*

[15] Sefton D. Temkin, *Bertram B. Benas: The Life and Times of a Jewish Victorian* (Albany, NY: State University Press of New York, 1978); *JC* 13 Dec. 1968, p. 39 (obituary of Benas); interview with Gabriel Sivan, 6 Aug. 1997.

[16] Interview with the late Eli Cashdan, 14 Aug. 1997; *JC* 4 Dec. 1998, p. 27 (obituary of Cashdan).

[17] Interview with the late Salmond Levin, 21 Jan. 1998.

[18] Interview with Montague Richardson, 16 June 1997; *JC* 24 Jan. 1997 (obituary of Temkin).

commented that Laski 'has enjoyed for some time a very extensive practice in Manchester, is a brilliant advocate and, I should say, a sound lawyer'.[19] He also defended Jewish clients in the Manchester courts, managing to have a charge of blackmail dropped against a professional boxer and a lesser charge of taking money by false pretences substituted; and representing a Mr Huller, who successfully appealed against an unduly harsh sentence of one month's hard labour for committing the technical offence of landing at a port of entry as an alien without the registration officer's permission. Huller had come to Britain as a child in 1890, had lived and worked in the country, and had served in the British army in 1917.[20]

After taking silk in 1930, Laski moved to London and built up a reputation as a formidable cross-examiner, building up 'a large practice in the King's Bench [Division of the High Court], particularly in commercial cases'.[21] 'Apart from the result, which of course is highly satisfactory,' a Blackpool solicitor informed Laski on 10 December 1932, 'I would like to congratulate you on the way the case was handled and the outstandingly able manner in which the witnesses were cross examined.'[22] Julius Elias (later Viscount Southwood), the managing director of Odhams Press, wrote to Laski on 29 January 1933 after his successful conduct of a case, saying

I prophesy very big things for your future—and you will not find that I am wrong. You are already being talked about. I have heard of you from many sources. In a year or two's time I venture to think that your difficulty will be to decide what briefs to accept and what to turn down. I shall certainly remember my promise in regard to introductions to pass some work over to you as soon as any Case is high up in the List.

H. Phillip Levy, his junior in another action in 1935, wrote to Laski pointing out that 'your clients lay and professional are highly satisfied with the result & your efforts which achieved it . . . I would like to add my own tribute & just say that your mastery of the case was complete & your conduct of it excellent'.[23]

However, between 1933 and 1940 Laski devoted so much time to the defence of the Jewish community as president of the Board of Deputies that he felt that his period in office 'had been "disastrous" from a professional point of view. It did not exactly help me much', he noted, 'when Jewish solicitors used to say that "Laski is quite a good man, but he is, of course, busy with communal affairs at the Board".' Because of the great stress engendered by the demands of his

[19] *JC* 13 Apr. 1928, p. 24, 21 Feb. 1930, p. 7.

[20] Rubinstein, *History of the Jews*, 233, 477 n. 44; press cuttings on the Huller case, Neville Laski Papers, London Metropolitan Archives, Acc. 3121 B5/1/1.   [21] *JC* 4 Feb. 1938, p. 10.

[22] Alfred Kidd Whitaker to Laski, 10 Dec. 1932, Neville Laski Papers, Greater London Record Office, Acc. 3121 B5/1/1.

[23] Julius Elias to Laski, 28 Jan. 1933, H. Phillip Levy to Laski, 25 Nov. 1935, Neville Laski Papers, Greater London Record Office, Acc. 3121 B5/1/1.

position he drank too heavily, and could be brusque and discourteous to clients at consultations. Thus, sadly, the reputation of one of the few star performers in court on the Anglo-Jewish scene became tarnished.[24]

David Weitzman QC (1899–1987) was born in Blackburn of Orthodox Jewish immigrant parents and was a strong adherent of traditional Judaism. After serving in the army during the First World War, he studied history at Manchester University, obtaining a first-class degree. He then moved to London and read for the Bar, where he was admitted in 1922. 'While David Weitzman struggled to establish himself as a lawyer he supplemented his livelihood by teaching in elementary schools by day and lecturing by night. He also acted as a "poor man's lawyer" at the Jewish Centre in the East End, then in Stoke Newington, which adopted him as its Labour candidate in 1931.'[25] Through his contacts in the Jewish world and his involvement in the labour movement, he was instructed by Jewish lawyers from immigrant families, such as Lewis Silkin and Morris Hart-Leverton. He built up a successful criminal and common law practice, particularly in the area of accident claims; among his pupils in the late 1930s was Chaim Herzog, the future president of Israel.[26] He was elected as an MP in the Labour landslide of 1945, but his career seemed doomed when he was tried with his brothers at the Old Bailey in 1947 on a charge of conspiracy for evading orders relating to the manufacture of cosmetics. However, the Court of Criminal Appeal quashed his conviction and later that of his brothers, not finding 'any shred of the evidence which pointed to the guilt of Mr David Weitzman'. Wonderfully resilient, he recovered from what proved to be a temporary setback and was elevated to the rank of QC in 1951.[27]

Weitzman appeared in a number of important cases which feature in legal textbooks. An early appeal conducted by him in the King's Bench Division was *Ratinsky* v. *Jacobs* (1928), where clarification of some inconsistent authorities was sought in a vain attempt to invoke Rent Act protection for a tenant. In *Robert Addie and Sons (Colleries) Limited* v. *Dumbreck* (1929) the House of Lords decided that no duty is owed by an occupier to a trespasser, apart from a duty not maliciously to cause him injury. The case involved a boy of 4 being killed when he was accidentally caught in the winding apparatus at a colliery where he was playing. In *Leaf* v. *International Galleries* (1950) the Court of Appeal decided that there can be no rescission of a contract after a reasonable time has elapsed because there has been an innocent misrepresentation. Here the plaintiff had purchased a picture from the defendants which both mistakenly believed had been painted by Constable. Weitzman also conducted an appeal in the House of

---

[24] *JC* 27 Sept. 1963, p. 15 (report of a talk by Laski); interview with the late Frederic Landau, 6 Aug. 1996. [25] *JC* 15 May 1987, p. 17 (obituary of Weitzman).
[26] Interview with Peter Weitzman QC, 8 May 1998.
[27] Iris Freeman, *Lord Denning: A Life* (London: Hutchinson, 1993), 186–8.

Lords in *Davies* v. *Director of Public Prosecutions* (1954) which established that where a person who was an accomplice gave evidence on behalf of the prosecution, it was the duty of the judge to warn the jury that although they might convict on his evidence, it was dangerous to do so without corroboration. True, Weitzman was unsuccessful in these appeals; yet this was not due to any lack of forensic skill on his part, and there were occasions when he was congratulated on the cogency of his argument for his client.[28]

Moss Turner-Samuels QC (1892–1957), like David Weitzman and a number of others from an east European Jewish background, saw his career in the law prosper through his involvement with the labour movement. Turner-Samuels was left an orphan at the age of 7 and, after attending elementary school, was apprenticed to a cabinet-maker in Newcastle upon Tyne; however, with the financial assistance of relatives he was articled to a solicitor and qualified in 1914. Selling his flourishing solicitor's practice in 1921, he studied for the Bar and qualified as a barrister a year later. He joined the Labour Party, becoming a city councillor and briefly MP for Barnard Castle in 1923. Defeated at Leeds Central in 1931 and Gloucester in 1935, he won the latter seat in 1945 and again in 1950. An admiring journalist wrote in the political periodical *MP*:

His practice at the Bar has increased steadily, through the vicissitudes of his political career, and through these years of activity there has accumulated a pile of those blue-bound House of Lord cases . . . *Radcliffe* v. *Ribble Motor Services* was one of these triumphs. Industrial lawyers recognize it as the leading case which changed the face of the infamous doctrine of common employment, now given its death-blow by the Law Reform (Personal Injuries Act), 1948. The Napier Will dispute, in which he was engaged was also a forerunner of legislation, for the Inheritance (Family Provision) Act of 1938 is considered to be an expression of the public opinion aroused by this case.

Among Turner-Samuels' publications were books on trade unions, industrial negotiation and arbitration, and the law relating to married women. He took silk in 1946 and became recorder of Halifax in 1948. Maintaining his Jewish identity, he was not only an active member of the West London Synagogue but represented a Newcastle congregation on the Board of Deputies.[29]

Julius Silverman (1905–96), who was brought up in Leeds, left school at 16 to become a warehouseman and provide for his family. He studied law in the evenings before entering Gray's Inn as a student and was called to the Bar in

---

[28] *Ratinsky* v. *Jacobs* (1928), *The Times Law Reports*, vol. xliv, pp. 548–50. *Robert Addie and Sons (Colleries) Limited v. Dumbreck* (1929), *The Times Law Reports*, vol. xlv, pp. 267–2; *Leaf* v. *International Galleries* (1950) 1 All ER, pp. 693–7. *Davies* v. *Director of Public Prosecutions* (1954) 1 All ER, pp. 507–15.

[29] *JC* 14 June 1957, p. 9, *The Times*, 7 June 1957 (obituaries of Turner-Samuels); 'M. Turner-Samuels KCM', *MP*, 1/1 (Apr. 1950), 11–15.

1931. His career pattern was similar to that of David Weitzman and Moss Turner-Samuels. He joined the Midland Circuit, where he built up a successful practice in landlord and tenant law. He entered politics as a Labour councillor for the City of Birmingham in 1934, but was not elected to Parliament until 1945; thereafter he represented a Birmingham constituency for the next thirty-eight years. In Parliament he was a champion of tenants' rights, criticizing Aneurin Bevan in his maiden speech for not giving sufficient protection to furnished tenants in his Furnished Houses (Rent Control) Bill (1945). During the 1950s he led the opposition to slum landlords and put the case for municipal housing. Silverman also led a parliamentary campaign to end breach of promise claims by women against men who refused to marry them. As a young councillor he represented a ward with a large number of Indian inhabitants, and when he became an MP he urged the case for Indian press freedom before the granting of independence. Between 1927 and 1947 he was secretary of the India League, of which he then became president. Tam Dalyell, who sat on the European Secondary Legislation (Scrutiny) Committee between 1974 and 1976, claimed that Silverman was a brilliant chairman, in the same league as Ian Mikardo and Harold Wilson. Unlike Weitzman and Turner-Samuels, he did not play an active role in Jewish affairs and, ignoring his mother's wishes that he should settle down 'with a nice Jewish girl', he married his non-Jewish secretary.[30]

Harold Lightman (1906–98) was the son of Louis Lightman, an Orthodox communal leader in Leeds who, after making furniture which was sold on barrows, later established a thriving furniture manufacturing business. Complaining of headaches as a schoolboy, Harold Lightman was examined by a specialist who stated that as he had a weak head he should leave school. He did so when he was 14 and went to work in his father's factory—whereupon it was discovered that his headaches were caused by the need to wear glasses. Motivated by a great love of reading, he educated himself by a correspondence course and by the time he was 21 had qualified as an accountant, written a book on company financing, and become a partner in the accountancy firm of Lightman & Sharp, where his dealings with many aspects of insolvency whetted his appetite to study law. After learning from an item in the *Jewish Chronicle* in 1928 that a Miss Sara Moshkowitz had been among the first half-dozen women to be called to the English Bar, Harold Lightman travelled to London to meet her; she recommended that he become a pupil in the chambers to which she was attached in Lincoln's Inn, which specialized in company law. Lightman was called to the Bar in 1932.[31]

[30] *The Times*, 23 Sept. 1996; *Independent*, 24 Sept. 1996; *Daily Telegraph*, 24 Sept. 1996 (obituaries of Silverman).

[31] *The Times*, 7 Oct. 1998 (obituary of Lightman); interview with the late Harold Lightman, 21 Mar. 1997.

As his funds were limited, Harold Lightman paid a fee of £50 for six months' pupillage (rather than £100 for a full year) and found accommodation at a Liberal Club. Shortly before he was due to return home at the expiry of his half-year, the head of chambers, Alexander Grant KC, had a difficult case involving accounts, and because of his background in accountancy Lightman was asked to look at the papers. At once he realized that the case was hopeless; Grant was so impressed by his advice that he insisted that he stay on. Contrary to protocol, Grant allowed him to remain in his room when he was discussing a case with juniors and pupils.[32] On 31 August 1932, Lightman persuaded Lord Romer to hear two or three urgent interlocutory appeals outside London in a case mainly concerned with a company which had gone into liquidation—the first time that this had happened in legal history.[33] With his background in corporate accountancy, Lightman attracted work in company law and personal and corporate insolvency; he also co-wrote, with Philip James Sykes and Stanley Borrie, the *Handbook on the Formation, Management and Winding Up of Joint Stock Companies* (1946). In 1936 he married Gwendoline Ostrer, the daughter of David Ostrer, a director of the Gaumont British Film Company and the General Theatres Corporation.[34]

Lightman appeared in over 100 reported cases, quite a considerable achievement. Nevertheless, he was hampered by the snobbery and class prejudice prevailing at the Bar. When called with another, public-school-educated, barrister in front of a judge in his chambers about some aspect of a case, the judge would address the former public schoolboy by his first name but simply address a question to Lightman. Certain judges made him read Latin legal phrases aloud in court, knowing that he could not pronounce them properly because he had not had the benefit of a classical education and that this would make him appear ridiculous. Again, many leading firms of City solicitors would not send instructions to Jewish barristers. Despite these handicaps, Lightman became a QC in 1955, head of his Chambers in 1966–7, and a Master of the Bench at Lincoln's Inn, a mark of the esteem of his colleagues.[35]

Lightman, who as a young man had stood as a Liberal candidate in local elections, also on occasions acted for the less privileged. In the *National Provincial Bank* v. *Hastings Car Mart Ltd.* (1964), heard in the Court of Appeal, a man called Ainsworth had left the matrimonial home, deserting his wife and children and forming a relationship with another woman. He then concocted an ingenious ruse whereby he turned his business into a limited company, to which he transferred the ownership of the matrimonial home and the business premises.

[32] Interview with the late Harold Lightman, 7 Oct. 1997.
[33] *Evening News*, 30 Aug. 1932; *Daily Mirror*, 1 Sept. 1932.
[34] *Yorkshire Evening News*, 4 Sept. 1936; *Daily Mirror*, 8 Sept. 1936.
[35] *The Times*, 7 Oct. 1998.

The company then borrowed money from the National Provincial Bank in return for which it charged the matrimonial home to the bank; the husband then decided not to repay the loan, causing the bank to enforce its charge and seek vacant possession of the home. Lightman acted for the deserted wife, who appealed against an order of the judge in the lower court that she did not possess an overriding interest in the property, so that she would have to give vacant possession of the matrimonial home. Lightman argued that 'A deserted wife has a right to retain possession of the matrimonial home as against the whole world except a bona fide purchaser for value without actual or constructive notice.' He relied on Denning's earlier judgment to this effect in *Jess B. Woodcock & Sons Ltd* v. *Hobbs* (1955), which was followed by a number of other authorities; and further claimed that the manager of the National Provincial Bank ought to have made the necessary enquiries that would have established that Ainsworth was not living with his wife at the matrimonial home. Although Denning presided over the Court of Appeal in the present instance and persuaded the court to allow the appeal, the decision was overturned by the House of Lords; the situation was rectified only by the Matrimonial Homes Act (1967), which gave spouses the right to register a caution against a property owned by the other spouse.[36]

Solicitors valued the close attention he [Lightman] paid to documents, and the early advice he gave on evidence, which often led to settlements. When cases did come to court, Lightman was a shrewd tactician and an efficient, often aggressive, advocate, with a puckish turn of phrase . . . In conferences, he often made do without a notebook, resorting instead to old scraps of paper he had salvaged and held together with a large paper clip.

Thus read the obituary of Harold Lightman in the *Daily Telegraph*, written by his grandson Daniel Lightman, which brilliantly conveyed the style of the man. Harold Lightman, like his father, participated in communal affairs, though in a slightly more Anglicized form, being president of the Central Synagogue's Orphan Aid Society and serving on the Council of the AJA.[37]

Fredman Ashe Lincoln QC (1907–98) was a pupil of Walter Monckton, being called to the Bar in 1929; both his father, Reuben Lincoln, and his brother, Ellis Lincoln, were solicitors. His first stroke of good fortune, which brought his name to public prominence, was the 'Guinea Gramophone' case heard by the Court of Appeal in May 1931. A businessman called Jacob Factor floated a company to market a gramophone which was sold for 1 guinea. He then went to

---

[36] *National Provincial Bank Ltd v. Hastings Car Mart, National Provincial Bank Ltd v. Hastings Car Mart (No. 2)* (1964) 1 Ch. [1964], pp. 665–703; Lord Denning, *The Due Process of Law* (London. Butterworths, 1980), pp. 215–19; Freeman, *Lord Denning*, 204–7.

[37] *Daily Telegraph*, 15 Oct. 1998; *JC* 16 Oct. 1998, p. 21 (obituaries of Harold Lightman by Daniel Lightman).

various provincial towns and put in bids for huge amounts of shares in the company to pump up the price. The shares soared in value; he sold them, making a killing on the stock market; then, with the police anxious to interview him, he fled to the United States. In the lower court Lord Darling and the jury found that there had been fraudulent misrepresentation by the company's directors, who were ordered to pay damages of £9,375 to the plaintiff.

An appeal was lodged against this ruling and Ashe Lincoln was to appear for the appellant. He had little time to prepare the case, as it was expected to be listed in the following week; but Lord Justice Scrutton, who was hearing the appeal, demanded that Ashe Lincoln speak first, as his client's surname (Abelson) began with the letter A. 'Young man, I have never seen you before; get on with it', remarked the judge. Ashe Lincoln read all the pleadings and a volume of correspondence to the court—which took up all of Wednesday afternoon—before plunging into legal argument on the next day and continuing into Friday morning to say why the verdict of the original trial judge was wrong. His legal submissions were adopted by the more senior counsel appearing for the other directors, and, despite the contrary arguments put forward over two and a half days by the silk opposing him, Lord Justice Scrutton found in favour of Ashe Lincoln's client and ordered a retrial. Scrutton declared that 'It appeared to be clear from the evidence that Factor's reputation in company matters was such that many respectable people would not deal with him. Dealing with him [however] was not necessarily either criminal or a breach of any contract.' The judge's assessment seems to have been accurate: a month later there was a share fraud trial at the Old Bailey in a completely different matter, in which Jacob Factor again figured.[38]

Another early success for Ashe Lincoln was attributable to his being in Chambers on a bank holiday in 1932, when the solicitor acting for the estate of Arthur Conan Doyle, who had died on 7 July 1930, was desperately looking for a barrister to represent Lady Doyle in court to apply for an injunction against the *Daily Mail*—which, not appreciating that the copyright was still in force, had stated that it was going to serialize the Sherlock Holmes stories. Having drafted the necessary affidavit, Ashe Lincoln appeared with his client and instructing solicitor before the vacation judge, Travers Humphreys, at his home in Ealing, and obtained an injunction forbidding publication.[39]

Ashe Lincoln went on to become a member of the chambers of Sir George Jones, who had a much better flow of work than Walter Monckton, especially in civil matters (he was particularly known as a libel expert). Jones was not only

[38] Interview with the late Fredman Ashe Lincoln, 19 Mar. 1996; *JC* 22 May 1931, p. 29, 26 June 1931, p. 27, 10 July 1931, p. 31.

[39] Interview with the late Fredman Ashe Lincoln, 19 Mar. 1996; *Guardian*, 28 Oct. 1998 (obituary of Ashe Lincoln).

instructed by Kingsley Wood, a solicitor and prominent Tory MP, but was on a permanent retainer from the *Daily Express* for libel matters; this connection brought instructions Ashe Lincoln's way, as did the success of his solicitor brother Ellis Lincoln in establishing a reputation as a criminal lawyer. Jones, occupied with his own parliamentary duties, handed over many briefs to Ashe Lincoln, who 'appeared in trials led by Norman Birkett—whom he regarded as the finest silk he ever heard—Patrick Hastings and Sergeant Sullivan'.[40] In 1933, however, Sir George Jones led Ashe Lincoln in the defence of Leopold Harris, who was charged with fraudulent fire insurance claims, while Ashe was also instructed by another one of the accused, Bowman, under the Poor Prisoners' Defence Act. This defence did not succeed. However, as a result of his earlier successes, Ashe Lincoln was instructed in a small claim against Charlie Chaplin in the Westminster County Court, which attracted more publicity for him; and gradually he started acting in more important cases.[41]

In February 1938 Ashe Lincoln defended John Christopher Mainwaring Lonsdale, who, with three other public schoolboys, was charged with conspiracy and robbery with violence in the 'Mayfair Boys' case. The young men had booked a suite of rooms at the Hyde Park Hotel and, on the pretext that one of them was engaged to be married, had invited Mr Etienne Bellenger of the famous jeweller Cartier's to bring them a tray of rings for inspection. As Mr Bellenger displayed the rings, one of the conspirators suddenly rushed in from another room and struck the unfortunate jeweller a series of blows to his head, fracturing his skull. Ashe Lincoln submitted that Lonsdale was nervous about the plot, so that when the jeweller was lured into the room, he had gone to the lavatory and did not participate in any violence. There was additional evidence against Lonsdale in that he had suggested the plan for the robbery, after reading a couple of months previously in the *Paris-Soir* that a thief had invited a jeweller to a hotel room in Paris and had absconded with some diamonds; but Ashe Lincoln argued that the inference to be drawn from this was that his client was not prone to violence. Whereas the other conspirators received lengthy prison sentences and two of them were also birched, Lonsdale escaped corporal punishment and was given a shorter term of eighteen months' imprisonment with hard labour by the presiding judge, Lord Chief Justice Hewart.[42]

Just after the outbreak of the Second World War, in October 1939 Ashe Lincoln represented Victor Hervey, a son of the marquis of Bristol, in an appeal against conviction for masterminding the theft of jewels from two society ladies. Having heard from a friend that a Mrs Daubny would be away for Easter,

[40] *Guardian*, 28 Oct. 1998 (obituary of Lincoln).
[41] Ibid.; Douglas G. Browne, *Sir Travers Humphreys: A Biography* (London: Harrap, 1960), 314.
[42] Interview with the late Fredman Ashe Lincoln, 19 Mar. 1996; Robert Jackson, *The Chief: The Biography of Gordon Hewart, Lord Chief Justice of England 1922–40* (London: Harrap, 1959), 314–21.

Hervey encouraged a group of burglars to break into her empty Mayfair home to steal valuable jewellery. He also arranged the theft of a diamond ring and clips from another acquaintance at a nightclub, by plying her with drink. Under the then applying rules, Ashe Lincoln appeared in court in a naval lieutenant's uniform; although he lost the appeal, the Lord Chief Justice wished him well and said that he should come back safely. During the war he commanded a minesweeper and rose to the rank of naval commander.[43]

Like Ashe Lincoln, Bernard Gillis (1905–96) came from a family that had emigrated to Britain from eastern Europe before the successive waves of immigrants after 1880. His grandfather had arrived in the 1860s, and his father, Rabbi Julius Kyanski, served the Newcastle Old Hebrew Congregation. After studying law at Cambridge, Gillis (who at some point early in his career Anglicized his name) became a pupil of Harold Simmons, a successful junior barrister and 'a recognised expert in the drafting of pleadings and on matters of procedure before Masters'; he was himself called to the Bar in 1927. To supplement his earnings, which totalled £76 in his first year and £180 in his second year at the Bar, Gillis lectured at the Regent Street Polytechnic and elsewhere, and regularly broadcast for the BBC on aspects of the law. Gillis's practice 'included the usual claims for personal injuries and various claims for breaches of contract, with an element of libel and slander, divorce and bankruptcy', but increasingly he appeared in the criminal courts. He successfully defended a vendor of cats' meat accused of murdering his wife after a quarrel in which she first struck him, and he then raised a knife to frighten her off; there was a struggle in which she unfortunately died. Acquitted of murder by the jury, the accused was given a sentence of five years by the judge for manslaughter. Gillis was less successful in defending an unemployed man who went berserk and killed his woman friend. He was led by Edward Hemmerde KC when defending a gentleman indicted for pushing valueless shares, and by Sir Patrick Hasting when acting for a widow who had been persuaded to sell her late husband's shares in a mine without the benefit of independent advice. In 1938 Gillis, like Ashe Lincoln, defended one of the accused in the 'Mayfair Boys' case, the assailant who struck the jeweller some blows on the head, for which he received a sentence of seven years' penal servitude. A year later he advised a woman who claimed to be the Grand Duchess Anastasia, daughter of Tsar Nicholas II of Russia, to sue a newspaper for libel.[44]

Gillis's greatest success was to make three Sunday newspapers pay thousands of pounds in damages to a woman called Mary whom they had libelled. She ran a domestic agency to supply servant girls from the north of England,

---

[43] Interview with the late Fredman Ashe Lincoln, 19 Mar. 1996; *The Times*, 2 May, 25 Oct. 1939.

[44] Bernard Gillis, 'Once Round Only' (unpublished memoirs), 2, 4, 9, 10, 16, 22, 23, 25–38.

where there was heavy unemployment, to London; the newspapers suggested that the girls were exposed to 'dangers and temptations' by such agencies, including Mary's, and that the agencies should be investigated. A few weeks before the trial was due to start, three eminent barristers acting for the newspapers requested a discussion with Gillis. One of them was Sir George Jones, who exclaimed, 'What about this procuress—this woman at King's Cross?' Gillis replied that she was 'the wife of an important clergyman in London who meets the girls when my client is absent' and that she was going to be called as a witness. When he stated that he had both an archdeacon's wife and a member of the diocesan charity board lined up as witnesses in support of Mary, the barristers acting for the press capitulated and the matter was settled. By 1940, Gillis's annual income at the Bar had risen to £1,500, a not inconsiderable sum.[45]

Frederic Moses Landau (1905–99) was another whose family had arrived in Britain from eastern Europe in the mid-nineteenth century; his father, Isaac Landau, was a well-known solicitor active in Jewish communal organizations, which he sometimes represented legally. Frederic was called to the Bar in 1927 and became a pupil of Herbert Garland, a general common law practitioner and a first-class pleader. Landau appeared frequently in criminal cases at the Inner London Quarter Sessions and at Kingston, although he also did a fair amount of civil work; he most enjoyed acting in defended divorce cases. He gradually built up a successful practice with the help of instructions received from his father and a number of Jewish solicitors, such as Jacques Cohen, Janus and Maurice Cohen, and Solomon Teff, and by dint of his own forensic skills. His busiest period as a barrister was during the Second World War, when a large number of his fellow practitioners were away on active service. In 1962 he was appointed chairman of a rent tribunal and a rent committee, retiring from these positions in 1977. For a number of years he was chairman of the Shops Act Appeal Tribunal which 'was concerned with exemptions from the Sunday Trading legislation' and operated under the aegis of the Board of Deputies.[46]

While some Jewish barristers between the wars held steadfastly to the Jewish tradition and were deeply involved in communal affairs, perhaps an equal number were indifferent and had few links with the Jewish community. Among the former was Alter Hurwitz (1899–1970), the son of Rabbi Hurwitz, who was spiritual leader of Leeds Jewry for thirty-five years. After attending Yeshiva Etz Chaim and London University, Alter Hurwitz qualified as a barrister in 1924 and rose to become recorder of Halifax in 1957. In addition to the many communal offices which he held, he founded the Leeds Mizrachi, the organization of religious Zionists, and helped to form the local *kashrut* commission, which

---

[45] Ibid. 38–40, 74.

[46] Interview with the late Frederic Landau, 6 Aug. 1996; *JC* 28 Jan. 2000, p. 25 (obituary of Landau).

determines licenses, and supervises businesses providing kosher food. He was also a book lover, amassing a library of 10,000 volumes.

Because Alter Hurwitz's Orthodox Jewishness dictated his radical approach to life and to a complete appreciation and yearning for egalitarianism and social justice, he never aspired to assimilate and become part of the Establishment . . . He never desired to become an Englishman of the Jewish faith and so attempt to out-county the county, as is the wont these days among Jewish professionals and business classes,

wrote Sir Karl Cohen.[47]

A similar figure in London was Elsley Zeitlin (1878– 1959), the son of Rabbi Dr Bernard Zeitlin, who retired as a barrister in 1939 to devote himself to communal affairs. He was chairman of the Shechitah Committee of the Board of Deputies for thirty years and an early advocate of the Weinberg casting-pen (a device to improve the procedure in the ritual slaughter of animals). In 1954 he toured the country to persuade local authorities to drop their support for the Crouch Bill which would have banned the Jewish ritual slaughter of animals, unless prior stunning had taken place. In 1938 Zeitlin brought to Britain a number of Jewish children of Polish parents who had lived in Germany but had then been deported by the Nazis, and after 1945 he interested himself in Jewish war orphans, especially those being brought up as Christians.[48] Among other barristers who took their communal obligations seriously was Louis S. Green (1872– 1940), a relative of the Revd A. A. Green (minister of the Hampstead Synagogue), who fought against antisemitism; Bernard Gillis and Arthur Diamond, (who were the children of ministers) and Frederic Landau were also communally active, Landau serving as chairman of the Law and Parliamentary Committee of the Board of Deputies and treasurer of the United Synagogue.[49]

Another outstanding provincial barrister and communal worker between the wars was Joseph Lustgarten (1878–1937) of Manchester, the father of the well-known barrister and writer Edgar Lustgarten. He originally qualified as a solicitor in 1903, being called to the Bar in 1917. He was generally regarded as the leader of the junior bar on the Northern Circuit and participated in many notable actions, including the Ministry of Health inquiry into the conditions at St Mary's Hospital, Manchester. He was president of the Higher Broughton Synagogue, but was also connected with the Jews' School, the Jewish Fresh Air Home and School (the Delamere Home), the Jewish Working Men's Club, and the Jewish Lads' Brigade.[50]

Captain Hermann Horace Roskin (1887–1960) was the Welsh counterpart of Lustgarten. He gained a B.Sc. from the University of Wales and an MA from

[47] *JC* 2 Sept. 1952, Leeds Supplement, p. iv, 30 Oct. 1970, p. 31 (obituary of Hurwitz).
[48] *JC* 17 Apr. 1959, p. 17 (obituary of Zeitlin).   [49] *JC* 28 Jan. 2000, p. 25 (obituary of Landau).
[50] *JC* 29 Oct. 1937, p. 13 (obituary of Lustgarten).

Oxford, and after war service was called to the Bar in 1922. He settled in chambers in Cardiff, where he had a wide practice in the South Wales Circuit. Before the Second World War he was appointed legal adviser to the Coal Commission and was later put in control of public utility undertakings. 'As a truly Orthodox Jew, he was a learned Talmudist.' He not only promoted the amalgamation of Cardiff synagogues, but was the President of the South Wales and Monmouthshire Zionist Society.[51]

Among the silks, only Lionel Cohen, Neville Laski, Cyril M. Picciotto, Phineas Quass, and Abraham Montagu Lyons had any extensive involvement with the Jewish community in the 1930s. Quass (1892–1961) gave useful service to the Central Jewish Lecture Committee. During the latter part of his career he specialized in overseas cases, in 1959 defending two Buddhist monks charged with the murder of the prime minister of Sri Lanka, S. W. R. D. Bandaranaike.[52] Cyril Picciotto (1888–1940) was educated at Cambridge, where he obtained first-class honours in the classical tripos and later in 1911 in the law tripos. He was called to the Bar in 1913, wrote several legal texts, served as referee under the Widows, Orphans and Old-Age Contributory Pension Acts (1930–2), and was made a KC in 1938. Of major importance were the zest and inspired leadership shown by Picciotto in fighting antisemitism at street level in the late 1930s, a campaign in which he was joined by a few brilliant young barristers such as Ingram Joseph Linder and Henry Burton. 'Here was a man of culture and distinction, who, from the inception of the anti-defamation campaign, did not deem it *infra dig.* to take his place on the street-corner platform in defence of his people against the Jew-baiting organisations', asserted Frank Renton, art publisher and member of the Defence Committee of the Board of Deputies.

His subsequent work as Chairman of the London Area Council was an inspiration to all who associated themselves with him. Would that other professional men in the Community, endowed with even a modicum of this great man's erudition and platform ability, had followed his example—we might then have had a more equitable distribution of the highly exhausting and onerous task imposed upon the public-spirited few. Unfortunately the oft-repeated appeal for speakers and workers failed to arouse the fighting spirit of the Community's host of able men.[53]

The minutes of the Co-ordinating Committee which later became the Defence Committee of the Board of Deputies show that Neville Laski sent a personal letter in October 1937 to each Jewish barrister, requesting them to speak at meetings; but he reported on 15 November 1937 that the response had

[51] *JC* 25 Mar. 1960 (obituary of Roskin).

[52] *JC* 6 Oct. 1961, p. 25 (obituary of Quass), 16 Feb. 1940, p. 10.

[53] *JC* 23 Feb. 1940, p. 7 (obituary of Picciotto).

been 'negligible'.[54] Equally, the Society for Jewish Jurisprudence founded by Herbert Bentwich in 1925 failed to flourish, as the organizers found themselves 'up against a good deal of apathy on the part of Jewish lawyers'. After six years of existence, the society, which had been established to revive research into Jewish law, could boast a membership of only eighty Anglo-Jewish lawyers; 'and if one may judge by the number of unpaid subscriptions, not a few of the members deem themselves to have accepted a very nominal obligation', commented the *Jewish Chronicle*. Attendances at meetings were denounced as 'despicable'.[55] Its chairman, Dr George Julius Webber, a barrister and academic who as reader in law at University College London educated many Jewish lawyers, and who later founded Jewish Book Week, struggled to keep the society afloat. On the other hand, it could be argued that the Jewish barristers were trying so hard to promote their own professional careers that they had no time for street oratory, which would have interfered with their commitments to their clients and the preparation of their presentations in court, and that in all organizations it was common occurrence for only a few persons to be motivated and actively engaged. Yet these were no ordinary times, and within the Anglo-Jewish communal leadership in 1938 there was increasing apprehension of the drift of public opinion and a genuine fear in sections of the communal leadership that within the space of a few years anti-Jewish legislation could be introduced in Britain.[56]

Moreover, many of the new KCs of the inter-war years were not from the old Anglo-Jewish families but of disparate origin (although hardly any were the children of the east European immigrants who had arrived between 1880 and 1920), and they tended to have a low level of Jewish involvement. Examples were men such as Vladimir Robert Idelson, Jacques Abady, Stanley Isaac Levy, Philip Vos, and Sylvain Mayer. Vladimir Robert Idelson (1880–1954) was born at Rostov-on-Don and educated at the universities of Kharkov and Berlin, and practised at the Russian Bar. Between 1914 and 1917 he was a member of the Council of the Russian and English Bank and of the Committee of the Union of Russian Banks. He left Russia after the Revolution and was called to the English Bar in 1926, where he practised as an expert in Russian and international law. He was made a KC in 1943.[57] Jacques Abady (1873–1964) was educated at Manchester Grammar School and studied engineering, afterwards inventing several scientific instruments. He then switched to the law as a career, being called to

[54] Board of Deputies, Minutes of Co-ordinating Committee, 7 Oct., 15 Nov. 1937, C6/1/1/1.
[55] Ernest Lesser to Herbert Bentwich, 2 Feb. 1930, Herbert Bentwich Papers, A100/16, Central Zionist Archive, Jerusalem; *JC* 25 Mar. 1932, p. 10; Society for Jewish Jurisprudence annual reports 1926–9.
[56] Board of Deputies, Co-ordinating Committee, memorandum of Gordon Liverman, Oct. 1938.
[57] *The Times*, 1 Dec. 1954, *JC* 3 Dec. 1954 (obituary of Idelson).

the Bar in 1905 and later taking silk; he continued to use his scientific training, specializing in patent cases. He also served for a time as Mayor of Westminster.[58] Stanley Isaac Levy (1891–1968) held a doctorate in chemistry from London University. 'He gave evidence as an expert witness in several important patent cases, and he used to tell us how on one occasion James Whitehead, then the leader of the Patent Bar (who had just cross-examined him without any success!) strongly urged him to consider taking up law, and making use of his abilities and qualifications as an advocate in patent matters', declared a colleague in *The Times*. He was called to the Bar in 1927, but did not start practising until 1935; after an interruption during the Second World War, when he served as assistant director of the Ministry of Supply, he became the leading junior in matters concerned with chemical patents. He was made a QC in 1957 at the age of 66.[59] Philip Vos was called to the Bar in 1921, taking silk in 1937. 'In later life, apart from the Lord Baldwin Fund [for refugees], Mr Vos had little active contact with the Jewish Community', remarked the *Jewish Chronicle* on his death.[60] Sylvain Mayer (1863–1948) had a distinguished career at the Bar, and also wrote several comedies for the theatre, as well as a novel.[61]

Just as Jews dominated the cheap end of the tailoring and fur trades, so Jewish barristers in the inter-war period were prominent as junior counsel in the criminal courts, the least prestigious sector of the Bar. All the principal performers, the leading KCs who appeared in the sensational murder trials, such as J. D. Cassels, Norman Birkett, and Sir Patrick Hastings, were non-Jewish. Whereas in the more open social environment of the late Victorian age and the period before the First World War the star Jewish names were often seen in the commercial courts and higher tribunals, in the inter-war years Jewish silks largely disappeared from view in these arenas; it was only in the period following the Second World War that names such as Sebag Shaw, Rose Heilbron, Alan King-Hamilton, Bernard Gillis, Fredman Ashe Lincoln, Richard Francis Levy, and Frederic Landau came to dominate the criminal courts.

Few men—and even fewer women—of east European origin entered the Bar during the 1920s and 1930s, lacking the right connections to obtain work which was in any case not very abundant; but a handful of such barristers with close ties to the Labour Party did see their careers prosper. A large proportion of those who joined the profession were the sons of rabbis, without openings elsewhere and brought up within a tradition of academic distinction and public service. Bernard Gillis, Arthur Sigismund Diamond, Alter Hurwitz, and Elsley Zeitlin were all Jewish 'sons of the manse'. However, the shortage of counsel

---

[58] *JC* 24 Apr. 1964, p. 39 (obituary of Abady).
[59] *The Times*, 19 Nov. 1968, *JC* 22 Nov. 1968, p. 22 (obituary of Levy).
[60] *JC* 16 Jan. 1948, p. 6, 23 Jan. 1948, p. 6 (obituary of Vos).
[61] *JC* 17 Sept. 1948 (obituary of Mayer).

during the Second World War enabled individuals such as Sebag Shaw and Rose Heilbron, both from east European families, to enter the profession and lay the foundation of eminent post-war careers. If Jewish barristers succeeded in other sections of the Bar, it was because they had specialist skills, in particular the combination of scientific training and legal knowledge essential in patent law claims, and here the names of Jacques Abady and Stanley Isaac Levy spring to mind.

Between the two world wars Jewish representation on the judicial bench declined precipitously. This was despite the fact that during the 1930s there were about 100 Jewish barristers to choose from, and that in 1922 there were seven Jewish King's Counsel out of a total of about 300, 'a higher proportion of Jewish as against non-Jewish silks relative to the proportion of the Jewish to the non-Jewish population'. In part this lack of representation in the higher courts was due to the almost complete political identification of Jews with the Liberal Party; for with the rapid decline of the Liberal Party in the early 1920s, its leaders no longer had access to the sources of patronage necessary to secure the appointment of Jews to high judicial office. Following the resignation on 7 March 1921 of the Lord Chief Justice Rufus Isaacs—a relic of the former political ascendancy—there were, with one exception, to be no more High Court judges of Jewish origin until 1943.[62] The sole exception was Sir Henry Slesser (born Schloesser, 1882–1979), who was Solicitor-General in the minority Labour government of 1924 and was subsequently appointed a Lord Justice of Appeal by Ramsay MacDonald in 1929. Both his parents were Jewish but agnostic, and, after attending Oundle public school, Slesser joined the Anglican Church until he converted to Roman Catholicism.[63] Although it has been suggested that the Jewish silks between the wars were not of sufficient calibre for high judicial office, the Lord Chief Justice between 1922 and 1940, Sir Gordon Hewart, may at times have been antisemitic, as is instanced by his constantly referring to the Lord Chancellor's secretary Schuster, a Christian from a family of German Jewish origin, as 'shyster', a crooked lawyer; certainly some influential judges, such as Sir Edward Acton and Rigby Swift, were antisemitic privately. So perhaps it was hardly surprising that Jews were not promoted to high office.[64]

The brilliant and flamboyant Gilbert Beyfus QC (1885–1960), one of the leading advocates of his day, was one partly Jewish candidate suitable for high office who was overlooked because of these antisemitic undercurrents. He had never faltered in his lifelong atheism. 'I may not be a very good Jew but I've

[62] Summerfield, 'Anglo-Jewry and the Law', p. iv.

[63] On Sir Henry Herman Slesser, see Joyce M. Bellamy and John Saville (eds.), *Dictionary of Labour Biography* (Basingstoke: Macmillan, 1993), ix. 258–65.

[64] Interview with Frederic Landau, 6 Aug. 1996.

no use for the Christian religion. I don't believe a word of it', he once told a colleague, declining his invitation to be a godfather of his child. Assisted by his father's law firm, Beyfus & Beyfus, he became an expert in moneylending transactions and bankruptcy claims, while his success after the First World War in *Dey* v. *Mayo* in the Appeal Court (1920) led to a steady flow of work in betting and wagering cases. Beyfus combined his predecessors' eloquence with a modern, simple, and direct style of speaking; and many have spoken of his capacity to absorb a myriad facts in a very short time. His complete mastery of the smallest details of a brief made him a devastating cross-examiner, and this, combined with a rare eloquence, made him notably persuasive with juries. On the other hand, his glamorous social life during the 1930s undermined his chances of promotion to the bench, and though there seemed to be an opportunity for him to fill such a vacancy in the early years of the Second World War, he was once again overlooked and his prospects of advancement faded altogether.[65]

If the Law List for 1939 is examined, it will be found that there were at this point few Jewish recorders (judges sitting in criminal courts), and that only three out of the sixty county court judges were Jewish: M. N. Drucquer, E. M. Konstam, and H. W. Samuel (a fourth, Sir Gerald Hurst, was descended from a German Jewish family called Hertz which abandoned any formal connection with Judaism in the mid-nineteenth century).[66] Whereas the Jewish county court judges associated themselves only minimally with the Jewish community, a different situation prevailed among the recorders. The careers of Samuel Henry Emanuel, the recorder of Winchester, and Adolph Max Langdon, the recorder of Salford, have been discussed earlier in this chapter; Abraham Montagu Lyons (1894–1961), the recorder of Grimsby and MP for East Leicester, participated in the deliberations of the Board of Deputies, sat on the Council of the AJA, and was a member of the committee set up by the Chief Rabbi in 1960 to inquire into the kosher meat trade.[67]

Sir Arthur Steibel (1875–1949) was educated at Clifton and Oxford, being called to the Bar in 1899. He was wounded during the First World War and lost a leg. The author of a standard work on company law, he was appointed Registrar in Companies (Winding Up) and Bankruptcy in 1920, and sixteen years later became the Senior Registrar, known for his courteous manner when presiding in court. He was also a warden of the West London Synagogue, treasurer of the Westminster Jews' Free School, chairman of the management committee of the West Central Jewish Lads' Club, and on the management committee of an old-age home. But the main focus of his energies was the Jewish Board of

[65] Ian Adamson, *The Old Fox* (London: Frederick Muller, 1963), 22, 23, 27–9, 87–96, 144–7; *The Times*, 31 Oct. 1960 (obituary of Beyfus).
[66] *The Law List 1939* (London: Stevens & Sons, 1939), pp. viii–xv.
[67] *JC* 1 Dec. 1961, p. 43 (obituary of Lyons).

Guardians, of which in 1912 he was elected vice-president and chairman of the Health Committee; later he presided over a number of other departments as well, and from 1920 until 1930 served the Board as president.[68] According to Vivian Lipman, his presidency was characterized 'by the same soundness of judgement and prudence' that he displayed in court, guiding the Board well through the financially difficult years of depression after 1920.[69] Between the wars, indeed, Jewish lawyers dominated the leadership of the Board of Deputies: H. S. Q. Henriques was president from 1912 until 1925, and Neville Laski served in the same capacity between 1933 and 1939.

In summary, then, the failure of Jews to reach the top tiers of the judiciary reflected in part the waning in the wealth and influence of the old Anglo-Jewish elite, in part the heightened antisemitism of the inter-war years, and in part the transitional nature of the period as one in which members of east European immigrant families were not completely accepted. Extensive communal involvement tended to be confined to certain committed individuals. Typically, Sir Benjamin Cohen KC, the son of Arthur Cohen, did 'not take any very active part in communal work'.[70] As in the Victorian age, it was easier for ambitious Jewish barristers to seek judicial appointments in the empire. B. L. Mosely became a judge in the Native Tribunals in Cairo, and during the First World War Dr Joseph Hockman resigned as minister of the New West End Synagogue to join the army, later becoming a barrister and a judge in an eastern British colony. Norman Bentwich's career prospered in the 1920s as Attorney-General of Palestine. Sidney Solomon Abrahams, the brother of the athlete Harold Abrahams, was made Chief Justice of Uganda in 1933, while Barthold Kisch rose to become a High Court judge in India, retiring in 1938.[71]

---

[68] *JC* 20 Mar. 1936, 25 Feb. 1949, p. 6 (obituary of Steibel).

[69] Lipman, *A Century of Social Service*, 178.   [70] *JC* 15 May 1931, p. 6 (on Cohen).

[71] *JC* 21 July 1916 (obituary of Mosely); Bentwich, *My Seventy Seven Years*, 20, 52–96; *JC* 27 Jan. 1933, p. 10 (on Abrahams), 2 Mar. 1962, p. 31 (obituary of Kisch).

SIX

Jews and the Courts
1900–1945

WERE Jews more active litigants in the English civil courts in the 1920s and 1930s than the bulk of the population, and did they appear more frequently in some of the criminal courts than is commonly believed? To both these questions, the answer appears to be yes. Did this hyperactivity in the law courts generate work for an increasing number of Jewish counsel and solicitors, and thus contribute to the expansion of the number of Jews in the legal profession during the 1930s? Again, the answer would have to be in the affirmative—but in this case a somewhat more qualified yes.

Woolfe Summerfield, an Anglo-Jewish barrister writing in 1924, asserted that immigrant Jews from eastern Europe were much more prone to resort to litigation than the more Anglicized sections of the Jewish community, although some of this litigation was concealed from public view because it was dealt with by a network of communal institutions set up to arbitrate in cases of dispute between Jews. Sometimes Jews went to Jewish courts run by rabbis; also, the Defence Committee of the Board of Deputies tried to keep cases out of the public domain by arbitration and by persuading parties to settle out of court. During the years between the two world wars Jews were more usually merchants, agents, and dealers rather than manufacturers and artisans. 'Thus it is indisputable', Summerfield remarked, 'that a very large proportion of those engaged in such businesses as money-lenders, credit drapers, suppliers of furniture and other commodities on the hire-purchase systems, are Jews. These types of business transactions involve the giving of credit over a period [of time] to the poorer members of the public in most cases.' When the payment of instalments fell into arrears, as it commonly did, Jewish claimants resorted to the county courts.

Thus it happens that the Jewish proprietors and members of the staffs of businesses of the type referred to so often display an extensive and peculiar knowledge of the highways and by-ways of the laws relating to the recovery of debts, promissory notes, bills of sale, distress, execution and the like; thus, it will be found that wherever there is an aggregation of Jews in any particular locality there a large proportion of the cases brought into the county courts are brought by Jews.

We have seen that a number of Jewish solicitors were the sons of moneylenders, and it is a reasonable inference that some of the children of these Jewish business-men frequenting the county courts also joined the legal profession to assist the family business. On the whole, Jews at this period did not resort so much to the High Court, although there were a number of notable communal cases involving Jewish charities and the regulation of *kashrut*, and the stipulation that claims involving sums over a certain level be heard in the High Court meant that the wealthier moneylenders utilized this venue.[1]

*

From 1911 to 1934 His Honour Judge Cluer sat in the Whitechapel and Shore-ditch county courts, which were thronged by Jewish litigants. Albert Rowland Cluer (1852–1942) was called to the Bar in 1877, was briefly recorder of Deal (1894–5), and then sat as a magistrate from 1894 to 1911 before being appointed to the county court bench.[2] Peeved by the volubility of these east European Jewish immigrants and their rapid flow of English expressed in an incompre-hensible Yiddish idiom, and suspecting them of nefarious stratagems whenever they were in financial difficulty, the judge quickly became irritated and tended to indulge in antisemitic quips to entertain an audience of unemployed workers sitting at the back of the Whitechapel court. Yet there was another side to Judge Cluer. To one English barrister, the judge stood out

in clear relief as an able, impartial, and courageous man with a single eye to the truth, with a strict sense of honour, and unvarying in his kindness towards the widow and orphan, the downtrodden and oppressed. No judge had a wider knowledge of life, or deeper sympathy with the trials of the poor . . . [He was always] a keen critic and a fear-less exposer of fraud and deceit. As a Police Magistrate, Judge Cluer was conspicuously broadminded and tolerant. He is . . . the last person in the world to insult Jew or Gentile, or to allow religious and racial questions to warp his judgment.[3]

Indeed, while sitting as the senior magistrate of the Old Street Magistrates' Court in October 1906, Cluer dealt in a most sympathetic manner with two young Jewish brothers found wandering around Old Montague Street in the East End without visible means of support. 'Jewish fathers are usually the best of fathers', he exclaimed,

and very, very rarely seek to escape their obligations in this way. They love their chil-dren too well. But there are exceptions to every rule, and [addressing the boys] you seem to have had a bad father unfortunately. You will both be sent to a Jewish boys'

---

[1] Summerfield, 'Anglo-Jewry and the Law', pp. iv, v.

[2] *Who Was Who 1941–1950* (London: A. & C. Black, 1967), 227.

[3] *JC* 30 June 1922, p. 15.

boarding school where you will live together, and be more happy and comfortable than wandering about the streets of London.[4]

Nor were these remarks unique; he consistently expressed such views about Jewish fathers. Commenting on the evidence when he was presiding over an interpleader case in the Whitechapel County Council in 1923, Judge Cluer stated 'that it appeared very strange to him that wives came complaining that their husbands were such brutes and outsiders. As far as Jewish husbands were concerned, he knew very well that no more devoted husbands or affectionate fathers were to be found.' The more tolerant and appealing side of Judge Cluer was shown again in September 1920, when he said 'He would not sit at White-chapel on Wednesday next, as it was the Day of Atonement, when no Jew would take part in litigation. "I must respect their principles", he added.'[5]

Nevertheless, there was undeniably a more boorish side of Judge Cluer, and this rankled with members of the Jewish community over a number of years, as is clear from an editorial in the *Jewish Chronicle* of 23 June 1922. 'Time after time attention has been drawn in the way in which he conducts himself, missing no opportunity for a vulgar display of rancorous prejudice against our people.' In one case,

After telling a judgment debtor, a Jew, that he had acted fraudulently and ought to be locked up, when the debtor said he was not now in the business he had carried on but his wife was, Judge CLUER proceeded to declare: 'that is another fraud and peculiarly characteristic of your race' . . . No-one in Judge CLUER's position has the right, and no-one ought to be allowed to employ that position to cast wanton offence upon a large section of the people who are under his jurisdiction.

The editorial suggested that the Board of Deputies should make represen-tations to the Lord Chancellor with the aim of either having the judge removed from the bench or at least having him transferred to some other county court.[6]

Instead, the Board took the easy option of arranging for a deputation of its president, H. S. Q. Henriques KC, himself a deputy county court judge, and its vice-president, Lord Rothschild, to call upon the judge on 18 September 1922 to voice the concern of the Jewish community about his behaviour in court. Judge Cluer 'frankly stated that it was quite possible that he had made the remark in question, but that if he did so he much regretted the occurrence. It was improper for him to have attributed any form of dishonesty to persons of a particular religion. He expressed his willingness to write a letter to that effect.' He wrote the letter, and the storm of protest duly abated—but at the same time he penned a second, separate letter to Henriques, in which he claimed 'that a

[4] *JC* 2 Nov. 1906.
[5] *JC* 12 Oct. 1923, 19 Oct. 1923, p. 31, 17 Sept. 1920.
[6] *JC* 23 June 1922, p. 8.

Russian defendant only last week denied that he had retained Mr Emanuel as his Solicitor & asserted that for the sake of £9 odd Mr Emanuel had committed perjury in making his claim. It is difficult not to speak severely in such cases.' Here Judge Cluer, as so often, imputed the basest of motives to a Jewish litigant who appeared before him, and speaking as one judge to a colleague who understood foreign Jewish foibles, asked him to sympathize with his conduct in court.[7]

The *Jewish Chronicle* returned to the attack against Judge Cluer on 10 May 1929, citing some new outrageous comments of the judge which had been quoted in the press. It asked,

Cannot some action be taken by some representative body such as the Deputies, who not long ago made formal complaints about this Judge, which would result in JUDGE CLUER in future giving his valuable services on the Bench in some Court where Jews are not likely so constantly to be litigants before him and, as evidently happens, to upset his judicial attitude? It is not right that Jewish witnesses, or those who bring their cases to the Whitchapel County Court, should be bullied and browbeaten by the one who is there first and foremost for their protection.[8]

On 31 May 1929 J. M. Rich, the secretary of the Board, wrote to Judge Cluer, objecting to two statements of his which were reported in the press. The first was: 'In the 34 years that I have sat in this district no Englishman has ever come to tell me falsehoods of this kind. It is always your people' (meaning Jews). This was surpassed by an even more outrageously antisemitic remark: 'Your only idea of a trial is to shout at the top of your voice so that the Judge shall not be able to hear the other side. That will never succeed with me. You did succeed once and you have paid for it for two thousand years.' Rich deprecated the statements and their reflections on 'a community which comprises many thousands of orderly and upright citizens'.

A few days later the judge replied, stating that no objection could be taken to a statement which he had made many times, namely 'that no English workman who has been paid his wages has ever sued his employer in my Courts and sworn that he did not receive them, whereas foreign Jewish workmen have in many cases taken such proceedings against their employers and supported their claims by perjury'. His remarks, he asserted, were not intended to reflect on the Jewish community. He ended by saying, 'If you were to spend some time in my Courts, I do not think you would identify yourselves with the individuals to whom my remarks were addressed.' When Rich wrote back, dwelling on the absurdity of his 'reference to the trial of Jesus as a present reproach to Jewish

---

[7] Report of an interview with Judge Cluer, 18 Sept. 1922, Acc. 312 B4/CL6 Board of Deputies Archive; Judge Cluer to Henry Henriques, 23 Sept. 1922, Acc. 312 B4/CL6, Board of Deputies Archive. [8] *JC* 10 May 1929, p. 8.

litigants', Judge Cluer fobbed him off with the reply that his letter contained nothing new which merited an answer.[9]

Having brushed aside these communal protests about his behaviour, Cluer became increasingly cantankerous in later years when confronted by Jewish litigants. A stream of letters from disgruntled Jewish businessmen flowed into the offices of the Board of Deputies. A Mr Paros wrote on 22 October 1930 that

Some people were in the witness box [in the Shoreditch County Court] who could hardly speak English and instead of helping them as a Judge should do he made a laughing stock of them and bullied them to such an extent that they could not answer. Furthermore when they answered he twisted the answers about in several ways and called the people liars . . . There were also other cases where he treated the Jews in the same way. Judge Cluer further made a remark that 'one could not expect a straight-forward deal in Shoreditch or Whitechapel and if one wanted a straight deal one would have to go elsewhere'. During the day he made such remarks as 'You can neither read nor write yet you come to a Heathen Court'.[10]

Earlier, in April 1928, the judge had sounded a similar refrain, exclaiming, 'But there is no defilement now attached to coming to a heathen Court, except by the most ignorant Russian Jews.'[11] A Mr Gershon Pick declared in 1931 that his own 'experience of him is as follows: My Jewish name he could not tolerate, on one occasion when I entered the plaintiff's box he remarked "Where do they come from? What names they come here with."' Moreover, Pick asserted that he had

an order for £35 against one man a builder, from the Registrar's court, and when I brought him to Cluer on a judgement Summons, he does all he can to prevent me getting the money. On a previous occasion the same builder with the same solicitor as I had was before him with a similar case and the judge made him pay immediately or alternatively go to prison, but on that occasion the plaintiff was a gentile, so he received justice.[12]

Next a Mr Samuel Zilesnick, a cabinet-maker from Bethnal Green, complained about a hearing at the Shoreditch County Court before Judge Cluer on 28 January 1932, where he was represented by a Jewish barrister and the other party, a Christian, by a non-Jewish counsel. Zilesnick took exception to two remarks of the judge. One was: 'If you and a Jury of your own Race were sitting there [pointing to the jury box] babbling for a number of hours, then you would win the case.' The other was an audible outburst of the judge, when Zilesnick's

---

[9] J. M. Rich to Judge Cluer, 31 May 1929, Judge Cluer to J. M. Rich, 5 June 1929, J. M. Rich to Judge Cluer, 11 June 1929, Acc. 312 B4/CL6, Board of Deputies Archive.

[10] W. Paros to the Secretary of the Board of Deputies, 22 Oct. 1930.   [11] *JC* 27 Apr. 1928, p. 33.

[12] Gershon Pick to the Secretary of the Board of Deputies, 4 Feb. 1931, Acc. 312 B4/CL6, Board of Deputies Archive.

daughter was giving evidence: 'How can we expect a Jew to tell the Truth in a Heathen Court?'[13] The judge's suspicion of the veracity of evidence given by Jewish witnesses is also evident in another matter which came before him later in the same year. A Mr Epstein complained of a case in which both the parties were Jewish and where the plaintiff, a poor Jewish girl, had four witnesses to corroborate her evidence, but where Judge Cluer preferred to accept the evidence of the defendant's only witness, who was not Jewish, although the plaintiff claimed she was committing perjury.[14]

As far as Zilesnick's case is concerned, Judge Cluer's misplaced utterances elicited a rebuke in the editorial columns of the *Jewish Chronicle* on 12 February 1932, which was hardly going to deter him from uttering fresh infelicitous remarks. Mr L. S. Green, a Jewish barrister who represented Mr Zilesnick at the hearing, privately admitted to the Board that it was

nonsense to take any notice of such remarks, which are the result of momentary irritation, and not intended to injure anyone's susceptibilities. Mr Green does not think that Judge Cluer is in any way antisemitic. On the contrary, he understands our people well . . . In Mr Green's opinion Judge Cluer has a good deal to put up with in the Whitechapel and Shoreditch Courts, and is a subject for sympathy rather than for condemnation.[15]

This was a view shared by the majority of Jewish barristers who appeared before Judge Cluer. 'The lawyers all assure me', continued the *Jewish Chronicle*, 'that he [the judge] displays a great commonsense, and that as a lawyer he is beyond reproach.' This view explains the muted response in the Jewish press and the unwillingness of the Board to take any forceful action. Under Judge Cluer and his predecessor a very competent Yiddish-speaking interpreter was attached to the Whitechapel County Court until 1919, by which time Cluer himself could grasp some of the Yiddish remarks muttered by litigants under their breath; and certain members of the Board seem to have sympathized with Judge Cluer's misgivings about the evidence given to him by Jews of east European origin, who lacked English manners and polish. Typical was a letter sent by the secretary of the Board to H. H. Haldin KC on 9 February 1931. 'As you know, these complaints against Judge Cluer have been repeatedly considered by the Law & Parliamentary Committee, but it has always been deemed inadvisable to take action.' Edward Abinger stated that 'Although some people do not like his mannerisms . . . his two courts are about the busiest in London, litigants knowing

[13] Samuel Zilesnick to the Secretary of the Board of Deputies, 8 Feb. 1932, Acc. 312 B4/CL6, Board of Deputies Archive.

[14] Epstein to the Secretary of the Board of Deputies, June 1932, Acc. 312 B4/CL6, Board of Deputies Archive.

[15] *JC* 12 Feb. 1932; note of telephone conversation with L. S. Green, compiled by B. A. Zaiman, 3 Mar. 1932, Acc. 312 B4/CL6, Board of Deputies Archive.

they will get a good hearing and justice.' Moreover, despite the judge's idiosyn-
crasies, Frederic Landau, a barrister whose own family had come from eastern
Europe in the mid-nineteenth century, felt that he was not antisemitic.[16]

For a balanced yet sympathetic view of Judge Cluer, we turn to the memoirs
of Bernard Gillis, a rising young Jewish barrister in the late 1920s and 1930s,
himself from an east European background. Gillis asserted that Cluer

required a high standard from those, counsel or solicitors, who practised there [in his
courts]. He was highly regarded, both as a sound lawyer and a judge of fact. He was a
classical scholar, too, and his judgments were excellent prose essays. He had a sharp
tongue for the evasive witness, and little patience for advocacy based on meagre or
trivial material. Many of us thought he expressed his views too quickly and gave insufficient allowance for the ordinary person who must have felt uneasy in an unusual place
. . . Many of the litigants were foreign Jews with little knowledge of English. Their
mannerisms were certainly not English; when giving evidence, some of them answered
by questioning the lawyer and avoiding difficult questions. There were times when
some of the remarks made by the judge were described as anti-Semitic. To the frank
and honest person, he showed no impatience; to the others, those especially he regarded
as untruthful, he made clear what he thought of them. To one witness, whom he did not
believe, he said, 'If I had the power, you would not go home in the motor car which is
kept in your wife's name, or to the comfortable house in Stamford Hill which she owns
to stop your creditors getting paid; if I had the power you would go to prison where all
perjurers go; if I had the power it would be for years.' Unperturbed the witness retorted,
'Your Honour, what's the good of talking "if"?'[17]

Some Jewish barristers, solicitors (for example, Edward Iwi; see Chapter 13),
and legal experts such as clerks and law reporters who were conversant with Judge
Cluer's ways, did regard him as antisemitic. Henry Cecil recalled that 'Judge
Cluer . . . did not like his Jewish customers. He would almost invariably prefer
the evidence of a witness who was not a Jew. I remember once appearing in a case
before him and confidently calling the next witness. "Call Mr Brown," I said.
The witness went into the box . . . "B-r-a-u-n," said Cluer, and he was right.' So
too, Serjeant A. M. Sullivan QC, a feared Irish advocate, claimed that

there is no doubt that he [Cluer] was addicted to making observations about the eastern
colony of Whitechapel that were uncomplimentary to their ancient race. 'Tell me', he
once said to a red-headed Irishman who was decorating his untruthful evidence with a
wealth of detail, 'did you put on your hat to be sworn [as was the Jewish practice]?' 'No,
your Honour.' 'But you know you are telling lies as if you did?'

---

[16] *JC* 12 Feb. 1932, p. 8; J. M. Rich to H. H. Haldin, 9 Feb. 1931, Acc. 312 B4/CL6, Board of
Deputies Archive; *JC* 25 Apr. 1924, p. 8 (obituary of Salo Rehfisch); Abinger, *Forty Years at the Bar*,
278, 279; interview with the late Frederic Landau, 6 Aug. 1996.
[17] Gillis, 'Once Round Only' (unpublished memoirs), 18, 19. Gillis's own career is discussed in
Ch. 5 above.

Morris Sellers, a law clerk and journalist, complained to the Board on 30 November 1929 that 'I hear the Judge passing his fantastical remarks without fear or discrimination—constantly.'[18]

A couple more examples of this practice will suffice. In March 1926 Judge Cluer exclaimed, 'It ought to be almost a capital offence, mutilating our fine, English language like this man [a foreign Jewish witness] is doing, but we must put up with it.' Two years later, when trying a case over whether a disputed discount should be allowed, the judge declared that 'we must go by ordinary English arithmetic not by abstruse Hebraic calculations'. What aggrieved Jewish litigants was a raw sense of injustice, 'for I have heard of litigants with impeccable cases who fear to commit themselves to the lash of his tongue', added a writer in the *Jewish Chronicle*. They were not alone; the Catholic Church, too, had been compelled to make separate representations to him about his obtuse remarks concerning Roman Catholics.[19]

For all his insensitivity on some occasions, on others Judge Cluer was notably sympathetic to the evidence of workmen, ridiculing the evidence of experts called to testify against them on behalf of their employers. When a steel splinter caused the loss of an employee's eye, Cluer reprimanded Sir Ambrose Woodall, a medical expert giving evidence on behalf of an insurance company. 'Excuse me, Sir Ambrose, what a pity you weren't advising the Almighty at the creation; and advised him that a workman could work as well with one eye as with two.'[20]

Even allowing for the evasions of some Jewish witnesses and the innocent misunderstandings of others, there was a class of respectable Jewish businessmen whom Judge Cluer treated with disdain and against whom he was consistently biased. Nor did these individuals always receive the support that was their due from the barristers who represented them in court, or from the communal institutions—pre-eminently the Board of Deputies—that were supposed to defend their right to fair play within the British legal system.

What is clear is that the Whitechapel and Shoreditch county courts were thronged by Jewish junior members of the Bar representing litigants who were co-religionists, while in other county courts many Jewish litigants appeared in person. Bernard Gillis confessed that he did not like attending county courts because of the nature of much of the litigation.

Here, one saw the struggles of the poor, landlords and tenants of slum properties in endless disputes over unpaid rents or houses unfit to live in; here were men and women

[18] Edward F. Iwi to J. M. Rich, 10 June 1929; Cecil, *Memories*, 53; A. M. Sullivan, *The Last Serjeant: The Memoirs of Serjeant A. M. Sullivan QC* (London: Macdonald, 1952), 286, 287; Morris Sellers to Major Brunel Cohen M., 30 Nov. 1929, Acc. 312 B4/CL6, Board of Deputies Archive.

[19] *JC* 19 Mar. 1926, p. 55, 13 Apr. 1928, p. 24, 12 Feb. 1932, p. 8.

[20] Interview with the late Frederic Landau, 6 Aug. 1996.

without work or enough for their ordinary needs offering to pay a shilling or two for the boots and clothes bought from the tally man on weekly instalments.[21]

*

While Jews seldom resorted to burglary or housebreaking, or crimes of personal violence, they were more regularly associated with such crimes as long-firm (credit) fraud (see p. 145 below), acting as fences, bankruptcy tainted by fraud, arson involving fraudulent claims against insurance companies, and sometimes company fraud. 'On a conservative estimate,' Summerfield declared in 1924, 'something like ten per cent of those charged with crime month by month at the Old Bailey Courts, the London Sessions, etc., are Jews, of whom something like ninety per cent are charged with those particular classes of offences against property and commercial stability.'[22] A High Court judge, Mr Justice Rowlatt, trying a civil dispute between two Jewish businessmen in 1929, ruled against a witness who objected to being questioned about his bankruptcy. The judge continued:

All the people in these cases have been bankrupt. All these people have their businesses carried on by companies, and all these people have their wives to conduct their businesses. So answer the questions. And there is usually a burglary in these cases as well . . . This is one of those squabbles between people who have come as strangers to this country and whose minds I don't understand. They trade with very little capital, and they can't settle the simplest business disputes without bringing them into the law courts which the people of this country supply to try the cases these foreign people bring.

So far from admonishing the judge for a biased expression of opinion, the editor of the *Jewish Chronicle* concurred with his viewpoint. 'Everyone who knows anything of some of our public courts and the Jewish cases that arise there, will agree that the learned Judge did not very much exaggerate the facts or draw unfair inferences from them. Our own law reports week by week are largely confirmatory of the Judge's remarks.'[23]

Let us turn first to an examination of the bankruptcy cases in which Jews were involved. Each week the *London Gazette* published details of receiving orders and other bankruptcy notices. In the week Summerfield wrote his article in October 1924, there were two lists of bankrupts comprising respectively twenty-one and seven names, the number of Jews totalling seven in the first list and five in the other one. 'When one recalls the proportionate Jewish population in the London area, one-third and five-sevenths respectively of the total number of

[21] Gillis, 'Once Round Only', 19; Gerald Hurst, *Closed Chapters* (Manchester: Manchester University Press, 1942), 141.

[22] Summerfield, 'Anglo-Jewry and the Law', p. ii.   [23] *JC* 1 Mar. 1929, p. 32, 8 Mar. 1929, p. 5.

bankrupts seems to be a proportion calling for explanation', commented Summerfield.[24] The discrepancy may be accounted for in part by the higher proportion of Jews than of the general population who were self-employed, and by the economic vicissitudes of the 1930s; but even so this still left a considerable percentage of Jewish businessmen prone to bankruptcy and sometimes to fraudulent insolvency practices. This may in part be attributable to Jewish immigrants from eastern Europe having grown up in countries where they were discriminated against in trading, tax, and educational matters, and where as a result they resorted to systematic chicanery and bribery in order to evade the restrictions of the repressive authorities. 'Licences and permits in czarist Russia, especially in governed Poland, were not issued in accordance with regulations. Reb Avigdor [David Ben-Gurion's father, who practised as an unqualified lawyer in Plonsk] had to flatter and bribe officials and justices; he participated in the conflicts between petitioners, who were quite capable of cheating on each other.'[25] Among a minority of second-generation immigrants to Britain there was a carry-over in these hostile attitudes to the state, and the *Jewish Chronicle* complained from time to time that certain fraudulent bankrupts among them, once out of prison, immediately became socially acceptable within the community and were even honoured. Charles Emanuel, the solicitor to the Board of Deputies, 'was convinced that bankruptcy was considered far less of a disgrace among the lower-middle-class Jews, than among the same class of Christians'.[26]

In Leeds in 1920 the Official Receiver castigated a Jewish debtor who, 'the day after the receiving order was made . . . was proved to have had his pockets full of money, which he spent freely in Leeds, boasting the while that he had plenty of cash, and did not care for the Official Receiver or anybody else in Leeds.' Again, in Liverpool in December 1923 a prosecution for perjury was instituted against an alleged Jewish bankrupt who forged an accountant's signature on a balance-sheet to obtain a loan from a bank, and who pretended to have negligible assets, but who, when he was arrested, was found to be in possession of £1,000 worth of certificates.

In October 1924 Sir Henry Dickens KC, the Common Serjeant, after trying a Jewish commercial traveller at the Old Bailey on a charge of obtaining goods by false pretences and bankruptcy charges, commented that 'These fraudulent bankruptcies are now getting almost insupportable. I have tried many of them, and I have found as a rule that the people who are fraudulent bankrupts are aliens.' So too, in 1925 at the Liverpool Bankruptcy Court, 'Mr Nield, the Registrar, said that some of the aliens, notably from Russia, abused the credit system, which was a necessity in British commerce. By some strange instinct

[24] Summerfield, 'Anglo-Jewry and the Law'; *JC Supplement*, 31 Oct. 1924, p. v.
[25] Shabtai Teveth, *Ben-Gurion: The Burning Ground 1886–1948* (London: Hale, 1987), 7.
[26] *JC* 3 Dec. 1926, p. 15.

they evaded bankruptcy offences and appeared in court with liabilities of thousands and assets mostly *nil*.' When a certain Jewish cabinet manufacturer applied to the London Bankruptcy Court for discharge from bankruptcy in 1929, the registrar said 'he had seldom read a worse report of conduct than that of the bankrupt . . . I wish I could send you back to Russia'. In his report the Official Receiver opposed the order for a discharge on grounds of the debtor's

continuance of trading with knowledge of insolvency; that the bankrupt had contributed to his bankruptcy by unjustifiable extravagance in living; that he had within three months preceding the bankruptcy order given undue preference to certain creditors; that he had been guilty of misconduct as a trader in disposing of stock in trade by way of sale at prices below cost; and that he had been guilty of misconduct in the proceedings by filing an inaccurate and misleading statement of affairs.[27]

When Jack Cooklin came before the Liverpool Bankruptcy Court in 1930, he was the seventh member of his family to appear there within ten years. 'The family's failures involved creditors in losses of £30,000. Mr Registrar Symond remarked that the appearances of members of this family were approaching the dimensions of a public scandal, and the Official Receiver . . . later said that all the circumstances of the debtor's failure pointed to nothing less than a swindle.'[28]

Arthur Stiebel, registrar of the Bankruptcy Court and president of the Jewish Board of Guardians, confessed in 1925 that there had been a wave of fraudulent trading in the Jewish community since the collapse of the wartime boom. During the 1920s Jewish businessmen were often indicted with an offence known as long-firm fraud—buying goods on credit and then selling them cheaply for cash, while not paying the people from whom they were bought. In December 1924 Sir Henry Dickens complained 'that fraud of this kind had reached such a pitch now in this country as to create almost a panic among manufacturers', causing him to pass harsh sentences on three Jewish cloth merchants. A month later, when sentencing some other Jewish traders for this offence at the Central Criminal Court, Dickens remarked that 'These kinds of frauds have to be put a stop to, and I intend to stop them. All over the country people are being defrauded of thousands and thousands of pounds, it goes to the root of all credit, and without credit business is impossible.' In another such case in March 1925, three Jewish cloth and woollen merchants were convicted of defrauding creditors and obtaining goods by false pretences. Until 1924 they had acted honestly and properly, but they had then purchased a great quantity of goods, for which it was alleged they never intended to pay, and the business collapsed with a deficit of £56,800. At a preliminary hearing a detective gave

[27] *JC* 3 Dec. 1920, p. 22, 23 Nov. 1923, p. 23, 31 Oct. 1924, p. 30, 3 Apr. 1925, p. 50, 5 Apr. 1929, p. 38.   [28] *JC* 13 June 1924, p. 27, 23 May 1930, p. 32.

evidence that he had found 500 one-pound notes, together with documents, stuffed between the mattresses of a director's bed. When sentencing the accused the same judge, Sir Henry Dickens, stated that 'People have no conception as to the stupendous losses sustained by traders. It has to be stamped out. I find [that a sentence] of penal servitude is the only way.'[29]

In yet another such case tried at the Old Bailey in February 1929 before Sir Ernest Wild KC, the recorder of London, Lewis Konskier, a manufacturing furrier at the cheap end of the trade, and his workshop manager, Mark Silverstein, were charged with conspiring to cheat and defraud trade creditors, and with obtaining a large quantity of furs with intent to defraud a number of firms. Roland Oliver KC and Mr H. Infield acted for the prosecution, while Norman Birkett KC and Mr Dobson represented Konskier, and Mr G. G. Raphael appeared for Silverstein. Because Konskier went into a property speculation in Houndsditch which he did not understand, his business was placed in a position of hopeless insolvency at the end of 1927. Instead of calling a meeting of creditors, Konskier—with his manager's assistance—let it be known that he was trading in a better class of goods and 'went into a perfect orgy of buying on credit £23,000 worth of furs in three months', ending up with a deficit close to £30,000. They then concocted a story that £20,000 worth of furs had been stolen from their cellar, but the jury found that this claim was bogus. Nor would the judge accept Mr Raphael's plea on behalf of Silverstein that he was in a subordinate position, without knowledge of his employer's true financial situation, and that, therefore, he had no case to answer. Taking into account Konskier's poor health, his previous good character, and his ill-fated venture into the property market, Sir Ernest Wild substituted a lesser sentence of twenty months' imprisonment, instead of five years' penal servitude. Silverstein was given a shorter sentence of fifteen months in prison.[30]

Jews also featured in two high-profile arson cases in 1923 and 1933. Apart from these two cases, there were a few other instances in the early 1920s and in 1930 of Jews setting fire to their business premises in order to file fictitious claims, for which the culprits received prison sentences.[31] Many fire insurance companies refused to insure Jewish businesses against the risk of fire because of the high incidence of Jewish claimants in such cases. Although some suspected that this attitude was due to antisemitism, Summerfield argued that this was not so: rather, insurance companies had made careful actuarial calculations of the

[29] *JC* 3 Apr. 1925, p. 9; Cecil, *Memories*, 49; Geoffrey Dorling Roberts, *Law and Life* (London: Allen, 1964), 98, 99; *JC* 26 Dec. 1924, p. 22, 23 Jan. 1925, p. 30, 30 Jan. 1925, p. 29, 6 Mar. 1925, p. 35.
[30] *JC* 8 Feb. 1929, p. 29, 22 Feb. 1929, p. 29.
[31] *JC* 8 Feb. 1924, p. 21 (*Goldblatt*), 4 July 1924, p. 29, 11 July 1924, p. 33, 18 July 1924, p. 29 (*Woolf Perkins*), 16 May 1930, p. 45 (*Benning and Garfield*); Roberts, *Law and Life*, 97, 98.

risk of insuring certain classes of people against fire damage and had concluded that it might not be profitable to insure Jewish businesses.[32]

Similarly, in Brooklyn, with the onset of the Depression the fire brigade made 10,181 calls in 1928 and 15,817 in 1932, and the insurance companies paid out $8 million in 1932 compared with $5 million four years earlier. Indeed, there was a common saying among Jews that 'two fires and a failure make a rich gentleman', and Robert Rice claimed that 'In such years [of economic contraction in the United States] one of the most popular methods of eluding bankruptcy . . . [was] to collect fire insurance.'[33] In any event, not all the claims under the English policies for fires were exaggerated. When Dombrofski Barnett sued a Lloyd's underwriter in the High Court in 1924 for non-payment on a claim, he was successful. The Lord Chief Justice severely reprimanded the underwriter, saying that it seemed to him a grave matter 'that when a respectable man claimed for his loss by fire he should be met by a defence consisting of a chain of charges of fraud, arson, and forgery, evidently based on trash'.[34]

In the autumn of 1923 Joseph Engelstein, Bernard Stolerman, and Julius Brust were charged at the Central Criminal Court with trying to defraud the Sun Insurance Company by setting fire to Stolerman's furniture-making workshop. Despite the fact that two eminent barristers, Sir Edward Marshall Hall KC and Sir Henry Curtis-Bennett KC, appeared for Engelstein and Stolerman, they were convicted by the jury along with the third defendant. Sir Ernest Wild, the judge, sentenced all three to penal servitude: six years in the case of Engelstein and lesser terms for the other two. Engelstein was known to the police as 'the King of the Fire Raisers' and had set fire to hundreds of premises in London and the provinces between 1920 and 1923, charging a fixed scale of fees for his fraudulent fires. Before Engelstein's appearance in court in 1923 the insurance companies had been forced to pay out many claims which they suspected were bogus, but were unable to prove that this was the case.[35]

In the summer of 1933 Leopold Harris, a Jewish fire insurance assessor, was tried with sixteen others for defrauding insurance companies by presenting bogus claims. After hearing news of a fire through agents, Harris would appear and offer to handle a claim on behalf of the insured for 5 per cent commission. Harris was disliked by the insurance companies because he invariably presented inflated claims. Not satisfied with his profits from this source, Harris became greedy and set up bogus businesses, in which he had a large stake, insuring the premises and stock for vastly inflated sums; after arranging for fires to be

---

[32] Summerfield, 'Anglo-Jewry and the Law', pp. ii, iii.

[33] Robert Rice, *The Business of Crime* (London: Gollancz, 1956), 21, 41–5, 62. Rice says that 'Sapphire was a specialist in burning Jewish businesses' in Brooklyn in the early 1930s, but there were also half a dozen Italian arsonists.

[34] *JC* 4 July 1924, p. 28.   [35] *The Times*, 25, 26, 27, 28 Sept. 1923; *JC* 5 Oct. 1923, p. 5.

started at the premises, Harris would submit a claim for an excessive amount. Harris was assisted by his brother David, brother-in-law Harry Gould (formerly Harris Goldstein), Louis Jarvis (formerly Jacobs), and others. Among counsel appearing for the defendants in 1933 were Sir George Jones, Sir Henry Curtis-Bennett, Norman Birkett, Walter Monckton, and Eric Sachs. Harris received a sentence of fourteen years' penal servitude, and again the others were given lesser sentences; but so accomplished a fire assessor was Harris that his services were utilized in assessing bomb damage during the Second World War.[36]

During the 1920s and the 1930s there was a spate of crimes in the City of London associated with share-pushing. 'A share-pusher', explains G. D. Roberts,

would rent an office at an address which suggested commercial probity: Gracechurch Street, perhaps, or Throgmorton or Broad Street. Then for several months he built up confidence by circulating ordinary Stock Exchange news to carefully chosen victims—clergymen, widows, spinsters and so on—living fifty or more miles away in the provinces. These victims were invited to . . . invest in shares recommended by the 'pusher'. At first the victims were allowed to make small profits on their dealings. Then came visits from touts: well-dressed aliens [a euphemism for Jews] usually, highly persuasive, earning 25 per cent commission, arriving at the door in expensive cars. They offered shares of the type which had already shown a profit, dazing the victims with promises of fabulous riches.[37]

The customers had to pay for these worthless shares by giving their own holdings of shares in blue-chip companies in exchange; but soon they realized that the shares which they had purchased were valueless.

Most of the principal company fraudsters, such as Horatio Bottomley, Jabez Balfour, Hooley, and Farrow, were in fact not Jewish. Clarence Hatry was of Jewish descent, though according to the *Jewish Chronicle* 'no longer Jewish', and was a brilliant reconstructer of companies; however, he came to grief in a bid to amalgamate steel companies, forging documents in the attempt to make up a £3 million shortfall and then seeing his shares collapse in the crash of 1929. Among the share-pushers, the most prominent, Edward Harold Guylee, was of impeccable English descent and a churchwarden in Surrey; and many of the share-pushing companies were staffed by non-Jews as well as Jews.[38]

Jacob Factor, who fled to the United States in the early 1930s, has already appeared in Chapter 5, as the prime mover in the 'Guinea Gramophone' case. It was estimated that nearly £800,000 passed through Factor's account in 1929,

---

[36] William Charles Crocker, *Far From Humdrum: A Lawyer's Life* (London: Hutchinson, 1967), 113–77; Browne, *Sir Travers Humphreys*, 302–19; Harold Dearden, *The Fire Raisers: The Story of Leopold Harris and his Gang* (London: Heinemann, 1934).   [37] Roberts, *Law and Life*, 100–6.
[38] A. F. L. Deeson, *Great Swindlers* (London: Foulsham, 1971), 126–35 (on Hatry); *JC* 13 Dec. 1929, p. 37.

and nearly twice that sum in 1930, when there was as yet no suspicion of fraud. In February 1931 Herbert John Spellen, Joseph Wise, Frederick Newbury, and Barnett Leon Elman were charged with conspiring with each other and others, including Factor (by this time out of the country), to obtain money and valuable securities from the general public by the false pretence that the Broad Street Press was carrying on a genuine business as stock and share brokers. In fact, the prosecution claimed that the accused were defrauding their clients by foisting worthless shares upon them in exchange for money and good securities. At the Old Bailey trial Newbury was given three years' penal servitude, and two others of the accused received lesser prison sentences. On appeal, however, the Court of Criminal Appeal later quashed the convictions of two appellants because Judge Holman Gregory had misdirected the jury.[39]

In another case a Mr Godfrey (alias Skylinski), who managed the Financial Telegraph Limited—a bucket-shop for gambling in stocks and shares, used to extract £500,000 from the public—was given a seven-year prison sentence for selling worthless shares.[40] Serge Rubinstein, the son of a Russian banker and a manipulator of company shares, became managing director of the Chosen Corporation, which owned mines in Korea worth over £2 million. He stripped the company of its assets in 1933 by exchanging its shares for worthless shares from the Banque Franco-Asiatic; only after prolonged litigation on both sides of the Atlantic did the shareholders settle in 1946 for half the value of the assets.[41]

An examination of these and other trials from the 1920s and 1930s seems to confirm that when Jews were charged with serious criminal offences, they would for preference invariably instruct their solicitors to brief the leading counsel at the Bar, such as Sir Edward Marshall Hall, Sir Patrick Hastings, Sir Henry Curtis-Bennett, and Norman Birkett, who were not Jewish. However, if they could not afford the fees, they might go to junior counsel, who might be Jewish. As we have seen, Mr G. G. Raphael appeared for Silverstein at the Old Bailey in 1929; and Philip Vos successfully defended a Jewish furrier against a charge of arson at the same court three years earlier. While it is relatively easy to discover who the counsel were in those cases which the press highlighted, it is much more difficult to find out whether any particular Jewish solicitors' firms were developing an expertise in this type of criminal work. It is apparent, though, that Jewish solicitors of east European origin, such as Hyman Fishman and Morris Teff, were beginning to appear both for the defence and the prosecution at the preliminary hearings in magistrates' courts.[42]

[39] Roland Wild and Derek Curtis-Bennett, *'Curtis': The Life of Sir Henry Curtis-Bennett KC* (London: Frank Cassell, 1937), 275; *JC* 27 Feb. 1931, p. 32, 26 June 1931, p. 27, 10 July 1931, p. 31.
[40] Roberts, *Law and Life*, 101, 102.
[41] Deeson, *Great Swindlers*, 136–42 (on Serge Rubinstein); *Financial Times*, 4, 5, 6, 9, 10 Nov. 1943.
[42] *JC* 5 Mar. 1926, p. 31.

Many of the business failures of the immigrant section of the Anglo-Jewish community, including some of the more marginal cases of long-firm fraud which ended in bankruptcy, also had a positive side. 'Jews are traders on their own account in a much greater proportion than the general public', suggested Mentor in the *Jewish Chronicle* in 1930.

That necessarily exposes them the more to the risks of offending under the laws of Bankruptcy. But they prefer to be independent traders—their own masters—because they are enterprising and 'go-ahead'. They are not content to go on all their lives working for others at just a living wage; they like to exercise their brains for themselves because they feel that every Jewish Jack is as good as his master, and if he be a Jacob he is ever so much better! But in addition Jews are a little more enterprising and are possessed of the urge to gamble so as to become rich if not quickly then the quicker. And in deploring the number of failures whose ghosts float around Carey Street in London, or the County Courts in the Provinces, we have to put against them . . . the number of those who have come through the fire of risk and adventure not alone unscathed but with fat material reward for their pains—the accumulation of which, without falling foul of the law, is often one of the things which gain for them the respect, the veneration and the honour of their co-religionists.[43]

It was also argued, as noted above, that the Anglo-Jewish community did not attach as much stigma to bankruptcy as the wider public.

The judiciary sometimes unfairly castigated these entrepreneurs, denouncing them as aliens and foreigners. But their successors, the Anglo-Jewish businessmen of the years after the Second World War, still taking risks and looking for new opportunities, dominated the property market, produced more goods for the affluent consumer, and perfected the techniques for taking over somnolent companies, thereby vastly increasing the wealth of the Jewish community—and, along with the newly expanded legal aid system, creating a financially secure base for supporting a much larger Jewish contingent in the nation's legal system. The trends in Anglo-Jewish business enterprise were all in place before the Second World War; they came to full fruition after it.

[43] *JC* 5 Sept. 1930, p. 11; see also *JC* 3 Apr. 1925, p. 9.

SEVEN

Jewish Solicitors
1890–1939

JOSEPH JACOBS found that in a London directory of 1883 there were forty-seven Jewish solicitors out of a total of 4,920; that is, slightly less than 1 per cent of solicitors were Jewish, a proportion smaller than the Jewish proportion of the population of London, where the vast majority of these Jewish practitioners would have been located. Manchester had four Jewish solicitors in 1871, and a similar number were practising in Birmingham in the 1870s and 1880s; the small Swansea Jewish community could not boast a single solicitor until the end of the 1880s, and that of Leeds not until 1890.[1]

At that time Jewish solicitors had been practising in England for a hundred years or more, the first Jews to be admitted as solicitors by the Society of Gentlemen Practitioners (later the Law Society) being Joseph Abrahams in 1770 and Joshua Montefiore, the uncle of the great philanthropist Sir Moses Montefiore, in 1784. In addition, Jews had frequently acted as notaries in London, where they were much in demand for attesting the validity of commercial and testamentary documents. Indeed, one of the oldest firms of notaries in London, H. de Pinna and John Venn, was founded by Jacob Sarfaty, who was granted a notarial faculty in 1772.[2]

The novelty of a Jew successfully establishing himself as a solicitor in an English provincial area at the beginning of the twentieth century is well illustrated in the career of Isadore Isaacs (1865–1901), who died prematurely, aged 36, from an illness brought on by overwork. 'Without any influence or substantial financial backing, Isadore Isaacs became one of the Town's [Sunderland's] leading solicitors, and was well known in the whole County of Durham; he had what is known as genius—"the infinite capacity of taking pains". He was a brilliant and fearless advocate, popular with his colleagues, and respected by the

---

[1] Jacobs, *Studies in Jewish Statistics*, 42; Williams, *The Making of Manchester Jewry*, 359; Zoe Josephs (ed.), *Birmingham Jewry*, 85; Tropp, *Jews in the Professions*, 5.

[2] Edgar Roy Samuel, 'Anglo-Jewish Notaries and Scriveners', *Transactions of the Jewish Historical Society of England*, 17 (1953), 131, 132, 143–5, 150–1; H. S. Q. Henriques, *The Jews and English Law* (Oxford: Oxford University Press, 1908), 205–6.

Bench', wrote his brother-in-law in a tribute. 'At first he elected to practise in the outlying districts of Sunderland, and though he had to combat considerable prejudice on account of his religion, he speedily made headway.' In 1894 he was elected as solicitor to the Durham Miner's Federation, carrying with it the responsibility for all their legal work, and rapidly built up a considerable practice. Although he was revered by the Durham miners for the way in which he stood up to the mine owners, he also enjoyed the confidence of the employers, who were impressed by his ability and fairness in negotiation. In the summer of 1900 he was appointed clerk to the Castle Eden Magistrates, beating a number of other candidates for the post. 'He was the first Jew in this country to hold the position of Magistrates's Clerk, and his success was all the more exceptional as it was achieved in a district where a considerable amount of ignorance and prejudice existed regarding the Jews.' He remained an Orthodox Jew, reciting a 'melodious' *haftarah* from the Prophets on the first day of the festival of Shavuot; despite his very busy life, he laboured unceasingly for the Sunderland Jewish community, helping them to acquire a new cemetery and also rendering them valuable legal and administrative assistance when the synagogue was renovated.[3]

Apart from the staple fare of solicitors' practices—conveyancing, probate, and litigation—these Jewish firms, which were closely connected by family and communal ties with the merchant and shopkeeping classes, specialized in commercial work, and, if need be, in guiding clients through the bankruptcy courts. In addition, there were a few firms which acquired a reputation by defending clients in the criminal courts, often the lowest class of legal work. For instance, the grandfather of Algernon Sydney (1834–1916), himself a distinguished solicitor, was Elias Isaacs of Jeffreys Square, St Mary Axe in the City of London, 'a well-known criminal lawyer in his day'.[4]

One of the Jewish bankruptcy experts, Hyman Montagu (1845–95), was articled to Messrs Linklaters, passing his law exams with distinction. After leaving their employment, he 'established himself as a bankruptcy lawyer, to which speciality he added a steadily augmenting practice'. He was an outstanding numismatist, the author of various standard works on this subject, honorary solicitor to the Industrial Committee of the Jewish Board of Guardians and to the Stepney Jewish Schools, and honorary secretary of Jews' College. 'He had not, however, taken an active part in the affairs of the community for several years', lamented the *Jewish Chronicle* on his death in 1895.[5]

---

[3] *JC* 9 Nov. 1900, p. 8, 31 May 1901, pp. 6, 19 (obituary of Isaacs); Arnold Levy, *History of the Sunderland Jewish Community 1755–1955* (London: Macdonald, 1956), 213, 214.

[4] *JC* 2 Jan. 1903, p. 10. Also worth noting is the early Victorian unqualified lawyer James Isaacs, who in 1830–1 defended Ikey Solomons, the chief of the London fences in the 1820s; see J. J. Tobias, *Prince of Fences: The Life and Crimes of Ikey Solomons* (London: Vallentine Mitchell, 1974), 64, 122.

[5] *JC* 22 Feb. 1895 (obituary of Montagu).

Henry Harris (1819–99), a relative of Sir George Jessel's mother, was born in Houndsditch, where his grandfather practised as an attorney, and was himself admitted as a solicitor in 1849. 'He soon had a large and important practice chiefly (in his early days) connected with the liquidation of Railway Companies and Banks. One such liquidation of the Royal Bank of Australia attracted much public attention.' As solicitor for the London Board for Shechitah he conducted the defence in *Schott* v. *Adler*, a libel suit brought by a butcher against the Chief Rabbi, where the former complained that he had been issued with a warning because he was not licensed for the sale of kosher meat, claiming that the Chief Rabbi had no right to exercise authority over him. Realizing that he may have been on shaky ground in English law, Harris managed to have the action stopped by the judge on a technicality, and the claim was dismissed. He assisted in drawing up the rules under the Common Law Procedure Act, and was offered the position of Chief Clerk in the Chancery Division, an offer which he refused. He was active in Jewish communal affairs and interested himself in the foundation of Jews' College, serving as honorary solicitor to the college as well as treasurer to the Morocco Relief Fund set up by the Board of Deputies for the relief of the community in Morocco, where in 1859 400 Jews were killed. Harris was strictly Orthodox and, as a friend of the Chief Rabbi, opposed the admission of Reform members to the Board of Deputies. He died childless, leaving a considerable estate estimated at £130,000.[6]

A third example of a Jewish bankruptcy specialist was Edward Lee (1839–1909), who qualified as a solicitor in 1873. 'His practice became an important one', commented his obituarist, 'and to this day the older officials of the public offices remember Mr Lee when a young man as a smart practitioner, more especially in bankruptcy, where his success as an advocate became well known.' Unlike Hyman Montagu and Henry Harris, he concentrated his energy on extra-communal activities, serving as a conscientious chairman of various committees of the Common Council, the local authority which governed the City of London, though he boycotted a reception held for the tsar. He was, however, buried in the United Synagogue's Willesden cemetery.[7]

The firm of Lewis and Lewis was founded in 1829 by James Graham Lewis (1804–73), who in 1834 was joined in the practice by his brother, George Coleman Hamilton Lewis. The family of Lewis were of Dutch Sephardi origin, their original name being Loew. James Lewis was clerk of indictments in the Midland Circuit for twenty-five years, 'and only resigned the appointment [in the mid-1850s] on account of increasing professional practice'. While he concentrated on building up the criminal work of the practice until it became one of the three leading firms in London specializing in this field, his brother George

---

[6] *JC* 27 Jan. 1899, p. 10 (obituary of Harris).   [7] *JC* 17 Sept. 1909, p. 9 (obituary of Lee).

was a bankruptcy expert, sorting out 'the insolvencies of gentlemen of the "leisured and professional classes"' as well as acting as solicitor for the Dramatic Authors' Society. George was also deputy clerk of the peace for over thirty years and clerk to the licensing justices for the Liberty of the Tower. Hence Sir George Henry Lewis (1833–1911), the son of James Lewis, who qualified as a solicitor in 1856, joined a thriving criminal law practice.[8]

George Henry Lewis was possessed of a prodigious capacity for hard work. Blessed also with an extraordinarily retentive memory, he could dispense to a very large extent with preparing laborious notes and data, enabling him to watch the changing facial expressions of the other participants in the case. Above all,

He specialised in the exposure of blackmailers, whether their means of extortion were by loans foolishly incurred, by libel actions or other unholy terrors. He reduced the employment of private detectives to a fine art, and the persons he assailed traded on the knowledge that their victims would be averse to having their monetary difficulties or peccadilloes exposed. Sir George often proved that he possessed information concerning their own practices, which they found very inconvenient to have drawn into the light of day.[9]

Lewis's first big case, which brought him to public prominence, was his successful application for the committal for trial on the grounds of fraud of the directors of Overend & Gurney's Bank (1869). He attracted more attention in the Bravo case in 1876; at the second inquest it was confirmed that Charles Bravo had been poisoned, and Lewis fixed suspicion on his wife, Florence (though she was never tried for his murder because there was insufficient evidence). He also prosecuted the fake medium Madame Rachel; in the Parnell affair of 1888–9 he persisted until he had exposed Pigott's letters which were published in *The Times* as forgeries, thereby helping to save Charles Parnell, the leader of the Irish Nationalist Party; and he successfully acted in the Baccarat scandal of 1891, in which the Prince of Wales was called as a witness.[10]

Lewis extended the bounds of the work open to Anglo-Jewish solicitors. He had an extensive society divorce practice, defending Lady Colin Campbell and the co-respondents in the divorce suit brought against her in 1883, and he acted on both sides in many newspaper libel actions. When Lloyd George was Chancellor of the Exchequer, he secured the retraction in open court of certain allegations made against him and damages of £1,000, with costs, for his client. Not all of Lewis's clients were innocent victims, and he could sometimes use quite unscrupulous means, including threats and monetary inducements, to

---

[8] *Solicitors' Journal*, 25 Jan. 1873 (obituary of Lewis), 22 Mar. 1879 (obituary of George Coleman Hamilton Lewis); John Juxon, *Lewis and Lewis* (London: Collins, 1983), 17–20.

[9] *JC* 8 Dec. 1911, p. 14 (obituary of Lewis).

[10] Juxon, *Lewis and Lewis*, 81–7, 115–39, 222–33, 242–8, 278–9; Michael Havers, Edward Grayson, and Peter Shankland, *The Royal Baccarat Scandal* (London: Kimber, 1977).

ensure that potential witnesses for the other side were bludgeoned into silence. In the Crawford divorce suit of 1886, in which Sir Charles Dilke was cited as the co-respondent, it was alleged that Lewis went to the house in Hill Street where the assignation between Mrs Crawford and Dilke was supposed to have taken place, and threatened the housekeeper that she would be indicted for keeping a house of ill fame if she gave evidence against his client; and that he had also bribed the housekeeper and her staff to remain silent. In the Campbell divorce case, Lewis gave the solicitor acting for the other side the clear impression during private negotiations that he wanted the dispute settled amicably, but then instructed his clerk to hurry to the Divorce Registry in order to ensure that his client's divorce petition was filed first, thereby giving her a tactical advantage.[11]

Lewis was married twice: first, in 1863, to Victorine Kann of Frankfurt-am-Main, who died in 1865 leaving a daughter; and secondly, in 1867, to Elizabeth Eberstadt of Mannheim, the German town from which his mother came. Elizabeth, who bore two daughters and a son, was a cultured woman with a particular interest in music. From the 1880s onwards the wealthy and hospitable couple entertained the leading figures from the artistic and theatrical worlds—men such as James McNeill Whistler, Henry James, Thomas Hardy, W. S. Gilbert, Arthur Sullivan, J. M. Barrie, and Edward Burne-Jones—in their new home at 88 Portland Place. Here they mingled too with celebrated politicians, lawyers, and financiers. Lewis attended to all the legal formalities when Richard D'Oyly Carte set up the Comedy Opera Company to stage the work of Gilbert and Sullivan; he also advised Thomas Hardy when the latter contemplated suing a playwright for plagiarism. Here again Lewis was a role model for other Jewish solicitors, many of whom subsequently cultivated clients from the world of the arts and the theatre.[12]

Despite his own lack of communal involvement and his somewhat lax membership of the Central Synagogue, which he attended infrequently, Lewis was a proud Jew and anxious that nothing should impair the good name and standing of the community. He informed the *Jewish Chronicle* that 'So far from wishing to disguise my race, I always make a point of acknowledging it in all the relations of my life.' His wife sat on the Ladies' Committee of the Council of the Anglo-Jewish Association, taking 'a keen interest' in its work.

Having started out as a criminal lawyer, and then acting increasingly for the impoverished sons of aristocratic families, Sir George Lewis at the peak of his career was the top society solicitor and a friend of the Prince of Wales. 'For more than a quarter of a century [he obtained] the practical monopoly of those cases where the seamy side of society is unveiled, and where the sins and follies

---

[11] Juxon, *Lewis and Lewis*, 198–202, 212–14; J. R. Lewis, *The Victorian Bar* (London: Hale, 1982), 138; G. H. Fleming, *Lady Colin Campbell, Victorian Sex Goddess* (Gloucestershire: Windrush Press, 1989), 194, 195, 220.   [12] Juxon, *Lewis and Lewis*, 290, 307.

of the wealthy classes threaten exposure and disaster.' Inevitably, given the aristocratic character of many of his clientele and their financial habits, he was constantly at odds with the chief West End moneylenders, notably Sam Lewis, the most important of them all.[13] Sir George was a lifelong and implacable enemy of the moneylenders, particularly the Jewish ones, who in his view brought the community into disrepute, telling a select committee of the House of Commons in 1898 that if they were swept away, commerce would flourish and the poor and younger sons of aristocratic families would be better protected. Of forty-one individual moneylenders or firms surveyed in a weekly journal called *The World* in 1874–5 by the radical MP Henry Labouchere, half were Jewish and two were solicitors in partnership who charged between 60 and 80 per cent; another was a former solicitor who had been struck off. When the proprietor of the journal was sued for libel by one of the moneylenders, Lewis, acting for the defence, succeeded through a masterly cross-examination and submission to the magistrate in having the summons dismissed. It was in part through his efforts that the 1900 Moneylenders Act was passed to ensure that the activities of the moneylenders were better regulated.[14]

Sam Lewis's solicitor and confidant was Algernon Sydney (1834–1916), an Anglo–Jewish communal heavyweight who was honorary solicitor to the Jewish Board of Guardians and the United Synagogue from their inception. In fact, Algernon Sydney's family were members of the legal profession for over five generations, from his great-grandfather through to his two sons, who were also solicitors. When Professor Jacob Waley, the conveyancer, and his pupil drafted the deed of Foundation and Trust of the United Synagogue, the largest organization of Orthodox synagogues in the metropolis, the indispensable Sydney was recruited to act as honorary solicitor and assist with the work; and, owing to the large amount of property owned by the institution, it subsequently made many calls on his time. He acted also for the substantial class of Jewish merchants, such as Rufus Isaacs's father, and the rising band of Jewish professional men, such as Dr Kisch—members of the small Victorian Anglo-Jewish middle class. For example, the case of the *Central Railway of Venezuela* v. *Kisch*, which went to the House of Lords, was won by Sir Roundell Palmer instructed by Algernon Sydney. He also handled difficult cases for landed gentlemen recommended by Sam Lewis.[15]

Sydney 'was so abundantly endowed with common sense that he was somewhat impatient with, and intolerant of, its absence in others, and when he

---

[13] Sidney Lee (ed.), *Dictionary of National Biography* (London: Smith, Elder & Co., 1912), Second Supplement, ii. 460.

[14] Gerry Black, *Lender to the Lords, Giver to the Poor* (London: Vallentine Mitchell, 1992), 101–4, 107–13, 238–53.

[15] *JC* 2 Jan. 1903, p. 10, 21 June 1907, p. 18, 7 Mar. 1919, p. 14. Isaacs, *Rufus Isaacs*, i. 36, 49.

thought any speaker was wasting the time of the [United Synagogue] Council he would on such occasions turn to his neighbours . . . to whom he would make some very caustic remarks as to the offender's intelligence'. He was prone to exclaim, 'When I hear a man talking foolishness, I just pop in a word and upset his apple-cart.' But it was said of him that 'he never rushed at a decision and his caution always gave his views, when they were expressed, very great weight'. He became a close friend of Sam Lewis, and could be relied on to give him quick advice on a difficult point of law if the occasion required. When the impecunious Sir George Chetwynd sued Hugh Lowther for libel over allegations about his racing stable, it appears that Sam Lewis recommended Sydney to act for Chetwynd. Through his links with Jewish organizations, and his friendship with Sam Lewis and other affluent Jewish businessmen, Sydney built up an extensive law practice, into which he was able to take his two sons in partnership.[16] Inevitably, Sydney's association with Sam Lewis, who epitomized everything that Sir George Lewis detested about the prominent Jewish moneylenders, led to a frosty rivalry between the two eminent solicitors and co-religionists.

Another Jewish solicitors' practice with close links to the moneylenders was the firm of Beyfus and Beyfus, popularly known as 'Fuss and Fuss': a partnership of Alfred and Philip Beyfus, whose elder brother Henry was an important moneylender and whose father Solomon sat on the Council of the United Synagogue. Alfred Beyfus (1851–1914), following in the footsteps of Sir George Lewis, also cultivated clients from the world of the arts and the theatre, but unlike Sir George he acted for the family moneylending business. 'Few men had a larger knowledge or a wider experience of the conditions of theatrical enterprise [than Alfred Beyfus]', pronounced the *Jewish Chronicle*,

and in the number of his clients he ranked many of the leading managers and actors of his time. It was he who helped to form the company known as the Palace Theatre (Ltd), after the failure of English Opera produced by Mr D'Oyly Carte. His firm also acted as solicitors for the Victoria Palace (Ltd). Some years ago he became one of a syndicate organised to build the Queen's and the Globe Theatres. To Mr D'Oyly Carte, also, he gave the benefit of his counsel and assistance at the time when the Savoy Theatre was founded by that gentleman.

Alfred Beyfus was the father of Gilbert Beyfus KC, one of the most brilliant barristers of the next generation.[17]

Many of the Jewish solicitors' firms which were situated in the City of London were run by men whose families were closely intertwined with those of the merchant, manufacturing, or retail elite. A good example was Herbert Bentwich

---

[16] *JC Literary Supplement*, 30 Mar. 1928, p. 3; *JC* 21 June 1907, p. 18, 21 July 1916, p. 15 (obituary of Sydney); Black, *Lender to the Lords*, 63, 149; Isaacs, *Rufus Isaacs*, i. 51.

[17] Black, *Lender to the Lords*, 103–33; Adamson, *The Old Fox*, 104; *JC* 27 Feb. 1914, p. 16 (obituary of Beyfus).

(1856–1932), the father of Professor Norman Bentwich, whose career was discussed in Chapter 5. Articled to Emanuel & Simmonds in 1873, having qualified as a solicitor in 1878 he opened a practice in Moorgate Street. Because of his friendship with Adolph Tuck, the driving force behind Raphael Tuck & Sons, manufacturers of greetings cards, he frequently acted for the firm in court, the first known action being against a tramway company for damage to a cart in 1879. Through his connection with the firm of Tuck, Herbert Bentwich began to act in a number of important cases involving the law of copyright. Under International Copyright Convention formulated in Berne in 1886, to which England adhered, registration of a copyright was not a necessary prior condition of action against those who pirated copies; and in the case of *Tuck* v. *Priester*, which went to the Court of Appeal, this principle was established in English law. Bentwich also acted for the German firm of Hanfstängl, publishers of engravings of pictures that they had acquired, who authorized their English agents to combat piracy. In *Hanfstängl* v. *Holloway* the defendants were enjoined to cease using one of the publishers' engravings in their advertisements. Between 1893 and 1895 Bentwich conducted a series of actions against the Empire Theatre, a famous music hall, and the *Daily Graphic* and the *Westminster Gazette* for infringement of copyright; the dispute went to the House of Lords, but although the main action was lost on an issue of the facts, the series of cases nevertheless established several vital principles with regard to copyright. As a result of his adroit handling of these copyright claims, Herbert Bentwich acquired the reputation of a specialist in this field and attracted a steady flow of clients between 1891 and 1900. He was invited to give evidence before a House of Lords Committee, and several of his recommendations were incorporated in the Copyright Act of 1911.[18]

The principal lawyers active in Jewish communal institutions in late Victorian and Edwardian England were Lewis Emanuel (1832–98) and his son Charles. Lewis Emanuel was admitted as a solicitor at the age of 21, having been articled five years earlier to Sampson Samuel, one of the few Jewish solicitors then practising in London. Samuel was solicitor and secretary to the Board of Deputies, a close associate of Sir Moses Montefiore, and an active participant in the early emancipation struggle. In 1845 a Jewish Disabilities Removal Act was passed, allowing Jews to sit on local councils, and in 1858, after a long campaign, Jews were finally permitted to become Members of Parliament. On Samuel's death in 1868 Emanuel took over his practice, replacing him as solicitor and secretary to the Board of Deputies; in 1875 he made Edwin Simmonds a partner, when the firm became known as Emanuel & Simmonds. Emanuel devoted most of his attention to conveyancing and was the confidant of many Jewish families.

---

[18] Margery and Norman Bentwich, *Herbert Bentwich: The Pilgrim Father* (Jerusalem: Hozaah Ivrith, 1940), 16–19, 132–5.

'Litigation was distasteful to him, and it is a fact that much of his work consisted in dissuading people from going to law.' Nevertheless, he triumphed in *Wallace* v. *The Attorney-General*. This case revolved around the will of Lord Henry Seymour, under which a large sum of money was bequeathed to 'the hospices of London'. When the Jewish asylums submitted a claim for a grant, the trustees rejected it, stating that the Jewish institutions were not covered by the words in the will. Emanuel 'displayed much ability in the various stages of the case, and in the end won the day, with the result that the Jewish asylums were declared entitled to receive the full benefits of the will, in the same proportion as the other London charities'.[19]

Lewis Emanuel was an individual of great public-spiritedness, both within and beyond the Jewish community.

Deeply attached as he was to his religion and his community, and prominent in every Jewish movement, . . . [Emanuel] felt that, as an English Jew, he ought to maintain a keen interest in the political, municipal and social life of his fellow citizens. He was one of the most ardent, as he was one of the earliest of Jewish volunteers [members of a military reserve force], and proficient in outdoor sports.[20]

Charles H. L. Emanuel (1868–1962) succeeded his father as secretary and solicitor of the Board of Deputies in 1898, holding the two positions for many years. His own successor A. G. Brotman remarked that 'He retained to the end of his life certain conventions and inhibitions characteristic of the Victorian and Edwardian age, in which he reached his middle years.' He inherited his father's interest in the City law firm of Emanuel & Simmonds, and through his connection with the Board of Deputies tended to act for litigants in high-profile cases which affected the Jewish community.[21]

In the divorce suit of *Friedberg* v. *Friedberg* (1908) Charles Emanuel acted for the wife, who was the petitioner, and instructed counsel, H. S. Q. Henriques, whom he frequently briefed in such cases, to ask the court to grant her a divorce on grounds of her husband's bigamy and adultery. Like Emanuel, Henriques was—as we have seen—a leading figure in the Board of Deputies, and the two men developed a close working relationship. The Friedbergs had married in Riga in 1902 and had then settled in England, where they lived together for a time before Mr Friedberg left his wife and in April 1907 presented her with a Jewish bill of divorce, a *get*, in the presence of Rabbi Schlossberg and other witnesses. On 4 May 1907 Mr Friedberg, assumed the surname of Frankenburg and married a Miss Pauline Stringer, who was expecting his child, in the Registry Office in Glasgow. According to Henriques, 'Whatever effect the [Jewish] divorce might have by Russian law, if it had taken place in Russia and

---

[19] *JC* 24 June 1898, pp. 22, 23.   [20] Ibid. 22.
[21] *JC*, 3 Aug. 1962, p. 29 (obituary), 17 Aug. 1962 (tribute by Brotman).

the parties had retained their Russian domicile, being pronounced here it could have no effect whatever.' Benjamin Grad who practised as an expert in Russian law in Moorgate Street in the City and was also a leading Zionist, was called by Henriques to prove the validity of the marriage in Riga in Russian law. Despite the hesitancies of the judge, Sir J. Gorrell Barnes, the president of the Probate, Divorce, and Admiralty Division of the High Court, over the question of the respondent's domicile, Henriques, after adducing evidence, managed to persuade him that Mr Friedberg had permanently settled in Britain; the petitioner was granted a decree nisi and custody of the two children of the marriage.[22]

Two years later Charles Emanuel again instructed H. S. Q. Henriques, in an appeal before the Lord Chief Justice and two other judges regarding the custody of three children, on behalf of their grandfather, a Mr Friedland, and a maternal aunt. While Mr Friedland, who was then living in Lithuania, was away on a short business trip, his home was pillaged and his daughter disappeared. He found her living with Casimir Minelga, a non-Jewish peasant farmer, in a nearby village. When Mr Friedland moved to Britain, he invited his daughter and her children to join him there, but unfortunately, while she was waiting in Germany for the tickets sent by her family to enable her to travel to Britain with her three children, she was taken ill and died. A custody dispute ensued, with both the grandfather in London and the father in Lithuania claiming rights over the children, who were brought to London.

Henriques argued that there was no evidence of marriage between Mr Minelga and Mr Friedland's daughter, and that in any case under Russian law a marriage between persons of different faiths was invalid. No documentary evidence of any marriage was produced to the court, although baptismal certificates for the children were available, but the Lord Chief Justice was aghast that the appellants persisted in maintaining that the children were illegitimate and, therefore, outside the father's control. For his part, Casimir Minelga maintained that the children's mother had converted to Catholicism and had married him: 'He had made all the necessary arrangements in his native village for his children's support, education and upbringing in the Roman Catholic faith.' The children's grandfather claimed that, after his daughter's disappearance, the villagers had threatened to kill him if he tried to take her back into his home, nor had he been asked to consent to any marriage. In an affidavit, the eldest daughter, Casimiera, stated that until she was 12 she had not been brought up in any religion, but that then her mother had told her that she wanted all the children to be brought up as Jewish and that she had encouraged them to practise Judaism in Germany. When Casimiera asked her father by letter what she should do after her mother died, he had said she should go to her mother's family in London.[23]

[22] *JC* 16 Oct. 1908, p. 17.   [23] *JC* 3 June 1910, p. 15.

Henriques claimed that the husband had, technically, deserted his wife, and that the respondent was not entitled to the custody of his three children. 'He urged that the only reason why the father had moved in the matter was that pressure had been brought to bear by the Roman Catholic Church.' It seems that the father was spurred into action to claim the custody of the children only after the intervention of a Lithuanian priest in London, who heard about the children from a Christian servant working for the children's aunt and uncle.

In his judgment, the Lord Chief Justice concluded that 'It was quite plain that this [case] was an attempt on the part of the Jewish community to override the wishes of the father . . . He commented on the attempt made by the appellants to cast doubt on the legitimacy of the children, which, he said betrayed a frame of mind which he could not understand.' Refusing a request by Henriques to allow the eldest daughter, who was almost an adult, to give evidence, the Lord Chief Justice declared without hearing her oral testimony that there had been no desertion by the father and 'The fact that the elder daughter wished to remain a Jewess was not sufficient ground for separating her from the others.' After he confirmed the award of custody to the children's father, 'The two elder children wept bitterly and took affectionate leave of the aunt, uncle and grandfather.'[24]

Unfortunately, the court had no understanding of the fraught, almost pogrom-like atmosphere in a Lithuanian village, while the motives and feelings of the children's Jewish family in London were incomprehensible to the highest judicial authorities. On the other hand, Emanuel and Henriques, notwithstanding their Oxbridge educations and privileged circumstances, had the greatest empathy for the plight of their co-religionists, and the case seemed to indicate that communal and ethnic solidarity could sometimes override both class divisions and the degree of Anglicization within different sections of Anglo-Jewry. Dismayed by what they felt was an unjust decision, some Jews in the East End decided to take their own action. The day before the children were to be returned to Lithuania, a nurse was taking one of them for a walk. She 'was surrounded by a crowd of Jews, who hustled her, and during the scuffle the child was taken away, and [had] not [been] since recovered'.[25]

A number of other leading Jewish solicitors benefited from their active involvement with communal institutions and charities, which attracted work into their offices. The point is illustrated by a case of 1909 involving a bequest of £5,000 in the will of Mrs Lewis Hill, the widow of the moneylender Sam Lewis, to the Jewish Maternity Institution. Unfortunately, no charity existed bearing that name; so the rightful recipient of the money became a matter of dispute. The adjourned summons in the action was heard before Mr Justice Eve sitting

[24] Ibid.   [25] *JC* 10 June 1910, p. 16.

in the Chancery Division of the High Court. Gilbert Samuel & Co. instructed Stewart Smith KC and Frank Samuel to appear for the Jewish Lying-in Charity, one of the claimants to the bequest, while Lindo & Co. instructed A. H. Jessel KC and Dr Judah Israel on behalf of the Beth Holim, a Sephardi charity. A. M. Langdon KC and Norman Bentwich, who were instructed by Albert Solomon, appeared for the Sick-Room Helps Society and Nurses' Home. Langdon argued that this 'charity was one of the greatest importance, and corresponded to the description in the will, and being, he contended, the only institution which was in a position to carry out the object of the request, was entitled, on the *cy près* principle [of adhering as closely as possible to the testator's intentions], to the legacy'. However, the judge stated that he could not decide which, if either, of the Jewish Lying-in Charity or the Beth Holim Mrs Lewis Hill intended to benefit, as she subscribed to both; in any event, the Sick Room Helps Society could not be substituted for them. He ordered the executors of Mrs Lewis Hill to draw up a scheme to apply the fund for the purposes intended by her, and for the costs of all parties to be paid out of the residuary estate.[26]

Other pre-1920 Jewish solicitors of whom something is known include several from old Sephardi families who had migrated to England in the eighteenth century: Herbert George Lousada (1846–1918), David Anijadar Romain (1861–1936), and the brothers Gabriel Lindo (1838–1908) and Arthur Lindo (1839–1905). Herbert George Lousada was the solicitor for the Anglo-Jewish Association and the West London Reform Synagogue, of which his father was one of the founding members. David Romain served as an elder of the Bevis Marks Synagogue and as a trustee of its real estate. He also assisted the Jewish bakers at the turn of the century, by successfully contesting a series of summonses for them when they were charged with infringing trading laws by baking on Sunday. His firm, Romain and Romain, absorbed the practice of Freke Palmer, which conducted many cases in the Marylebone Magistrates' Court and which frequently instructed Marshall Hall and Sir Henry Curtis-Bennett in celebrated criminal cases. Both the Lindo brothers were articled to their father Nathaneel Lindo, a City solicitor, before being admitted into partnership in his firm, Lindo & Co. It had long acted as solicitors for the Spanish and Portuguese Synagogue and the Italian Consulate, a tradition which the brothers continued. Arthur 'enjoyed the reputation of being a very sound lawyer and conveyancer. In the old days of the Metropolitan Board of Works the firm acted for some of the contractors under the Board. In this capacity Mr Arthur Lindo had charge of several legal cases in which the Board of Works was involved. He conducted every one of them personally without the assistance of Counsel, and never lost an action.' Unfortunately, the strain of this work, plus the loss of his eldest

---

26 *JC* 29 Jan. 1909, p. 16.

son at the point when he was about to celebrate his bar mitzvah, undermined his health, forcing him to retire prematurely. Both brothers served as legal advisers of the Sephardi congregation, holding office in its various charitable organizations.[27]

*

Before the Second World War, Jewish solicitors in London were overwhelmingly concentrated on the fringes of the East End, along Bishopsgate, and in the City in such places as Finsbury Square and the London Wall. By the 1920s there were about 100 Jewish solicitors catering for the needs of a prosperous, compact, but numerically relatively insignificant Anglo-Jewish bourgeoisie. Up to the 1960s most Jewish solicitors' firms were small, being run either by a single practitioner with the aid of a managing clerk or jointly by two partners. The exceptions were the few larger firms such as Herbert Oppenheimer, Nathan & Vandyk, and Bartlett & Gluckstein, which handled a large volume of company and other commercial matters and supervised the trusts and settlements of families belonging to that group of elite Anglo-Jewish families known as the Cousinhood.[28]

Herbert Oppenheimer has been described as possessing 'an incisive mind with a shrewd and practical knowledge of commercial and financial business . . . including taxation'—expertise which was rare among solicitors' firms in this period. Harry Louis Nathan (1889–1963), later the first Lord Nathan, joined him as a litigation partner on 1 August 1913. After service in the army during the First World War, Nathan returned to his law practice, attracting Lord Londonderry, one of the largest mine owners, and Sir Alfred Mond MP, the chairman of Brunner, Mond & Co., the forerunner of ICI, as clients. Mond became a friend as well as a client of Oppenheimer and Nathan, introducing the latter into the Zionist movement.[29] Arthur Vandyk was injured during the First World War and did not play a prominent role in the firm. Leslie Cork became a partner in Herbert Oppenheimer, Nathan & Vandyk in 1933, working closely with W. H. Cork, an insolvency practice started by his father, and extending the activities of the law firm into a new area. By the early 1960s, the firm had grown 'from two partners with a couple of clerks and a typist to one of sixteen partners and a total staff of 150'.[30]

---

[27] Anne J. Kershen and Jonathan Romain, *Tradition and Change: A History of Reform Judaism in Britain 1840–1995* (London: Vallentine Mitchell, 1995), 110; Wild and Curtis-Bennett, *'Curtis'*, 9, 82, 274; *JC* 12 Dec. 1902, p. 19, 2 June 1905, p. 14 (obituary of Lindo), 10 Apr. 1908, p. 10 (obituary of Lindo), 7 June 1918, p. 9 (obituary of Lousada).

[28] This estimate is based on an analysis of the names in *The Law List 1919* (London: Stevens & Sons, 1919), 453–679.

[29] H. Montgomery Hyde, *Strong for Service: The Life of Lord Nathan of Churt* (London: Allen, 1968), 29, 30, 76, 77.   [30] Kenneth Cork, *Cork on Cork* (London: Macmillan, 1988), 16.

Through his connection with Mond, Nathan became a friend of Chaim Weizmann and legal adviser to the Zionist Organization and the Economic Board of Palestine, which was responsible for the electrification of the country and the foundation of the Palestinian Potash Company in 1930. Weizmann was at first not uncritical of Nathan, whom he feared showed insufficient tact in dealing with some of his influential contacts—for example, the banking family the Kadoories, who had been prepared to finance the establishment of a school in Palestine, and wanted separate Hebrew- and Arabic-speaking institutions to be built. 'The old gentleman [Elly Kadoorie] is rather upset,' Weizmann wrote to Mond on 4 June 1922, 'and I don't think from all I hear that Nathan had handled the matter very seriously or very skilfully. It is a thousand pities. K. is very wealthy and very well disposed.'[31] Later Weizmann's confidence in his adviser grew, and in 1929 Nathan briefed various counsel to represent the Jewish Agency at a government commission of inquiry into the recent disturbances in Palestine and took counsel's opinion on the merits of lodging an appeal to the Privy Council on behalf of Yosef Urphali, a Jew whom the British had sentenced to death.[32] Nathan also acted as lawyer to Moses Novomeysky, a Russian Jewish industrial chemist and mining engineer, and handled a complex series of negotiations from 1921 to 1930 which resulted in Novomeysky being granted the concession by Britain to extract potash from the Dead Sea. To achieve this, Nathan had to circumvent the legal complications resulting from the revival of a concession granted by the Turks to another party; to see off the bids of gigantic American corporations such as General Motors and Du Pont; to counter parliamentary opposition to the concession being granted to a foreign Jew; and to obtain the assent of the authorities in Jordan and Palestine.

In May 1929 Nathan was elected as the Liberal MP for Bethnal Green, though he later crossed the floor of the House and joined the Labour Party. Nathan, who allied himself to a new, growing, and modernizing middle class in Anglo-Jewry with a Zionist outlook, developed an expertise in the promotion of large commercial operations and capital investment overseas. Because of this orientation, which involved him in international negotiations with various states, he had plenty of opportunity to polish his diplomatic skills, and the firm was soon acting for the Swiss, American, and Czech governments.[33]

During the 1930s Herbert Oppenheimer, Nathan & Vandyk represented the Russian Bank for Foreign Trade and claimants (including White Russians and the Bank of England) to assets in the English branches of other defunct Russian banks. Nathan was ably assisted in this work by a bright Cambridge graduate and protégé of Oppenheimer named Walter Eric Wolff, who was both fluent in

[31] *The Letters and Papers of Chaim Weizmann* (Jerusalem: Israel Universities Press, 1977), vol. xi, ser. A, ed. Bernard Wasserstein, 110.   [32] Ibid., vol. xiv, ser. A, ed. Camillo Dresner, 52, 53, 280.
[33] Hyde, *Strong for Service*, 90–8, 113.

German—the language of many Czech Jews since the days of the Habsburgs—and a specialist in commercial and international law. From the 1920s onwards the firm had also acted as solicitors for the Petscheks of Prague, a family which owned major business concerns in Czechoslovakia. Nathan informed a parliamentary select committee of the close connection between his own firm and a company in which the Petscheks had a majority holding in Britain, explaining 'that one of my partners from the beginning until a few months ago has been a director, together with Dr Petschek for some part of that time; that my partners and I are their nominees, and that when my partners used to go to Czechoslovakia they always enjoyed the hospitality of the Petscheks'.[34]

During the 1930s Nathan gave advice to many more Czechs with business interests in Britain, and when, after the German invasion of Czechoslovakia in March 1939, the Treasury froze the assets of the Czech government in Britain to prevent their falling into the hands of the Germans, a committee was set up in Nathan's office to represent Czech claimants and to urge a speedy settlement of their claims. Nathan asserted that because his firm had been acting for the Czech government for a number of years, 'It was quite obvious that the Czech Legation would send anybody to my Firm, and equally obvious that a large number of Czecho-Slovaks, the great majority of whom would know of my Firm, would come to my Firm'. Nathan did not charge the committee for his services, nor did he bill Robert Boothby, a Conservative MP who was chairman of the committee. Initially the Petscheks, who purported to have a large individual claim that they wished to pursue separately (it turned out to be illusory), were reluctant to join the committee, which placed Boothby in a difficult position. After a complaint from Boothby, Nathan wrote a somewhat clumsily phrased letter to Dr Petschek on 1 August 1939 in terms which could be misconstrued to suggest that undue pressure was being exerted by Boothby to compel Petschek to join the committee with the other Czech claimants. When he was asked by a parliamentary body whether such a construction could be placed on his letter, Nathan replied 'that as a solicitor of very long standing and no inconsiderable practice (I would even say, important practice) I greatly resent any such suggestion'.[35] In 1940 Nathan became the first practising solicitor to be raised to the peerage, taking the title of Baron Nathan of Churt.[36]

The elite of interconnected families called the Cousinhood still had a great influence in Anglo-Jewry during the inter-war period. Apart from Herbert

[34] *Russian Bank for Foreign Trade, In re* (1933), Bankruptcy and Company Reports, pp. 157–69; *Russo-Asiatic Bank, In re* (1934–5), Bankruptcy and Company Reports, Law Society Library, pp. 71–84; *Select Committee on Conduct of a Member (Mr Boothby)*, PP 1940–41, II Q1322A.

[35] Richard Rhodes James, *Bob Boothby: A Portrait* (London: Hodder & Stoughton, 1991), 197–283; *Select Committee on Conduct of a Member (Mr Boothby)*, PP1940–41, II Q1296.

[36] Hyde, *Strong for Service*, 136.

Oppenheimer, Nathan & Vandyk, two firms in particular acted for these families: Gilbert Samuel & Co. and Bartlett and Gluckstein. Gilbert Ellis Samuel (1859–1926) was the son of a banker, and the brother of Lord Samuel (Herbert Samuel, Liberal MP and Home Secretary) and Sir Stuart Samuel (also a banker). He 'was in his day one of the ablest solicitors in London. His more lucrative work was in the region of international finance, but he grudged no effort to the humblest client . . . Part of his success in negotiation may have been due to his genius as an amateur actor. His features were quite sphinx-like when serious work was at hand.'[37] Gilbert Samuel was the honorary solicitor to a large number of Jewish and other charities, including the Federation of Synagogues, the London Board of Shechitah, the Jewish Provincial Ministers' Fund, and the East London Apprenticeship Fund. Through his connection with these organizations work poured into his office, as it did into other similar Jewish solicitors' firms. On his death he was succeeded as senior partner by Walter Louis D'Arcy Hart, a grandson of the first Lord Swaythling and a Law Society prize-winner. In addition to drawing up the trusts and settlements of the Swaythling and Montagu banking families, the firm was heavily engaged in commercial work and acted for various banks, including the Russo–Asiatic Bank.[38]

At the end of the 1930s there was one large Jewish solicitors' firm in Piccadilly: Bartlett and Gluckstein, with six partners—half of whose income was possibly derived from acting for J. Lyons & Co., a firm owned by the Salmon and Gluckstein families which ran a famous chain of teashops and later branched out into the manufacture of food products. Lyons also opened some larger Corner House restaurants as well as the Trocadero in Piccadilly. As Lyons owned the premises on which these restaurants and cafeterias were situated, there was a considerable amount of conveyancing work flowing into the family law practice. The firm also handled the trusts and settlements of the Salmon and Gluckstein families.[39]

While the second Sir George Lewis (1868–1927), a rather shadowy figure who shunned publicity, did not have the allure of his father, he ensured that the firm of Lewis and Lewis continued to have its share of 'sensational litigation—society *causes célèbres*, big newspaper libels and the like. Those who knew him were aware that, for every scandal or dispute in which the firm was concerned, and which came into public notice, a very large number were disposed of without attracting public attention.' According to the *Solicitors' Journal*, 'When the late Baronet appeared as a witness in the *Dennistoun Case* [in 1925], Counsel

[37] *The Times*, 26 Oct. 1926 (obituary of Samuel).

[38] Ibid.; *JC* 29 Oct. 1926, p. 11 (obituary of Samuel); *JC* 29 July 1927, p. 11 (will of the second Lord Swaythling).

[39] Private information; Stephen Aris, *The Jews in Business* (Harmondsworth: Penguin, 1973), 154–62.

referred to him as the greatest living expert in the practice of divorce laws.' Mrs Dennistoun, for whom Sir George acted, claimed that her former husband Colonel Dennistoun had at the time of their divorce entered into an agreement to support her; this was denied by the defendant, Colonel Dennistoun, who had since married her friend, the wealthy Lady Carnarvon. Although the jury believed Mrs Dennistoun and awarded her damages of £5,000, the trial judge overruled them, concluding that the terms of the agreement were too vague to be enforceable.[40]

Among the most interesting libel cases in which Sir George Lewis was involved was his conduct of the defence when Lord Alfred Douglas, the former lover but later adversary of Oscar Wilde, sued the *Morning Post* for libel in July 1923. The cause of the alleged libel was a letter written to the *Morning Post* by the editor of the *Jewish Guardian*, containing the words: 'It must no longer be a paying proposition to men like Mr T. W. H. Crosland and Lord Alfred Douglas to invent vile insults against Jews.' Comyns Carr appeared for Lord Alfred Douglas, while Sir George Lewis instructed Sir Patrick Hastings for the defendants and other counsel represented the executors of Sir Ernest Cassel, whose honesty had been impugned by malicious statements made by Douglas.[41]

Comyns Carr opened for Lord Alfred Douglas, stating that the newspaper held high Tory opinions and believed that 'there was a world-wide conspiracy to promote the dominance of the Jewish race, and among the people who believed in the existence of such a conspiracy were the plaintiff and the *Morning Post*'. Carr asserted that it was the practice of the Jews 'in Syria and elsewhere to indulge in human sacrifice—what were called ritual murders', saying that his client would be relying on an unpublished manuscript of the explorer Sir Richard Burton. Afterwards Sir Patrick Hastings cross-examined Lord Alfred, who declared that a telegram from Admiral Beatty forged by Winston Churchill allowed the German fleet to escape after the Battle of Jutland; that Churchill acted in this manner because he was financially indebted to a group of Jewish financiers, particularly Sir Ernest Cassel, who made £48 million out of speculating in the financial markets in connection with the Battle of Jutland; and that Churchill drafted the report on the Battle of Jutland, although it nominally appeared under Balfour's name. Hastings asked Lord Alfred Douglas: 'Do you believe that Lord Balfour has forged the document [the report on the Battle of Jutland] which appears in his own handwriting?'

'No', replied Douglas, 'I don't see why I should say that, but I think that it is very likely that Lewis and Lewis [the solicitors for the *Morning Post*] forged it.'

[40] *Solicitor's Journal & Weekly Reporter*, 13 Aug. 1927 (obituary of the second Sir George Lewis); H. Montgomery Hyde, *Norman Birkett* (London: Reprint Society, 1965), 133–56.
[41] *JC* 20 July 1923, p. 33.

Douglas was further questioned: 'Do you mean to say that the Jews caused the death of Lord Kitchener in the *Hampshire?*'

'Certainly . . . Kitchener was murdered to prevent him from reaching Russia, because, if he had arrived there, the revolution would not have taken place and the war would have been shortened by two years.'[42]

Winston Churchill, called by the defence as a witness, was taken through his evidence by Hastings. 'Is there a single word of truth in the suggestion', asked Hastings, 'that you were ever in the hands of any man, Sir Ernest Cassel or any-one else, Jew or Gentile?'

'No, never at any time.'

'Is there any truth in the suggestion', reiterated Hastings, 'that you entered into a plot with Jews or anybody else in relation to reports of the Jutland Battle?'

'There is no truth in it.'

'Is there any truth in the statement', posed Hastings, 'that after the battle Sir Ernest Cassel or anybody else paid you a farthing in any shape or form in regard to anything you had done in connection with the Jutland battle?'

'It is an absolute lie.'

Churchill then told the court that he had decided not to prosecute Lord Alfred Douglas for libel after these articles first appeared, on the advice of Hewart, the then Attorney-General.

His view was that the status of the paper [*Plain English*] was so obscure and contempt-ible that it would only give a needless advertisement and notoriety if a State prosecution or an action for libel were started. Lastly, he considered that the character of Lord Alfred Douglas made it unnecessary for me to take any notice at that stage of these very gross and cruel libels; but he assured me that if at any time the question was raised and I was asked why I had not taken action to clear my honour, he would himself testify to the advice he had given me and the reason for doing so.[43]

In his summing up, the judge remarked that

having listened to the plaintiff for some time it was rather difficult to say what he believed and did not believe, and what he considered to be true and what not. He thought that he was a man who got into such a state of violent and unreasoning opinion that he published accusations of the gravest character without taking any sort of pains, and without knowing whether they were true.

Although this was a clear hint for the jury to dismiss the claim, they decided that Lord Alfred Douglas genuinely believed his spurious charges and awarded him contemptible damages of one farthing.

[42] *JC* 20 July 1923, pp. 33, 34.
[43] Ibid. 34; H. Montgomery Hyde, *Sir Patrick Hastings: His Life and Cases* (London: Heinemann, 1960), 110–16.

In an editorial the *Jewish Chronicle* regarded the case as a defeat for Anglo-Jewry because Douglas had been given a magnificent platform to air outrageous antisemitic propaganda. 'Allegations against the Jews so astoundingly false, so viciously malignant, have never before been paraded in the columns of the press, and it is impossible to believe, though the evidence of their falsity . . . was so overwhelming as to be palpably indisputable, but that some of the mud flung on our people will stick.' If anything, it was a hollow victory for the tiresome Lord Alfred Douglas, who six months later was charged with criminally libelling Churchill in a pamphlet entitled 'The Murder of Lord Kitchener and the Truth about the Battle of Jutland and the Jews'. For this he was sentenced to six months in prison.[44]

Towards the end of his life Sir George Lewis, the second baronet, went to a Swiss clinic to recuperate from overwork and a subsequent breakdown; his death on 9 August 1927 may have been an accident, or may possibly have been suicide. At his death, unlike his father, he showed a highly ambivalent attitude to the Jewish faith. His body was cremated, which is contrary to Jewish law; on the family's instructions, his ashes were interred in the local churchyard at Rottingdean which adjoined his own garden. The vicar, who was a personal friend, conducted a non-denominational service at the burial, consisting of a few passages from Scripture and a short address. A separate memorial service led by Rabbi Dr Mattuck was held at the Liberal Jewish Synagogue. The marquess of Reading, a close friend, claimed that 'Sir George Lewis was at the time of his death, so far as I know, of the Jewish faith. From intimate conversations with him before he went abroad, I have no doubt about his faith; and from all I have ascertained there is absolutely nothing to indicate any change in his belief.'[45] To the *Jewish World* this apologia was nonsensical, and it riposted:

But it is altogether a different matter when the interment is in a Churchyard. That is a definite indication either on the part of the deceased . . . or on the part of the relatives responsible, that the deceased had renounced attachment—even as slight as shown by Jewish burial—to the Jewish Community. The indication is made all the stronger when the burial is accompanied by the good offices of the Vicar of a church.[46]

Perhaps unsurprisingly, coming as they did from such an equivocal background, one of Sir George's daughters married in a Roman Catholic church a year after his death.[47]

We have seen how Sir George's father, the first baronet, and Alfred Beyfus developed the connection between Jewish solicitors and distinguished personalities from the world of the theatre and the arts before the First World War.

---

[44] Hyde, *Sir Patrick Hastings*, 117; *JC* 20 July 1923, pp. 8, 35, 9 Nov. 1923, p. 29, 14 Dec. 1923, pp. 22, 23, 21 Dec. 1923, pp. 9, 24.   [45] *JC* 19 Aug. 1927, pp. 8, 11.
[46] *JC* 26 Aug. 1927, p. 11, 2 Sept. 1927, pp. 7, 8.   [47] Endelman, *Radical Assimilation*, 198.

Between the wars and in the period after 1945 this tradition was continued by the firm of Rubinstein, Nash & Co. The founder of the firm was Joseph Samuel Rubinstein (1852–1915), who was born in Dublin and 'was an active, able, and energetic man, never afraid to utter his own opinions, as a speaker and writer of no mean ability'.[48] Not all his views were constructive, and he led an ill-judged campaign against the compulsory registration of land, by speaking at Law Society meetings and by writing pamphlets which enjoyed an extensive circulation. Despite his opposition, the nationwide registration of land was implemented after his death in 1925.[49] He was also the author of a pioneering *Articled Clerks' Handbook* (1876), separate volumes on the Conveyancing Acts and costs, and a guide to the Married Women's Property Act. 'He was also much devoted to music, and was associated professionally with the Queen's Hall at the concerts at which he was an almost constant attendant.' This taste led him into a close contact with members of the musical profession, many of whom became personal friends, while his wife's 'musical receptions in Addison Road brought together many artistic celebrities'.[50] Here was the beginning of the firm's association with the artistic world, an association much developed by Rubinstein's sons. He was also the founder of the Fireproof Fibre Company, which made non-inflammable partitions—much in demand for temporary buildings during the Great War. An Orthodox Jew, Rubinstein was a member of the New West End Synagogue and a committee member of the Home for Jewish Incurables.[51]

Joseph's practice was taken over by his eldest son, Stanley Rubinstein (1890–1976). Like his father, Stanley was passionately interested in music, and assisted in the administration of a number of musical organizations. Among his clients were the pianists Mark Hambourg, Benno Moiseiwitsch, and Myra Hess, together with the violinist Jascha Heifetz and the conductor Sir Henry Wood, the founder of the Promenade Concerts. Because Sir Henry Wood's wife refused to divorce him, Stanley Rubinstein arranged to have the name of Wood's companion changed by deed poll to Lady Jessie Wood. He was joined in the practice by his brothers Harold and Ronald. Harold (1891–1975), a talented dramatist, 'was a mild-looking man, immensely courteous, immensely gentle, but with vehement opinions, as I found afterwards', wrote Arnold Goodman, who was articled to him. 'He was a lover of liberty, and I would think in his political views a Liberal, but a passionate opponent of communism and anything to do with systems of government which were antagonistic to human liberty.' His brother Ronald Rubinstein (1896–1947) was considered to be the ablest lawyer

[48] *JC* 19 Mar. 1915, p. 11 (obituary of Rubinstein).
[49] *JC* 11 Oct. 1901, p. 12 (speech against land registration); J. Stuart Anderson, *Lawyers and the Making of English Law* (Oxford: Clarendon Press, 1992), 204, 205.   [50] *JC* 19 Mar. 1915, p. 11.
[51] Hyman, *The Jews of Ireland*, 134; *The Jewish Year Book 1910*, ed. Isidore Harris (London: Greenberg & Co., 1910), 411.

of the three, running the firm's extensive litigation department in libel and other matters related to the publishing trade. He also wrote the classic *John Citizen and the Law* (1947), which lucidly explained the various facets of the civil law which the average person was likely to encounter in his daily life. Sadly, he died prematurely.[52]

Harold Rubinstein 'was a quiet and gentle man'; not over-enamoured with the niceties of the law—he had returned to legal practice reluctantly, finding himself unable to make a living as a playwright. He was nevertheless trusted and used as an adviser by many distinguished literary personages and publishers, and dutifully grappled daily with the issues of libel law, copyright, and passing off which concerned them. Although he could not make the stage his full-time profession, one of his plays was put on in the West End; most of his works were one-act dramas and were frequently performed by amateur dramatic societies. At Covent Garden Harold Rubinstein met Victor Gollancz, a fellow opera lover; they became great friends and married two sisters. After a serious setback in a libel action in 1931, Gollancz ensured that 'every manuscript was read for libel by Harold Rubinstein, who received in return a modest fee and access to enough manuscripts to keep him reading happily at home every evening. (And long after Gollancz had abandoned the *genre*, Rubinstein's plays were published, because Victor could not bear to hurt his feelings.)'

When Radclyffe Hall's lesbian novel *The Well of Loneliness* was prosecuted for obscenity in 1928, Harold had Virginia Woolf, E. M. Forster, and a host of other public figures lined up to give evidence in the book's favour, but the magistrate would not allow them to be called, and banned the book as obscene. Harold was also secretary of the British League of Dramatists, spending almost every afternoon in a basement office in Gower Street dealing with their affairs. By the early 1930s the practice of Rubinstein, Nash & Co. 'attracted all the literary and dramatic talent in the country [including novelists of the stature of Graham Greene, Evelyn Waugh, and J. B. Priestley], and a large portion of the musical talent and not a few painters, although there was less emphasis on that side of the artistic scene than on the literary side'.[53]

Another interesting Jewish lawyer in the inter-war period who acted for musicians was Philip Emanuel. Having started out as a barrister's boy in the Temple, he went on to work as the managing clerk of a solicitor called Captain W. R. Bennett, who because of his respect for Emanuel's abilities gave him articles, enabling him to qualify as a solicitor in 1927, when he was in his forties.

[52] Interview with Joan Rubinstein, 3 Dec. 1996; Goodman, *Tell Them I'm On My Way*, 27; Stanley Rubinstein, *John Citizen and the Law* (Harmondsworth: Penguin, 1947), 5th edn. 1963.

[53] Goodman, *Tell Them I'm On My Way*, 29, 86, 89, 90; Ruth Dudley Edwards, *Victor Gollancz: A Biography* (London: Gollancz, 1987), 180–4; interview with Michael Rubinstein, 20 Jan. 1997; Michael Baker, *Our Three Selves: A Life of Radclyffe Hall* (London: Hamilton, 1985), 232–7; Sally Cline, *Radclyffe Hall: A Woman Called John* (London: Murray, 1997), 254–5.

Invariably they [the managing clerks] started their careers as office boys in solicitors' offices, and without any tuition other than such guidance as they might receive from their seniors, the partners and, when they were consulted, members of the Bar, they built up a store of legal knowledge and of practice and procedure which frequently far exceeded that of the solicitors who employed them. Certainly this was true of practice and procedure . . . as was the case with Philip Emanuel

recalled David Napley, who in turn became his articled clerk in 1932. 'Although his knowledge of the law was limited, this presented no special difficulty for him, since it was compensated by a dynamic personality, a keen wit, a lively intelligence and a superabundance of confidence.'[54]

Emanuel was the legal adviser and friend of the conductor Sir Thomas Beecham for thirty-seven years; together they formed the London Philharmonic Orchestra and later the Royal Philharmonic Orchestra, of which Emanuel was chairman. Beecham's extravagant lifestyle led him into constant financial diffi-culties, and because of this his inheritance had been placed in a discretionary trust, from which his trustees could dole out payments when they deemed it wise. Much of Emanuel's time was spent fending off the bankruptcy petitions which had been filed against Beecham by moneylenders who had not been paid promptly, or saving him from the unwelcome solicitations of his mistresses. Once, when the Official Receiver traced an unco-operative Beecham to an orchestra rehearsal, the latter exclaimed: 'Gentlemen; I must bring this rehearsal to an end. I am given to understand that the Official Receiver is here and insists upon seeing me. For what he is about to receive may the Lord make him truly thankful.' Through his friendship with Beecham, Emanuel was introduced to the composer Delius, after whose death he was appointed a trustee of the Delius Trust. In *In re Delius decd. Emanuel v. Rosen* (1957) the court granted an appli-cation of Emanuel that, since the trusts in the will of the composer's wife for promoting Delius's music were charitable, the money should continue to be used by Beecham for this purpose, instead of passing to the residuary legatee.[55]

In its obituary of Philip Emanuel, the *Jewish Chronicle* paid tribute to his con-tribution to communal life, noting that 'Mr Emanuel was commended by the Willesden Magistrates' Court for the many cases he undertook to represent there, purely from the goodness of heart and generosity, for nearly fifty years.' He served on several committees of the United Synagogue, helping them to acquire the site of the Willesden Synagogue; later in life, however he seems to have moved away from Orthodoxy and become active in the West London Reform Synagogue, following a pattern of acculturation and assimilation common among professionals.[56]

[54] Napley, *Not Without Prejudice*, 15.

[55] Ibid. 17–19; *JC* 3 Jan. 1975, p. 8 (obituary of Emanuel); *Re Delius decd. Emanuel v. Rosen* (1957) 2 Weekly Law Reports, pp. 548–55.   [56] *JC* 3 Jan. 1975, p. 8.

Between the two world wars there was a steady drift of solicitors from the older Jewish families out of the community. Increasingly, these solicitors were concerned primarily with their professional ethos or with their social circles outside Judaism, mixing with the artistic and theatrical elites, and their Jewish affiliations shrivelled and withered away to nothing. Apart from the second Sir George Lewis, other prominent solicitors of Jewish origin who severed their links with the Jewish community were the brothers Edward Simmons and Sir Percy Coleman Simmons, the founders of Simmons & Simmons, a City firm which acted for the big insurance and industrial companies. Edward married in a register office in 1904; Sir Percy married the daughter of a High Court judge in a society wedding at St Clement's Dane in 1931.[57] As far as the Jewish commitment of the second generation of Rubinsteins was concerned, only Ronald was a member of a synagogue; his son celebrated his bar mitzvah and he was for a time honorary secretary of the Jewish Blind Society. Harold had an uncertain identity, not knowing whether he was a Jewish Christian or a Christian Jew. Nevertheless, all three sons went to their mother's house for the Friday night dinner, which still had some religious meaning—at least for their mother, who recited her prayers daily.[58]

Throughout the 1920s and 1930s a number of Jewish solicitors continued to act for moneylenders. This is clear from a discussion at a Board of Deputies meeting on a proposal to amend its constitution to ban delegates who were moneylenders. 'And talking of lawyers,' proclaimed the *Jewish World* in 1919, 'is the Board [of Deputies] going to vomit forth the moneylender and swallow incontinently the solicitor who aids and abets him in the very art of his calling which gives it the bad name? Everyone must know there are solicitors who virtually confine their practice to the lucrative field of the registered moneylender.' When it was pointed out that there was little moral difference between the moneylenders and the 'pawnbrokers, tallymen, hire-system furnishers, [and] reversion brokers (to name only a few who lend money at rates far above the Bank price for the time being)', it was decided to drop the proposal to exclude moneylenders from membership of the Board in the amended constitution. In 1925 a military man committed suicide at the United Services Club, leaving a note in which he claimed to have been 'hounded to death by Jew lawyers and moneylenders', although the *Jewish World* wondered whether the victim had been treated harshly, or whether he was at fault himself.[59]

On 13 August 1926 the columnist Mentor in the *Jewish Chronicle* renewed the attack on Jewish solicitors who were too closely associated with the money-

[57] Teresa Henry, *Partnership: The Story of Simmons & Simmons* (London: Granta, 1996), 24–31, 36.
[58] Interviews with Joan Rubinstein, 3 Dec. 1996, Michael Rubinstein, 20 Jan. 1997; Endelman, *Radical Assimilation*, 198.   [59] *JC* 10 Jan. 1919, p. 11, 31 Jan., p. 5, 27 Feb. 1925.

lending business, revealing that some solicitors were using the moneylender as a front for their own nefarious practices: 'But unhappily we Jews do provide a quota of those who leaven the lump with their evil ways and the "Shylockism" which they practise. Some of them are really money-lenders under the guise of being solicitors.' That is, they would tell a client that they do not do these things themselves, but that they know a friend who can arrange a loan.

The subsequent transaction often becomes a joint one between money-lender and solicitor. Sometimes when the almost inevitable day of disaster for the creditor comes, the solicitor will pay out the money-lender on the transaction partnership, so that the solicitor may have longer odds for success in squeezing the poor debtor. I am assured that nine cases out of ten of harsh and unconscionable conduct that occur nominally on the part of the money-lender, in regard to financial dealings, are the work not of the money-lender but of the solicitor who sets himself to bring the law into the matter as a vast engine, not of Justice, but of oppression.[60]

Under the 1900 Moneylenders Act—strongly supported by the first Sir George Lewis—moneylenders had to register their own names, and the courts were empowered to look behind the transaction to see if it was 'unconscionable', in which case judges could fix a fair rate of interest. Conditions were tightened still further under the Moneylenders Act 1927, which required moneylenders to obtain a licence from the local magistrates' court on payment of an annual fee of £15, and to put all present or past names of the company's directors on letters and circulars; it further laid down that 'The court should presume the interest excessive and the transaction harsh and unconscionable . . . if the rate charged exceeds 48 per cent a year'. During the 1920s Jewish moneylenders frequently sued debtors who had fallen behind with their payments, particularly in the King's Bench Division of the High Court. In 1921 Lewis Schaverein, a registered moneylender of 6, 7, and 8 Old Bond Street, dealt harshly with a borrower 'who, not having paid the second of a series of monthly instalments on the exact day, was forthwith served with a writ for the whole amount of the debt together with the interest which had been fixed for several months more credit'; but the borrower was granted relief by the court because he had not been allowed the three days' grace to which he was entitled. When Schaverein sued the Earl of Rosslyn for £340 in 1928, he instructed the well-known London firm of solicitors Isadore Goldman & Son to act for him. Again, after part of the case was heard and after further discussion between the parties, the plaintiff decided that it would be wisest for him to withdraw the action.[61]

[60] *JC* 13 Aug. 1926, pp. 7, 8; James Arthur Dunnage, *The Modern Shylock* (London: E. J. Larby, 1926), 12, 13.

[61] *JC* 4 Mar. 1921, p. 14, 26 Oct. 1928, p. 33; Dorothy Johnson Orchard and Geoffrey May, *Moneylending in Great Britain* (New York: Russell Sage Foundation, 1933), 137–9, 143.

Isadore Goldman & Son, besides acting for moneylenders, carried on a thriving practice in the related field of bankruptcy work. The firm had been established in 1885 in Sunderland, where Isadore Goldman's father ran a jewellery and pawnbroking business which produced a considerable amount of county court litigation. In 1895, after a short interlude in Australia, Isadore moved to London and rapidly built up a flourishing agency and bankruptcy practice, acting in such cases as *Evans, In re: Salaman, ex parte* (1916). After the First World War he was joined by his son Joseph Goldman (1893–1978), who developed his skills as an advocate while participating in court martial work in France. Joseph Goldman attended daily before the registrars in the bankruptcy courts, and by the 1920s the firm was being instructed in some high-profile bankruptcy cases—including that of Horatio Bottomley, who had received one of the greatest numbers of petitions ever presented against a debtor. Joseph Goldman also acted in a series of actions involving Maundy Gregory, who was convicted of having sold honours for cash. As in the Bottomley case, Joseph Goldman acted for the trustee in bankruptcy, vainly pursuing Gregory to Paris in the attempt to elicit answers to questions.[62]

Another firm which acted regularly for moneylenders was Messrs Woolfe and Woolfe, which had offices at 13A Old Burlington Street in the West End. They were said to have employed a very capable managing clerk who was a frequent visitor to the bankruptcy courts, where, it was rumoured, he so insinuated himself into the favour of the registrar that he was able to extract whatever orders he asked for. In *Garde* v. *Kerman and Others* (1925) the judge allowed the plaintiff relief under the Moneylenders Act 1900 and halved the rate of interest payable by her on a series of loans to 30 per cent, not accepting the defence proffered on behalf of Messrs Woolfe and Woolfe's client, Hyman Kerman 'that he was unaware of facts material in determining the fair terms of the bargain'. In *Reading Trust* v. *Spero* (1929), Messrs Woolfe and Woolfe successfully acted for the respondent moneylender when the Court of Appeal dismissed the appeal of Mr Spero, a Bond Street dealer in antiques. Lord Justice Slesser suggested that

The terms were very stiff and his [Spero's] business was extraordinarily speculative, but he was making very large profits—this was a true matter of business embarked upon by a gentleman who struck me as being . . . a man of great intelligence . . . carrying on a

---

[62] Angela Thirlwell, *A Century of Practice: Isadore Goldman & Son 1885–1985* (London: Isadore Goldman & Son, 1985), 1–26; *Law Society's Gazette*, 24 May 1978 (obituary of Joseph Goldman). *Evans, In re; Salaman, ex parte* (1916) Bankruptcy & Companies Winding-Up Cases, pp. 111–15; *Maundy Gregory, In re; Trustee* v. *Norton (No. 1)* (1934) Bankruptcy & Companies Winding-Up Cases, pp. 57–62; *Maundy Gregory, In re . . . Trustee* v. *His Beatitude Louis II, Barlassina, Patriarch of Jerusalem (No. 2)* (1934–5) Bankruptcy & Companies Winding-Up Cases, pp. 62–4; *Maundy Gregory, In re; Trustee* v. *Norton (No. 1)* (1934–5) Bankruptcy & Companies Winding-Up Cases, 165–73.

high class of business, simply finding that his business is so speculative that he cannot get finance from the banks, but so profitable in his skilful hands that he can make profits which can pay 60 or 80 per cent interest . . . The policy of the [1927 Moneylenders] Act was to enable the Court to prevent oppression, leaving it to the discretion of the Court to weigh each case upon its own merits.[63]

On the whole, though, the courts were more sympathetic to debtors and frequently hostile to moneylenders. In the Whitechapel and Shoreditch county courts, Judge Cluer boasted that he kept 'moneylenders away from his court by his judgments'. A moneylender called Ellis Rosenthal had a summons dismissed in 1929 in the Welshpool County Court when he tried to obtain a committal order against a defendant for a debt of £38. In his judgment, Judge Ifor Bowen stated that

You have persecuted this man in a scandalous manner. There are things which you have done which the defendant's solicitor knows nothing about. Your solicitor, who is your nephew, sold up this man lock, stock, and barrel, and then you apply for an order to send him and his wife to prison for the balance . . . The defendant should consider whether he has not a case against you and your solicitor.[64]

Not only did the Jewish moneylenders create business for solicitors, they were often represented in court by Jewish barristers. Harold Simmons became a successful barrister by acquiring expertise in the law of moneylending. Some other members of his chambers at 4 Elm Court Temple, including R. F. Levy and Bernard Gillis, also worked from time to time in this field. Gillis was of the opinion that 'moneylenders . . . were the last persons to whom anyone turned, and their terms were often hard because there was a great risk of getting nothing back. I found that, almost without exception, they kept strictly to their contracts and would readily agree to easier arrangements if there was genuine hardship.' In 1928 A. M. Langdon, the recorder of Salford, allowed two appeals under the Moneylenders Act and decided that a man could apply for a certificate under the name by which he was generally known, apart from a trade name which he did not use in private life; in both instances, the appellants were represented by Joseph Lustgarten, a Jewish barrister from Manchester.[65]

Apart from the Jewish solicitors acting for moneylenders, there was one outstanding City lawyer in the inter-war period: Barry (Baruch) Cohen of Messrs

[63] Interview with Lucien Isaacs, 6 Oct. 1997; *Garde* v. *Kerman and Others* (1925) *The Times Law Reports*, vol. xli, 1924–5, pp. 597, 598; *Reading Trust Limited* v. *Spero* (1929), *The Times Law Reports*, vol. xlvi, 1929–30, pp. 117, 118. Orchard and May, *Moneylending*, 144.

[64] Gershon Pick to the Secretary of the Board of Deputies, 4 Feb. 1931, Acc. 312 B4/CL6, Board of Deputies Archive (on Judge Cluer); *JC* 13 Dec. 1929, p. 37.

[65] Aylett, *Under the Wigs*, 14; Gillis, 'Once Round Only', 17; *JC* 13 Jan. 1928, 33, 30 Jan. 1925, report of *British Finance Company* v. *Barbu Jonesco*.

Cohen and Cohen, who followed in the tradition of the first Sir George Lewis in acting for impecunious members of both the aristocracy and the middle class, including professional men such as doctors, against the moneylenders. Among his landed clients was the Lowther estate. Cohen often saved these gentlemen from bankruptcy by arranging cheap loans from alternative sources, such as banks and insurance companies. The existence of a different element in the firm's clientele is suggested by the fact that in 1924 Messrs Cohen and Cohen successfully sued the society magazine the *Sphere and Tatler* over an article by Michael Arlen alleging that they had a lady in their pay to enable them 'to arrange collusive divorces'. For his advice, Cohen could attract fees of 500 or 1,000 guineas—substantial sums during the 1930s. Yet, again like Sir George Lewis, Barry Cohen on occasion gave an hour or two's gratuitous advice to solicitors who were in financial difficulties and in danger of a disciplinary hearing before the Law Society.[66]

Cohen, who was admitted as a solicitor in 1891 and practised for over fifty years, was a brilliant litigation lawyer. His articled clerk, Ariel Solomon, who had a desk in his room,

noticed the tenacity he had in dealing with cases. He never gave up [even in a bad case] . . . he would keep on if people were writing to him and saying there is no further object in continuing this correspondence but that did not deter him until he got what he wanted to know from them. I still remember how he eventually won on that because they made an error and slipped up and gave him information which he wouldn't have got otherwise. He was marvellous really . . . I learned a lot from him.[67]

The action for which Barry Cohen is best remembered is *Tolley* v. *Fry & Sons Limited* (1929), a leading case in the law of libel, in which he acted as the solicitor for the plaintiff, Cyril Tolley, the reigning British amateur golf champion. Tolley recalled that 'A member of my [stock exchange] firm suggested that I employ Mr Barry Cohen, a very enterprising solicitor. He in his turn suggested Rayner Goddard [as counsel] because he was good and not expensive. His fee was, I think, 30 guineas whereas [Norman] Birkett's was 150 guineas with Monckton as junior.' In June 1928 Fry's, the chocolate manufacturers, ran a series of advertisements in the national press showing a caricature of Tolley, without his knowledge or consent, with a packet of chocolate protruding from his pocket. Next to him was a caddy, also depicted with a packet of chocolate bulging from his pocket. Underneath was a caption with the following limerick:

[66] *Report of the Joint Committee of the House of Lords and the House of Commons on the Moneylenders Bill*, PP1924–25, vol. viii, Qs 1060, 1062, 1098; *JC* 26 Dec. 1924, p. 22; *Report of the Joint Committee of the House of Lords and House of Commons Appointed to consider the Solicitors Bill 1939*, PP1938–9, vol. viii, Qs 794, 801, 805, 836.   [67] Interview with Ariel Solomon, 21 Nov. 1992.

The caddy to Tolley said: 'Oh, Sir!
Good shot, Sir, that ball see it go, Sir.
My word, how it flies
Like a Cartet of Fry's
They're handy, they're good, and priced low, Sir.'

The plaintiff alleged that the defendants' advertisement implied that he had allowed his portrait to be exhibited for the purpose of advertising their chocolate, that he had done so for gain, and that he had thus prostituted his status as an amateur golfer. Goddard called evidence from golfers to show that an amateur who consented to such an advertisement tarnished his reputation, and could be called upon to resign his membership of his golfing club; and he produced correspondence between the defendants and their advertising agents to demonstrate that the latter were aware of the possible effect of the advertisement on Tolley's amateur status. For the defendants, Birkett denied that the advertisement could bear any such defamatory meaning. The jury found for Tolley, awarding him £1,000 damages, but the Court of Appeal overturned this decision, stating that the advertisement was not defamatory and that the damages were excessive. Goddard appealed to the House of Lords on the first point as to whether the advertisement could be construed as being capable of having a defamatory meaning, and in 1931 was successful. Thus it was established in libel law that language which might in its ordinary sense be considered innocuous could be regarded as defamatory because it contained an innuendo. While Goddard has received the credit for his presentation of the case in court, the masterly preparation of the case and the series of appeals bear the hallmark of Barry Cohen's characteristic dogged tenacity.[68]

A number of Jewish solicitors in the period between the two world wars established a reputation by undertaking work for Jewish communal institutions. William Telfer Leviansky (1860–1936) succeeded Algernon Sydney as honorary solicitor to the United Synagogue in 1916; his articled clerk, Jack Gaster, remembered issuing dozens of summonses at the nearby City and Mayor's Court for unpaid synagogue fees.[69] Leviansky was a tough negotiator, as became clear when he represented the Shechitah Board in a dispute with the inventor of the Weinberg pen, a device for improving the procedure of ritual slaughter. The latter chose Samuel Landman (1885–1967), a former general secretary of the World Zionist Organization and another well-known communal personality, as his solicitor.[70] Hyman Isaacs (1874–1961) was the founder of the firm Hyman

---

[68] Fenton Bresler, *Lord Goddard: A Biography of Rayner Goddard, Lord Chief Justice of England* (London: Harrap, 1977), 63–8; Hyde, *Norman Birkett*, 272–4.

[69] *JC* 4 Apr. 1930, p. 12, 1 May 1936 (obituary of Leviansky); interview with Jack Gaster, 11 Nov. 1997.

[70] *JC* 21 Apr. 1967, p. 27 (obituary of Landman). Landman remained an important figure in Zionist circles: he participated in the Board of Deputies and served on the Council of the Jewish Health Organization.

Isaacs, Lewis & Mills; he succeeded Leviansky as the solicitor to the United Synagogue and also acted for various building societies. For many years he was vice-president and chairman of the Board of Managers of the Jews' Free School. 'Of outstanding intellect,' recalled its headmaster, Dr E. Bernstein, 'his high financial gifts skilfully conserved the funds of the school and enabled it to make an impressive contribution to the London Jewish Educational Foundation, which aided substantially in the construction of the new J.F.S. in Camden Town'.[71]

Isaac Landau (1874–1954) was a member of the Committee of the Jews' Temporary Shelter; he was also on the council of Jews' College and was active in the Board of Deputies. In 1910 he was employed by the First Lodge of the B'nai B'rith, the international organization dedicated to charitable and educational purposes and to the combating of antisemitism, which was later joined by the Board of Deputies in representing distressed Jewish refugees who could not gain admission into Britain, and he became a specialist in immigration law, successful in all five such appeals he handled in 1911. By 1916 it was estimated that 'many hundreds of poor emigrants were saved from repatriation through the [joint] Committee's activities'.[72]

All of these solicitors active in communal work came from older Ashkenazi families who had migrated to Britain no later than the mid-nineteenth century; they were not representative of the renewed and large-scale influx of east European immigrants after 1880.

During the inter-war period there were relatively few Jewish solicitors' firms in the West End in comparison with the situation prevailing after the Second World War. Of those there were, some worked closely with the nearby offices of the Jewish moneylenders; others, such as Hyman Davis, assisted the fashion trade which was located in the streets around the Middlesex Hospital from the 1920s; yet others were enterprising lawyers, such as Lionel Wigram, ready to move in new directions, notably into the property market. Another West End firm was Lazarus, Son & Hart, whose partners included Louis Albert Hart and Bernard Lazarus. Hart was a very go-ahead solicitor with a dashing appearance who had built up a big conveyancing practice and acted for a few people on the fringes of society. Careful to cultivate the right tone, he used to put on a silk hat and attend Royal Ascot. He 'had [as] a client, a man called Henry Brandon, who was quite a big property owner, a Sephardic Jew. He owned a big building

---

[71] *JC* 15 Sept. 1961, p. 16, 29 Sept. 1961, p. 26 (obituary of Isaacs).

[72] *JC* 23 Sept. 1910, p. 5, 21 Oct. 1910, pp. 5, 6, 17, 28 Jan. 1916, p. 16, 19 Nov. 1954 (obituary of Landau). In 1910 Herbert Bentwich was the driving force behind setting up the B'nai B'rith's voluntary legal aid scheme to assist immigrants, modelling it on the work of the East London Tenants' Defence Committee, with which he was connected. See Walter M. Schwab, *B'nai B'rith. The First Lodge of England: A Record of Fifty Years* (London: Wolff, 1960), pp. 23, 24.

called Arcade House, which had two addresses, it ran from Bond Street to Albermarle Street.' The granting and renewal of leases generated much conveyancing work. Eventually Hart became very active in the financial world and joined the merchant bankers Ansbacher & Co. Bernard Lazarus, whose father had been a solicitor, did a great deal of work with a firm which specialized in reversions: he would buy either a reversionary interest in an estate subject to a life interest or an endowment policy payable on death, and then sell them. He was the first solicitor of Sir John Cohen of the Tesco supermarket chain, who remained a loyal client.[73]

From the beginning of the twentieth century Jewish law firms (notably Simmons & Simmons) began to be associated with small and medium-sized Jewish property owners, and this trend gathered momentum throughout the inter-war years. Maitland Kisch established a property company called Town Investments, which brought in a considerable amount of conveyancing work for his solicitor brother Ernest Royalton Kisch (1886–1967). The latter was married to an heiress and was a pillar of the Anglo-Jewish establishment, being the energetic honorary secretary of the Education Aid Society, which sponsored bright Jewish students from impoverished families, and a stalwart member of the Liberal Synagogue. 'He had a spare and elegant frame and was always immaculately dressed,' declared Lord Goodman, 'and his strong aquiline features and particularly alert and gleaming eyes savoured of the Bedouin, but in voice and gesture he was impeccably public school. He had himself been educated at St. Paul's and Clare College, Cambridge.' His hobby was rose-growing and he was president of the National Rose Society.[74]

The law practice of Alexander Rubens & Co. was based on a partnership of two brothers, Alexander and Charles Rubens; they did a considerable amount of commercial and conveyancing work, as their father was an estate agent and small-scale property developer, who died suddenly in 1918. Alexander Rubens (1886–1932) had a noteworthy case on the efficacy of a notice to repair, *Jolly* v. *Brown and Others* (1912), which went to the Court of Appeal. He was an important communal figure; a prominent member of the Board of Deputies and the Council of the United Synagogue, he was also the founder in 1910 and honorary secretary of the Sabbath Observance Bureau, which obtained employment for Orthodox youths. Charles Rubens (1900–99) worked as a City solicitor from the years after he graduated from Cambridge with a first-class degree in law into his eighties; during the 1930s he gave free or low-cost advice to hundreds of German Jewish refugees. Like Alexander, he was active in Anglo-Jewish life, serving as warden of the West London Synagogue and founding the Cambridge and Bethnal Green Jewish Boy's Club. Another brother, Alfred Rubens

---

[73] Interview with Lucien Isaacs, 6 Oct. 1997.
[74] Goodman, *Tell Them I'm On My Way*, 33, 34; *JC* 21 July 1967, p. 39 (obituary of Royalton Kisch).

(1903–98), left school at 14 and helped his mother run the family business. Together with another brother, Harry, and Montie Arnold, Alfred Rubens later floated the Property and Reversionary Investment Corporation to develop commercial property, in which they made their fortunes; and he played a vital role in the resuscitation of the Jewish Museum and its relocation to new and more suitable premises. In 1931 three of the Rubens brothers, Alfred, Harry, and Charles, teamed up with two other partners to form a smaller, private concern, the Copthall Property Company. No doubt the expansion of the family property business assisted the buoyancy of the associated law practice. When Charles Rubens died in 1999, he left a net estate of £3,943,108.[75]

In the early part of the twentieth century tenants had very little protection against summary eviction by their landlords, and inevitably conflicts arose. In the East End of London in March 1939 the owners of a block of flats contemplated issuing possession proceedings against nine tenants whose cases were being supported by the Stepney Strikers' League, a tenants' organization supported by the Communist party. Both the owners and some of the tenants were Jewish, and the Jewish solicitor acting for the owners told Basil Henriques—a leading figure in East End Jewry who served as chairman of the East London Juvenile Court and also as a club leader—that he was not adverse to negotiations and 'was equally anxious to avoid proceedings which might lead to undesirable publicity'. Behind the scenes the Board of Deputies encouraged the Jewish owners of other buildings in the East End where tenants were striking to enter into negotiations with their tenants. In the north of England 'The number of Jewish landlords and property owners . . . was comparatively large', but 'very few of the landlords can be described as being harsh or ruthless; the number of distraints during the year being comparatively small'. In south Wales, however, Jewish moneylenders dabbled in property speculation, buying up the tail-ends of leasehold properties and then treating the tenants badly. What is obvious is that this new property-owning stratum among immigrant Jewish families meant more conveyancing work for solicitors who were related or family friends.[76]

Among Jews the movement from property ownership into active property development was slow until the late 1940s and 1950s. J. S. Salaman, a solicitor practising in Cheapside, purchased and rebuilt freehold premises in nearby Tokenhouse Yard which he was unable to let at the anticipated rent; as a conse-

[75] Interview with the late Charles Rubens, 22 Sept. 1997; *Camden New Journal*, 13 Jan. 2000; *JC* 31 Mar. 2000, p. 31 (obituary of Charles Rubens); *JC* 26 Feb. 1932, p. 10 (obituary of Alexander Rubens). *Jolly* v. *Brown and Others* (1912) 2 King's Bench, pp. 109–31; *Independent*, 29 June 1998, *JC* 3 July 1998, p. 27; *Jewish Historical Studies*, 35 (2000), pp. xix–xxi (obituary of Alfred Rubens); *The Times*, 26 May 2000.

[76] Board of Deputies Defence Committee, C6/1/1/1, memorandum on landlordism [Apr. 1939]; private information.

quence he was made bankrupt in 1884.[77] In the first decades of the twentieth century Abraham Davis was chairman of the Central London Building Company, the umbrella organization for many subsidiary companies set up to erect houses and flats, while in the inter-war years Leo Meyer became the most prolific of the London property developers and Ellis and Lawrence Berg developed houses in south London.[78] Perhaps the most outstanding pre-war Jewish property developer was the lawyer Lionel Wigram (1907–44), described by the West End estate agent Edward Erdman as 'a tall, handsome young solicitor with a forthright and fearless character and an obvious flair for property. His legal practice, Wigram & Co., was established [in the 1930s] first in Langham Street and then in a Georgian House in Queen Street, Mayfair . . . Wigram was first in the news in 1938 as a result of a large deal he carried out with the Bute Estate in Cardiff'—a deal worth some millions of pounds. He worked closely with Henry Denton and Francis Winham, who 'purchased, developed and let many shops to multiple firms'.[79] As the director of a number of companies he had an income of £30,000 per annum, and one of his clients was the property developer Joseph Aaron Littman.[80] Lionel Wigram revolutionized the battle training techniques of the British army during the Second World War, instituting the use of live ammunition; unfortunately, he died in action in 1944.

During the inter-war period the economic fortunes of British Jews, which had peaked in the Edwardian period, declined; and this was especially true of a number of prominent City of London commercial and banking families. Nevertheless, members of the Cousinhood remained linked to a few select Jewish law practices: Herbert Oppenheimer, Nathan & Vandyk; Bartlett & Gluckstein; Gilbert Samuel & Co.; and perhaps Lewis and Lewis. These apart, the only distinctive Jewish law firms were those with connections to the moneylenders or the world of the arts; the few practices which specialized in bankruptcy law, such as Herbert Baron & Co. and Isadore Goldman & Son; and a small number of Jewish firms associated with communal figures. Most of the other Jewish law firms were small family practices many of which (like King-Hamilton & Green) handled little litigation.[81] Meanwhile, the movement of some members of old Ashkenazi families and the east European immigrants into the property market and into diverse forms of enterprise was gathering pace. Wigram & Co. was perhaps the prototype of the post-Second World War Jewish law firm associated

[77] *In re Salaman, ex parte Salaman* (1885) Morrell's Bankruptcy Reports, pp. 61–70.

[78] *JC* 1 Feb. 1924, p. 11 (obituary of Davis); Alan A. Jackson, *Semi-Detached London* (London: Allen & Unwin, 1973), p. 107.

[79] Edward L. Erdman, *People and Property* (London: Batsford, 1982), 34, 35; Denis Forman, *To Reason Why* (London: Deutsch, 1991), 214–16.

[80] *Broadstairs Picture House Limited* v. *Littman* (1940) 1 Chancery 860–3.

[81] W. D. Rubinstein, *Men of Property: The Very Wealthy in Britain since the Industrial Revolution* (London: Croom Helm, 1981), 92–3, 156; King-Hamilton, *And Nothing but the Truth*, 15.

with property companies. Before examining the full impact of this development on the legal profession after 1945, we must first examine the growing attraction of the solicitors' profession to the second generation of east European immigrants in the 1920s and 1930s.

EIGHT

The Entry of East European Jews into the Law between the World Wars

PRIOR to the First World War, Jewish entrants into the solicitors' profession and the medical schools in England were confined to a small proportion of the upper and middle classes. During the First World War and into the 1920s, it appears, children of east European Jewish immigrants to England began to train as doctors in increasingly large numbers; but few became solicitors, and even fewer barristers, until the late 1920s and 1930s. Why was this? Cost was one highly significant factor. If a young man aspired to become a solicitor, his parents were required to pay a premium of between 300 and 500 guineas in the 1930s and 1940s, together with a stamp fee of £80, and a salary was paid to a trainee only in exceptional circumstances. This meant a long period of non-earning work, for articles were usually for five years—though if the articled clerk had passed his higher school certificate examination the period was reduced to three years, and if he was a university graduate it was four years. When Ariel Solomon (1908–2001) became articled to Messrs Cohen and Cohen in 1929 his mother had to sell her jewellery to raise the money for his premium of 500 guineas. Lucien Isaacs (1907–2001), whose father was a commercial traveller of modest means, was fortunate to be taken on in 1924 as an articled clerk by Mr Dolman, who not only set the premium at a lower figure of 300 guineas but agreed to accept a payment of 150 guineas with the balance to follow; he also provided his articled clerk with a wage of 10 shillings a week. From various sources, it is clear that most parents paid the solicitor to whom their son was articled a premium of 300 guineas, though if the solicitor knew the boy's family well the premium was sometimes waived altogether.[1] In contrast, a medical student in the late 1920s had to pay fees of only £35–£40 per annum for a five-

---

[1] Summerfield, 'Anglo-Jewry and the Law', p. vi; Brian Abel-Smith and Robert Stevens, *Lawyers and the Courts* (London: Heinemann, 1967), 181; Silman, *Signifying Nothing*, 59, 63, 64; interviews with Ariel Solomon, 21 Nov. 1992, Lucien Isaacs, 6 Oct. 1997, Sidney Jaque, 14 July 1998, Jack Gaster, 11 Nov. 1997; Goodman, *Tell Them I'm On My Way*, 27.

year programme of studies at medical school, and many of the brighter students won scholarships which covered the cost of their training in part or in whole.

As noted in the Introduction to this book, Tony Kushner has argued that there was discrimination against Jews applying to enter the professions in England in the late 1930s and during the Second World War, and that numerical limits were placed on Jewish entrants to the legal and medical schools.[2] I have in earlier chapters cast doubts on the efficacy of any such quota in respect of the medical schools; similarly, there is no evidence that in practice the law schools of England limited the number of Jewish students. In the United States the situation was quite different. 'During the late nineteenth and early twentieth centuries,' declared Robert W. Gordon, 'some universities maintained quotas on Jewish applicants. Certain leaders of the bar also spearheaded campaigns to upgrade entry requirements in the hope of screening out those with immigrant or lower class backgrounds.'[3] In 1874 George T. Strong, an American lawyer, supported the idea of 'a college diploma, or an examination including Latin [for admission to Columbia Law School]. This will keep out the little scrubs (German Jew boys mostly).'[4]

In the absence of special entrance requirements devised to suppress the number of Jewish solicitors admitted to the profession in England, there were economic rather than social barriers that impeded their entry. During the mid-1920s A. G. Hughes reported that 'Commerce attracts Jews of good intelligence, men of calibre, who if they were non-Jews, would probably enter the professions.'[5] As Vivian Lipman pointed out,

It is likely that the middle-class element of London Jewry was between 40 and 50 per cent by 1930, and that it would rise even higher with increasing living standards and the immigration of the socially bourgeois Central Europeans, by the end of the 1930s . . . The rise in real earnings increased demand for employment in the service and distributive trades and consumer-orientated industries.[6]

The obverse of Lipman's statement, of course, is that in 1930 between 50 per cent and 60 per cent of London Jewry was still working-class. Thus, on the one hand, there was a delay in the inter-war years before Anglo-Jewry adjusted its occupational distribution to its economic restructuring; on the other hand, there were still many Jewish families too poor to support their children through the lengthy and costly legal training process necessary for them to become

---

[2] Kushner, 'The Impact of British Anti-Semitism', 201.

[3] Geoffrey C. Hazard and Deborah L. Rhode (eds.), *The Legal Profession: Responsibility and Regulation* (Westbury, NY: Foundation, 1988), 40, 50.   [4] Quoted ibid. 50.

[5] A. G. Hughes, 'Jews and Gentiles: Their Intellectual and Temperamental Differences', *Eugenics Review* (July 1928), 92, 93.

[6] V. D. Lipman, *A History of Jews in Britain since 1858* (Leicester: Leicester University Press, 1990), 203–13.

solicitors. An even smaller number of the children of east European Jews could hope to establish themselves as barristers, as this was a career for only those who were both exceptionally gifted and exceptionally resilient.

All the factors discussed above explain why there were relatively few Jewish lawyers from immigrant families prior to the Second World War. Most of those who did embark on the study of law, like most of the medical students, came from families with a steady income; they were the children of successful shop-keepers, clerks, workshop and factory proprietors, rabbis and cantors. For the children of synagogue officiants, there was no family business to go into and they often chose a career in the professions because of their family tradition of scholarship combined with service on behalf of the community.[7]

Several other factors were also at work in attracting talented Jewish youths to the medical and, to a lesser extent, the legal professions. American research has shown that Jews tend to prefer self-employment to employment by others, and Joseph Zelan writes 'the image (though perhaps not the reality) of . . . [this] is found' chiefly in the free professions of medicine and law, which have not been subject to guild-type regulation. Zelan has further suggested that 'the patterns of occupational choice . . . can in part be explained by a model in which each indi-vidual strives to attain an occupational status equal or higher than that of his father, but with Jews tending to restrict their choices to law and medicine'.[8] Since the prestige of doctors was higher than that of lawyers in both America and Britain, more Jewish youths would incline towards the medical rather than the legal profession; but in England the greater expense of a legal training and the better employment prospects for those graduating from medical school encouraged many more young men and women to study medicine than law. In addition, during the inter-war years in England, young Jews found it difficult to enter other professions such as teaching and engineering. As the 1937 report of the Education Aid Society noted, 'The difficulty confronting a young Jew, even if he possesses an honours degree and a teaching diploma, in obtaining a teach-ing post in Secondary Schools has been experienced over and over again by the Society's students.'[9] As far as engineers were concerned, Joseph Shlosberg obtained a B.Sc. before he was 20 years old and worked for a world-famous firm of engineers, but he encountered such difficulties over obtaining time to observe the sabbath that he switched to a career in medicine.[10] Even 'in the case of ordinary businesses, it seems to be difficult for Jewish boys from Central Schools to obtain posts through the official Employment Bureaux'.[11]

   [7] Jacoby, *Journey*, 19; interview with Montague Richardson, 16 June 1997.
   [8] Wakov, *Lawyers in the Making*, ch. 3 by Joseph Zelan, esp. p. 50.
   [9] Endelman, *Radical Assimilation*, 194, 195; Education Aid Society, *Annual Report* (1937), 8, Parkes Library, Southampton University.   [10] *JC* 13 Feb. 1953.   [11] *JC* 2 Sept. 1932, p. 9.

To examine the situation in more detail, let us focus on one town, Leeds, in the 1930s. According to the leadership of the Jewish community there, 'There was locally a known aversion on the part of non-Jewish employers of labour from giving employment to Jews or Jewesses.' Hence employment opportunities within the local Jewish community were considered to be of vital significance by the Leeds education authority. F. R. Worts, the head of one of the largest secondary schools in Leeds,

was of the opinion that it was those [important] Jewish employers [of labour] who should be the first to come forward with offers of employment to those of their own race. He was, however, aggrieved to say that this did not happen. Most of those young men were far above the average as regards their scholastic attainments and their general mental and personal capacity, and he felt assured that with an intellectual equipment of this kind they could certainly render a great service in the field of industry.[12]

His views were supported by a Mr M. Sclare, himself Jewish, who claimed that 'It was common knowledge that there were numerous young men who were unable to find posts either in business or the professions.' To these complaints, Jewish leaders responded by saying 'that the number of vacancies for Jewish boys and girls [within the community] were not really so great as it was imagined to be by the Education Authority', and that if Jewish employers employed only Jewish youths, this would create ill feeling.[13]

Squeezed between an unfriendly local community and Jewish employers with limited absorptive capacity, many of these highly educated Jewish youths gravitated towards the medical and legal professions. At a discussion at the Leeds B'nai B'rith in 1934, the feeling was expressed that the medical and legal schools at Leeds University were 'over-weighted with an undue proportion of Jewish students'. Moreover, there was 'always a floating taunt that there are too many Jewish doctors and lawyers in Leeds'.[14] These comments reflected a tension within the Leeds Jewish community between members of the middle class, represented in the B'nai B'rith, who wished to curb the entry of Jews into the professions, and the poorer sections of the community, who wanted entry to be more open. A letter signed 'Hard-Hit Parent' to the *Jewish Chronicle*, printed on 24 August 1934, clearly enunciated the latter viewpoint:

The majority of members [of the Leeds B'nai B'rith] consist of the so-called 'well-to-do *baalei-batim* [householders]'. Almost all of them could well afford to retain their sons in their own business, and still most of their children have gone in for the professions. In fact, some well-to-do members of the B'nai B'rith have even allowed their children to go in for scholarships, thus depriving the poorer boys to whom a profession would not be a luxury but a vital necessity. There must be at least fifty young doctors and solicitors who could have a very comfortable career by following their father's business. That

[12] *JC* 3 Feb. 1933, p. 29.   [13] *JC* 15 July 1932, p. 23.   [14] *JC* 17 Aug. 1934, p. 6.

would give a chance to more brilliant boys not so fortunately placed, whose only career outside a profession would be an under-presser or some similar trade, which is now also getting filled up by female labour and machinery.[15]

The employment situation in Leeds had parallels in other towns, in respect of both Jewish–Christian relations and class friction within the Jewish community. Everywhere, financial problems among would-be lawyers from poor families are a common theme. 'Cases have occurred fairly frequently where students, having successfully become LL.B's, find themselves without the resources to pay the necessary fees to enable them to qualify and pass the examinations as barristers or solicitors', wrote an anonymous correspondent to the *Jewish Chronicle* in 1936. 'The students or their parents have endeavoured to raise funds by donations from those appealed to on the ground that the student had successfully obtained his LL.B. degree but is unable to make use of it professionally because of lack of means for the further qualifications.'[16] Henry Cohen (1900–77), the youngest in one such poor immigrant family of five children in Liverpool, chose to study medicine with the aim of becoming a criminal lawyer, but later decided that a career in medicine was interesting enough in its own right.[17]

The one Jewish charitable body, that might have assisted poor Jewish law students to qualify, the Education Aid Society, tended on the whole to concentrate its efforts elsewhere, particularly in aiding those training to become doctors. It also had a rigid policy of not offering

any encouragement to the numerous class whose abilities might be sufficient to enable them to make a living of some sort in one of the professions, but who, from lack of means to procure the necessary training, are destined to become clerks and artisans. It is no part of the Society's functions to deplete the ranks of trade and industry in order to turn out second-rate professional men. The Society has therefore from the outset pitched its standard consistently high and has confined its assistance to those whose natural qualifications are such as to ensure their passing the highest educational tests and practising with distinction the art or profession of their choice.[18]

In exceptional cases, nevertheless, the society made a small grant to impoverished students in urgent need of funds to complete a course. Thus one young man who had passed his solicitor's finals was voted a grant of £35 to obtain formal admission to the profession and to take out a practising certificate; but Asher Fishman, later a well-known communal figure who served as president of the Shechitah Board and was an important influence in Jewish education, requested and was refused an allowance of £1. 10s. 0d. a week towards his main-

[15] *JC* 24 Aug. 1934, p. 29.   [16] *JC* 2 Oct. 1936, p. 8.
[17] Blake and Nicholls (eds.), *The Dictionary of National Biography 1971–1980*, 161 (on Henry Cohen).
[18] Education Aid Society, *Objects, Methods and Progress* (London: Education Aid Society, 1930), 4.

tenance and the payment of the premium of £150 in eight instalments, for which he applied when his father's business was in difficulties.[19]

As noted above in the case of Philip Emanuel, a number of capable young men with limited financial resources started as solicitors' managing clerks and then went on to qualify as solicitors themselves; others who took this route into the profession included Lewis Silkin and Solomon Levy. In addition, a group of bright young men from immigrant families, among them Jacques Cohen (1900–49), Solomon Teff (1892–1979), Janus Cohen (1900–84), and Samuel Magnus (1910–92) studied Semitics at Jews' College in order to gain a degree, thereby securing a shorter period of service in articles to become solicitors or, in the case of Magnus, to provide him with the necessary preliminary qualifications to start his barrister's training.[20] This tactic caused some resentment among the communal elite when the young men abandoned their training for the Anglo-Jewish ministry in this way; but although there was a suggestion that they should repay the tuition fees advanced to them by the college, it was not enforced, and it has been asserted, for example by Eli Cashdan, that they more than repaid any sum expended by their service within the Jewish community. Magnus, who had been offered and refused jobs as a minister, attracted the particular ire of Sir Robert Waley Cohen, a communal magnate, who had no hesitation in vetoing the fledgling lawyer's application to the Education Aid Society in 1937 for a grant of '£205 to cover his call fees [to the Bar] and the expenses of reading in chambers for six months'.[21] Not all those who trained for the ministry as a stepping-stone to the law made the transition immediately: Reuben Lincoln served as minister of a number of congregations in Britain and the United States before concentrating on his career as a solicitor; and Benjamin Benas Lieberman was for some years the minister of the Brighton Synagogue before qualifying as a solicitor in 1929 and leaving the ministry in the following year.[22]

Writing in 1922, Woolfe Summerfield claimed that 'It is difficult to estimate the numbers of Jewish barristers and solicitors; in the provinces there are but few, and even in London . . . there are not nearly so many eminent practitioners as could be desired.'[23] Nevertheless, it seems that by 1919 there were over 100 Jewish solicitors practising in London, and by 1939 approximately 290, out of a total of about 3,530. In other words, by 1939, 8.2 per cent of London's solicitors

[19] Education Aid Society, Minute Book, General Committee, 14 Apr. 1937, 30 Dec. 1937, Parkes Library, University of Southampton, MS 135 AJ/35/5.

[20] *JC* 9 Sept. 1949, p. 9 (obituary of Cohen), 28 Sept. 1979, p. 31 (obituary of Teff); *The Times*, 18 Apr. 1992 (obituary of Magnus); interview with the late Eli Cashdan, 14 Aug. 1997.

[21] Education Aid Society, Minute Book, General Committee, 19 July 1937, Parkes Library, University of Southampton, MS 135 AJ/35/5.

[22] *JC* 31 Jan. 1969, p. 9 (80th birthday tribute to Lieberman), 11 Oct. 1957, p. 25 (obituary of Reuben Lincoln).   [23] Summerfield, 'Anglo-Jewry and the Law', p. vi.

were Jewish.[24] Thus the number of Jewish solicitors practising in London in the two decades between the world wars almost trebled; and the majority of these new recruits to the profession came from east European immigrant families.

To discover when the influx of Jews from a second-generation east European immigrant background into the legal profession commenced, it is best to look at the situation in Leeds, Liverpool, and Manchester, for in these smaller cities the trends are easier to discern. In a B'nai B'rith Vocational Advisory Committee Report issued in September 1934, it was stated that

In Leeds, only seven Jewish solicitors were in practice prior to 1925. Since 1925 the number has risen to 27, while one third of the students in the Law faculty at Leeds University are Jews. It is understood that steps are already being taken by the local community with a view to counteracting this tendency. We were informed that the position in Manchester University 'could not be regarded as healthy' from this point of view and in Liverpool there has been a noticeable increase in the last few years in the number of Jewish solicitors.[25]

As well as law students, some Jewish graduates from other faculties entered solicitors' offices and many young Jews became articled clerks without attending university.

In Leeds the growing tension between the Jewish law students and the general body of the Law Students' Society, rooted in the fear of future competition for clients arising from increased numbers of Jewish solicitors, came to a head in 1927. 'Although not affiliated to the Law Society,' wrote a correspondent in the *Jewish Chronicle* early in this year,

it [the student body] is fostered and encouraged by the qualified members of the legal profession who give it their financial support and act as chairmen of its weekly meetings. The anti-Jewish attitude became noticeable during the session 1925–1926, when a Jewish student, articled to one of the leading firms of solicitors in the city, failed to secure a requisite majority [for admission into the society]. As the rejection of any applicant was an unprecedented fact in the history of the Society, it appeared likely that the underlying motive was anti-Jewish. Shortly afterwards four Jewish students were nominated for membership, but were all rejected.

Other Jewish students who were nominated for membership, were also rejected; one application from a Jewish candidate was blocked, but then accepted when he reapplied under an Anglicized variation of his own name. As a result of this

---

[24] This estimate is based on an analysis of the names in *The Law List 1939* (London: Stevens & Sons, 1939), 449–741, together with interviews with Lucien Isaacs (admitted 1929), 6 Oct. 1997 and Barnett Saffron (admitted 1939), 12 May 1997. The total Jewish population of London stood at about 200,000 in 1920.

[25] Report of the Vocational Advisory Committee of the B'nai B'rith First Lodge of England [Sept. 1934], 2, Board of Deputies Archive, Acc. 3121 B4/PM/42.

treatment of their co-religionists, almost every Jewish member of the society resigned. 'In view of the fact that membership of a society of this kind forms such an invaluable part of the training for the profession of Law,' continued the correspondent, 'it seems unfair that such a bar should be placed in the way of Jewish aspirants to the legal profession.'[26] None of the other English university student law societies discriminated against Jews in so blatant a manner, more characteristic of the countries of central Europe; nor was the ban on Jewish students in Leeds enforced for long, as Julius Silman was admitted as a member in the following year (though he did not attend its meetings, boycotting it out of unease at its attitude to Jews).[27]

By the mid-1930s there was a growing awareness among Jewish families in the provincial towns that there was a surplus number of solicitors available for the work that was open to them; this was followed by a decline in the number of first-year law students. 'Liverpool, Leeds, Cardiff and Cambridge all report that there are fewer Jewish Law students in the first year than there are in their final year.' In a survey of a representative group of 788 Jewish students in 1936–7, seven were found to be studying law in Leeds, though the numbers in the law faculties in Liverpool and Manchester were appreciably greater, at sixteen and twenty respectively.[28]

In Liverpool there were two Jewish solicitors before 1919—John Davis, who was admitted in April 1888, and Sydney Walter Price, who was admitted in 1913—as well as Henry Samuel Oppenheim, who qualified as far back as 1868 and was probably Jewish.[29] By 1925 there were five Jewish solicitors practising in the city, possibly six, again if we include Oppenheim.[30] By the outbreak of the Second World War the number had risen sharply to twenty-four in 1939.[31] The bulk of this increase occurred during the 1930s, but six individuals— Samuel Dean, Samuel Sydney Silverman, Geoffrey Isadore Compton, Nathan Silverbeck, Stanley Masheder, and Alfred Beiber—qualified in the years 1927– 9.[32] Thus the pattern of recruitment for Jewish solicitors in Liverpool much resembled that already encountered in Leeds, with a sharp rise after 1925 and a steady increase throughout the 1930s; and it is reasonable to infer that the trends among Jewish solicitors in London were similar.

According to Brian Abel-Smith and Robert Stevens, 'The total number [of solicitors] in practice rose during the thirties more rapidly than the work available for them. Thus whereas solicitors seeking work through the Law

---

[26] *JC* 7 Jan. 1927, p. 38.
[27] Silman, *Signifying Nothing*, 67, 68.
[28] Blok, 'Jewish Students', 188.
[29] *The Law List 1919* (London: Stevens & Sons, 1919), 969–85.
[30] *The Law List 1929* (London: Stevens & Sons, 1929), 1037–53.
[31] *The Law List 1939* (London: Stevens & Sons, 1939), 1083–1106.
[32] Interview with Dr and Mrs Mervyn Goodman, 18 Oct. 1997.

Society's Employment Registry in 1928 expected salaries of £250 or more, by 1938 most applicants were prepared to accept salaries of £200.' In the year 1937/8 there were 24,000 solicitors, 16,899 of whom held practising certificates (the remainder included retired and unemployed solicitors, as well as some working in other business areas), and at this time there was a fresh intake of about 400 newly qualified solicitors a year. 'Moreover the Law Society informed a Parliamentary Committee in 1939 that the average net income of a solicitor was "not more than £400 a year". The average solicitor, having arrived socially, was seldom wealthy', Abel-Smith and Stevens concluded.[33]

Even in the 1920s it was not always easy for solicitors to make a living. In 1924 William Marcus Pyke was struck off the register by the Law Society for improperly retaining money paid to him for arrears of alimony. He had recovered the sum of £5. 2s. 6d. on behalf of a poor client, but instead of paying the sum forthwith he paid it to her in small instalments. On an appeal to a divisional court, it was said on Pyke's behalf that he was almost 70 and had practised without any complaint being made against him for forty years; in these circumstances the court decided to reduce the penalty, by suspending him from practice for twelve months. It could be argued that Pyke may have been suffering from a cashflow problem in his office as a result of his advancing years and consequently depleted energy and activity, and that this induced him to eke out the repayment of instalments to his client.[34] In 1924 Joseph Nunes Nabarro was suspended from practice for two years by the Law Society for making payments to a clerk in the Public Trustee Office as an inducement for introducing new clients to him. In this case, despite an appeal, the court would not interfere with the length of the sentence, even though it was stated on Nabarro's behalf 'that the appellant was a man of high character, who had conducted a reputable business for many years'. It is possible that Nabarro was under pressure to make enough income to provide for his growing family, and as a result took desperate measures to gain new business; one of the judges found the sentence unduly harsh. Financial pressures could be severe: in 1927 two London-based Jewish solicitors, Edward Henry Coopman and Ralph Livermore, went bankrupt.[35]

As the competition for work among the new recruits to the profession intensified, there were widespread accusations of price undercutting and ambulance-chasing to attract clients, accusations from which Jewish solicitors were not immune. In 1934 A. D. Pappworth, the editor of *The Jewish Academy*, the journal of Inter-University Jewish Federation (IUJF), wrote to Neville Laski, the president of the Board of Deputies, complaining that 'In Leeds young

[33] Abel-Smith and Stevens, *Lawyers*, 210. *Report of the Joint Committee of the House of Lords and House of Commons to Consider the Solicitors Bill 1939*, PP1938–9, vol. viii, Qs 133, 134, 1048.

[34] *JC* 4 July 1924, p. 28, 31 Oct. 1924, p. 30.

[35] *JC* 23 May 1924, p. 29, 22 July 1927, p. 32, 29 July 1927, p. 48, 23 Dec. 1927, p. 25.

Jewish solicitors were cutting rates and in other ways not observing professional standards.' Similar complaints were ventilated privately in the Coordinating Committee, the forerunner of the Defence Committee of the Board of Deputies, on 12 January 1938. 'Mr Harry Samuels raised the question of the conduct on the part of certain Jewish solicitors in Liverpool and Manchester, and wondered whether it would be possible to suggest some means of bringing home to them the seriousness of such behaviour as it affected the Community at large.'[36] So too, in a Board of Deputies survey of the 'Internal Causes of Anti-Semitism' produced at the beginning of 1940, it was claimed that certain

professional men, particularly solicitors . . . have acquired a bad name for the manner in which they conduct their practice and the way in which they treat their clients . . . [This resembled the complaints made against Jewish traders for indulging in price-cutting, which was lawful but regarded as morally dubious.] Some time ago a meeting of solicitors was held not only for the Defence Fund but also to discuss the question of checking malpractice and it was suggested that Jewish solicitors might set up a committee for this purpose somewhat on the lines of those already set up by the trades. Strong opposition to this from senior members of the profession of the highest reputation and integrity made it clear that the suggestion could not be accepted. The argument against this proposition . . . was that there was already in existence a disciplinary Committee which dealt with offences of the kind complained of, and that it would be invidious to create a special committee to deal with offences committed by members of the Jewish faith alone. The remedy was . . . in bringing these offences to the attention of their own professional disciplinary Committees, which also met the criticism that we were attempting to hide our own faults.[37]

American research by Reichstein showed that lawyers from small firms 'resent the way in which (they feel) the professional elite seeks to control them using the ethical code as an instrument',[38] and it could be argued that some members of the old professional elite within Anglo-Jewry were exaggerating the faults of the new class of lawyers in an attempt to control them and to curb the additional competition they represented.

The number of Jewish solicitors either struck off or suspended by the Disciplinary Committee of the Law Society between 1936 and 1940 was not large. Of twenty solicitors struck off in 1936 only one was Jewish, and no Jewish solicitors were suspended in that year. In the following year serious infractions by Jewish solicitors reached a peak: three (out of sixteen) were struck off for professional

[36] A. D. Pappworth to Neville Laski, 18 Jan. 1934, Board of Deputies Archive, Acc. 3121 B4/ PM/42; Board of Deputies Co-ordinating Committee, Minutes, 12 Jan. 1938, Board of Deputies Archive, C6/1/1/1.

[37] Board of Deputies, 'Memorandum on the Internal Causes of Anti-Semitism', 3, 6, Cambridge University Library, Redcliffe Nathan Salaman Papers, Add. MS 8171, Box 14.

[38] Quoted in David Podmore, *Solicitors and the Wider Community* (London: Heinemann, 1980), 25, 26.

misconduct, and one more was suspended for two years. In 1938 none of the sixteen solicitors who were struck off was Jewish, but one Jewish solicitor was suspended for three years and three were penalized for minor breaches of the solicitors' accounts rules. In 1939 only one Jewish solicitor, from Manchester, was struck off out of the eighteen who suffered this fate; one solicitor from Leeds was suspended for four years because of breaches of the solicitors' accounts rules; another London-based Jewish solicitor was fined; and Samuel Landman, a leading figure in the Zionist movement, was suspended for three years for professional misconduct. In 1940, out of the seven solicitors who were struck off one was Jewish; Ellis Lincoln, a rising criminal lawyer, was suspended for five years, and two more of the solicitors who were suspended were probably Jewish. Thus the evidence suggests not only that the fears expressed privately within the Board of Deputies about the misconduct of certain Jewish solicitors appear to have been exaggerated, but also that—contrary to the view of their detractors—few of these rogue lawyers came from the provinces.[39]

In fact, it was later discovered, when he died, that one of the worst defaulters was Robert Nathaniel Eichholz (1896–1957), who was from an old Anglo-Jewish family and was a member of the City firm of Adler & Perowne. His victims were mostly Jewish refugees from Nazi Germany in the 1930s, whose money disappeared into his account. After the Second World War, Eichholz offered elderly ladies 'quick, tax-free capital gains. He brought property with their money and offered bogus papers as proof of ownership. Records show that at one time five of his clients "owned" the same property.' His second wife was an Italian maid, for whom he bought a Tudor manor in Kent from Sir Thomas Overy. Eichholz misappropriated at least half a million pounds; most of these losses were covered by the Law Society compensation fund, but the scandal led to accountants making more rigorous enquiries before issuing solicitors with the necessary clearance to obtain their annual practising certificate.[40]

There certainly were some Jewish lawyers among the ambulance-chasers and those accused of dubious practices. In the leading case of *Wiggins* v. *Lavy* (1928), a Mr Wiggins sued Frederick Lavy, a Jewish solicitor of High Holborn, for 'maintenance and champerty'. 'Maintenance' in this sense means giving a defendant in an action money or some other inducement to maintain his plea; 'champerty' is 'the unlawful maintenance of a suit in consideration of some bargain to have . . . some profit out of it'. Wiggins contended that Lavy procured

---

[39] These figures are based on an analysis of the names in the *Law Society's Gazette*, 1936–40.

[40] *New York Law Journal*, 1 May 1967, 17; Quintin Johnstone and Dan Hopson, *Lawyers and their Work: An Analysis of the Legal Profession in the United States and England* (New York: Bobbs-Merrill, 1967), 507; *Re: Eichholz (deceased)* 1 All ER 1959, pp. 166–79. Elkan Nathan Adler (1861–1946), son of Chief Rabbi Nathan Marcus Adler, a bibliophile and Jewish historian, formed a partnership with Perowne, the son of a bishop.

Miriam Schneider and her infant son by his father to bring an action against him in the Shoreditch County Court for damages for personal injuries caused by him or his employees.[41] The case was heard in the High Court before a judge and jury. Sir Patrick Hastings KC, who represented Wiggins, said that while the action was for a sum of only £70,

it was an important case, because the person sued was a solicitor, and because of the issue necessarily involved. There was in existence . . . an organisation with the high sounding name of the Legal Aid Society . . . but he thought that he would be able to show that the organisation was closely associated with Mr Lavy. It seemed that if a person had the misfortune to be involved in an accident, the society, by some means, received a report, and then approached the sufferer with the suggestion that it was desirable to bring an action for compensation, at the same time indicating that if an action was brought the person injured would not be liable for any legal expenses, but that the solicitor would deduct a percentage of whatever amount might be recoverable. In the case of a Mrs Isaacs, who had met with an accident, she had kept the documents. One of these was a form bearing a figure of Justice, which asked whether she would claim compensation, and intimated that the society would obtain evidence 'without the least worry or trouble to you'. The form added that no fees would be made for the society's assistance, but if any compensation was obtained 'you are expected to pay two shillings in the pound towards the working expenses of the society'. A form was enclosed for Mrs Isaacs to fill up, appointing Mr Lavy as her solicitor. Sir Patrick added that he would be able to show that there were many cases which had come to Mr Lavy in precisely the same way.

After further evidence, the jury found for Mr Wiggins on both counts and awarded him damages of £29. 14s. 2d. together with costs.[42]

The defendant then appealed on the grounds that Wiggins had 'failed to prove that Mr Lavy was the society, or that he had received any part of the 2s. in the pound'. In giving judgment Lord Hanworth, the Master of the Rolls, stated that in so far as the Legal Aid Society carried on business,

it had been admitted by a [Mr] Osborne that when an accident occurred he had introduced the person involved to the appellant [Lavy] 'who took up the case for him'. A book had been kept by the appellant showing the transactions which had taken place. Sometimes the persons threatened paid up without fighting. Two shillings in the pound were deducted from the amounts received, but the appellant, a solicitor of 35 years' standing, had not kept any record of those accounts.

To suggest that the appellant's case was similar to *Ladd* v. *London Road Car Company* or *Rich* v. *Cook* in that a solicitor might take up a speculative case for a poor client was, said the judge, 'a travesty' in the circumstances of the present case; and 'There was, therefore, clear evidence of maintenance.' Because the

[41] J. A. Jolowicz and T. Ellis Lewis, *Winfield on Tort* (London: Sweet & Maxwell, 1963), 717.
[42] *JC* 18 May 1928, 37.

Yorkshire Insurance Company had instructed their own solicitor on Mr Wiggins's behalf 'to defend the proceedings, and the costs of the solicitor were the subject matter of the claim in the action. There was, therefore, no case of any special damage to Mr Wiggins, the plaintiff in the action, and on that technical ground the appeal would be allowed.'[43] Although he won his appeal, Lavy was clearly shown by these proceedings to be connected with the Legal Aid Society, an ambulance-chasing organization, and to have failed to keep proper accounts of his earnings.

Another case involving what some would regard as sharp practice, *Orpen v. Haymarket Capitol Limited and Others* (1931), was instigated by Jacques Cohen, a solicitor with offices in Bishopsgate who, as noted above, was a graduate of Jews' College. Cohen arranged a conference with Herbert Garland and Frederic Landau, who had recently been called to the Bar, in order to bring a claim on behalf of Miss Offenheim, a clerk in his office, as a common informer under the Sunday Observance Act 1781 with regard to Sunday cinema sessions. She was claiming over £25,000 from cinema owners for opening on Sunday. Cohen's main contention was that the Haymarket Capitol Cinema and a number of other West End cinemas were in breach of the Sunday Observance Act because they were giving only a tiny proportion of their takings to charity—this being the sole basis on which they were allowed to open on Sunday. He wanted his secretary to collect penalties from the cinema and its directors, while he would be entitled to collect the costs of a successful action. At the conference Garland said it was inconvenient that the plaintiff in the intended action was Jewish, as the authorities would take unkindly a Jew defending the Sunday observance legislation. When Cohen asked what he should do, Garland suggested that Miss Offenheim should change her name, which she duly did by deed poll, taking the new surname Orpen. On Garland's advice, Sir Thomas Inskip KC, whose brother was the bishop of Norwich, was briefed to appear for Miss Orpen in court, while Sir Patrick Hastings KC appeared for the cinema company. Lionel Cohen KC was counsel for the defendant directors, a number of whom were Jewish, including Maurice Ostrer, whose brother Isidore, a merchant banker, had laid the foundation of the Gaumont-British Picture Corporation and was one of the key figures in the British cinema industry during the 1930s.[44]

Hastings's first and only question to Miss Orpen was: 'Isn't your real name Millie Offenheim?'

In response the young woman said, 'My name is Millie Orpen and here is the deed poll', producing the document from her handbag.

This exchange seemed to undermine the effectiveness of the rest of Sir Patrick's presentation. Lionel Cohen successfully argued that no case had been

---

[43] *Wiggins v. Lavy* (1928) 44 *The Times Law Reports*, pp. 721–3.
[44] *JC* 19 Dec. 1930, p. 33; interview with the late Frederic Landau, 6 Aug. 1966.

made out against any of the directors on the evidence.[45] In his judgment Mr Justice Rowlatt declared that 'In the present case the plaintiff was [a] clerk to a solicitor. Two days before the issue of the writ she changed her name by deed poll from Offenheim to Orpen, under which designation, perhaps, she could more colourably come forward as the champion of the English Sunday. No claim could come before the Court in less attractive circumstances.' Despite this distaste for the claim, he found in favour of Miss Orpen, awarding her the sum of £5,000 against the cinema company; but he also gave judgment against her in favour of the defendant directors with costs.[46]

The cinema owners would not take this rebuff lying down. Garland warned Jacques Cohen that the Home Secretary would 'remit all the penalties [i.e. order their payment to a particular individual or charity], but he has no power to remit costs'. Lord Knutsford, though nearing death, sent a message through to Jacques Cohen to ask him if he would agree to the penalties going to the London Hospital, of which he was chairman. Cohen consented to this, but the Home Secretary would not allow it, and the money went to the Inland Revenue.

Three months later Charles Doughty KC and Garland appeared for Miss Orpen in another similar action, *Orpen* v. *New Empire Limited and Others* (1931), which could not proceed to a full hearing as Parliament had in the meantime passed the Sunday Performances (Temporary Regulation) Act 1931 which rendered the action void in respect of penalties, though the judge still had the power to make an order for costs. Mr St John Field submitted on behalf of the defendants that the court 'had consistently set its face against common informers' and complained that 'the plaintiff was a Jewess who attended a synagogue and was hardly a person who should come forward as a champion of the Christian Sunday'. Mr Justice Rowlatt gave the plaintiff her costs, but also ordered her to pay the directors their costs. So Jacques Cohen made some money out of the action and Miss Orpen ended up with nothing, sadly dying from tuberculosis while still only in her twenties.[47]

*

As early as the mid-1920s doubts began to surface within the ranks of the immigrant Anglo-Jewish community about the wisdom of providing their children with a university education. Some claimed that such a training alienated these children both from their parents and families and from their cultural roots. In

[45] *Orpen* v. *Haymarket Capitol Limited and Others* (1931) 47 *The Times Law Reports*, pp. 575–7; interview with the late Frederic Landau, 6 Aug. 1996.

[46] *Orpen* v. *Haymarket Capitol Limited and Others* (1931) 47 *The Times Law Reports*, pp. 576, 577.

[47] Ibid. 575–7; *Orpen* v. *New Empire Limited and Others* (1931) 48 *The Times Law Reports*, pp. 8, 9; interviews with the late Frederic Landau, 6 Aug. 1996, Mrs Ethel Levine, 24 Nov. 1997.

1926 Sol Goldberg, a Jewish man living in Chapeltown, the centre of the Leeds immigrant community, penned a series of sketches in the *Jewish Chronicle* describing how, in one such family, the parents pawned jewels and took loans to buy their son a surgery, only for him to fail his exams; how Reb Samuel, a poor grocer, undertook deliveries by hand, only to see his daughter, having obtained her BA, marry in church; how another father, the owner of a small drapery and furniture shop, after spending thousands on the education of his son, explained that 'he has left us, and lives in a hotel, where he eats *trefah* [non-kosher food], and it doesn't suit him to come and see us. He is ashamed of us.' Mr Goldberg bemoaned what he saw as parents' desire to use education as a means of making 'their son a professional man, a doctor, solicitor, etc. Even the cobbler dreams of nothing else but that his son should become a doctor, and when they do become a doctor they are lost to our people and to their parents.'[48] Some parents, however, clearly took a view similar to Goldberg's. Around 1916, in London, Henry Bloomstein was determined that none of his children should become doctors or lawyers. 'To the headmaster's dismay', he 'removed one of his most talented sons from the Cowper Street School at 14 years, although this youth was at the top of his class in a grammar school, fearing that if he became a professional man, he would rapidly become assimilated and lose his religious zeal. Similar episodes occurred in other orthodox families.'[49]

In answer to Sol Goldberg, a Mr Arnold Rosenthal stated that

The tragedy of inter-marriage and of the children outgrowing the parents is as prevalent in business circles as in academic circles . . . there has been formed a sub-section of the Manchester Jewish students (a good percentage of whom are medicals) which holds a weekly class for the study of the Talmud . . . While admitting that a few individual instances exist of the frustration of parents' hopes in the education of their children, we must recognise that in the vast majority of cases the sacrifice of parents has met with its due reward in the enhanced social and intellectual status of their children and in the enrichment of our Jewish public life.

He was supported by Dr Maurice Sourasky of Leeds, who declared that 'I have the privilege of counting among my friends and acquaintances many university-trained Jews: I do not know of a single instance where Mr Goldberg's characterisation would hold true.' So far from the young Jewish doctors and lawyers becoming alienated from their people, according to Dr Sourasky Jewish students tended to be 'intensely nationalistic'.[50] Within the ranks of the immi-

---

[48] *JC Supplement*, 29 Jan. 1926, p. iii.

[49] John Cooper, 'The Bloomstein and Isenberg Families', in Aubrey Newman (ed.), *The Jewish East End 1840–1939* (London: Jewish Historical Society of England, 1981), 68.

[50] *JC* 5 Feb. 1926, p. 14. Maurice Sourasky's career, after he changed his surname to Sorsby, is discussed above in Chapter 3.

grant community, there was a division between a small section of the Orthodox, who were opposed to their children's embarking on professional careers, and a larger group, imbued with a modernizing or secular Zionist ethic, who whole-heartedly approved such a career choice for their children.[51]

Earlier chapters of this book have described how, during the First World War and with increasing momentum in the 1920s and 1930s, Jewish youths from immigrant backgrounds enrolled in the British medical schools. By the mid-1920s and throughout the 1930s there was a similar upsurge, albeit on a considerably smaller scale, in the number of young men from such families becoming solicitors. Not everyone was happy with this trend. Dr Selig Brod-etsky, professor of mathematics at Leeds University and later president of the Board of Deputies, announced in 1928 that while he 'admired all the Jewish passion for study',

there was one suspicious feature about it—its aims were too obvious. He wished Jews had less professional men and more genuine students. The rush into the professions was one of the most alarming symptoms of modern Jewish life. In England, Jewish doctors were beginning to stumble over one another, Jewish lawyers were beginning to compete unpleasantly with one another. The lucky young Jew was he who found a pitch that had not yet become crowded with Jewish stalls. He admired the student who went into industry more than him who drifted into a so-called learned profession.[52]

Four years later, the *Jewish Chronicle* voiced similar reservations. 'There is, and has been for some time, an increasing influx of Jews in this country into various professions—medicine, the law, and now . . . accountancy', wrote 'Watchman' on 5 February 1932. 'To be sure, young Jews and Jewesses have as much right as any other citizens to embrace these occupations. The question is whether, seeing how crowded some of these professions are, they are doing the best thing for themselves.' 'Watchman' went on to cite a number of instances of young Jews who had obtained the qualifications necessary to become teachers and dentists but had been unable to find suitable employment. 'I was told of a young Jew who had graduated as a dentist with great distinction. But having obtained his diploma, he found himself up against a brick wall. His people were very poor. They could not give him the money to set up in practice in the pro-fession for which he had so determinedly and bravely qualified.' In conclusion, he wanted 'to ask the Jews of this country to pause for a moment and to consider whether the trend to the professions is a healthy one, whether the road to a pro-fessional occupation is necessarily paved with either money or glory'. He sug-gested that many talented Jewish boys should seek alternative careers in industry and agriculture rather than the professions.[53]

[51] Cooper, 'The Bloomstein and Isenberg Families', 68.   [52] *JC* 20 Jan. 1928, p. 16.
[53] *JC* 5 Feb. 1932, p. 11.

Again, this article elicited a robust response from Dr Maurice Sorsby (Sourasky), who repudiated the suggestion that Jews were overcrowding the medical profession in England:

The dread that the medical profession is getting overcrowded is probably as old as medicine itself . . . If, for example, Vienna Jewry has produced great physicians, it must not be forgotten that medicine in Vienna is almost a Jewish monopoly. The general population of Vienna is about a quarter that of London; the Jewish population of the two cities is about equally strong (200,000 souls); yet Vienna has 4,000 Jewish doctors as against London's about 500 . . . if I may express a personal opinion, I should say that the saturation point of Jews in British medicine is far from reached.[54]

All these fears about the eagerness of Anglo-Jewish youths to seek careers in the professions were eclipsed by the coming to power of the Nazis in Germany in 1933 and what Saul Friedlander describes as Hitler's 'war-cry against Jewish professional monopolists'. Friedlander has argued that while the majority of ordinary Germans were moderate rather than extreme antisemites, the German elites, including the universities, the churches, and the professions, colluded with Hitler by becoming active supporters of his attempt to curtail the allegedly inordinate influence of Jews over German life. Hitler early adopted the aim of segregating Jews from Germans, as he told an inner group of party members in 1935: 'Out of all professions, into the ghetto enclosed in a territory where they can behave as becomes their nature, while the German people look on as one looks at wild animals.'[55] Hence from March 1933 official measures were introduced in Germany to debar Jewish doctors from practising. Under a government decree of 22 August 1933 only Jewish doctors who had been active combatants in war or had been employed in hospitals for infectious disease could treat patients belonging to the national health insurance scheme; there were also exemptions for Jewish doctors admitted before 1 August 1914. 'Today it is a rare thing to find a Jewish doctor or medical student in any German hospital', wrote Fritz Seidler in 1934. Similarly, officials of the Nazi party started a campaign to oust Jewish judges and lawyers, a campaign to which the government later gave legal sanction. Again, under a law of 1 August 1933 exemptions were permitted for Jewish lawyers who had begun to practise before 1 August 1914, who had fought for Germany in the First World War, or whose fathers or sons had fallen in combat. 'By means of an organised boycott, special regulations imposed by the authorities, and pressure from the Nazi factory "cells"', the Jewish lawyers who were still allowed to practise were intimidated and in many instances compelled to stop working.[56]

[54] *JC* 12 Feb. 1932, p. 12.

[55] Saul Friedlander, *Nazi Germany and the Jews: The Years of Persecution, 1933–1939* (London: Weidenfeld & Nicolson, 1997), 143.

[56] Fritz Seidler, *The Bloodless Pogrom* (London: Gollancz, 1934), 209–38.

Outside Germany, Jewish communal leaders in both the United States and Britain became alarmed at the overcrowding of Jews in certain professions,[57] and in England there was a series of reports and articles in the Jewish press coloured by the German experience. Under the impetus of events in Germany, 'Watchman' repeated his warnings about the unhealthy eagerness of Jews to seek careers in the professions in the *Jewish Chronicle* on 3 November 1933. 'Meanwhile . . . the number of Jewish students grows apace, here and on the Continent. The vistas that stretch before them when they graduate are . . . of overcrowded professions in which men and women are struggling for their daily bread.' A. D. Pappworth remarked in the December 1933 issue of the *Jewish Academy* that

The conditions of Jewish professional workers on the Continent should be a warning. In Eastern Europe, and to a greater extent in Germany . . . a transformation, is taking place. The Jews, it is recognised, cannot maintain their large proportion of doctors and lawyers and other professional workers. They must turn to a simpler and more productive life; they must adopt a more normal distribution of employment.

Privately Pappworth wrote to Neville Laski, the president of the Board of Deputies, on 18 January 1934 that although the Jewish Students' Federation had passed a resolution critical of Jews devoting themselves to a small number of occupations and professions, it was likely to remain a dead letter as there did not exist among the students a 'serious realization of the nature of the problem'.[58]

Among the leadership of the B'nai B'rith, which represented prosperous Jewish businessmen—many of them of east European origin—and a sprinkling of professionals in major communities, such as London, Leeds, and Manchester, there was growing alarm at the situation on the Continent, which was interpreted as a warning sign to British Jewry to slow down the pace of their advance into the professions. At a conference in London in October 1933 attended by many delegates from the provinces, the Revd M. L. Perlzweig referred to the situation in Germany and the coming catastrophe in Poland. He declared that 'The community must be made alive to the fact that it cannot deal with the German-Jewish problem in isolation. The whole economic structure of Jewry must change. The professions were overcrowded and there must be a movement for occupational readjustment.' His solution was the opening of training centres to equip countless thousands to emigrate to Palestine.[59] During 1934 the undue concentration of the Jews in the professions in England was much discussed, as noted above, by the B'nai B'rith in Leeds, and in Manchester as well.[60]

---

[57] Beth S. Wenger, *New York Jews and the Great Depression* (New Haven: Yale University Press, 1996), 29, 30.

[58] *JC* 3 Nov. 1933, p. 11; A. D. Pappworth, 'The Professions', *Jewish Academy*, 1/2 (Dec. 1933), 3, 4. A. D. Pappworth to Neville Laski, 18 Jan. 1914, Board of Deputies Archive, Acc. 3121 B4/PM/42.

[59] *JC* 27 Oct. 1933, p. 23.   [60] *JC* 3 Aug. 1934, July 1934 *Supplement*, p. iv, 17 Aug. 1934, p. 25.

In 1935, when Dr George Webber was installed as president of the First Lodge of the B'nai B'rith, he spoke on the need to give young Jews vocational guidance at the time of their bar mitzvah, rather than at the university stage, when it was already too late. He suggested:

many lawyers and doctors might well have gone into business. For when a man merely regarded his work as a means for making money, he should be engaged in business . . . one sphere to which Jews might betake themselves was agriculture . . . Then there were not many Jewish engineers, while accountancy was a profession which Jews did not frequent, and architecture as a profession could very well be supplemented by more of their people. With regard to industry, Jews preferred to distribute goods rather than manufacture them, and he had often wondered why there were not many Jewish mill-owners in Lancashire or mill-operatives.

Webber's remarks were echoed by Harry Samuels (b. 1893), a communally active barrister 'with a specialised practice in trade union law and industrial injuries'. He declared in a speech to the First Lodge of the B'nai B'rith in 1938 that 'The number of Jewish youths entering into the professions of medicine and the law were out of all proportion to the number of Jews who entered into other professions. Too narrow a choice of professions was unhealthy for the individuals themselves.'[61]

Earlier, during January 1935, the *Jewish Chronicle* shifted the emphasis of its campaign against the maldistribution of Jews in the professions to focus on the problems of American Jewry. 'This question has been sharply underlined', it commented,

by the President of one of the Eastern colleges [stating] that the Jews must come to expect a virtual *numerus clausus* in medical schools . . . Many Jews have come to realise that they must face this question realistically, that there is palpable overcrowding of the professions, especially the medical and law professions, by Jews, and that this situation must be stopped.

A fortnight later Neville Laski asserted that

There are, as is known, social inhibitions in America which do not exist in this country. There is the difficulty of the entry of Jews into the professions, and of Jewish youth into the larger businesses, problems as to the numbers of Jewish youth desirous of entering into the law and medical schools and the number of Jews who are practitioners in both of these professions . . . I think it is . . . [a problem] which ought in every Jewish community to engage the attention of its leaders. We cannot wait until it has assumed dimensions which may become unmanageable. Our policy must be one of prevention and not of cure.

[61] *JC* 18 Oct. 1935, p. 26, 7 Jan. 1938, p. 12, 15 Nov. 1963, p. 18. Dr Webber was himself from Manchester; his father had in fact established a factory there (Pifco) that manufactured electrical goods.

By 1938, indeed, the discriminatory policy of American medical faculties had driven 540 American Jewish medical students from the United States to Edinburgh and Glasgow.[62]

At a conference on 'the Jewish Student' organized by the Federation of Zionist Youth in April 1938, Professor Norman Bentwich surveyed the number of Jews in the professions in Germany, Austria, Poland and England.

He found that in all cases, particularly in the big towns, the Jews were very prominent in the medical and legal professions, and in all professions they were entirely out of proportion to their numbers in the general population. 'By common consent of the leaders of German Jewry', he said, 'that had caused violent anti-Semitism'. The position of the Jews in Germany had changed fundamentally and the young people were being trained in agricultural and technical schools with the hope of emigration. Palestine was the one country in which they had a fairly normal vocational distribution.[63]

On 28 April 1939 'Watchman' returned to the topic of the overcrowding of Jews in the medical and legal professions—now one of his favourite themes—and the dire consequences which could follow:

From time to time, during recent years, I have felt it my duty to direct attention to the urge which exists in the Community for enrolling in certain specific trades and professions . . . The successful attack upon German Jewry was largely based on a similar weakness. The popular mind was influenced by tales, often highly coloured, of the numbers of Jews in this or that occupation—medicine, the law, and all the rest of them. It was said that the Jews had gained a mastery—which had to be smashed—of the national life. And the campaign, which had become the foundation of the movement to clear out Jewish racials and restore the country to its 'Aryan' ownership, was the chief factor in carrying the Nazi colours to victory . . . Only four months ago I quoted our leading journal [*The Times*] as saying that many German Jews had acquired positions in the post-War years which gave them too strong a hold on the social life of the country.[64]

Fears that these events might be repeated in Britain were very strong among the Anglo-Jewish communal leadership; Gordon Liverman admitted in October 1938 that a prominent member of the Deputies' Defence Committee had warned 'that within three years we may be faced with anti-Jewish legislation in this country'.[65]

Among the majority of Jewish students, however, there were doubts as to both the acuteness and the accuracy of the communal leaders' analysis of the situation. 'The problem of general overcrowding (both by Jews and Gentiles) of

[62] *JC* 11, 25 Jan. 1935, pp. 7, 20, 21 Jan. 1938, p. 11; Collins, *Go and Learn*, 99–132.
[63] *JC* 8 Apr. 1938, p. 14.
[64] *JC* 28 Apr. 1939, p. 11; see also 'Watchman', *JC* 21 Jan. 1938, p. 11.
[65] Board of Deputies Co-ordinating Committee, memorandum of Gordon Liverman, Oct. 1938, Board of Deputies Archive.

certain professions has been overlooked', pointed out two students of the London School of Economics, C. J. Israel and Louis Phillips, on 1 February 1935,

by those who criticise the numbers of Jews in the professions. No parent will send his child into an occupation without making enquiries and fully considering the prospects of that occupation. Jews have concentrated in certain professions, notably medicine and law, because these are to a great extent professions where the individual is his own master . . . Many graduates attempt to obtain employment in trade and industry, but latent anti-Semitism plays its hideous role; and they turn to the professions if possible.[66]

The barrister and communal activist Frederic Landau, after discussing the issue with other Jewish graduates, came to a similar conclusion: 'There is no problem of overcrowding in the professions in so far as this can be said to constitute a Jewish problem as alleged. It is a general problem affecting the country as a whole.' Further,

It has never been suggested that there is overcrowding by Jews in the fur, furniture or tailoring trades, in each of which trades there are more Jewish employers and employees than in any other trade or profession . . . It is difficult to see how the younger generation can be prevented or restricted from entering trades or professions. They may be persuaded to alter their minds when they experience the fact that certain professions or trades are not by any means as lucrative as they imagined them to be.[67]

In fact, a resolution was passed at the IUJF conference in 1935 stating on the part of the students 'That the present attitude of the Jewish communal leaders and of the Federation (I.U.J.F.) which is to dissuade Jews from entering the professions is futile and mischievous, in that it implies the existence of a problem which in fact does not exist, and which gives the outside world an impression which tends to increase anti-Semitism.'[68]

Professor A. V. Hill, a leading British physiologist and Nobel Prize winner, told Selig Brodetsky that he 'did not like Jewish academic refugees being admitted to British academic life, because Jews had the habit of filling their departments with Jews'.[69] Similarly, when Sir Henry Dale, the director of the National Institute of Medical Research, addressed the annual meeting of the London Jewish Hospital Medical Society in December 1937, he upset his audience, many of whom were young recruits to the medical profession from an east European Jewish background, when he referred to

his good fortune into coming into intimate contact with such Jews as Paul Ehrlich, Carl Weigert, and Rudolf Magnus, all of whom were intensely loyal to the country of their birth . . . It was largely a product of history, he thought, and the restrictions and persecutions of the past, that, in certain countries especially, Jewish ability was abnormally

---

[66] *JC* 1 Feb. 1935, p. 27. Cecil Israel qualified as a solicitor in 1938 and Louis Phillips in 1939.
[67] *JC* 1 Mar. 1935, p. 36.   [68] *JC* 1 Feb. 1935.
[69] Selig Brodetsky, *Memoirs: From Ghetto to Israel* (London: Weidenfeld & Nicolson, 1960), 161.

concentrated and unhealthily predominant in certain professions and callings. He could never sufficiently acknowledge what he had received from Jewish men of genius with whom he had studied . . . He did not believe that it would be more healthy for a nation or a city of predominantly non-Jewish people to leave all or most of their medical research to Jews or to receive all or most of their medical attention from Jews than it would be for a Gentile nation to be subjected to a wholly Jewish Government.[70]

Dr Laurence Phillips recalled that

The dead silence betokened the acute distress of the audience, to whom the implications and the associations of the advice were only too familiar . . . Those who were present will remember the patient urbanity and the polish of phraseology with which Professor Henry (now Lord Cohen) courteously apprised the distinguished guest of the need for caution in accepting the plausible, and exposed to the politically naive scientist the lamentable implications of his attitude. The crash of applause marked both the relief and the approbation of the listeners.[71]

Sir Henry was also rebuked for his remarks by the *Jewish Chronicle*.

But when, in the course of his speech, Sir Henry began to cast doubts on the wisdom of a 'disproportionately large' number of Jews in Vienna and New York entering certain professions—particularly medicine—and when he went on to ask, in effect, whether it would be a good thing if all the doctors or lawyers, or members of the Government, were Jews, then we think that some at least of his audience must have begun to feel a little restless and uncomfortable. For while the speaker was not moved by anti-Jewish animus . . . one cannot forget that his utterances . . . could be used as justification by the advocates of the *numerus clausus* and the ghetto benches, and for the terrible oppression of the Jewish professional men in Germany.[72]

As a result of the communal concern with the problem of the overcrowding of the professions by Jews, the First Lodge of the B'nai B'rith assembled a committee to examine the question. In its report, issued in September 1934, the committee recommended that the alleged maldistribution of Jews in the professions be ameliorated by the provision of Jewish scholarships for the encouragement of research in medicine, science, and agriculture, the distribution of leaflets written by vocational guidance experts, and the establishment of a vocational guidance centre with an adviser trained by the staff of the National Institute of Industrial Psychology. Dr Charles Myers, the principal of the institute, assisted the committee in its deliberations.[73]

The B'nai B'rith inaugurated a programme of lectures on choice of careers at two secondary schools in London with a preponderance of Jewish pupils, and

---

[70] *JC* 17 Dec. 1937, p. 12.
[71] Laurence Phillips, 'Presidential Address to the London Jewish Hospital Medical Society', 22 Oct. 1964 (London: privately published, 1964), 7.   [72] *JC* 17 Dec. 1937, p. 8.
[73] Report of the Vocational Advisory Committee of the B'nai B'rith, 1–3.

Harry Samuels 'instanced what had happened in Germany as the most convincing argument for the necessity of such action in this country, particularly with regard to the medical and legal profession, where the percentage of Jews was high'. In response to his urging, on 24 January 1939 the Defence Committee decided to give the B'nai B'rith a grant of £50 as an experiment to expand such work in schools; at the same time, the *Jewish Chronicle* and the B'nai B'rith together established a career guidance service in the newspaper in June 1939.[74]

*

As far as the legal profession was concerned, during the inter-war years Jewish solicitors' firms associated with the Cousinhood or the world of the arts and business all throve, whereas many others, especially those from an east European background, struggled to make a living. Just as in the United States during the 1930s, so in Britain there may well have been a sizeable legal underclass among newly trained lawyers.[75] The touting for work and ambulance-chasing among Jewish lawyers, the sometimes dubious litigation undertaken by individuals, and the undercutting of conveyancing costs by some Jewish law firms all point to the conclusion that it was sometimes difficult to earn more than a modest living. When in 1939 a young Liverpool solicitor named Baskin lost his position through no fault of his own, he was prepared to go anywhere, even as far as New Zealand, to find an appropriate post.[76] Abraham Kramer, who qualified as a solicitor in 1932, and Barnett Saffron, who qualified in 1939, have stressed how hard it was for a Jewish solicitor in London to find a place as an assistant in a law firm, and that this was why many Jews opened their own offices. Both Kramer and Saffron came first in the Law Society final examinations in their year, but, as Kramer acknowledged, 'The legal establishment was [then] very much public school and a young Jewish boy was not their ideal recruit.'[77] The well-known media lawyer Oscar Beuselinck, the son of a Belgian sea-cook, confessed that 'I got articles because my firm, with its Jewish clients, wanted someone who looked Jewish without having to employ a Jew.'[78] Yet some Jewish solicitors from an east European background had a completely different experience: Sidney Jaque, for example, was articled to Jesse Allan Nickinson and eventually became a partner in this long-established London firm which had moved to Bedford Row and had a good conveyancing and trust account practice.[79]

---

[74] Board of Deputies, Jewish Defence Committee, Minutes 24 Jan. 1939, C6/1/1/1, 6 Feb. 1940, C6/1/1/2, Board of Deputies Archive.   [75] Auerbach, 'From Rags to Robes'.

[76] Education Aid Society, Minute Book, General Committee, 27 Feb. 1939, Parkes Library, Southampton University, MS 135 AJ/35/5.

[77] Iris Freeman interview with Abraham Kramer, 20 Feb. 1996.   [78] *Lawyer*, 12 Aug. 1997.

[79] Interview with Sidney Jaque, 14 July 1998.

Despite the opposition of the Jewish communal magnates and the new business and professional leaders represented in the B'nai B'rith, and despite the ambivalent attitude of top British scientists, Anglo-Jewish students were not deterred by their gloomy prognostications. They continued to opt in substantial numbers for careers in medicine and law, thus laying the basis of their own future prosperity in the post-Second World War conditions of full employment. So, too, in the United States, Beth S. Wenger has noted that, in spite of the economic crisis,

young Jews continued to aspire to professional and white-collar careers, but such positions were in short supply and almost half of all Jewish youth looking for work failed to find jobs [in the 1930s] . . . As it turned out, Jews of the post-World War II era benefited greatly from their occupational preferences, but in the midst of the Depression, some Jews began to doubt the economic path they had chosen . . . many social workers and community leaders attempted to guide young Jews away from overcrowded white-collar fields.[80]

In Britain, however, the flood of refugee academics, lawyers, and doctors from central Europe lent the problem of overcrowding in the professions a new dimension.

[80] Wenger, *New York Jews*, 29, 30.

NINE

Jewish Refugee Doctors

WITH the advent of the Nazis to power in Germany in 1933, the harassment of Jewish professionals intensified and there began an exodus of Jewish doctors from Germany, which accelerated when laws were passed to exclude Jews from the German medical service. In May 1934 non-Aryan physicians were debarred from participating in the state health insurance scheme; from April 1937 Jews were no longer entitled to take exams to qualify as doctors; and from 30 September 1938 all Jewish medical licences were to be revoked, even if in certain cases Jews were to be permitted to provide medical treatment for other Jews. Already by the end of 1933 578 doctors had left the Reich, and by mid-1934 1,100 had fled abroad. There were also 311 persons dismissed from medical research institutes in the mid-1930s because they were Jewish or partly Jewish. Robert N. Proctor has quoted a source which suggested that by December 1936 4,000 of Germany's 7,500 Jewish physicians had emigrated, but another source estimated that these figures were not reached until the middle of 1938. It is possible, too, that Proctor's figure for the number of Jewish physicians in Germany may be too low, as the highly influential Dr W. M. Kotschnig, an official of the High Commission for Refugees, put the total number of Jewish and non-Aryan doctors in Germany in 1934 at 9,000; and Paul Weindling has suggested that of Vienna's 4,900 doctors, some 3,200, or 60 per cent, were Jewish.[1]

A report of the academic registrar of London University prepared in April 1933 pointed out that

[a] serious problem has arisen owing to the influx of Jewish students from Germany. Already during the past three or four weeks over a hundred of these students have applied for admission to the University. Most of them are medical students in various stages of their courses. Many of them are within six months of Final qualification. The remainder are mostly Engineers.

---

[1] Proctor, *Racial Hygiene*, 152, 153, 374 nn. 74, 85; memorandum of the High Commission for Refugees coming from Germany, prepared for the conference in London on 4–5 July 1934 by Dr W. M. Kotschnig, pp. 5, 6, Central Zionist Archives, Norman Bentwich Papers A255/785; Paul Weindling, 'Jews in the Medical Profession in Britain and Germany: Problems of Comparison', in Michael Brenner, Rainer Liedke, and David Rechter (eds.), *Two Nations: British and German Jews in Comparative Perspective* (Tübingen: Mohr Siebeck, 1999), 400.

The unqualified medical students, even those 'within six months of their final qualification', would have to take the ordinary British students' courses, studying from three to five years. There was already a 'limitation of entry . . . enforced in the London Medical Schools on two classes of British subjects, namely women students and students of non-European parentage'. Thus some London medical schools were unable to take all the British students who applied, and were consequently unwilling to take foreign students; others were willing to take a limited number of foreign students provided they had comparable entry qualifications to British entrants; still others were willing to select a limited number of foreign students on their merits without any proviso. It was urged on behalf of the German Jewish medical students that they would probably be able to find work in the British empire. The board of the Faculty of Medicine, however, doubted this, partly because 'The Dominions are now able to educate sufficient doctors to supply their needs', and partly because there was little work available in the smaller colonies outside the Colonial Medical Service, which was now full.[2]

At the meeting of the Committee of Vice-Chancellors and Principals of the Universities of the British Empire held in London on 24 June 1933, Dr Deller, the delegate for London University, declared that whereas the medical schools 'might be able to take about 12 postgraduate' students, they 'would deal with applications from undergraduates on their merits but he thought that the total number admitted would be inconsiderable. No modification of the existing regulations was proposed and the students who were admitted would be required to take at least a three year course.' Delegates from the other universities spoke in a similar vein, or suggested even harsher terms. Sir Thomas Holland, representing Edinburgh University, said that 'On the medical side they had no vacancies [for students].' Sir James Bailee, on behalf of Leeds University, confirmed that 'They had no room for medical students and he thought that as far as the medical profession was concerned, they were approaching the saturation point.' The negative attitude of Leeds University was somewhat surprising, given that there was a large contingent of Jewish medical students of east European origin already studying there, and that the Jewish Refugees Committee in London had approached the board of the Leeds medical faculty on behalf of the German Jewish students. Dr Moberley, for Manchester University, said that they had a fund to provide two or three fellowships but that the appointments would not be permanent, while as far as medical students were concerned, 'they had no room for more than one or two'. Summing up the consensus reached, Sir Charles Grant Robertson, the chairman, proposed to write to the International Student Service, a body acting on behalf of the refugee students, to the effect

[2] University of London, Report of the Board of the Faculty of Medicine, 1 June 1933, pp. 1–3, Bodleian Library, Society for the Protection of Science and Learning, archive box 1/8.

that 'the number of medical students who could be admitted [to British univer-
sities] was small'.[3]

At a further meeting of the Committee of Vice-Chancellors and Principals
held on 14 December 1935, Sir Charles Grant Robertson again raised the question
of admission to university medical schools of German refugee undergraduates.

Most of the Members present informed the Chairman that only a few such Undergraduates were now being admitted. Mr Eason, [the representative of London University, mentioned] . . . that such Undergraduates, as they arrive in this country, were
informed by the Home Office that after completion of their degree course they would
not be permitted to remain in this country. In these circumstances, it was agreed that no
joint action was called for.[4]

By excluding these German Jewish medical students altogether or by accepting
them only in very small numbers (University College London medical school
decided to take just three every year), the English medical schools limited the
influx of these refugee students to negligible numbers. Despite the funds the
Anglo–Jewish elite bestowed on the London hospitals through large charitable
donations, its members were reluctant to press the claims of the refugee doctors
on the medical establishment in too forceful a manner. For instance, P. S. Waley
and Anthony de Rothschild tried to find a place at St Mary's Hospital for Dr
Rosendahl (Rossdale), a young Jewish doctor from Cologne who Anglicized his
name after requalifying in Britain. Rothschild's secretary wrote to the dean,
thanking him for his help, and added that 'He quite appreciates the necessity for
restricting the number of students who can be admitted to the schools in the
various hospitals.'[5] In all, fifty to seventy-five refugee students, who had received
some of their medical training in Britain, were allowed in 1940 to practise there
on a temporary basis; but a group of younger students, who had completed the
whole of their medical training in Britain, were permitted to follow the occupation or profession of their choice with no time limit.[6]

To cope with the influx of qualified German Jewish doctors and dentists into
Britain, the Jewish Medical and Dental Emergency Association was set up on 23
April 1933 as an offshoot of the London Jewish Medical Society. David Eder was
then serving as president of the society and naturally assumed a similar position
in the new body. By March 1934 the number of German Jewish medical

---

[3] Committee of Vice-Chancellors and Principals, Minute Book, 24 June 1933; Board of the Faculty
of Medicine, Leeds University, Minute Book, 2 May 1933, University of Leeds Archive.

[4] Committee of Vice-Chancellors and Principals, Minute Book, 14 Dec. 1935; Mann, *Reflections*, 28.

[5] On Dr Eric Rosendahl (Rossdale), see *Ham & High*, 21 Feb. 1997, S. Waley to Dr Wilson, 9 July
1933, V. Buckeley-Johnson to Dr Wilson, 2 Aug. 1933, Moran Papers, Wellcome Library, PP/
CMW/A4/1.

[6] Minutes of the Home Office Medical Advisory Committee, 21 Aug. 1940, British Medical Association Archive.

refugees had reached between 180 and 200, after which, according to the Emergency Association, the position rapidly 'stabilised, for very few are now arriving to seek British qualifications'. Eder possessed an authoritative presence and was a tough negotiator, with diplomatic skills honed by his dealings with the Mandatary authorities in Palestine. These abilities were now to be sorely needed. An approach to the General Medical Council to relax the regulations for foreign doctors seeking to requalify had been rebuffed, and the disquiet of the British Medical Association at the threatened competition of refugee doctors had to be dispelled. Under Eder's guidance, the executive of the Jewish Medical and Dental Emergency Association decided that he should approach the council of the BMA informally 'with a view to securing their co-operation or at least forestalling unfavourable intervention on their part—a conceivable possibility'. According to C. O. Hawthorne, writing to Eder on 1 June 1934, 'The pressure to which the B.M.A. is subject is less from home members than from members in the Dominions & especially South Africa.' In the latter country, doctors with foreign qualifications had to undergo three years of clinical study as well as passing the local examination before they could practise; but if doctors took the Scottish Board examination, they would gain a British qualification after one year and thus short-circuit the South African medical regulations. A short while later Eder informed the secretary of the Emergency Association after his interview with Sir Henry Brackenbury, the chairman of the BMA council, and Dr Anderson, secretary of the BMA,

that they at once explained there would be no opposition, so far as the B.M.A. is concerned, to the Home Office granting permission to our refugee German doctors, when qualified here, to practise in Great Britain. The B.M.A. is chiefly concerned that no one should proceed to the Dominions—South Africa, Australia, New Zealand, Canada. Sir Henry said it would be impossible for the B.M.A. to contemplate the sending back to Germany of medical practitioners who have been forced to leave their home.[7]

When the matter was discussed at the BMA council, there were no dissenting voices raised against the views of the leadership.

While most of the refugee doctors enrolled in the extra-mural colleges at Edinburgh and Glasgow to take the Scottish triple qualification (the final medical examination for those studying outside the universities), from 1935 onwards a rising number also studied in London to sit for the shorter examinations designed to allow refugee doctors to requalify in Britain.[8] In 1933, after being refused admission by St Mary's medical school, Dr Rosendahl proceeded to

---

[7] Dr Laurence Phillips to Dr Wand, 22 May 1934, C. O. Hawthorne to Dr David Eder, 1 June 1934, Dr David Eder to Dr Laurence Phillips, 12 June 1934, and Dr Laurence Phillips to Dr Wand, enclosing a copy of a memorandum: London Jewish Hospital Medical Society Records in the possession of Dr Charles Daniels.   [8] Collins, *Go and Learn*, 133–46.

Edinburgh, where his fellow students included two other refugees, Dr Freddy Himmelweit and Dr Otto Kohnstamm.[9] By June 1935 (presumably after a contemplated approach to the Home Office had been followed up), 125 of the German doctors and a smaller number of dentists had obtained British qualifications, while forty-one were still completing qualifying courses. In addition, thirty-four foreign students were taking a full medical course and five a full dental course. Of the German Jewish doctors, thirty-three had established themselves as general practitioners, twenty had set themselves up in independent practice as specialists, eighteen obtained positions in hospitals (mostly as assistants), ten became assistants of general practitioners, twelve purchased existing practices, three were doing research work, and two were acting as *locum tenens*.[10] The doctors were found positions by the Jewish Refugees Committee, chaired by Otto Schiff, though much of the work on behalf of these medical men was undertaken by Eder himself, assisted by Dr Bernard Homa.[11] At the same time, the Emergency Association tried to persuade Jewish doctors and dentists in Britain to boycott German drugs and spas, by suggesting various alternatives. By the middle of 1936 the total number of refugee medical practitioners who had obtained British qualifications was 147, while about ninety dentists also passed the British examinations.[12]

Maurice Sorsby, the honorary secretary of the Emergency Association, praised Eder for doing

most of the work in placing 250 of them [the doctors] in the way of new self-supporting and self-respecting professional careers. He saw all of them, some of them several times over, and must have given, say, a thousand interviews in moments snatched from his own busy consulting hours. He took upon himself to arrange the one-year post-graduate hospital (clinical) studies required as a preliminary, and 200 were placed in such schools. The B.M.A. and the Royal College of Physicians had to be assured against their first fears of opening a flood of rival foreign doctors; and here the risk of latent anti-Semitic prejudice emerging had to be overcome by tactful persuasion. Eder found the Home Office reasonably open-minded, but this delicate and detailed work was a great strain on his feelings and his physical energy.

Exhausted by his efforts on behalf of the refugee doctors from Germany and physically weakened, Eder died in 1936.[13]

In February 1938 Germany invaded Austria, causing a new exodus of Jewish refugees. Sir Samuel Hoare, the Home Secretary, met with representatives of the BMA, the universities of Oxford, Cambridge, and London, and the Royal Colleges of Physicians and Surgeons in July 1938, and it was agreed 'that it would be possible to admit only a limited number [of refugee doctors], and that

---

[9] Interview with Mrs Olga Rossdale, 19 Mar. 1997.
[10] Jewish Medical and Dental Emergency Association Annual Reports, 1934, 1935.
[11] Homa, *Footprints*, 93.   [12] *JC* 24 July 1936, p. 21.   [13] Eder, *Memoirs*, 132, 133.

any such admissions must be the subject of careful selection. A Committee representing the medical profession should be set up to assist in the selection.' Through delicate negotiations with the Home Office and the BMA, the Jewish Medical and Dental Emergency Association (now led by Professor Samson Wright) arranged for fifty Austrian doctors to enter Britain, where they would study for two years, after which they would be allowed to practise.[14]

Opposition to the refugee doctors emanated principally from the Medical Practitioners' Union (MPU), which had 5,857 members in 1938, but the BMA, with a much larger membership of 37,000, took a more conciliatory line, despite the hostility of some of its membership at grass-roots level. Frank Honigsbaum noted that during the Depression in the mid-1930s, one-third of the panel practices in Britain were in debt to either moneylenders or insurance companies. The leadership of the MPU, which had been infiltrated by fascists, whipped up their members' resentment against both Jewish moneylenders and the admission of refugee doctors into Britain. As there was an upsurge of public support for Oswald Mosley's British Union of Fascists between 1934 and 1936, so the MPU saw its membership climb from 2,816 in 1929 to a peak of almost 6,000 because of the popularity of its antisemitic campaigning. The MPU 'threatened a "stay-in" strike [in the summer of 1938] if the Government does not take steps to prevent alien doctors from practising', though this never happened. The MPU claimed that, by putting pressure on the BMA and alerting sections of the national press, it had thwarted the Home Secretary's original intention to allow 500 Austrian doctors into Britain.[15] In all, from the beginning of 1934 until July 1938, a total of 264 non-nationals had been admitted to the British Medical Register. With the coming of the war and the waning support for fascism in Britain, the strength of the MPU gradually ebbed.[16]

In May 1933 the Academic Assistance Council was set up to find employment for refugee academics and scientists; later, in 1937, this body became the Society for the Protection of Science and Learning (SPSL). Jews were not only kept off the council of the SPSL to emphasize that the problem of discrimination against certain classes of academics affected people of all nationalities, but were encouraged to keep a low profile in the organization so as not to stir up an antisemitic backlash. Nevertheless, behind the scenes Jews (notably Professor Charles Singer) served on the executive committee, and much of the society's financial support came from a Jewish charity, the Central British Fund,

[14] *JC* 8 July 1938, p. 15, 22 July 1938, p. 20, 23 Dec. 1938, p. 19; *BMJ* 12 Aug. 1938, 7 Oct. 1938, 16 Dec. 1938; Collins, *Go and Learn*, 142–6.

[15] Frank Honigsbaum, *The Division in British Medicine* (London: Kogan Page, 1979), 167, 169, 170, 275–8, 312; *JC* 15 July 1938, p. 19.

[16] Paul Weindling, 'The Contribution of Central European Jews to Medical Science and Practice in Britain: The 1930s–1950s', in Werner E. Mosse (ed.), *Second Chance: Two Centuries of German-Speaking Jews in the United Kingdom* (Tübingen: Mohr, 1991), 245; *BMJ* 23 July 1938, *Supplement*, pp. 54–6 .

Although Singer was dedicated to relieving the plight of the refugees, he told a co-worker that he could not possibly agree to support another refugee doctor 'because I have long been spending far more than my income on refugees and have guaranteed seven others'.[17] A number of prominent non-Jewish supporters of the SPSL had a curiously ambivalent attitude towards Jews. Professor A. V. Hill had been awarded a Nobel Prize for physiology in 1923 which he shared with Otto Meyerhof, while Sir Henry Dale, the director of the National Institute of Medical Research, was also awarded a Nobel Prize with a Jewish colleague, Otto Loewi. As we have seen, both Hill and Dale criticized Jews for allegedly bringing too many co-religionists into British university departments and for overcrowding the medical profession. So too, Professor Major Greenwood of the London School of Hygiene was against refugee doctors being allowed to practise; he also noted that some of the Continental Jewish health experts were inordinately proud and psychologically difficult. Even Dr Norman Haire of the Jewish Emergency Association wrote in exasperation to Singer that 'When one is seeing refugees all day as I am, and discovers how difficult and *anspruchsvoll* [difficult to please] many of them are, one has to get a little hard hearted in self-defence.'[18] Thus Home Office policy, which was opposed to the entry of rank-and-file refugee doctors and dentists and favourable to those with high scientific qualifications, neatly coincided with the attitudes of the British medical scientists, who welcomed able young Continental researchers into their laboratories; at the same time, the British directors of medical research agreed with the views of the hospital consultants in impeding the entry of high-flying refugee specialists into the clinical side of the hospital system.[19]

A further wave of Jewish refugees followed Germany's invasion of Czecho-slovakia in March 1939. After consultation with the medical profession, the government agreed that fifty Czech refugee doctors might be allowed to practise in Britain, provided they obtained a British medical qualification. Between 500 and 600 doctors applied to fill these positions, from which the required number was selected by an Advisory Sub-Committee for Medical Research set up by the Society for the Protection of Science and Learning. The committee, of which Dr D. N. Nabarro and Dr Philip D'Arcy Hart were members, gave preference to specialists aged between 30 and 55, the principal grounds for selection being merit, personality, and family responsibility and to general practitioners between the ages of 30 and 50 who were married with children, with special preference being given to those under 35 with children. Dr D'Arcy Hart 'explained that an attempt had been made to keep the balance in the selec-

[17] Professor Charles Singer to Dr Norman Haire, 15 Feb. 1939, Charles Singer Papers, Wellcome Library, PP/CJS/A6/Box 1.

[18] Dr Norman Haire to Professor Singer, 21 Feb. 1939, Charles Singer Papers, Wellcome Library, PP/CJS/A6/Box 1. [19] Cooper, *Refugee Scholars*, 37; Weindling, 'Contribution', 243–52.

tion between Sudeten Germans and Czechs and between Christians and Jews'.[20] Although the English Conjoint Board of the Royal Colleges of Physicians and Surgeons reduced the period of clinical study from three years to two, the examination requirements could be fulfilled in a shorter time in Scotland and the bulk of the refugee doctors continued to study there.[21] The absorption of these Austrian and Czech doctors proceeded slowly, and by 30 May 1940 only four, all Austrians, out of a total of 100 Austrian and Czech doctors, had gained their British medical qualifications.[22]

Whereas the leadership of the BMA was prepared to make concessions as regards the admission of refugee practitioners, most of the leaders of the Royal Colleges of Physicians and Surgeons were much more hostile to the potential competition of foreign medical specialists. At a meeting with the Home Secretary in November 1933, Lord Dawson of Penn, the president of the Royal College of Physicians, conceded that there were places in Britain for refugee doctors of distinction, though he declared that 'the number that could be usefully absorbed or teach us anything could be counted on the fingers of one hand'. Esther Simpson, the secretary of the Society for the Protection of Science and Learning, recalled that she was 'bitterly disappointed that in 1938 this country did not take the opportunity of inviting the Viennese medical school to come here *en bloc*; I knew from my stay in Vienna how medicals from all over the world went there to do research'. The Home Secretary stated in his memoirs that he 'would gladly have admitted the Austrian medical schools *en bloc*', but that the antagonism of the medical profession was too difficult to overcome.[23] The otolaryngologist Professor Heinrich Neumann (1873–1939), one of the stars of the Viennese medical school, who had examined Edward VIII in 1936, wanted to settle in Britain; 'but Neumann's wish to be put on the Medical Register without examination, so that he could practise, was a difficulty that could not be overcome'. Indeed, in December 1938 Dr Robert Hutchinson, president of the Royal College of Physicians, declared that 'He had been made indignant . . . by the insistence of some of his colleagues on some years of probation being served here in England by refugee professors and teachers from whose knowledge English medicine had benefited greatly in the past.'[24]

During 1939 Dr D'Arcy Hart worked with colleagues in the Advisory Sub-Committee for Medical Research to promote a scheme to recreate a Viennese

[20] Minutes of the Advisory Sub-Committee for Medical Research of the Society for the Protection of Science and Learning, 24 July 1939, and Minutes of the Home Office Medical Advisory Committee, 19 Jan. 1940, 1 Feb. 1940, in the possession of Dr Philip D'Arcy Hart.

[21] Collins, *Go and Learn*, 144.　　　　　　　　　　　　　　　[22] *BMJ* 8 June 1940, p. 958.

[23] R. M. Cooper (ed.), *Refugee Scholars: Conversations with Tess Simpson* (Leeds: Moorland, 1992), 38; A. J. Sherman, *Island Refuge: Britain and Refugees from the Third Reich 1933–1939* (London: Frank Cass, 1994), 48, 124.

[24] *JC* 9 Oct. 1936, 23 Dec. 1938, p. 19, 10 Nov. 1939, p. 10, 17 Nov. 1939 (obituary of Neumann).

school of medicine in India. By 1936 there were already about twenty German Jewish medical men in India, including a small number of dentists. Despite the opposition of the local medical establishment, most of them 'succeeded in making a fair living, while several of them do very well indeed. On the other hand, the non-acceptance by the [medical] Corporations means a serious handicap for surgeons and gynaecologists, since they are barred from city hospitals and must make arrangements for their patients at private nursing homes.'[25] Sir B. N. Rau and Sir Ramaswami Mundeliar offered to finance the project for the Viennese medical school and it was envisaged that the centre would be established in Bangalore. Much time was spent in interviewing between twenty-five and fifty prospective staff, in some cases by visiting them in their homeland which they had not yet left. If Austrian and Czech specialists were unavailable, German refugee doctors were considered in their stead. At first the scheme was supported by the Indian government and the India Office, but when in July 1939 the India Office suddenly withdrew its support, probably because of the resistance of local doctors to the proposed settlement of more refugee practitioners, the scheme collapsed.[26]

Throughout 1940 the BMA worked strenuously to preserve the restrictions on the employment of refugee doctors. As late as 21 August that year the Home Office Medical Advisory Committee decided that selected doctors from other countries should not be allowed to obtain British qualifications in the same way as the Austrians and Czechs, partly because it was expected that the war would soon be over and partly because the 'introduction of new foreign groups into British practice might lead to difficulties after the War'. Nor would the committee consent to filling any vacancies that occurred in the Austrian and Czech quota lists. Further, it condemned the employment of alien doctors as psychotherapists. Colonel J. R. Rees, the medical director of the Tavistock Clinic, protested at this because he was employing seven experienced refugee psychiatrists as psychotherapists, who had agreed to be supervised by British doctors.[27] Another difficulty was that the Home Office was suspicious that the refugees had been infiltrated by Nazi spies, resulting in many of these exiles being interned in May 1940, though as a result of interventions by supporters they were gradually released.

Because so many British doctors were serving in the Royal Army Medical Corps, eventually the government had reluctantly to utilize the services of the

[25] *JC* 22 May 1936, p. 34.

[26] Minutes of the Advisory Sub-Committee for Medical Research of the Society for the Protection of Science and Learning, 1 Feb. 1939, 3 Mar. 1939, 24 Apr. 1939, 15 May 1939, 23 June 1939, 24 July 1939; Dr D'Arcy Hart to D. G. Vaisey, 16 July 1984, 2 Aug. 1984.

[27] Minutes of the Home Office Medical Advisory Committee, 21 Aug. 1940, 31 Oct. 1940, British Medical Association Archive.

refugee doctors. Towards the end of 1940 the Medical Register (Temporary Registration) Order was made to empower the General Medical Council to admit British subjects and Americans holding American or Canadian qualifications to the register. This was closely followed in January 1941 by a further Medical Register (Temporary Registration) Order which permitted the employment of refugee practitioners who did not hold American diplomas, but restricted their employment to approved hospitals, institutions, or services not involving the attendance of patients in their own homes.

A considerable number of medical officers serving with the Czech, Polish and other Allied Forces in this country have been so registered, and a few alien doctors who have been appointed to emergency commissions in the R.A.M.C. The majority of temporary registrations under the 1941 Order, however, have been in respect of civilian medical appointments. Nearly 500 doctors with overseas qualifications have obtained approved civilian employment . . . most of them in comparatively junior hospital appointments.

This left another 500 refugee doctors unemployed on account of 'their seniority or the specialised nature of their experience'. It was soon found necessary to amend the 1941 order by adding doctors who had qualified in Egypt, Spain, and Hungary to those eligible to register, and by allowing temporarily registered practitioners to engage in private practice. In no circumstances could a temporarily registered practitioner practise privately on his own account or conduct a single-handed practice as a *locum tenens*, while the right to perform this type of work would be withdrawn at the end of the war. The regulations were later relaxed still further to allow particularly the smaller hospitals to use the services of the refugee practitioners.[28]

During the Second World War the BMA worked through the Aliens Committee of the Central War Medical Committee, the successor body of the Home Office Medical Advisory Committee, which was set up on 26 September 1941, to prevent the refugee doctors from establishing too firm a foothold either in private practice or in the hospital system.[29] The understanding was that, at the end of the war, the services of these practitioners would be dispensed with and they would return to their countries of origin. In keeping with this general policy the fifty Austrian and fifty Czech doctors who were allowed into Britain were scattered throughout the provincial cities rather than being allowed to settle in London. It was also agreed that no additional alien doctors would be allowed to set up in private practice in London, except in exceptional circumstances. Dr Benno Silberger, an ear, nose, and throat surgeon from Czechoslovakia who had a post as a part-time assistant at St Bartholomew's Hospital as a result of his

[28] Aliens Committee of the Central War Medical Committee, Minutes, 24 Nov. 1941, with an appended historical note, and 9 Mar. 1942, British Medical Association Archive.

[29] Minutes of the Home Office Medical Advisory Committee, 28 May 1941.

work with the Czech Research Institute, was informed that he could open a private practice in London for the duration of the war. Another Czech, Dr J. V. Mandel, a urinary surgeon at the Fulham Hospital, was also allowed to establish himself in private practice in the capital, while the German-born ophthalmologist Oscar Fehr, a widower with two teenage daughters, who was 72 years old in 1943 and in poor financial circumstances, was exceptionally allowed to practise as an ophthalmic surgeon in central London. Moreover, in 1943 the Aliens Committee amended the Medical Register (Temporary Registration Order (No. 2)) of 1941 to block the appointment of temporarily registered practitioners to the honorary visiting staffs of hospitals, unless the local medical war committee had been consulted first.[30]

At the end of 1944 there were 3,171 alien doctors on the Temporary Medical Register, of whom 1,185 were in civilian medical employment and 1,986 were attached to the British or Allied armed forces. At one time there were 500 alien doctors serving in the British army, of whom 192 were commissioned in the United Kingdom and 308 overseas. Another ninety-five had obtained security clearance but had not yet obtained employment in a medical capacity, and an additional group of twenty-nine doctors were working in a non-medical field; none of these 124 was eligible for temporary registration. When registration in the Temporary Register ceased in 1946, there were 3,553 foreign doctors registered, of whom a large proportion were serving 'with the Allied Forces and have now been repatriated'. If we estimate the number of Jewish refugee doctors who migrated to Britain from Germany and Austria at between 1,080 and 1,200, the total number of such Jewish practitioners, including those from Poland, Hungary, Czechoslovakia, and Italy, would not be in excess of 1,500.[31]

On 28 May 1946 Professor Samson Wright, who had become president of the Jewish Emergency Association on Eder's death in 1936 and who had also been a long-serving member of the Aliens Committee, was elected chairman of the latter. He shifted the balance of power in the committee to one more in sympathy with the aspirations of the refugee doctors. As early as 5 June 1945 he had voiced his concern 'that many German and Austrian doctors would be completely destitute when they were no longer allowed to practise in this country by reason of the cancellation of temporary registration in the Medical Register'. Within the Home Office, planning started for the situation envisaged in the post-war world and in November 1944 its representative on the Aliens Committee, Mr Prestige, stated that 'although a large number of aliens would be willing to return to their own countries, there would be a considerable proportion

---

[30] Aliens Committee of the Central War Medical Committee Minutes, 5 June 1942, 17 June 1942, 9 Oct. 1942, 17 Feb. 1943, 15 June 1943.
[31] Ibid. 17 Apr. 1945, 10 Dec. 1946; Weindling, 'Contribution', 243.

who would not want to go back and who . . . could stake a moral claim to remain'.[32] In addition, the general election of 1945 had brought into office a Labour administration with a new Home Secretary, James Chuter Ede, who was more willing to assist the refugee doctors and who encouraged his civil servants' radical thinking on this issue. Chuter Ede 'had come to certain conclusions of what was right in his view', after which he had approached Aneurin Bevan, the health minister, who did not take issue with his approach.[33] At a meeting of the Aliens Committee on 10 December 1946, Mr Prestige asserted that

an entirely new situation had arisen from that contemplated at the beginning of the war, owing to the fact that, the war having continued for so long, alien doctors who came to this country as refugees had now been here for many years—some as long as ten years. There was, therefore, considerable difficulty in repatriating them now . . . There was a discussion as to whether it was a fact that all these doctors could not return to their own countries. It was felt that Jewish doctors particularly would dread the thought of returning, in view of the bitter experiences of many of them, and it was doubtful whether they would be welcomed in their own countries.[34]

Conditions in the central European countries from which many of these refugee practitioners came were unsettled. The 3,000 doctors in Vienna were superfluous to the needs of a shrunken and impoverished population; German-speaking doctors in Czechoslovakia were disliked. Some practitioners who did attempt to return had unhappy experiences and trickled back to Britain.

In contrast, in Britain there was a post-war shortage of doctors, and the plans for a National Health Service encouraged the expansion of the medical profession. The Aliens Committee recommended that an estimated 2,000 refugee doctors, who were temporarily registered, be put on to the permanent Medical Register subject to their being able to provide a certificate of competence from their employer. Under the Medical Practitioners and Pharmacists Act 1947 the refugee doctors were granted the opportunity of so registering and by May 1948 approximately 1,000 doctors had availed themselves of this opening.[35] They were advised, however, in June 1948 that even if they had been naturalized as British subjects, they should not purchase a practice or partnership share until they had obtained permanent registration in the Medical Register.

As some of the refugee doctors left Britain after the war to return to central Europe or to seek better employment opportunities in the United States, by 1953 the number remaining in this country, chiefly concentrated in London, had contracted sharply to about 450. Of these, 150 had studied in German universities and seventy-six were Austrians; most of these were Jewish, as were

---

[32] Aliens Committee of the Central War Medical Committee Minutes, 15 Nov. 1944.
[33] Ibid. 6 June 1945, 26 Sept. 1945, 9 Jan. 1946, 28 May 1946.   [34] Ibid. 10 Dec. 1946.
[35] Ibid. 26 Sept. 1945, 10 Dec. 1946, 26 Feb. 1947, 23 Jan. 1948, 4 May 1948.

many members of the sizeable Czech contingent of just over fifty. To these must be added a smaller group of twenty-four mainly Jewish physicians who had studied in Italy, which had reciprocal arrangements with Britain as regards medical qualifications, ten from Switzerland, sixteen from France, four from Lithuania, and two from Romania. Most of the 100 or so Polish doctors working in London were not Jewish. Kenneth Collins has estimated that Jewish students made up about 9 per cent of the total number of graduates from the Polish medical school in Edinburgh, which gives us a rough-and-ready guide to the percentage of Polish doctors who were Jewish.[36] Taking all these factors into account, it is possible to estimate that in 1953 there were between 300 and 320 Jewish refugee doctors located in London.

Of those doctors who chose to stay in Britain, the clinicians among them obtained positions as consultants in the smaller hospitals in the Greater London area or the provinces, or opened consulting rooms in Harley Street. One of the gynaecologists, Stephen Westman, had gained his MD in Berlin in 1920, rising to become an assistant gynaecologist at the University of Berlin and an obstetrician at its postgraduate medical school. Because of his liberal viewpoint and the fact that he had a Jewish grandmother, he left Germany in 1933; Otto Schiff of the Jewish Refugees Committee directed him to study in Scotland, where he was awarded his triple qualification in 1934. He slowly built up a practice among the aristocracy, successfully treating the wife of the heir of one of the oldest titled families, who was then able to conceive, and in 1935 he used a new German sulphonamide drug to combat two cases of childbed fever; this was the first time this drug had been tried in Britain. In 1943 he became a fellow of the Royal Faculty of Physicians and Surgeons of Glasgow. Until then, he ruefully declared,

I repeatedly had the experience that, when I applied for the post of an honorary gynaecological surgeon in a back-alley hospital . . . the Board of Governors cast my application aside straight away . . . Decades of practice or scientific achievements apparently did not count: they only looked for the magic letters . . . Instead they chose someone who hardly had any practical experience . . . Even some of the larger nursing homes at first refused to admit patients of mine, as Matron did not find in the Medical Directory the awe-inspiring letters.

When the obstetrician Professor James Young was appointed director of the British Postgraduate Medical School in Hammersmith, he invited Westman from time to time to lecture in his department, and after the war Westman ran a prosperous Harley Street practice; but he never gained entry into the British hospital system.[37]

    [36] *Medical Directory 1953*, i. 1–363; Collins, *Go and Learn*, 133, 154.
    [37] Stephen K. Westman, *A Surgeon's Story* (London: Kimber, 1962), 175, 179, 217, 235, 237, 253–6; *Medical Directory 1953*, i. 345.

Alfred Alexander Loeser (1888–1962) was another upper-middle-class German Jewish gynaecologist—'with a handsome face deeply marked by old duelling scars'. He had acquired his MD from the University of Berlin in 1913, later acting as an assistant at the gynaecological clinic at Rostock, where he gained experience in obstetrics and gynaecology. He moved to the gynaecological clinic of the Charité Hospital in Berlin, afterwards becoming director of the gynaecological and obstetrics department of the Jewish Hospital in the city and a consultant at the Municipal Hufeland Hospital. Trained also as a scientist, he was a pupil for a short while of Otto Warburg, under whom he investigated the influence of hormones on cancer cells. 'His concentrated clinical research in this field led to his epoch-making discovery of the inhibitory effect of testosterone on breast carcinoma, first described by him at the International Gynaecological Congress in Amsterdam in 1938, and since accepted as the standard practice throughout the world.' Like Westman, he was awarded a Scottish triple qualification during the 1930s, having emigrated to Britain. He opened consulting rooms at 2 Devonshire Place in the West End, 'where his international reputation soon enabled him to establish himself, and where his skill and personality rapidly built up a considerable practice'. He was a very good surgeon, adept at reconstructive tubal surgery, which he practised with marked success in infertility cases. Despite a busy life caring for his patients, he yet managed to produce some ninety scientific papers.[38]

Emanuel (Uly) Schleyer-Saunders (1897–1984) was the eldest child in a working-class Viennese family. After his father's early death forced him to seek employment at the age of 16, he continued his medical studies on a part-time basis, qualifying as a doctor in 1923. He was a member of the staff of the University Clinic for Gynaecology and Obstetrics in Vienna and had a considerable practice. After Hitler's annexation of Austria Schleyer-Saunders rapidly made arrangements to leave Vienna, but before moving to Britain he baptized his family, though he never attended church again thereafter. He passed the Scottish triple qualification in 1939 and spent the war years building up a gynaecological practice in Wimpole Street. 'He was of the old school, never expecting an assistant to prepare his patients or his ward sister to remove sutures. He was often seen at breakfast time in the London Clinic complete with red carnation, having sat all night at the bedside of a labouring mother.' His chief medical interest was in the menopause and the prevention of ageing. He was one of the first to suggest treatment to prevent cancer of the uterus by combining progestogens with oestrogens; and he carefully studied the effects of such prescriptions on patients, even without the resources of an academic department behind him. Schleyer-Saunders suffered 'only one real disappointment, which

---

[38] *BMJ* 22 Dec. 1962, p. 1692 (obituary of Loeser); *Medical Directory 1953*, i. 196.

was that he could not get the British medical establishment to give him a hospital appointment, even on an honorary basis'. Eventually he did secure such an appointment in the small Italian Hospital in Queen Square, for which he subsequently raised funds.[39]

Westman, Loeser, and Schleyer-Saunders were all men of remarkable attainment, combining surgical dexterity with scientific distinction; yet as refugees they were not considered eligible for consultant positions in any of the major hospitals. It did not seem to count that Loeser had made an important discovery in the treatment of breast cancer and had pioneered innovative surgical techniques, that Westman was a brilliant surgeon and teacher and probably the first person in the country to use sulphonamides to overcome puerperal sepsis, or that Schleyer-Saunders 'developed new approaches to operating techniques and post-operative care' as well as the treatment of the menopause.[40] So too, Julius Joel Handler, who obtained his MD from Berne in 1938 and his English qualifications ten years later, rose to become senior registrar in the Obstetric and Gynaecological Unit of the Farnborough Hospital in Kent, but as a refugee could not obtain a consultant position.[41]

Professor Bernhard Zondek (1892–1967), a gynaecologist and endocrinologist, was appointed associate professor at Berlin University in 1926, the year he discovered the female sex hormone and gonadotrophic hormones. With Professor Selmar Aschheim he devised the first biological pregnancy test, the 'Aschheim–Zondek test', in 1928, and in 1929 he became head of the department of obstetrics and gynaecology at the Spandau Municipal Hospital. In 1933 he stayed for a short while in Manchester as a refugee, but later that year moved to Sweden, where he worked until 1934 as a member of the Biochemical Institute at the University of Stockholm. In 1935 both he and his brothers Hermann and Samuel, also distinguished medical men, were persuaded by Chaim Weizmann (who was friendly with Bernhard Zondek through the Zionist movement) to emigrate to Palestine. Later, Zondek accepted an invitation to become professor of obstetrics and gynaecology and head of the Hormone Research Laboratory at the Hebrew University and Hadassah Medical School, positions he held until his retirement in 1961.[42]

It is necessary to see the careers of these doctors in context, for as foreigners and Jews they were working under a double handicap. Even English Jews after the Second World War were only slowly securing consultant positions in major hospitals, facing particular difficulties in surgery and gynaecology, both because of the vestiges of discrimination which remained in the higher reaches of the

---

[39] *BMJ* 1 Sept. 1984, p. 563 (obituary of Schleyer-Saunders); James Saunders, *Nightmare: Ernest Saunders and the Guinness Affair* (London: Arrow, 1990), 1–8; *Medical Directory 1953*, i. 291.

[40] Saunders, *Nightmare*, 1.   [41] *Medical Directory 1953*, i. 136 (on Handler).

[42] *BMJ* 7 Jan. 1967, p. 58 (obituary of Bernhard Zondek); *JC* 6 Oct. 1933, p. 26, 20 July 1951, p. 6.

medical profession and because of the fear of competition from Continental medical experts with new methods and new techniques. It was also difficult for middle-aged refugee practitioners to pursue further studies in order to gain qualifications from the Royal Colleges when they had pressing family obligations; yet a fellowship of one or other was a precondition for advancement on the hospital career ladder. Paul Weindling has shown that the same pattern applied in other medical fields: the talents of the refugee paediatricians with advanced clinical and scientific skills and the equally innovative public health experts were inadequately exploited, even though English medicine lagged behind in these sectors.[43]

Pre-eminent among the refugee cardiologists who migrated to England was John (Janos) Plesch (1878–1958), who qualified as an MD in Budapest in 1900 and requalified in Germany in 1909, going on to become professor of internal medicine in the University of Berlin. Arriving in England in the summer of 1933, Plesch was awarded the Scottish triple qualification in the following year. 'Thanks to colleagues with whom I cooperated in this country,' remembered Plesch,

to diplomats who had consulted me in Berlin and to my many English patients who had come to Berlin to place themselves in my hands, it soon became known that I was in circulation again, and before long my flat [in Park Lane] became too small for my practice . . From the really sick people to the 'lion-hunters' who spend their lives collecting specialists, they all streamed into my consulting-rooms, until my main problem came to be how best to dam the stream.[44]

Among Plesch's patients was the economist John Maynard Keynes, who thanked him for the enormous improvement in the condition of his heart and in a later letter described the treatment, telling Plesch that 'The arsenic, the opium, the thyroid, the [hot] bath and the wash out have all been performed according to instructions.' In 1939 Plesch restored Keynes 'back into active life' by treating a serious throat infection with Prontosil, a new German sulphanilomide drug, and was praised by his patient for being 'very fertile and ingenious in ideas, trying out every sort of thing imaginable until he finds something useful'.[45]

During the 1920s and 1930s wealthy English patients were fascinated by foreign doctors. 'The European spas, clinics and sanatoria obtained their main contingents from this country. Carlsbad, Bad Ems, Kissingen, the sanatoria of the Black Forest and Switzerland, Aix-les-Bains, Vittel and Vichy were

[43] Weindling, 'Contribution', 250–2; David A. Pyke, 'The Great Insanity: Hitler and the Destruction of German Science', *Journal of the Royal College of Physicians of London* (May/June 1995), 199–206.

[44] John Plesch, *Janos: The Story of a Doctor* (London: Gollancz, 1947), 403, 408, 409; *Medical Directory 1948*, i. 260.

[45] Copy letters John Maynard Keynes to Professor Plesch, 13 Apr. 1939, 18 Apr. 1939, Plesch Papers, Wellcome Library, GC/32/2; Robert Skidelsky, *John Maynard Keynes: Fighting for Britain 1937–1946* (London: Macmillan, 2000), iii. 40–3.

English colonies.' Plesch confessed to learning new things in England as well as imparting medical knowledge unknown to his colleagues. Now his patients could see a world-renowned physician in London, and their enthusiasm for him stirred 'a certain amount of disagreeable professional jealousy'—but other refugee cardiologists suffered from worse than resentment.[46]

Dr Wilhelm Neumann (1885–1940), who had practised at Baden-Baden and the Riviera and was the author of thirty books on heart and rheumatic disease, died at Leamington after only four months' sojourn in England—just one example of the many doctors who died young as a result of the upheaval involved in starting out on a new career in a new country in middle age.[47] Dr Gertrude Goldscheider (1902–86), who had held positions in the university department of paediatrics and a children's hospital in Vienna, became a research officer at the Marie Curie Hospital in London and a clinical assistant at the National Heart Hospital before joining her husband in a general practice in London.[48] Dr Paul Rothschild (1901–65), after carrying out research in Otto Meyerhof's laboratory at the renowned Institute of Physiology in Berlin and into heart problems under Sir Thomas Lewis in London in 1930, requalified in Scotland in 1934. Forced to abandon a career in research because he had a wife and two children to support, on Lewis's advice he moved to a Welsh mining valley, where he became an assistant in a general practice. Later he opened a surgery in Fulham, serving as a consultant physician to the Persian and Iraq Force during the Second World War and was made a lieutenant-colonel in the RAMC. After the war he moved the principal location of his practice to Kensington, where he numbered distinguished individuals such as Professor A. V. Hill, Chaim Weizmann, and the Sieff family among his patients.[49]

The largest specialist group within the ranks of the refugee doctors, and the one which had most impact on British medicine, were the psychiatrists and psychotherapists. In 1910 Georg Dobrick, a German asylum doctor, asserted that 'We know a lot and can do little', but in the following decades Continental psychiatrists developed a whole series of measures to assist the mentally ill. In England, in contrast to Germany, 'neurology and psychiatry were regarded as separate specialities and neither was a university subject. Apart from the Maudsley Hospital, research and post-graduate teaching in psychiatry featured in only one or two mental hospitals.' The influx of the refugee doctors was to contribute to changing this state of affairs and to the transformation of British psychiatry.[50]

[46] Plesch, *Janos*, 409, 414.   [47] *JC* 5 Jan. 1940, p. 6 (obituary of Neumann).

[48] *BMJ* 21 June 1986, p. 1678 (obituary of Goldscheider).

[49] Cooper, *Refugee Scholars*, 74; *BMJ* 27 Nov. 1965, p. 1315 (obituary of Rothschild).

[50] Roy Porter, *The Greatest Benefit to Mankind* (London: Fontana, 1999), 513; *Independent*, 12 July 1991. Nervous disorders and insanity were also alleged to be 'Jewish diseases', and this may have influenced specialization by Jewish doctors.

Dr Eric Guttman MRCP (1896–1948) had an international reputation as a neurologist in Germany before 1933. When the Maudsley reopened after the war, he was given the task of reorganizing clinical teaching there. The Maudsley had been first opened in 1923 on lines advocated by Emil Kraepelin (1856–1926), who prepared a classification of mental illness by distinguishing between manic-depressive psychoses and *dementia praecox*, the forerunner of schizophrenia. Like the German asylums, it was to be both a research centre and a training hospital for psychiatrists. Both here and during the war at the Neurosis Centre at Mill Hill Emergency Hospital, 'he was the mainstay of teaching and [a] dominating influence among his junior colleagues. He was a first-rate clinician.' Guttman carried out fundamental research into the psychiatric aspects of brain injuries and suggested 'the possibility of analysing symptoms into those directly due to a basic organic process and those which represented a reaction of the personality'. He also introduced the use of amphetamines in psychiatry. But finally, when he seemed on the point of reaching the position his merits deserved, his health failed.[51]

Dr Willy Mayer-Gross (1889–1961) was not only a psychiatrist with an international reputation and an authority on schizophrenia, which he treated with insulin, but the senior author of a magisterial survey entitled *Clinical Psychiatry* which was translated into a number of European languages. With Guttman, Mayer-Gross 'constituted the department of research at the Maudsley, which became a precedent and a model for similar departments in other hospitals'. Having worked as a research fellow of the Maudsley Hospital in London and a consultant psychiatrist at the Royal Mental Hospital in Dumfries, he spent some years as a senior fellow in the department of experimental psychiatry in the Birmingham medical school and as the director of a clinic. Despite being elected FRCP, the handicap of coming to Britain as a middle-aged foreigner impaired Mayer-Gross's chances of 'attaining the highest positions in Britain'.[52]

Erwin Stengel (1902–73), another FRCP, was appointed to the consultant staff at the Bethlem Royal Hospital and the Maudsley in 1949 and was also reader in psychiatry at London University. Professor Stengel became the head of the department of clinical psychiatry at Sheffield University and the first holder of such a chair in Sheffield. He carried out important research into suicide and, having known Freud in Vienna, was sympathetic to the psychoanalytic approach to mental illness.[53] Although Mayer-Gross and Guttman obtained higher medical qualifications in Britain and despite their undoubted talent, both failed to

[51] *JC* 7 May 1948; *BMJ* 8 May 1948, p. 908 (obituary of Guttman).

[52] *JC* 24 Feb. 1961, p. 14, *BMJ* 25 Feb. 1961, p. 596 (obituary of Mayer-Gross); Collins, *Go and Learn*, 148.

[53] *JC* 16 July 1971, p. 23; *BMJ* 16 June 1973, p. 668 (obituary of Stengel); Erwin Stengel, *Suicide and Attempted Suicide* (Harmondsworth: Penguin, 1964).

reach the front rank of the medical hierarchy. Their younger colleague Stengel was more successful, as was Alfred Meyer (1895–1990), who contributed to the transformation of British psychiatry 'from an asylum based practice to the scientifically orientated psychiatry of today'. After studying neuroanatomy and neuropathology, Meyer was in charge of a laboratory in Bonn by 1924 and then worked with Professor Spielmeyer in Munich. Leaving Germany in 1933, he was welcomed into the central pathological laboratory at the Maudsley Hospital, where he published papers on the 'selective vulnerability of different brain regions to disease and the anatomical basis of psychiatric disorders'. At first holding the position of neuropathologist to the Maudsley Hospital, he was appointed professor of neuropathology at the Institute of Psychiatry of London University in 1949, but was forced to retire in 1956 because of ill health. During his active years he carried out a study of prefrontal leucotomy, throwing fresh light on the functioning of the frontal lobes of the brain, and conducted other research that elucidated the changes in the brain associated with epileptic seizures.[54]

Dr Samuel Last (1902–91), another refugee from the Continent (in this case Romania), trained in British psychiatric methods and joined the newly built Runwell Hospital in Essex, where he ran an electro-encephalography department. By recording the electrical changes taking place in different parts of the brain, the electro-encephalogram served as a useful tool in the diagnosis of brain tumours and in understanding a variety of brain disorders, including epilepsy. Later, as its director, Last transformed the Buckinghamshire County Mental Hospital from a slum into a first-rate institution, before moving to the London Hospital to create a professorial psychiatric department, where he became a consultant psychiatrist and physician.[55]

The influx of Jews into psychiatry came about partly because it was thought to be a 'Cinderella' profession, where there were plenty of openings for Jews, and partly because, as one experienced psychoanalyst put it, 'Jews have an awareness of pain and a desire to alleviate it . . . To be in touch with pain and emotion is very Jewish.'[56] While it is true that the galaxy of Continental stars who migrated to Britain lent lustre to the profession in the 1940s and 1950s, there was also an important contingent of Jewish psychiatrists who were born there or whose parents were born in English-speaking countries. One of these was Eric Benjamin Strauss (1894–1961), a convert to Catholicism at Oxford, who pioneered electric shock treatment in London and used it on his out-

---

[54] *The Times*, 30 Oct. 1990; *BMJ* 1 Dec. 1990, p. 1273 (obituary of Meyer).

[55] *Independent*, 12 July 1991; *BMJ* 7 Sept. 1991, p. 577 (obituary of Last).

[56] Stephen Brook, *The Club: The Jews of Modern Britain* (London: Pan, 1989), 314. See also Aubrey Lewis, 'Psychiatry and the Jewish Tradition', in *The Later Papers of Sir Aubrey Lewis* (Oxford: Oxford University Press, 1979), 227–37.

patients at St Bartholomew's Hospital. He had a busy practice in Wimpole Street, where he was consulted by 'the oddest specimens of the aristocracy' and stalwarts of the Catholic Church, including Evelyn Waugh. Strauss stressed a multiple causal approach to mental illness, taking into account 'the mind, the body, the inherited constitution, and the social environment of the sufferer'.[57] Hyam Joseph Shorvon (1907–61) was an acknowledged expert in the physical treatment of mental illness and a key member of the St Thomas and Northern Hospital psychiatric teams. Endowed with a phenomenal memory that enabled him to recall all the personal and clinical details of an individual when provided with just a name, he was extremely devoted to his patients; seriously overworking himself, he died at the age of 54.[58] Dr Hertzl Kaufman (1917–71), who was on the psychiatric staff at Guy's Hospital, also died young.[59]

Jews tended to be concentrated in posts at the Maudsley Hospital or the Tavistock Clinic into the 1950s and 1960s, with none reaching consulting rank in the main London teaching hospitals (apart from Emanuel Miller, to whom we shall shortly turn). Despite his reputation, Eric Strauss was merely a lecturer in psychological medicine at St Bartholomew's Medical College, while Hyam Shorvon was an assistant psychiatrist at St Thomas's Hospital. But in the Tavistock Clinic in the mid-1960s three-quarters of the staff were Jewish, though since then the numbers have declined.

Until the end of the 1940s the prescribing of barbiturates or insulin therapy, the administration of electric shocks (ECT), and leucotomy remained the principal forms of treatment for the seriously mentally disturbed. The introduction of chlorpromazine in Britain in 1953, followed by other 'wonder drugs', helped to transform psychiatric practice, by alleviating the symptoms of some schizophrenics and permitting many others to be released from hospital. The pharmacological revolution of the 1950s entailed upheavals in the administration of mental hospitals which were radically altered by the implementation of an open-door policy, allowing patients to come and go more freely, the establishment of therapeutic communities, and the freeing of many inmates.[60]

An important figure who helped to implement the revolution in psychiatric practice was Dr Isaac Sutton (1909–2001). He was the son of the Revd Suchanitsky, an immigrant from Russia who served as minister of an Orthodox synagogue in Manchester. A brilliant scholar, Sutton qualified as a doctor at the age of 21, gaining a diploma in psychological medicine in 1938 and his MD in

[57] *The Times*, 13 Jan. 1961, 17 Jan. 1961, p. 15 (obituary of Strauss); Flora Solomon and Barnett Litvinoff, *Baku to Baker Street: The Memoirs of Flora Solomon* (London: Collins, 1984), 175–6; William Sargant, *The Unquiet Mind* (London: Heinemann, 1967), 80.

[58] *JC* 21 Apr. 1961, p. 11; *Lancet*, 27 May 1961, pp. 1177–8 (obituary of Shorvon).

[59] *JC* 29 Oct. 1971 (obituary of Kaufman).

[60] Jonathan Andrews *et al.*, *The History of Bethlem* (London: Routledge, 1997), 695–700.

1947. On demobilization after the Second World War, he was appointed medical director of a 2,000-bed Victorian psychiatric hospital in Yorkshire. In 1957 he became chief medical superintendent of the Friern Barnet Mental Hospital, a major institution, where he modernized treatment of patients with the new 'wonder drugs' and opened locked wards. A devout Jew and fluent Yiddish speaker, he assisted Jewish communities in Britain and abroad with mental health work.[61]

Sir Aubrey Julian Lewis (1900–75) was the most distinguished psychiatrist of his generation. Born and educated in Australia, where he qualified as a doctor in 1923, between 1926 and 1928 he studied with Adolf Meyer in Baltimore, in London at the National Hospital, and with Karl Beringer and Karl Bonhoeffer in Germany, having been awarded a Rockefeller travelling fellowship for training in psychiatry. As he could not find a suitable position in Australia, he settled in London, joining the staff of the Maudsley Hospital and becoming its medical director in 1936. Here he was joined by a brilliant coterie of German and Austrian Jewish refugees whose careers have already been outlined—Eric Guttman, Willy Mayer-Gross, Alfred Meyer, and Erwin Stengel—as well as celebrated younger psychiatrists such as Sir Martin Roth (b. 1917), the son of an East End synagogue cantor, who worked at the Maudsley with Mayer-Gross and rose to become professor of psychiatry at Cambridge.[62] When Lewis succeeded Edward Mopother as director in 1946 after an interregnum, he was appointed professor of psychiatry and implemented his plans for improving the training of psychiatrists and research workers; he also expanded the Institute of Psychiatry, creating new departments of psychology and neuroscience. He instituted a new three-year training course for psychiatrists, rotating the trainees through the various departments. When the Social Psychiatry Unit was established by the Medical Research Council, he was made its first honorary director. Sufficiently flexible in his approach to include psychoanalysts on the staff, Lewis appointed S. H. Foulkes and Willi Hoffer, even though he felt that their hypotheses needed further testing.

Lewis had both an extraordinarily retentive memory for all that he had read and a remarkable quickness of mind, enabling him 'to combine clinical judgment with scholarship and common sense'. According to Neil O'Connor, after the war 'Lewis accomplished two important aims: he transformed psychiatry from a clinically orientated study to a respectable academic discipline and he

---

[61] *JC* 11 Jan. 2002, p. 23.

[62] Michael Shepherd, 'The Career and Contributions of Sir Aubrey Lewis', Adolf Meyer Lecture, delivered at the 129th annual meeting of the American Psychiatric Association, 1976. *Lancet*, 1 Feb. 1975, 1 Jan. 1977; Blake and Nicholls (eds.), *Dictionary of National Biography 1971–1980*, 504, 505 (on Aubrey Lewis).

established a group of research workers in psychiatry and associated disciplines which became a model for similar hospital groups in other parts of the world'.[63]

Willy Mayer-Gross pointed out in the mid-1950s that during the last thirty years the focus of psychiatry had shifted 'from the major psychoses, statistically relatively rare occurrences, to the milder and borderline cases, the minor deviations from the normal average'.[64] This encouraged the use of medication and the explosive growth of psychotherapy rather than long-term residential hospital care as the preferred form of treatment.[65] Once again, refugee practitioners played a prominent role in the spread of psychotherapy through and alongside the hospital system. Joshua Bierer (1901–84) came to England from Vienna and in 1938 was appointed 'the first psychotherapist in a public mental hospital (Runwell). He founded the first therapeutic community.' After war service in the RAMC, in 1946 he set up 'the first community hospital—the social psychotherapy centre that was later named the Marlborough Day Hospital, the first hospital of this kind in the world. That was the start of the day hospital movement.' A man endowed with deeply held Jewish communal and socialist ideals, Bierer was convinced that psychiatric hospitals should be replaced by self-governing communities, so that mental patients with chronic disabilities could be rehabilitated.[66]

Sigmund Heinrich Foulkes (formerly Fuchs, 1898–1976), in addition to receiving a thorough training in neurology and psychiatry, worked in Germany with the leading psychologist Kurt Goldstein, who introduced him to the Gestalt school of psychology. He later trained as a psychoanalyst in Vienna and was the director of a clinic in Frankfurt. Foulkes was posted to the Military Neurosis Centre at Northfield in 1942, where with a group of colleagues he devised 'the basis of the therapeutic community approach to hospital psychiatry . . . and group analytic methods', starting his first analytic group in Exeter in 1944. After the war he founded the Group Analytic Society and the Institute of Group Analysis, serving for some years as a consultant psychotherapist to the Maudsley Hospital.[67] Dr Walter Schindler (1896–1986), after working at the Tavistock Clinic until 1946, became a consultant at the Marylebone Hospital and later the Paddington Day Clinic, practising mainly as an analytical group therapist. Dr Franz Max Greenbaum was a psychiatrist and Jungian therapist at the Salford Royal Hospital and the Hope Hospital, combining the techniques

[63] *JC* 3 Dec. 1971, p. 23 (on Martin Roth).   [64] Porter, *The Greatest Benefit*, 521.   [65] Ibid.
[66] *BMJ* 12 Jan. 1985, p. 163 (obituary of Bierer).

[67] Paul Weindling, 'Austrian Medical Refugees in Great Britain: From Marginal Aliens to Established Professionals', *Wiener Klinische Wochenschrift*, 110/4–5 (27 Feb. 1998), 158–61; *BMJ* 21 Aug. 1976, p. 483 (obituary of Foulkes); Jeff Roberts and Malcolm Pines (eds.), *The Practice of Group Analysis* (London: Routledge, 1991), 32–54.

of psychotherapy with the latest physical developments in psychiatry. He also evolved his own form of group therapy for dealing with anxiety neuroses.[68]

The outstanding figure in psychiatric provision for children is Emanuel Miller (1893–1970), the son of a furrier from an Orthodox Lithuanian Jewish family. Miller was educated at Cambridge and the London Hospital, where he qualified in 1918, adding a diploma in psychological medicine a year later. Before the Second World War he became director of the East London Child Guidance Clinic, which was opened by the Jewish Health Organization in 1927 to combat juvenile delinquency—the first such centre in England. He also worked at the Tavistock Clinic, where he pioneered family therapy. Some years later, in 1959, he founded the *Journal of Child Psychology and Psychiatry*, and in 1967 he edited a volume entitled *Foundations of Child Psychiatry*. As child guidance clinics proliferated, quite a number of Jewish doctors found positions in them. Miller 'always remained a psychotherapist at heart, convinced of the power of reason and gentleness, not so convinced that the brutal mental clashes which Freud constantly likened to battle were all important in human nature'. Meanwhile, prompted by his interest in juvenile delinquency, he qualified as a barrister and decided to specialize in psychiatry, gaining his fellowship of the Royal College of Physicians in 1946. He was appointed physician in child psychiatry to St George's Hospital and was later senior physician in psychotherapy at the Maudsley, 'where he helped to mould the minds of a brilliant group of young psychiatrists who now occupy posts in teaching and research at universities and hospitals throughout the world'. As part of the band of psychotherapists assembled at the Maudsley by Aubrey Lewis he 'found the grand rounds especially satisfying, exemplifying as they did the holistic approach he had always advocated'. Like many of the staff at the Maudsley, Miller tried to link the findings of psychiatry 'with the teachings of general biology, neurology, and the relevant social sciences'. Widely read in European literature and well stocked with Jewish learning, Miller could as easily quote Shakespeare as the Talmud, or analyse the poetry of Baudelaire and Verlaine.[69]

Dr Kate Friedlander (1902–49), who emigrated to England from Austria in 1933, did important work in West Sussex in child guidance and with juvenile delinquents, but died just as she was beginning 'to assemble a group of co-workers, and to make a name for herself'.[70] The Austrian Dr Liselotte Frankl (1911–89) was appointed consultant psychiatrist and later medical director of the famous Hampstead Child Therapy Clinic under Anna Freud, besides working in the East End. Paul Weindling noted that Georg Stroh (1919–79) was

---

[68] *BMJ* 29 Mar. 1986, p. 904 (obituary of Schindler); *Lancet*, 16 Dec. 1961 (obituary of Greenbaum).

[69] *The Times*, 30 July, 4 Aug. 1970; *JC* 7 Aug. 1970, p. 31, *Lancet*, 8 Aug. 1970, p. 318 (obituary of Miller). Black, *Lord Rothschild*, 104, 105.

[70] Elisabeth Young-Bruehl, *Anna Freud* (London: Macmillan, 1991), 254, 332–3.

head 'of the High Wick Hospital for Emotionally Disturbed Children, pioneering family therapy and research on the effects of sensory deprivation on infants, and autism'.[71] Arthur Zanker (1890–1957), who was born in Czechoslovakia but practised in Austria before coming to England, with a background in paediatrics and Adlerian child psychiatry, worked mainly in a child guidance clinic, but was also a pioneer of music therapy. Another Austrian, Erich Wellisch (1898–1954), specialized in child psychiatry and from 1947 onwards was director of the Crayford Child Guidance Clinic in Kent.[72]

Whereas the German Jewish psychiatrists brought hope to the inmates of the asylums, many of whom had previously been regarded as untreatable, another refugee doctor, Sir Ludwig Guttmann (1899–1980) brought solace and hope to another class of patient: the paraplegics. 'Today, it is difficult for us to comprehend the ingrained attitudes of hopelessness towards disabled people which existed in 1944', noted Susan Goodman. 'A medical student in a London teaching hospital in the 1950s, now a consultant physician, still remembers a paraplegic patient confined to a corner of the ward, dying of septic sores.'[73] Guttmann trained as a neurosurgeon in Breslau under Otfrid Foerster, whose neurosurgical techniques were not highly regarded in Britain. After he came to England as a refugee, Guttmann carried out research in Oxford into nerve regeneration, but felt so frustrated by the lack of suitable clinical opportunities that he was eager to start his own centre for paraplegics; this he did at Stoke Mandeville in 1944. Guttmann's combination of a rather authoritarian personality and total dedication to his work enabled him the more easily to implement his revolutionary ideas on the treatment of paraplegic patients. To begin with, patients were turned over in bed every two hours to permit bedsores to heal; antiseptics were dispensed with, as they failed to assist the healing process; instead, dead tissue was excised and replaced by skin grafting, and penicillin was used to control urinary and other infections. At first the hospital staff were extremely sceptical of the new methods of treatment advocated by Guttman; so, to ensure that his instructions were obeyed, he made sudden inspections in the hospital at all hours of the day or night. Patients were urged to sit up, to walk with calipers, and to participate in wheelchair basketball, archery, and table tennis. Hitherto paraplegics had survived for only a year or two, but Guttmann's methods revolutionized their treatment and life-chances. He became an FRCS in 1961, FRCP in 1962, and FRS in 1976.[74]

Another outstanding innovator among the refugee doctors was Joseph Dallos

[71] Ibid. 333, 373–5; *BMJ* 21 Jan. 1989, p. 182 (obituary of Frankl).

[72] Weindling, 'Austrian Medical Refugees', 160; *BMJ* 15 June 1957, p. 1432 (obituary of Zanker), 29 May 1954, p. 1269 (obituary of Wellisch).

[73] Susan Goodman, *Spirit of Stoke Mandeville: The Story of Sir Ludwig Guttman* (London: Collins, 1986), 95.

[74] Blake and Nicholls (eds.), *Dictionary of National Biography 1971–1980*, 369–71 (on Guttmann).

(1905–79), the inventor of the modern contact lens, who was born in Budapest. By using a soft dental moulding substance, Negocoll, Dallos made exact replicas of the eyeballs, to which he adapted glass lenses which were further modified by hand grinding and polishing until a good fit had been obtained. He designed a lens with channels which allowed the natural tear ducts to flow, thereby permitting it to be worn for up to twelve hours. This method enabled Dallos to dispense with the artificial fluids which had hitherto been used with lenses to act as a cushion for wide corneal clearance. Obrig and Salvatori, US experts on contact lenses, claim that 'The original work of Dallos in discovering and proving the use of Negocoll . . . has done more than anything else to make modern contact lenses a reality.'[75] Meanwhile, in Hungary Nazi influence was growing. When Ida Mann, a British ophthalmologist, visited the country in 1937, she was so impressed with the work of Dallos that she persuaded him to leave his native land in 1938 and open a contact lens centre in London.[76] Dallos duly took clinical charge of a centre in Cavendish Square financed by Theodore Hamblin, the owner of a chain of dispensing optical outlets, and guaranteed under charter by a group of leading British eye surgeons. It was an institution for dispensing, developing and researching contact lenses, not primarily a profit-making organization. During the war, Dallos assisted RAF personnel who needed contact lenses, and tested the use of contact lenses under pressure for the navy. After the war he worked for a time at Moorfields Eye Hospital before transferring to the Western Eye Hospital. His widow, Dr Vera Pinter, stated that in 1964 he set up an independent practice, where he developed precise corneal impressions for plastic corneal lenses.[77]

The inauguration of the National Health Service in 1948 created a huge demand for specialist medical personnel, allowing the refugee doctors to fill a wide range of jobs; but, despite the new procedures for appointing staff, the refugees still failed to obtain the most prestigious positions. Dr Walter Weiner (1899–1967) was given a post in the Birmingham Regional Blood Transfusion Service; later, as its director, he supervised the building of the new Blood Transfusion Service building and stayed in post until it was running smoothly, while at the same time carrying out research into haemolytic anaemia and classifying auto-immune anaemias.[78] Robert Heller (1908–80) became the acting tuberculosis officer at the Hounslow Chest Clinic and in 1948 consultant physician to the West Middlesex and Ashford hospitals. Dr Alfred Fessler (1897–

[75] A. G. Sabell, 'The History of Contact Lenses', in *Contact Lenses: A Textbook for Practitioner and Student* (London: Butterworths, 1985), 17.

[76] Elizabeth Beckley and Dorothy Usher Potter (eds.), *Ida and the Eye: A Woman in British Ophthalmology from the Autobiography of Ida Mann* (Tunbridge Wells: Parapress, 1996), 155–7.

[77] Sabell, 'The History of Contact Lenses', 1–33; *BMJ* 21 July 1979, p. 217 (obituary of Dallos); letters from Dr Vera Pinter, the widow of Dallos, to the author, 20 July, 6 Sept. 1999.

[78] *BMJ* 7 Oct. 1967, p. 59 (obituary of Weiner).

1956), having done a stint as a dermatologist in child welfare clinics and the school health service, was in 1948 appointed a venereologist by the Manchester Regional Hospital Board.[79] Dr Paul Kiewe, who had performed a corneal graft for the first time on a patient suffering from a congenital disease, was employed at the Institute of Ophthalmology. Dr Martin Bodian MRCP (1910–63) joined the permanent staff of the Great Ormond Street Children's Hospital in 1946, rising to the rank of consultant pathologist and producing impressive research on childhood cancer.[80]

The only refugee doctors whose careers truly flourished were some of the consultant psychiatrists, the occasional maverick who abandoned a previous specialty to try new ventures, such as Ludwig Guttmann, and the younger generation of high-flying scientists born after 1900, most of whom were medically qualified and who conducted research in biochemistry, physiology, pharmacology, and genetics. William Grossman (1912–71), who had gained his MD in Prague and had become a major figure in English dentistry, failed to become dean of the University College Dental School, even though the previous holder of this office supported his appointment;[81] and, despite often acting as the head of the endocrinology unit at St Bartholomew's Hospital, Cornelius Medvie, an Austrian Roman Catholic of Jewish origin, was not made a consultant. On the other hand, Carl Eisinger (1895–1956), formerly on the staff of the Vienna medical school, spurned two offers of a professorship in Austria after the war in order to stay as a surgeon in the Metropolitan Ear, Nose and Throat Hospital.[82]

With the departure of the refugee scientists, Germany lost its pre-eminence in medical research to Britain and America.[83] 'In the last years before the war', remarked Sir Arthur Hurst, 'very little work of scientific or clinical importance was published in Germany.'[84] Despite their often ambivalent attitude towards Jews, influential figures in the British scientific establishment found places for the most brilliant of those evicted from their laboratories in central Europe. The influx of so much talent from the Continent augmented the ranks of Anglo-Jewish scientists, so that from being at the very periphery of innovative medical research before the Second World War they had by the 1950s and 1960s moved into its centre.

[79] *BMJ* 21 June 1980, p. 1547 (obituary of Heller), 22 Dec. 1956, p. 1493 (obituary of Fessler).
[80] *BMJ* 5 Oct. 1963, p. 873 (obituary of Bodian). *AJR Information*, Mar., May 1962; *JC* 16 Feb. 1962, p. 6 (on Paul Kiewe).
[81] *BMJ* 22 Jan. 1983, p. 313 (obituary of Grossman); private information; Pyke, 'The Great Insanity', 203.   [82] *BMJ* 4 Feb. 1956, p. 295 (obituary of Eisinger).
[83] Weindling, 'Contribution', 252, 253; id., 'The Impact of German Medical Scientists on British Medicine: A Case Study of Oxford, 1933–45', in Mitchell G. Ash and Alfons Sollner (eds.), *Forced Migration and Scientific Change* (Cambridge: Cambridge University Press, 1996), 86–114.
[84] Hurst, *A Twentieth Century Physician*, 75.

Sir Hans Adolf Krebs (1900–81) FRS, a medically trained scientist who had worked in Cambridge since his arrival in England, elucidated the chemistry by which the liver produced urea and then explained 'the chemical steps by which muscle and other cells oxidize sugars to carbon dioxide and water'.[85] He shared the Nobel Prize for Physiology and Medicine in 1953 and was appointed to the chair of biochemistry at Oxford in the following year. Apart from Krebs, who had gone to Cambridge because Sir Frederick Gowland Hopkins (1861–1947), Nobel Prize winner and professor of biochemistry, was well acquainted with his early preliminary findings, there were four other refugees working in the laboratories there, including E. Friedmann, Rudolf Lemberg, Hans Weil-Malherbe, and Ernst Chain. Sir Ernst Boris Chain FRS (1906–79), a German-trained chemist and physiologist, participated with Florey at Oxford in the testing and production of penicillin, for which he shared the Nobel Prize for physiology and medicine in 1945; he later held the chair of biochemistry at Imperial College London.[86] Werner Jacobson (1906–2000), after completing his medical training in Heidelberg, moved to Cambridge, where he pointed to folic deficiency in pregnant women as a cause of spina bifida in their babies; after some spells at Harvard medical school, he returned to Cambridge as professor of experimental medicine.[87] Hermann Lehmann FRS (1910–85) began his career as a research assistant for Otto Meyerhof, who sent him to Cambridge, where he worked for a time with Gowland Hopkins. After the war he based himself in Uganda, where he demonstrated that the common form of anaemia was due to hookworm infection and where he became interested in sickle-cell anaemia. Returning to England, he became reader in chemical pathology at St Bartholomew's, carrying out an experiment which laid the foundation for much subsequent work on genetically determined variation in drug responsiveness. His area of research interest shifted to abnormal haemoglobins and, with Max Perutz FRS—a refugee from Austria—at Cambridge, he studied the effect of haemoglobin amino-acid sequence changes on the three-dimensional configuration of the molecule. In 1967 Lehmann was appointed as the first professor of clinical biochemistry in Cambridge.[88] Max Perutz himself (b. 1914) worked on the structure of an oxygen-carrying protein, haemoglobin, by using X-ray crystallography, for which he was awarded the Nobel Prize for chemistry in 1962. Albert Neuberger FRS (1908–96) professor of chemical pathology at

[85] *Dictionary of National Biography 1981–1985* (1990), 229, 230 (on Krebs); Hans Krebs, *Reminiscences and Reflections* (Oxford: Clarendon Press, 1981), 88, 92; Pyke, 'The Great Insanity', 201; Jean Medawar and David Pyke, *Hitler's Gift: Scientists who Fled Nazi Germany* (London: Richard Cohen, 2000), 102–7.

[86] *Dictionary of National Biography 1971–1985*, 132, 133 (on Boris Chain); Medawar and Pyke, *Hitler's Gift*, 114–20.   [87] *The Times*, 31 Jan. 2000 (obituary of Jacobson).

[88] *Lives of the Fellows of the Royal College of Physicians of London*, viii. 274–6; *Lancet*, 3 Aug. 1985, p. 284 (obituary of Lehmann); Medawar and Pyke, *Hitler's Gift*, 113–14.

St Mary's Hospital, having studied medicine and chemistry, was one of the first to use isotopes as precursors for the study of metabolic processes, showing, for instance, how the red pigment of the blood was formed; later he became interested in the structure of proteins, particularly in the properties of glycoproteins.[89]

Wilhelm Feldberg FRS (1900–93) was reader in physiology at Cambridge and later the distinguished head of the physiology division at the National Institute for Medical Research, where he made 'fundamental contributions to the physiology and pharmacology of chemical transmission in the nervous system'.[90] As a young medically trained scientist, he was invited by Sir Henry Dale to join his laboratory in 1933; here, by use of eserine, Feldberg was able to detect the acetylcholine released during nerve stimulation and assist Dale in winning the Nobel Prize for medicine in 1936.[91] Even so, Feldberg had to wait until after the war, for recognition in his homeland, when the title of emeritus professor was eventually conferred on him by the West German authorities.[92] Hugh Blaschko FRS (1900–93), an MD from Freiburg and a research assistant of Meyerhof, went to Oxford to work on transmission in the nervous system. Bernard Katz FRS (b. 1911), another German-trained doctor, held the chair of biophysics at University College London from 1952 to 1978 and was the winner of the Nobel Prize for physiology and medicine in 1970. He extended the physiological researches of Dale and Feldberg, the investigation for which he is best known involving the transmitter acetylcholine: 'the findings of his research group have brought a better understanding of how such agents are passed across the narrow gap . . . separating nerve cells. It is important to understand this mechanism because poisonous agents or disorders which block the action of acetylcholine can lead to paralysis of muscles.'[93]

Edith Bülbring FRS (1903–90) was the daughter of a professor of English at Bonn; her mother belonged to a Dutch Jewish banking family. Having qualified as a doctor in 1928, she moved to England to work in a pharmaceutical laboratory and settled in Oxford in 1938, where she undertook research into the physiology of smooth muscle (visceral or involuntary muscle), such as the gut. She was appointed to the Oxford chair of physiology in 1967, having been appointed reader in 1960.[94] After Hans Gruneberg FRS (1907–85) qualified in medicine

[89] Horace Freeland Judson, *The Eighth Day of Creation: Makers of the Revolution in Biology* (London: Penguin, 1995), 504–7; *The Times*, 22 Aug. 1996 (obituary of Neuberger); Medawar and Pyke, *Hitler's Gift*, 102–20.   [90] *The Times*, 8 Nov. 1993 (obituary of Feldberg).

[91] W. Feldberg, 'The Early History of Synaptic and Neuromuscular Transmission by Acetylcholine: Reminiscences of an Eye Witness', in A. L. Hodgkin *et al.* (eds.), *The Pursuit of Nature: Informal Essays on the History of Physiology* (Cambridge: Cambridge University Press, 1977), 65–83; Medawar and Pyke, *Hitler's Gift*, 97–100.

[92] Pyke, 'The Great Insanity', 202, 203.   [93] *The Times*, 16 Oct. 1970 (on Katz).

[94] *Dictionary of National Biography 1986–1990*, 51, 52 (on Edith Bülbring); Medawar and Pyke, *Hitler's Gift*, 100–2 (on Blaschko), 121–3 (on Katz), 128–9 (on Bülbring).

in Bonn, he went to Berlin to study in one of the finest European centres for animal genetics. On moving to University College London in the 1930s, he carried out experiments which showed 'a wide range of pathological mutants in the mouse and other laboratory animals, many with similarities to human conditions'.[95]

Erica Wachtel Gordon (1912–80) was almost the only refugee doctor apart from the psychiatrists to achieve academic distinction and to rise to the rank of consultant in a major hospital. She graduated as an MD in Vienna in 1937 and emigrated to England a year later, where she was employed in various capacities until she was able to resume her medical career in 1941. In 1947 she worked as a part-time assistant in the infertility department of the Hammersmith Hospital before being put in charge of the new department of cytology (the study of cells). She was appointed a consultant in the hospital in 1964 as well as becoming senior lecturer in the Institute of Obstetrics and Gynaecology. In 1976 she was promoted and made the first professor of gynaecological cytology in the United Kingdom. She was a commanding personality, and 'the Hammersmith Hospital became a meeting place for international experts and trainees in cytology from all over the world. The clarity of her teaching and her dry wit that accompanied it left a lasting impression on all who knew her.'[96] Another important figure of Austrian origin was Robert Steiner (b. 1918), who was educated at the University of Vienna and University College Dublin, and who became professor of diagnostic radiology at the Hammersmith Hospital, where he promoted the introduction of scanners.[97]

The introduction of so many foreign-born specialists into the smaller National Health hospitals, the transformation of the practice of psychiatry and the care of paraplegics by refugee practitioners in this country, and the achievements of the refugee scientists, who were an overpowering presence in the world of medical research in the 1950s and 1960s, all gave an enormous boost to the prestige of the home-grown Jewish doctors, enabling them after an institutional revolution to climb to the highest positions after the Second World War.

[95] *BMJ* 8 Jan. 1983 (obituary of Grüneberg); Medawar and Pyke, *Hitler's Gift*, 60–1, 97–100.
[96] *BMJ* 5 July 1980, p. 67 (obituary of Gordon).   [97] Interview with Stuart Carne, 10 Feb. 2000.

Jewish Refugee Lawyers

W HEREAS refugee doctors were given the opportunity of taking up their profession again because of urgent wartime needs, German Jewish lawyers faced a much more difficult task in attempting to integrate themselves into the British legal system. Barristers with German accents felt unwelcome, so that few refugees tried to make a career at the English Bar. Refugees could not become solicitors unless they were naturalized, something that was difficult to achieve during the war, and only a small number qualified as solicitors after the war, as the English common law and Continental legal systems were so divergent. Nevertheless, some German Jewish lawyers settled in England and helped to create and staff the international restitution organizations; others opened practices which specialized in these claims or joined law firms as clerks to handle such work. As these lawyers found a wholly new way of reactivating their legal skills and of protecting the rights of other refugees, I thought that they merited inclusion in this chapter.

The migration of German lawyers in the 1930s was preceded by an earlier upheaval among Russian Jewish professionals. On the whole, the ethos of the Russian Bar under the tsarist regime of the late nineteenth century was more liberal and more tolerant than that of the population at large. In 1896, 389 out of 2,149 Russian lawyers (18.1 per cent) were Jewish, and of lawyers in training 42.6 per cent were Jewish. However, in the 1890s the tsarist regime imposed a quota of 10 per cent as the percentage of Jews who could be admitted to the Russian Bar, citing in defence the alleged morally dubious qualities of the Jew. The Russian *Journal of Civil and Criminal Law* claimed in 1889 that 'Jewish lawyers are more talented, have more knowledge and are more attentive to their duties than the Russians; they defend their clients by all means . . . and that competition with Jews is dangerous and even impossible for them [the Russians].'[1] Because of the restrictions imposed on Jews practising at the Russian Bar, one of the most talented jurists of the period, A. Y. Passover (1840–1910), qualified for the English Bar, though he reluctantly decided to return to Russia. After the Russian

---

[1] Samuel Kucherov, *Courts, Lawyers and Trials under the Last Three Tsars* (New York: Praeger, 1953), 273–80.

Revolution of 1917–18, however, many Jewish luminaries of the Bar dispersed overseas, principally to the United States and France, but also in some cases to England.[2] Among those Russian lawyers who requalified for the English Bar were M. Wolff, A. J. Halpern, and V. R. Idelson (1880–1954), who, as noted in Chapter 5, became a QC. Most of these gentlemen tended to specialize in international and banking law.[3] Dr John Mackover (1880–1971), a member of the team which defended Beilis against false accusations of ritual murder in Kiev in 1913, also migrated from Russia to Britain, where he became chairman of the Federation of Jewish Relief Organizations, though he does not appear to have practised at the English Bar.[4]

'The professional crisis of the 1920s [in Germany], marked by hyper-inflation, overcrowding and the impoverishment of one-third of practitioners to below subsistence level', declared Konrad Jarausch, 'made desperate attorneys grope for neo-Conservative solutions', including a campaign by an antisemitic minority within the German lawyers' association to disbar all Jewish attorneys.[5] It was estimated that in mid-1934 there were 5,000 Jewish and other non-Aryan lawyers in Germany, of whom 1,650 had been disbarred from practising. Of these, 300 had already emigrated, while another 300 who were still free to practise took the precaution of joining their colleagues overseas. Of the 3,350 left at the Bar, only 1,500 were still earning enough to support themselves and their families, and even they could not expect to continue to be able to do so; the rest were impoverished, partly because of the shrinkage of legal work and partly because, after Hitler came to power, the state would no longer instruct them when it had to pay for the services of a lawyer. To these 3,350 lawyers had to be added another 500 individuals, who were completing their training, making the total number of lawyers in need of assistance in the region of 4,000. By the end of 1938 the pressure of the Nazi lawyers' association had resulted in the elimination of most Jewish lawyers from active practice in Germany. There was also a high percentage of Jewish lawyers in Austria, particularly in Vienna, where in 1938 there were 1,674; these too had to follow their German Jewish colleagues into exile—the only alternatives being suicide or the concentration camps.[6]

Only a few of the refugee lawyers who arrived in Britain were admitted to the

---

[2] A. D. Margolin, *The Jews of Eastern Europe* (New York: Seltzer, 1926), 33–7; O. O. Gruzenberg, *Memoirs of a Russian-Jewish Lawyer*, ed. Don C. Rawson (Berkeley and Los Angeles: University of California Press, 1981), 1–25, 33–43, 217.

[3] *The Law List 1955* (London: Stevens & Sons, 1955), 862; *The Law List 1935* (London: Stevens & Sons, 1935), 117.   [4] *JC* 11 June 1971, p. 33 (obituary of John Mackover).

[5] Konrad H. Jarausch, 'Jewish Lawyers in Germany, 1848–1938: The Disintegration of a Profession', *Leo Baeck Institute Year Book*, 36 (1991), 171–90.

[6] Memorandum of the High Commission for Refugees Coming from Germany prepared for the conference in London on 4–5 July 1934 by Dr W. M. Kotschnig, p. 5, Norman Bentwich Papers, Central Zionist Archives, A255/785; Seidler, *The Bloodless Pogrom*, 209–25.

English Bar or became solicitors; more returned to the law after the Second World War, when they joined the United Restitution Organization or took up other restitution work. The first to establish himself as a lawyer in England was Professor Ernst Joseph Cohn (1904–76), who at the time he emigrated to Britain in 1933 was the youngest professor of civil law in Germany. 'Cohn managed to maintain himself by giving advice on German law, mainly to other German refugees, while at the same time he . . . studied English law.' He was called to the Bar in Lincoln's Inn in 1937, and after war service in the artillery served for four years as legal consultant to the Foreign Office on German law, publishing a *Manual of German Law* (1950). According to an obituary in *The Times*, this work 'marries a deep understanding of the Common and of the Civil law with a brilliant use of the Comparative method. It has been widely acclaimed as authoritative and is frequently cited in England and elsewhere as evidence of what German law is.' Moreover, 'In 1950 he went back into legal practice and, within a short time, he became a leading practitioner in matters relating to the conflict of laws, arbitration, and in matters involving a mixture of English, German and Swiss law', appearing in a number of notable trials in these specialist areas. In *Oppenheimer* v. *Cattermole (Inspector of Taxes)* (1970) Cohn gave expert evidence on behalf of the Crown, suggesting that the German federal constitutional court had declared that a 1941 decree depriving German Jews of their citizenship was void from its inception, but that a 1913 decree which stated that citizens who did not reside in Germany lost their nationality on acquiring a foreign one still applied. Therefore, when Mr Oppenheimer became a naturalized British subject in 1948, he forfeited his German nationality. Although Cohn practised at the Bar he remained in many respects an academic, whose primary interest was in the comparative law of procedure. He was not only an honorary professor of Frankfurt University but also a visiting professor of European law at King's College London.[7]

During the 1930s the City solicitors' firm of Herbert Oppenheimer, Nathan & Vandyk provided accommodation for Dr Drucker, a distinguished Czechoslovakian lawyer, to assist them with their Continental clients, while Denton Hall & Burgin relied on the services of Dr Walter Schoenhof, a German Jewish lawyer, for work of this nature. Lord Kissin (1912–97), a merchant banker with a doctorate in law from Basle, 'worked as legal adviser to Paul Winn, a produce company which had traded with his father's grain firm'. A number of Continental lawyers, including Ernst Cohn, Franz Paul Jacques, and Reinhold

---

[7] Marion Berghahn, *Continental Britons: German-Jewish Refugees from Nazi Germany* (Oxford: Berg, 1988), 87–8; *The Times*, 10 Jan. 1976; *AJR Information*, Feb. 1976 (obituary of Cohn); *Oppenheimer v. Cattermole (Inspector of Taxes)*, *Nothman v. Cooper (Inspector of Taxes)*, *Simon's Tax Cases 1975* 91–126. Cohn's point about the continuing effect of the 1913 decree was adopted by the House of Lords, and Francis Mann thought that his argument was valid.

Lachs, were called to the English Bar before the Second World War, but because of the time it generally took to become naturalized—a process required of would-be solicitors (possibly because they were often required to handle large sums of money), though not of barristers—only two refugees were admitted as solicitors before the end of the war: Dr Feist and Dr Kaufmann. Their cases may have been exceptional owing to their knowledge of English and rapid naturalization. The *Law Lists* for 1949 and 1955 show that there were at least nineteen Continental lawyers practising as solicitors in London who were of partially Jewish origin.[8] The list is as follows, with the year of admission in England given in brackets:

Philipp Cromwell (English Bar 1937, solicitor 1949)

Rudolph Edler, Dr Jur. Bonn (1946)

H. J. Feist, Dr Jur. Cologne (1942)

Owen Emil Franklyn (1948)

Marie Louise Froehlich, Dr Jur. Vienna (1954)

Walter Richard Moritz Furth, Dr Jur. Vienna (1947)

Rudolf Graupner (1948)

Frank Gerrard Holland, Dr Jur. Heidelberg (1946)

John Horitz, Dr Jur. Prague (1954)

Hans Jakobi, LLD Cologne (1947)

Ernst Arthur Kaufmann, LLD Leipzig (1940)

Seweryn Karol Maria Kon, Mag. Jur. Lvov (1952)

Victor Lehmann, LLD Rostock (1945)

Dr E. H. Loewenfeld (1948), based in Cambridge

Herbert Edgar Lorch, Dr Jur. Frankfurt-on-Main (English Bar, 1946)

Eleonore Mann, Dr Jur. Berlin (1953)

Frederick Alexander Mann, Dr Jur. Berlin (1946)

Hans Herbert Marcus (1948)

Frederic Alan Gustavus Schoenberg, Dr Jur. Vienna (1948).

To these names must be added Dr Rita Lehmann (1910–75) and G. A. Baracs, DL Budapest, who were both admitted as solicitors in 1958. There was also Gerard John Reyburn (formerly Rebenwurzel, 1914–81), who, having migrated from Austria in 1933, gained his LLB with first-class honours from London University and was placed at the head of the Law Society's honours list for

---

[8] *Select Committee on Conduct of a Member (Mr Boothby)*, PP1940–41, vol. ii, Q 1298; Lord Fletcher of Islington, *Random Reminiscences* (London: Bishopsgate, 1986), 32. *AJR Information*, Dec. 1984 (obituary of Lachs); *JC* 26 Dec. 1997, p. 17 (obituary of Lord Kissin); *The Law List 1949*, 216, 1869; *The Law List 1955*, 1–233.

November 1939, after which he became senior partner of Charles Crocker, a City law firm. Another well-known refugee solicitor was Johann Ferdinand Beer, a commercial and tax lawyer, who was an Austrian Catholic, but who possibly had some Jewish ancestry.[9]

During the Second World War Dr George Weis, a Czech refugee lawyer, researched the historical precedents for restitution, while Dr R. Callmann presented a memorandum to the Assembly of the United Nations in 1945, outlining claims to compensation on behalf of Jewish refugee organizations from central Europe. After serving in 1946 as the legal adviser of the Jewish Committee for Relief Abroad, based in British-occupied Germany, Dr Weis convened a conference of 200 Jewish lawyers from Germany and elsewhere on the Continent at Detmold in the British zone to discuss the restitution issue. The meeting was hailed as a symbol of professional recovery for Continental Jewish lawyers. In 1947 the Americans passed a restitution law for their zone of Germany and set up a trust body to claim heirless and Jewish communal property; they were followed by the British and the French, who instituted similar schemes in their zones. Further, in 1952 Chancellor Adenauer of the German Federal Republic enacted a law to pay DM 3 billion to Israel and DM 450 million to Jewish communities outside Israel in compensation for Nazi crimes. Former state employees, such as teachers and judges, and civil servants of the Jewish community, including rabbis and directors of charitable organizations, received generous pensions. Under amending legislation, east European subjects who had been persecuted or uprooted from their countries of origin were also given the chance to claim compensation. As a result of the persuasiveness and negotiating skills of Dr Nehemiah Robinson, a senior official of the World Jewish Congress, in 1959 Austria undertook with reluctance to establish a property restoration fund to compensate victims of the Nazis. Pressure from former judges and advocates in the ranks of the Council for the Protection of the Rights of German Jews, an international body based in London, for the setting up of a legal aid body to assist the various categories of claimant resulted in the establishment in Britain in 1948 of an international body, the United Restitution Organization (URO).[10]

The URO opened offices in Israel, the United States, France, Britain, and the three Allied zones in West Germany. At the peak of its activity it employed a staff of 1,026 full-time and 106 part-time workers, of whom 223 were practising lawyers. While most of the assistant lawyers and clerical staff in Germany were

---

[9] *Solicitors' Diary and Directory 1975* (London: Waterlow, 1975), 159, 240; *AJR Information*, Apr. 1985 (obituary of Lehmann); *Law Society's Gazette*, 9 Dec. 1981 (obituaries of Beer and Reyburn).

[10] Margot Pottlitzer, 'Restitution through the Ages', *AJR Information*, Aug. 1975; F. Goldschmidt, 'Restitution and Compensation', *AJR Information*, Oct. 1962; *AJR Information*, Feb. 1964 (obituary of Robinson); Norman Bentwich, *They Found Refuge* (London: Cresset, 1956), 145; id., *The United Restitution Organisation 1948–1968* (London: Vallentine Mitchell, 1968), 7–27.

non-Jewish, the URO offices both inside and outside Germany were headed by Jewish lawyers trained on the Continent. The organization 'had to find German Jewish lawyers, who had practised in Germany before the Hitler persecution, to man all these offices, because the work required expert knowledge of the German law. Some were recruited in Palestine, others in Germany itself, where a remnant of the Jewish legal fraternity had returned, others in England and America.' Dr George Weis, for instance, moved on from his efforts on behalf of those in the British zone of Germany to play a leading role in the American restitution organization. The sum claimed by the URO between 1949 and 1968 on behalf of claimants for compensation, as distinct from restitution, was $547 million; the total value of the amount awarded in the same period as restitution for seizure of immoveable and moveable property was another $40 million. At the same time the restitution claims provided a considerable amount of work for refugee lawyers in private practice in Britain.[11]

Among the refugee lawyers based in Britain who worked for the restitution institutions was Dr Kurt Alexander (1892–1962), an experienced lawyer who during the 1930s had built up a substantial clientele, particularly among the local silk manufacturers in his region of Germany. From 1939 to 1949 he lived in Britain, and was a Jewish communal leader in both countries. While in Britain he helped to set up the Association of Jewish Refugees (AJR), becoming its general secretary in 1943 and then one of the founders of the Council for the Protection of the Rights of German Jews and the URO, moving in 1949 to take over as the secretary of the latter's New York restitution office. Dr Hans Reichmann (1900–64) had worked as a lawyer in Germany and had joined the Berlin office of the Centralverein, the chief organization of pre-war German Jewry, before emigrating to England in the 1930s. When Alexander left for the United States, his responsibilities as secretary of the URO and secretary of the Council of Jews from Germany were jointly shared between Reichmann and Dr Frederick Goldschmidt. Dr Goldschmidt had been an assistant judge of the Berlin Court of Appeal when in 1933 the Nazi regime deprived him of his position; he fled to Britain in 1939. After the war, partly because of his excellent contacts with judicial circles in Germany and partly because at the same time he had the confidence of his Jewish colleagues, Goldschmidt was chosen by them to negotiate with German ministers. Between 1953 and 1963 Reichmann also acted as chairman of the AJR. He 'was relentless in his fight for restitution of recovered assets not only for the individual victims but also for the organisations which represented the remnants of German Jewry'. Thanks in part to his efforts in claiming a share of heirless and communal German Jewish property, the

---

[11] Bentwich, *The United Restitution Organisation*, 31, 33; Berghahn, *Continental Britons*, 89; Bentwich, *They Found Refuge*, 146, 188.

Council of Jews from Germany was able to provide its affiliate organizations with the wherewithal to support a network of welfare institutions. On Reichmann's death, Goldschmidt became head of the London office of the URO as well as legal adviser to the whole organization.[12]

Dr Reinhold Lachs (b. 1894), another German lawyer, qualified for the English Bar in 1937 and from 1945 to 1947 was legal adviser to the Foreign Office, after which he spent three years as legal adviser to the Control Commission in Germany. From 1950 to 1956 he was chief executive of the Jewish Trust Corporation for Germany in Hamburg, recovering much heirless and unclaimed Jewish property which was used to establish homes for the Jewish elderly in Britain. Dr Charles Kapralik (1895–1993), formerly a lawyer and deputy manager of a large insurance company in Vienna, was associated with Lachs in the activities of the Jewish Trust Corporation and succeeded him as its chief executive. As well as being vice-chairman of the URO in London and Frankfurt, he successfully negotiated on behalf of a New York committee with the Austrian government to recover social insurance benefits for 30,000 Jewish claimants dispersed all over the world.[13]

Of the refugee lawyers in private practice, most of those solicitors named above from the 1949 and 1955 *Law Lists* were heavily involved in restitution work. Hans Marcus (1921–97), who had three Jewish grandparents but was brought up as a Lutheran (though he later repudiated his upbringing, becoming a Buddhist) was partly educated in Britain, qualifying as a solicitor in 1948. He specialized in international law in London, at the same time opening a legal office in Hamburg as a sponsored civilian at the behest of the British military authorities.

[He] was one of the world's leading legal experts on German restitution claims arising both from postwar compensation schemes and the reunification of Germany. In recent years he represented Holocaust victims and their families, many of whom had failed to register their claims with the Jewish Claims Commission. He also championed the cause of the children of Holocaust victims who left Germany on the *Kindertransport*, pursuing their interests against Swiss banks that retained gold and other assets plundered by the Nazis, arguing that there was insufficient evidence of succession.

Marcus was also a masterly divorce lawyer and was involved in many film projects because one of the partners in his legal practice pioneered film completion guarantees.[14]

---

[12] Bentwich, *The United Restitution Organisation*, 28, 29; *JC* 2 Mar. 1962, p. 31; *AJR Information*, Mar., Apr. 1962 (obituary of Alexander); *AJR Information*, July 1964 (obituary of Reichmann).

[13] *AJR Information*, Dec. 1984 (90th birthday tribute to Reinhold Lachs), Dec. 1993 (obituary of Kapralik); C. I. Kapralik, *Reclaiming the Nazi Loot: The History of the Work of the Jewish Trust Corporation for Germany* (London: privately printed, 1962).

[14] *The Times*, 24 Sept. 1996, 31 Oct. 1997 (obituary of Marcus).

Not all the Continental refugee lawyers requalified in English law. Dr George Cohn (1892–1965)

was one of the first German lawyers who established a legal practice in London for restitution and compensation from Germany, and he built it up to become one of the largest of its kind in this country. Through his untiring efforts, which hardly allowed for any holidays, many renowned personalities as well as poor and needy victims of Nazi persecution received the full amount of indemnification due to them according to the German laws.[15]

Dr Erich Julius Goldstein (d. 1984), having worked as a lawyer in Germany, lived for twenty-two years in Palestine, where he tried to promote reconciliation between Arabs and Jews while he eked out a meagre living doing clerical work. After moving to London in 1955, he worked in the URO office and then in the practice of Dr George Cohn. Dr Andrew Michael Kraft (1900–65), a German-trained lawyer, worked for a number of years in a solicitor's office in England before in 1952 setting up his own practice to deal with restitution and compensation claims.[16]

Again and again the less fortunate of the refugee lawyers who migrated to Britain found themselves having to abandon their profession and seek out any means of employment. One worked as a welder until the strain of this heavy labour undermined his health; another damaged his hands while working in a hat factory. That was why restitution work proved to be such a splendid opportunity in allowing these practitioners to re-enter their chosen profession, and that is why a larger number of lawyers returned to Germany than any other class of Jewish professional.[17]

One refugee lawyer who did manage to practise in England—and indeed, reached the top of the profession—was Francis Mann (1907–91), hailed as 'one of the leading litigating solicitors of this century'. Born in Frankenthal in Germany, he studied and worked as an assistant in the Berlin University law faculty, but migrated to England in 1933 when a career as an attorney in Germany was closed to him. Although Mann was tempted to become a barrister, he did not pursue this career choice as he thought clients would be reluctant to accept someone with a thick German accent. For a time Mann and his wife practised as German lawyers in London; then he decided to become a solicitor and was articled to a member of the firm of Swann Hardman & Co., but could not be admitted as a solicitor until 1946. After the war Mann stayed in Berlin for a time as a British member of the legal division of the Allied Control Council to assist in the denazification of German law. Back in London, when his law partner was

---

[15] *AJR Information*, Oct. 1965 (obituary of Cohn).
[16] *AJR Information*, Feb. 1984 (obituary of Goldstein), Feb. 1965 (obituary of Kraft).
[17] Berghahn, *Continental Britons*, 89–92.

killed in an accident in 1955 he decided to merge his practice with that of Herbert Smith, which he helped build into one of the outstanding City law firms.[18]

Mann's area of specialization was that between international public law and international private law, but he also acted for Nubar Gulbenkian, who sought to modify his father's will, and for Somerset Maugham in a dispute with his daughter. Like Professor Cohn, Mann combined his career as a practitioner with rare academic expertise, being a frequent contributor to law journals and the author of the authoritative *The Legal Aspect of Money* (1938), which went through many editions. Under Lord Denning's guidance the Court of Appeal accepted Mann's view that a creditor could demand payment in the relevant foreign currency, not just in sterling, at the rate of exchange at the date of actual payment; the House of Lords confirmed this decision in *Miliangos* v. *George Frank (Textiles) Ltd.* (1976). In 1973 Mann wrote a seminal article in the *Law Quarterly Review*, setting out a masterly interpretation of Article 116(2) of the German Basic Law and subsequent cases in the German Federal Constitutional Court in 1958 and 1968. This resulted in the House of Lords reconsidering the arguments in *Oppenheimer* v. *Cattermole (Inspector of Taxes)* (1975) and deciding that the taxpayer concerned had ceased to be a German citizen.

Kurt Lipstein declared that Mann's 'influence was partly indirect through his writings and partly direct by his active conduct of cases involving an international element. This resulted in decisions of the House of Lords which constitute milestones in the development of English private international law.'[19] Many judges treated Mann's views with deference, Lord Justice Lloyd referring to him as 'a learned author whose views are happily not yet authoritative but are, nevertheless, entitled to great respect'.[20] Another judge remarked that 'a member of the House of Lords confessed to me that he felt nervous at seeing him listening to argument in the Committee Room. He could foresee that any shortcomings in his judgment would be remorselessly exposed in the next number of the *Law Quarterly*.'[21] Moreover, 'Mann's flinty virtue did not make him an easy man.'[22] Denied the chair of international law at London University which he coveted, he lectured frequently at German universities and was made honorary professor of law at Bonn.[23]

Other refugee solicitors from Germany with flourishing practices were Dr Erwin Loewenfeld (1888–1979) and Dr Rudolf Graupner (1907–99). Loewen-

---

[18] *Independent*, 25 Sept. 1991; *Daily Telegraph*, 2 Oct. 1991 (obituaries of Mann).

[19] Kurt Lipstein, 'The History of the Contribution to Law by German-Speaking Jewish Refugees in the United Kingdom' in Mosse (ed.), *Second Chance*, 225.

[20] Lawrence Collins, 'Dr F. A. Mann: His Work and Influence', in *British Year Book of International Law* (1993), 55   [21] Ibid. 109.   [22] *Daily Telegraph*, 2 Oct. 1992 (obituary of Mann).

[23] Lawrence Collins, 'Francis Alexander Mann 1907–1991', *Proceedings of the British Academy*, 84 (1994), 396–7.

feld was a successful international lawyer based in Cambridge; his father, a prominent Berlin lawyer, had acted for members of the former German imperial house and other important clients. Gradually Loewenfeld retrieved some of the vestiges of his father's practice, including clients such as members of the Opel family, the motor manufacturers, and sent instructions to Kurt Lipstein, then a member of the Cambridge law faculty, to advise on merits. Graupner, after staying for a time as a partner in the London firm of Buckeridge & Braune, moved to the better-known firm (also in London) of Pritchard Engelfield & Tobin. He was involved in a number of leading cases, including *Schorsch-Meier GmbH* v. *Hennin*, when—unusually at that time—Dr Mann's book *The Legal Aspects of Money* was quoted in court, and *Thyssen Edelstahl* v. *Armour*, which concerned the retention of title.[24]

Erstwhile German Jewish lawyers who could not find an opening in the legal profession in England went into a wide range of occupations and often enjoyed a good measure of worldly success. As Marion Berghahn has pointed out, 'Some went into banking or commerce, where they became involved either in management or accountancy. Others again took to journalism or publishing.'[25] Dr Julius Netter (1884–1964) built International Addressing Ltd. into one of the most important publicity agencies in the United Kingdom. Dr Jacob Braude (1902–77), a leading Jewish educationist, was a hog-bristle merchant with a large export trade. Dr Vernon Peter Ackerman established a high-class confectionery business patronized by the royal family. Dr Fritz Levy (1907–84) entered merchant banking, becoming a partner in Henry Ansbacher & Co. Dr William Guttman (1904–86) wrote a wartime feature in the *Observer* called 'The Voice of the Axis' as well as setting up a multi-language archive for the newspaper. After the collapse of his printing business in Slough as a result of the outbreak of war, Dr Walter Zander (1898–1993) in 1944 became secretary of the British Friends of the Hebrew University in Jerusalem. Isidor Grunfeld (1900–75) switched from reading for the English Bar to studying for the rabbinate in order to use his legal experience as a member of the London Beth Din, the highest Jewish court in the country. Refused admission by the Law Society in 1945, as he had not yet been naturalized, Dr Frank Falk (b. 1907) qualified as an accountant, specializing in taxation; in 1986 he obtained 'complete exemption from UK taxation for all German social security payments and civil servants' pensions'. Both Grunfeld and Falk applied their legal training to new areas of competence, and Dr Zander was much concerned with the search for justice between Arab and Jew, so that all three men put their legal knowledge to good use.[26]

---

[24] Interview with Professor Kurt Lipstein, 3 Aug. 1999; obituary of Graupner.

[25] Berghahn, *Continental Britons*, 88, 90–1.

[26] *AJR Information*, June 1964 (obituary of Netter), Apr. 1985 (obituary of Levy), Sept. 1986 (obituary of Guttman), Sept. 1991 (on Falk); *JC* 5 Feb. 1960, p. 6 (on Ackerman), 28 Oct. 1960, p. 13 (profile of Dayan Grunfeld), 23 Dec. 1977, p. 21 (obituary of Braude); *Independent*, 20 Apr. 1993 (obituary of Zander).

Once the initial handicap of being classified as an 'enemy alien' had been overcome by applying for naturalization, it was possible for refugee attorneys to advance rapidly as solicitors. In contrast, it was much harder for the older generation of refugee lawyers to make much headway as barristers, that most English of professions, with the notable exception of Professor Cohn (1904–76) and perhaps Frederick Honig (b. 1912) and Brian Grant (b. 1917), two Germans who became circuit judges. At least two of the refugee barristers, Philipp Cromwell and Herbert Edgar Lorch, later requalified as solicitors, which is some indication of their lack of progress as counsel. On the other hand, the younger generation of barristers of central European origin, who had been partially educated in England, advanced further. Sir Michael Kerr, born in Germany in 1921, having been head of prestigious commercial chambers, rose to become a lord justice of appeal.[27] Two of the younger generation stood in the front rank as barristers. Arriving in England at the age of 14, John Wilmers (1920–84) attended a Quaker school, and, after serving in the commandos, was called to the Bar in 1948. He acquired 'a reputation in Libel and Contract, and in the complex litigation which straddles the border of Common Law and Chancery'. A brilliant cross-examiner, Wilmers, who took silk in 1965, appeared in many cases concerning the press, particularly *The Times*, and acted for the BBC as well as businessmen from Hong Kong and the Near East. He also sat as a judge of the Court of Appeal of Jersey and Guernsey. Though influenced by Quaker principles, Wilmers never became a practising Quaker; he was one of those German Jewish refugees who found the question of identity problematic, refusing either to return fully to their Jewish roots or to embrace fully their Christian upbringing. George Shindler (1922–94) acted as an interpreter in the war crimes trials at Nuremberg; he was determined to make a career for himself as an actor, but was persuaded that he had a gift for law and was called to the Bar in 1952. From 1965 to 1970 he was standing counsel to the Inland Revenue, acting as a criminal prosecutor. After taking silk in 1970 he appeared for the defence in a string of famous trials, including those of the Parkhurst prison rioters and the Angry Brigade. A bout of ill health led Shindler to decide to ease his workload and in 1980 he became a circuit judge.[28]

The refugee lawyers who made arguably the greatest impact on the English legal system were the German-born academics, particularly if Ernst Cohn and Francis Mann, who never found their rightful place in the university world, are included among their number; this would parallel the position in the medical world, where the refugee scientists rather than the foreign-born doctors had

[27] Lipstein, 'The History of the Contribution to Law', 226; *Who's Who 1996* (London: A. & C. Black, 1996), 763, 933, 1072 (for Grant, Honig, and Kerr).

[28] *The Times*, 21 Dec. 1984 (obituary of Wilmers); *Daily Telegraph*, 17 Dec. 1994, *JC* 20 Jan. 1995, p. 19 (obituary of Shindler).

the most influence. Sir Otto Kahn-Freund (1900–79), who had studied labour law at Frankfurt University under Hugo Sinzheimer, joined the law faculty of the London School of Economics, where he inspired his students with his functional analysis of the law in action, going beyond arid instruction in the legal rules. K. W. Wedderburn claimed that Kahn-Freund had the linguistic ability

to paint upon a canvas denied to others, one which encompassed so many various systems of foreign law and, more lately, of European Community Law, to which he had a special devotion. In all of them, especially perhaps in his contributions to family law and matrimonial property and to labour law, he held firmly within his focus the needs of ordinary people which, he felt passionately, it was the task of law to serve . . . The most outstanding example of the direct effect of his published work was, perhaps, the acceptance by the High Court in 1969 of his analysis of the non-contractual status of British collective agreements [*Ford Motor Co.* v. *A.E.F.*].

Able to lecture fluently in four languages and understand the nuances of each, Kahn-Freund was called from the LSE to the chair of comparative law at Oxford at the age of 63, remaining there beyond retirement age until he was 70. At Oxford, remarkably, he widened the syllabus to include comparative law, family law, labour law, and European Community law.[29]

While the refugee scholars advanced the exploration of European and comparative law, they above all enriched the study and practice of international law. Georg Schwarzenberger (1908–91) taught in the law faculty at University College London from 1962 onwards, being promoted to the chair of international law in 1975. He wrote a series of volumes entitled *International Law as applied by International Courts and Tribunals*, often subjecting the decisions of the International Court of Justice to piercing criticism from a perspective of power politics.[30] Clive Macmillan Schmitthoff (1903–90) was a successful advocate in the Berlin Court of Appeal when he was forced to leave Germany in 1933, and was called to the Bar in England in 1936. Not having sufficient connections to make a full-time living at the Bar, he lectured in law at the City of London College and was appointed to the Gresham Chair in Law at City University in 1976. He created a new area of study, international trade law, and his book *The Export Trade* (1948) was translated into several languages. At the behest of the United Nations he prepared a report which led to the creation of a commission 'devoted to the harmonization of international trade law; and it is he who is credited with first propounding the new *lex mercatoria*, the transnational law of international trade'.[31] Kurt Lipstein was professor of compara-

---

[29] K. W. Wedderburn, 'Professor Sir Otto Kahn-Freund' (obituary), *Modern Law Review*, 42/6 (Nov. 1979), 609–12. *Dictionary of National Biography 1971–1980*, 457 (on Kahn-Freund).

[30] *The Times*, 30 Oct. 1991 (obituary of Schwarzenberger).

[31] *Dictionary of National Biography 1986–1990*, 399, 400 (on Schmitthoff).

tive law at Cambridge from 1973 to 1976; he not only introduced European law into the curriculum, but participated in the drawing up of the International Convention on the Recovery Abroad of Maintenance (1956) and the Hague Convention on the Administration of Estates of Deceased Persons (1973).[32]

Sir Hersch Lauterpacht (1897–1960), a refugee from earlier conflicts, was educated in Lvov and Vienna, coming to England in 1923 to undertake further study with the intention of settling in Palestine. But he was persuaded by Norman Bentwich and Professor McNair to stay in Britain and, after holding various positions in the law faculty at the LSE, was elected Whewell Professor of International Law at Cambridge in 1938. He edited the standard textbook on international law by L. F. L. Oppenheim (now called Oppenheim–Lauterpacht) as well as the *British Yearbook of International Law* and the international law reports. At the same time as pursuing his academic career he was called to the Bar in 1936 and took silk in 1949. As an international lawyer, he was associated with the continental shelf arbitrations aimed at resolving disputes over territorial rights, and acted as counsel for the United Kingdom in the *Corfu Channel* and the *Anglo-Iranian Oil Company* (interim measures cases) at the International Court of Justice. As a judge of this court from 1955 until his premature death, he held that countries such as France and the United States, which accepted the compulsory jurisdiction of the International Court, could not exclude certain matters as falling within their domestic jurisdiction. In a child custody dispute between Sweden and the Netherlands, he similarly decided that an agreement made between two states could not be vitiated by an internal law passed by one of the contracting parties. In a dispute as to whether the Mandate of South Africa continued in South-West Africa, he reached the same verdict as his colleagues, but unlike them set out in full the reasons for his decision.

Lauterpacht served on the British War Crimes Executive in 1945–6. Like many Polish Jewish lawyers interested in international law, he wanted to devise new means of protecting minorities after the Second World War, given the evident failure of the existing minority rights treaties (some of his relatives were killed in the Holocaust). In 1945, encouraged and assisted by the American Jewish Committee, he published a universal bill of rights which had some influence on the framing of the Universal Declaration of Human Rights (1948), notably in the form of article 35 which protected persons belonging to 'ethnic, linguistic or religious minorities'. Although he played little part in Anglo-Jewish life, he remained concerned about Jewish issues, visiting Jewish student summer schools, and was consulted by the Jewish Agency on the interpretation of the Palestine Mandate. Throughout his work, he was 'inspired by a moral earnestness, and a belief in right and justice, and that right and justice will pre-

---

[32] Lipstein, 'The History of the Contribution to Law', 223–6.

vail'.[33] One of his successors on the bench of the International Court was Judge Manfred Lachs (1914–93), another Polish Jewish polymath, who spent the war years in Britain before being elected president of the International Court in 1973. He tended to follow the majority of his colleagues in his judgments, favouring consensus-building.[34]

How Jewish were these refugee doctors and lawyers in their identity? From reading the accounts of their lives, one gathers the impression that on the whole lawyers, apart from those in the universities, had a much higher level of synagogue affiliation and a closer connection with the Association of Jewish Refugees and Zionist bodies than the generality of doctors. Even so, Professor Kurt Lipstein and Sir Michael Kerr were brought up as Christians, while John Wilmers QC was influenced by the Quaker principles of the school he attended. The medical specialists and scientists tended to be much more secular in orientation, many of them having non-Jewish wives. Speaking of Professor Fritz Jacoby (1902–91), an expert on tissues, a colleague wrote that 'No one who attended the Jacobys' Christmas parties will ever forget the warmth of the welcome and the happy family atmosphere in their Cardiff home.'[35] Yet there were exceptions, such as Professor Neuberger, who was warden of an Orthodox synagogue; Dr Himmelweit and Professor Chain, who were enthusiastic Zionists; and Professor David Daube (1909–99), the Regius Professor of civil law at Oxford and an authority on Greek, Roman, and Jewish law, who waited until middle age to loosen his adherence to 'a strictly observant Jewish life'. Although he was the founder and first president of the World Union of Jewish Students, Lauterpacht played 'little or no part in the Jewish life of England'.[36]

The influx of the refugee doctors and lawyers altered the standing of Anglo-Jewry in the professions. While the impact of the refugee solicitors and barristers was negligible—with the exception, perhaps, of Francis Mann—the infusion of the Continental academic lawyers into the universities revitalized the study of European, comparative, and international law. Similarly, the American Arthur Lehman Goodhart (1891–1978), who settled in England, through his notes on cases in the *Law Quarterly Review* helped to persuade judges after the Second World War to consider the views of living academic authorities on the issues before the court.[37] This was a wholly new practice. Before the war, academic

---

[33] *Dictionary of National Biography 1951–1960*, 611–13 (on Lauterpacht); Dorothy Stone, 'Sir Hersch Lauterpacht; Teacher, Writer and Judge: A Presidential Address', *Transactions of the Jewish Historical Society of England*, 28 (1984), 102–10.

[34] *Independent*, 16 Feb. 1993 (obituary of Lachs).

[35] *The Times*, 24 Oct. 1991 (obituary of Jacoby).

[36] *JC* 25 Mar. 1977, p. 30 (obituary of Himmelweit), 30 Aug. 1996, p. 17 (obituary of Neuberger); Chaim Weizmann, *Trial and Error* (London: Hamish Hamilton, 1949), 549; *Independent*, 5 Mar. 1999; *JC* 12 Mar. 1999, p. 31 (obituary of Daube); Stone, 'Sir Hersch Lauterpacht', 109.

[37] Goodhart's influence was assessed in the *Law Quarterly Review*, 91 (Oct. 1975), 457–71.

lawyers with immigrant parents from east Europe encountered considerable prejudice in English university circles, particularly during the 1930s; it is noteworthy that Coleman Phillipson became a professor in Adelaide and Julius Stone moved to a chair of law in Sydney.[38]

[38] See *JC* 8 July 1910, 10 Dec. 1920, p. 25 on Coleman Phillipson. Leonie Star, *Julius Stone: An Intellectual Life* (Melbourne: Oxford University Press, 1992), 14, 15, 43, 44.

ELEVEN

Jewish Consultants after the Second World War

I N the years immediately after the Second World War there was a shortage of
places in British medical schools, and in the intense competition for admission between recent school-leavers and returning soldiers priority was given to
those who could show evidence of military service. As a result there were instances of prejudice being shown against Jewish applicants and refugees, some
of whom were of Jewish origin; but it should be stressed that the antisemitism
displayed by the Leeds medical school was relatively isolated, not a general
occurrence, and that the refugee plight was of short duration. Several Jewish
students failed to gain places at the Leeds medical school in 1945 and turned to
dentistry instead, but they were reluctant to complain, fearing that there could
be further repercussions for them if they were vocal about their rejection. 'One
student, however, whose qualifications were better than many who were accepted', declared Gerald Wootliffe, a spokesman for the Leeds Jewish students
who himself became a dentist,

was asked whether he was an orthodox Jew (the excuse being whether he was prepared
to attend on *Shabbos* [Saturday] . . . Another student with an excellent University
Scholarship, specifically for the study of Medicine was rejected, but after making a fight
of the case through the Education Authorities of the City of Leeds and through the
University Authorities he was finally accepted on the first day of term. Incidentally, this
student on application had rather a foreign sounding name, but before entering the
School, changed his name to one more anglicised, yet the Sub-Dean, upon whom all
acceptances depend, delights in referring to him by his former name before his fellow
students. This is quite a common practice with regard to other students who have also
changed their names.[1]

As far as refugee students were concerned, Danuta Waydenfeld reported
that her application for admission was rejected by a number of medical schools
after the war and that she was unable to understand the reason for this until a
professor from Manchester enlightened her. 'Our boys are coming back from the

---

[1] Gerald Wootliffe to M. J. Roston, 20 Feb. 1945, Board of Deputies Defence Committee,
C6/4/2/22, Board of Deputies Office.

war', he explained; 'you are a woman, a foreigner, you have zero chance of gaining a place.' Her husband Stefan also failed to find a place initially, but after waiting until 1948 'secured an ex-serviceman's grant and a place at the Royal College of Surgeons in Dublin'.[2] Female applicants generally were discriminated against in the post-war period. 'In 1945, University of London policy obliged each of the London medical schools to admit a minimum quota of women amounting to 15 per cent of the total entry', noted James Stuart Garner. 'It was not until the late 1960s that this policy was discarded in favour of more meritocratic selection criteria.'[3]

Within the Medical Practitioners' Union (MPU) there was a last splutter of antisemitism directed against the employment of the refugee doctors who stayed in Britain after the war. A typical example was a letter from a Dr R. E. Illingworth which appeared in the *Medical World* on 10 August 1945. 'So far as British medicine is concerned, a position is arising in this country analogous to that which existed in Germany in 1930. One loathes Hitler and all he stood for, but there can be no doubt that there was in Germany a question which demanded a drastic solution.' This letter fortunately drew a sharp riposte from several individual practitioners. So, too, the local medical war committee in Salford tried in 1946 to prevent Dr Fritz Rothenberg from working as an assistant to Dr J. Libman, protesting that 'we have far too many alien doctors in Salford who have established themselves whilst the British doctors have been in the Forces. Why can't these alien doctors return to their own countries to alleviate the sufferings of their fellow countrymen?' When Dr Bruce Cardew took over as secretary of the MPU in 1948, he finally rid it of both its last vestiges of antisemitism and its anti-scientific bias.[4]

Because of the shortage of consultants at the inauguration of the National Health Service in 1948, hospitals had to employ a large number of refugee doctors, many of whom were specialists; but, as we have seen, most of them ended their careers in provincial hospitals or in the smaller London hospitals and in private practice. At the same time, some of the doctors who had held important hospital posts during the war were eased out of their positions to make way for returning consultants who had been serving in the army or air force medical service.[5] Norman Maurice Jacoby, a South African, having been sponsored by the eminent surgeon Robert Davies-Colley and having specialized in paediatrics, was appointed registrar in the children's department at Guy's just before the war; when hostilities began in 1939, the children's department was evacuated to

[2] Stefan Waydenfeld, *The Ice Road* (Edinburgh: Mainstream, 1999), 395.

[3] Garner, 'The Great Experiment', 70.

[4] Honigsbaum, *The Division in British Medicine*, 312, 313; Aliens Committee of the Central War Medical Committee, Minutes, 28 May 1946, British Medical Association Archive.

[5] Honigsbaum, *The Division in British Medicine*, 313.

Pembury Hospital in Kent, where Jacoby became a consultant in the Emergency Medical Service, undertaking the teaching of paediatrics and holding various children's clinics. Notwithstanding this record, at the end of the war Guy's abruptly dispensed with his services.[6]

While the post-war period saw an expansion of the number of Jewish doctors practising in London, the increase over the late 1930s was not dramatic. If we follow the assumption general among Anglo-Jewish sociologists that by 1950 the number of British-born Jewish doctors in London had at least reached its pre-war level of 800, then we must add to this number the additional influx of 300–320 refugee doctors. This would bring the total of Jewish doctors to around a figure of 1,100; allowing for a certain amount of overlapping between the refugee doctors and the 800 pre-war doctors, the total number may be put at no more than 1,050. This calculation can be checked using a method employed by Asher Tropp, based on noting certain distinctive Jewish surnames which occur regularly in professional directories and then multiplying this figure by 14.26 to arrive at a total for the number of Jewish doctors.[7] In the *Medical Directory* for 1953 there were sixty-eight doctors in London with such distinctive surnames, which when multiplied by 14.26 gives us a figure of 970; but we should exclude from the list of sixty-eight one woman with a Jewish surname but a non-Jewish maiden name, and a group of South African Jewish doctors who for personal reasons decided to stay registered on the British list without practising there.

For the 1990s we have more helpful information, particularly data collected in June 1991 by Dr Martin Sarner, a consultant at University College Hospital and secretary of the London Jewish Medical Society, relating to doctors in the Greater London area affiliated to Jewish organizations. Sarner arrives at a total of 1,123 such doctors, which drops to 1,000 when we exclude doctors located outside the London area and certain individuals who were dentists, historians, or widows of medical practitioners. If this smaller figure is multiplied by 30 per cent to include doctors who were not affiliated to Jewish organizations, the total number of Jewish doctors in the London area comes out at 1,300. It could also be argued that doctors had higher incomes than the Jewish population as a whole, and that consequently more doctors than other Jews tended to be affiliated to Jewish associations; if this were so, perhaps it would be more correct to say that only 20–25 per cent of the Jewish doctors were unaffiliated. This would give us a total of 1,200–1,250 Jewish doctors in the London area. To check the accuracy of this figure, I applied the methods devised by Asher Tropp by concentrating on the distinctive Jewish surnames listed in the *Medical Directory* of

    [6] Jacoby, *Journey*, 36–43.
    [7] Tropp, *Jews in the Professions*: the multiplier of 14.26, used to arrive at the total number of Jews by means of the number of Jewish names, is discussed on pp. 95–7.

1990 for the London area and arrived at a figure of 108 practising and five retired doctors, which when multiplied by 14.26 gives a total of 1,540 doctors together with seventy-one retired doctors. The two figures added together yield a total of 1,611 doctors. I would conclude that Martin Sarner's figures for 1991, based on lists of actual doctors associated with specific synagogues and Jewish charities, are more likely to be accurate than the figures produced by following Tropp's more conjectural method.[8]

Until the advent of the National Health Service in 1948 the appointment boards of hospitals, in the words of Dr Maurice Silverman, 'were relatively private affairs with an interviewing committee more or less limited to the individual hospital', in which, as we have seen, all kinds of prejudices could be safely aired and which were sometimes nothing more than a closed shop. According to another informant, until the 1960s the London medical schools remained White, Anglo-Saxon, and Protestant in character, inbred, and imbued with an emphasis on students who were rugger players and skilled oarsmen. Under ministerial regulations introduced shortly after the establishment of the health service the appointment of consultants and senior registrars was transferred from the hospital management committees to regional hospital boards. To quote Dr Silverman again,

the new Advisory Appointments Committees were essentially effective from the start in view of the much wider field the members were drawn from and the resultant more democratic process. This, of course, does not exclude the fact that the old die-hards still formed part of these committees and in this sense there was also a measure of gradual change as the old die-hards were progressively replaced.[9]

For teaching hospital appointments, the selection committees included outside assessors—representatives of the university and the Health Service. At the same time, many registrars had been trained either in general medicine or general surgery, and for each vacancy in these areas there was a glut of applicants, while trainees were reluctant to move into the less glamorous specialties of psychiatry, anaesthetics, pathology, and radiology, where there was a shortage of recruits.[10]

One of the major changes introduced by the NHS was the classification of specialists into separate grades, partly for the purposes of remuneration and partly to create a career ladder. Before the Second World War, doctors having passed the examination for membership of the Royal College of Surgeons or the Royal College of Physicians ultimately applied for positions as honorary consultants in the teaching hospitals, where they worked hard and acquired a

[8] *Medical Directory 1990*, 2 vols., *passim*.
[9] Letters from Dr Maurice Silverman to author, 20 July 1997, 4 Aug. 1997; private information.
[10] Charles Webster, *The Health Service since the War*, vol. i (London: HMSO, 1988), 307, 308.

reputation, thereby ensuring a ready flow of private patients. Thus, because many aspiring consultants had to face a long, practically unpaid apprenticeship, recruits were drawn in the main from the upper or upper-middle classes, and doctors without private means had to undergo considerable hardship and delay marriage to achieve such goals.[11] Partly for this reason, there had formerly been a wide class gulf between the consultants and doctors from modest east European Jewish families. Now, in the new health service, consultants were offered paid contracts, either full-time or, if they wished to retain some of their private patients, part-time.[12] During the early 1950s there was a rapid recruitment of junior hospital medical staff, resulting in the creation of a surplus of registrars with little hope of advancement; and while the government wished to reduce the number of registrars by 1,100, it was able to secure the dismissal of only about a hundred of them.[13] It is against these changes in the structure of the appointment committees and the radical overhaul of the recruitment system for specialists that the rise of the post-war Jewish consultant must be seen.

In the late 1950s and during the 1960s, all those seeking appointment as consultants—not just Jews—faced great difficulties. Martin Sarner recalled that

There were not a lot of consultant posts, and there were graduates coming up through the consultant programmes, who had graduated after the war. There were also people whose careers had been interrupted by the war and were coming back from being in the war, and either resuming their medical studentship or starting off from where they left off, already graduated. There were people quite long in the tooth, forty plus, still looking for consultant jobs. There was, of course, a great shortage of consultant jobs and a great number of people trying [for] them; and as a result, people went off into general practice because they couldn't get appointed or they went abroad.[14]

Discouraged in part by the lack of opportunities in Britain, a significant number of highly trained medical personnel sought employment overseas, and shortly after the foundation of the State of Israel in 1948—in some cases earlier—a handful of specialists imbued with Zionist ideals settled there. One of these was Eli Davis (1908–97), deputy medical superintendent and senior resident physician at St Andrew's Hospital in Bow, which was one of the major institutions under the control of the London County Council. When Dr Haim Yassky, the director of the Hadassah Hospital in Jerusalem, was killed in an Arab ambush in 1948, he was succeeded as director-general by Dr Davis for three crucial years, but in 1951 Davis resigned from this position to resume his

---

[11] Harry Eckstein, *Pressure Group Politics: The Case of the British Medical Association* (London: Allen & Unwin, 1960), 114–25; Jacoby, *Journey*, 44, 45.

[12] Honigsbaum, *The Division in British Medicine*, 318; Charles Webster, *The National Health Service: A Political History* (Oxford: Oxford University Press, 1998), 26.

[13] Eckstein, *Pressure Group Politics*, 117–25.   [14] Interview with Martin Sarner, 24 Nov. 1999.

career as a physician.[15] Dr Myer Makin, a student Zionist leader from Liverpool, after becoming a Fellow of the American College of Surgeons, was chosen as the first head of the Hadassah Hospital's orthopaedic department.[16] Professor Marco Caine was so frustrated by the lack of opportunity for promotion to the rank of consultant in a central London Hospital, which he was told was beyond his reach as a Jew, that he left for Israel with his family in the late 1950s and set up the department of urology at the Hadassah Hospital.[17]

Quite a few doctors migrated to the United States, others to Canada and beyond. Alexander Gol, after reading medicine at Cambridge and training at Guy's, moved to the Children's Memorial Hospital, Chicago, in the late 1950s. He died in 1989. Victor Rosenoer became associate clinical professor of medicine in the University of California, where he specialized in liver disease and metabolism; Tony Tavill, a gastroenterologist, moved as a professor to Cleveland, Ohio. Alan Harris Levy (1925–82), a gold medallist at Bristol, took up an appointment as president of the medical staff at St Joseph's Hospital and director of the Peterborough Clinic in Canada. G. J. Fraenkel, the surgical tutor at the Radcliffe Infirmary, Oxford, under Hugh Cairns, became professor of surgery at the University of Otago in New Zealand before moving to Australia as dean of the School of Medicine, Flinders University. Perhaps the most interesting migrant was Joshua Samuel Horn (1914–75), once a tutor in anatomy at Cambridge, who became a surgeon in the Birmingham Accident Hospital in 1948, and afterwards spent fifteen years in China until his career as a doctor was threatened by multiple sclerosis. While in China, he established an accident hospital and pioneered the attachment of severed limbs. He spent his retirement in England.[18]

Jews were sometimes not appointed to positions during the 1950s for well-meant but slightly odd reasons. Maurice Garretts was trained in dermatology by William Goldsmith, his departmental head at University College Hospital; Goldsmith, who incidentally was from an old Anglo-Jewish family, established in England since at least the nineteenth century and possibly earlier, was editor of the journal of his specialty and author of the authoritative *Recent Advances in Dermatology*. Having reached the rank of senior registrar, Garretts was looking for a vacancy in a teaching hospital. 'I was very well trained, though I say it myself', remarked Garretts:

[15] Interview with Professor Eli Davis, 22 Aug. 1996; *Korot*, 12 (1996–7), 202–4 (obituary of Davis); *Medical Directory 1943*, i. 73; interview with Dr Davis in Manfred Wasserman and Samuel Kottek (eds.), *Health and Disease in the Holy Land* (Lampeter: Edwin Mellen, 1996), 361–87.

[16] *JC* 28 June 1957 (on Dr Makin).   [17] Interview with Professor Marco Caine, 19 Aug. 1996.

[18] *Lives of the Fellows of the Royal College of Surgeons 1983–1990*, 132 (on Alexander Gol); interviews with Martin Sarner, 24 Nov. 1999, and Sir Leslie Turnberg, 14 Mar. 2000. *Lives of the Fellows of the Royal College of Surgeons 1974–1982*, 230 (on Alan Harris Levy), 187 (on Joshua Horn); Joshua S. Horn, *Away With All Pests: An English Surgeon in People's China* (London: Hamlyn, 1969), 14, 15, 25; G. J. Fraenkel, *Hugh Cairns: First Nuffield Professor of Surgery* (Oxford: Oxford University Press, 1991), preface.

I was primed for a good job; and I applied to Cambridge and the dermatologist was a very nice man called Arthur Rook . . . he was looking for a junior colleague . . . and he said, 'Maurice, I don't know if you have thought this through, we have a fine Cambridge University Jewish Society, but this is a passing flock, they come and they go . . . and the number of people who are Jewish who live in Cambridge, you can count on one hand, do you think you'd be happy with me at Cambridge? . . . I would advise you, though I would very much like you as my colleague, I would advise you if Judaism means anything at all to withdraw from this appointment. I don't think it would suit you'; and I thanked him very much . . . and I withdrew.[19]

Dr Joseph Jacobs, who held house appointments at the London Jewish Hospital in 1956–7, declared 'that even then there was a great deal of prejudice in the teaching hospitals when it came to appointments', but this was a somewhat exaggerated account of the position, as Jews could gain good appointments in hospitals as registrars. In fact, the difficulties these registrars encountered during the late 1950s and 1960s when they applied for promotion to consultant posts had more to with the overproduction of qualified trainees chasing too few vacancies than any widespread covert antisemitism.[20]

Following the Race Relations Acts of 1965, 1968, and 1976, a more tolerant climate of opinion gradually evolved which assisted Jews and others when they applied for medical scholarships and appointments as specialists.[21] An example of this change in attitude was the refusal in the mid-1960s of the Royal College of Surgeons to accept an endowment for students which was framed to exclude Roman Catholics and Jews. While Mr Justice Buckley agreed that 'racial and religious discrimination is nowadays widely regarded as deplorable in many respects', he was reluctant to delete the offending phrase from the trust until the college stipulated that the gift would be unacceptable unless these discriminatory words were removed.[22] N. M. Jacoby, who sat on an appointments committee for hospital posts, stated that these boards often leaned over backwards to be fair, even when a candidate for a vacancy was aggressive and had a 'colonial' accent which made him difficult to understand, and appointed an individual despite the fact that some prejudicial remarks had been made against him.[23] Later there was a tendency to rely on the recruitment of medical practitioners from India and Pakistan, who had been partially trained in Britain, to fill the shortages of specialist staff. Whereas in 1958 there were 2,500 overseas doctors working in England and Wales, in 1999 there were 25,000 such doctors employed in the National Health Service.[24] There was still, however, a residual

[19] Interview with Dr Maurice Garretts, 24 Feb. 1999.
[20] Interview with Dr Alex Saluka, 10 Apr. 2000; Black, *Lord Rothschild*, 97.
[21] Anthony Lester and Geoffrey Bindman, *Race Law* (London: Longman, 1972), 68.
[22] *Re Lysaght* 1 Chan. 1966, p. 191.   [23] Jacoby, *Journey*, 45, 46.
[24] Webster, *The Health Service since the War*, 309; *The Times*, 8 Nov. 1999.

degree of prejudice and a suspicion that Jewish candidates for some specialist posts were occasionally favoured over their Asian colleagues, though in the case of a contretemps at the Royal Free Hospital this was strongly denied.

I turn now to a detailed examination of how the new machinery set up for the selection of senior hospital staff enhanced the opportunities for Jewish candidates to make successful applications, beginning with the area of surgery. It is a commonly held view that, despite the swelling numbers of Jews in the medical profession, there were relatively few Jewish surgeons. Jonathan Miller explained in 1989 that 'Surgery has always been associated with the rather patrician side of the profession. It's been associated with a sort of stylish metropolitan grace— it's a craftsman's job . . . Because the emphasis among Jews has always been on learning rather than handwork, they tend not to go into surgery.'[25] While Jews may have preferred to join the ranks of the Royal College of Physicians, it would be wrong to suggest that the number of Jewish surgeons in the post-war period was sparse. What is also overlooked is that Jews were drifting into areas of the hospital system where there were vacancies and avoiding a career in surgery, where there were fewer such openings.

Most of the Jewish surgeons born in Britain in the closing years of Queen Victoria's reign and the opening two decades of the twentieth century, or even a little later, were the children of immigrant parents. However talented, they still tended to end their careers in the smaller outer London hospitals or in the provinces; some of them, frustrated over promotion, joined the staff of the London Jewish Hospital or migrated overseas. That is why, despite their large numbers, they have escaped proper notice. The career prospects for Anglo-Jewish surgeons remained bleak during the 1950s, improving only slowly during the 1960s.

Joel Gabe (d. 1989) was the consultant urological surgeon to the Greenwich, Deptford, and other south London hospital groups, while Solomon Lewis Citron (1920–87), the son of a tailor, became a senior registrar at University College Hospital and the Royal Ear Hospital, after which he was appointed a consultant in Enfield. Mendel Gordon (1902–83), the winner of a gold medal in medicine and surgery at the Charing Cross medical school, became the registrar in ear, nose, and throat surgery at the Royal Free Hospital. During the war he worked with Sir Archibald McIndoe in plastic surgery, and later held appointments at, among other institutions, the National Temperance Hospital. Harry Isaac Deitch (1903–90) moved in the 1930s to Yorkshire, where as surgeon superintendent at the Halifax General Hospital he carried out gynaecological, orthopaedic, ENT, and general surgery; following the reorganization of health provision under the NHS he was appointed consultant to the Bradford Royal Infirmary. Gerard Erwin Stein (1916–86; born in Germany but trained in

---

[25] Quoted in Brook, *The Club*, 313.

England) was an ear, nose, and throat consultant to the Whittington, Royal Northern, Hornsey, and Teddington memorial hospitals. Solly Morris Cohen (1904–89) entered Guy's Hospital, where his ability attracted the attention of Sir Heneage Ogilvie, after which he went back to South Africa, where he had been born, and acquired an expertise in surgery connected with stab wounds and fractures of the skull caused by weapons. On his return to Britain in 1939 he became a superintendent at the Southern Hospital in Dartford, where he treated many casualties among the soldiers evacuated from Dunkirk. An expert on vascular injuries, after 1948 he was appointed consultant surgeon to the Medway and Gravesend group of hospitals and surgeon to the peripheral vascular centre in Dartford. So great was his reputation that he was described as 'a consultant's consultant'. Stanley Rivlin (1923–98), a *bon viveur*, 'confined his surgery to operating on varicose veins' and developed 'a huge international practice', opening a clinic in Battersea.[26]

Jewish orthopaedic surgeons included the South African-born Woolf Herschell (1903–77), who became the resident surgical officer at the Royal National Orthopaedic Hospital, Stanmore. After being awarded his FRCS in 1949, he was appointed consultant orthopaedic surgeon to the Windsor group of hospitals. Eric Martin Kupfer, having served as registrar to the East Suffolk and Ipswich Hospital, became the consultant in orthopaedic surgery to the Chester and District hospital group. Because of the continuing difficulty Jews had in obtaining appointments as specialists in Leeds, many were compelled to leave the city and look for work elsewhere. Geoffrey Hyman ran a rehabilitation unit in Wakefield with a colleague during the Second World War, after which he was appointed orthopaedic surgeon to the Halifax hospital group and the Leeds Jewish Hospital.[27] When Max Harrison decided to become a surgeon, he was advised by medical colleagues to quit Leeds; he moved to Birmingham, where he became consultant surgeon to the General Hospital and the Royal Orthopaedic Hospital and part-time lecturer in orthopaedic surgery at the university.[28]

Among the Jewish eye surgeons, Eugene Wolff (1896–1954) attended University College medical school, winning the Lister Medal for clinical surgery in 1918 and serving as ophthalmic registrar. In 1928 he was appointed ophthalmic surgeon to the Royal Northern Hospital and eight years later to the Royal Westminster Ophthalmic Hospital, besides becoming a member of the staff of the London Jewish Hospital. He was a consulting surgeon to the London County

[26] *Lives of the Fellows of the Royal College of Surgeons 1983–1990*, 123 (on Joel Gabe), 69 (on Solomon Lewis Citron), 133 (on Mendel Gordon), 92 (on Harry Isaac Deitch), 347 (on Gerard Erwin Stein), 75 (on Solly Morris Cohen), 115 (on the neurosurgeon Bernard Fairburn); *Lancet*, 5 May 1990 (obituary of Cohen); *The Times*, 16 Jan. 1998 (obituary of Rivlin).

[27] *Lives of the Fellows of the Royal College of Surgeons 1974–1982*, 182 (on Herschell), 225 (on Kupfer), and 195 (on Hyman).   [28] Private information, *Medical Directory 1993*, ii. 1548 (on Harrison).

Council and after the war taught at the Institute of Ophthalmology.[29] Isidore
Spiro (1898–1978) trained as an eye surgeon at Wolverhampton and then at Uni-
versity College Hospital under the eminent Sir John Parsons. After the Second
World War he held the position of consultant ophthalmologist to Queen Mary's
Hospital for the East End, the Hillingdon Hospital, and Lister Hospital in
Hitchin.[30] Mark Tree (1898–1984), the son of an outfitter, was educated at the
Central Foundation School in Whitechapel before qualifying and becoming a
consultant ophthalmologist to the Birmingham Regional Hospital Board.[31]
Joseph Minton (1900–61) was born in Lublin and came to England as an adult
in 1920, qualifying in the Middlesex Hospital in 1926. While working as a
general practitioner in Highbury, he developed an interest in eye diseases and
took his FRCS in 1932, a remarkable achievement; in 1936 he was appointed
consultant to the Hampstead General Hospital and later to a number of other
hospitals, including the London Jewish Hospital. Leonard Lurie (1911–85),
who was born in Russia, 'revolutionised cataract surgery and pioneered the use
of intra-ocular implants', a technique which he taught both in Britain and overseas.[32]

It was probably in the medical schools that Jewish surgeons made the swiftest
advance in the post-war years. Ralph Shackman (1910–81), after serving as a
surgical specialist in the RAF during the Second World War, joined the staff of
the postgraduate medical school at the Hammersmith Hospital, where he was
made a consultant and was later appointed professor of urology, the first holder
of the title at London University. Earlier he had been sent by Ian Aird to the
United States to learn the techniques of 'blue baby' operations, and 'performed
several of the rare mitral-valve operations which British surgeons were attempting at the time'. Shackman then switched his attention from heart surgery to
kidney grafting. 'He became an accomplished academic and clinical urologist
and made early and important contributions in the field of renal failure, renal
dialysis and renal transplantation. In 1960 with W. J. Dempster he carried out
Britain's first kidney transplant.'[33] Equally important contributions were made
by Benjamin Milstein (b. 1918), who was the senior surgical registrar at Guy's
Hospital before becoming a consultant at the Papworth Hospital near Cambridge, where he successfully performed the first open-heart operation in 1958.
'His patient was immersed in a bath of ice-cold water so that her heart would

[29] *Lives of the Fellows of the Royal College of Surgeons 1952–1964*, 449, 450.

[30] *Lives of the Fellows of the Royal College of Surgeons 1974–1982*, 374.

[31] *Lives of the Fellows of the Royal College of Surgeons 1983–1990*, 364.

[32] *Lancet*, 25 Mar. 1961; *JC* 24 Mar. 1961, p. 46 (on Joseph Minton); *JC* 19 July 1985, p. 11 (obituary of Lurie).

[33] *Lives of the Fellows of the Royal College of Surgeons 1974–1982*, 360 (on Shackman); Hugh McLeave, *A Time to Heal: The Life of Ian Aird, the Surgeon* (London: Heinemann, 1964), 139, 152, 209, 245, 246; *JC* 24 Aug. 1962, p. 6.

stop beating. At the time this was an essential procedure before the operation could take place, and one that gave the surgeon only ten minutes to complete his work. Nowadays a heart–lung machine takes over vital functions while surgeons work on a still heart.'[34] John Wallwork, the director of Papworth, declared that 'Without the pioneering work carried out by Ben Milstein in the late 1950s we would not be able to do the surgery we do today. Transplantations grab the headlines, but the earlier surgery set the scene for these later developments.'[35]

Harold Ellis (b. 1926) went to St Olave's School in south London, where he excelled at biology and opted for a career in medicine. Having graduated from Oxford BM, B.Ch. in 1948, he served as surgical tutor at the Radcliffe Infirmary in Oxford and held other resident positions in Sheffield, Northampton, and London. In 1960 he was appointed senior lecturer at the Westminster medical school and was rapidly promoted, holding the position of professor of surgery from 1962 until 1989. Among his numerous publications are *Principles of Resuscitation* (1967), *Intestinal Obstruction* (1982), *Varicose Veins* (1982), *Wound Healing for Surgeons* (1984), *Maingot's Abdominal Operations* (1985), and *Problems in General Surgery; Wound Healing* (1989).[36]

Sir Roy Calne (b. 1930) studied medicine at Guy's Hospital, where he was taught by Ben Milstein; later Harold Ellis, another one of his teachers, became his colleague at the Westminster Hospital. Calne recalled that when he was a student he saw one of his patients, a young boy called Jonathan, dying of kidney failure, and that this event, along with a number of similar occurrences, triggered his interest in organ transplantation. After qualifying in medicine in 1953 he took the membership examination for the Royal College of Surgeons, which he passed in 1958.[37] He then applied for the position of registrar at various London teaching hospitals until he was invited to join the staff of the Royal Free medical school, a teaching hospital for female students, which began to admit men after the Second World War. 'Although by now the staff and students were mixed,' wrote Calne, 'women still predominated, and the hospital was not regarded as a first choice by most young surgeons.' Here he carried out laboratory experiments on organ transplants using animals and secured a Harkness fellowship to work at the Peter Bent Bingham Hospital at Harvard medical school. A dog with a kidney graft, which Calne treated with azathioprine to prevent the rejection of the organ, was still alive after six months and doing well.[38] On his return to Britain, he became lecturer in surgery at St Mary's, where he remained for eighteen months before joining the Westminster Hospital in 1962.

---

[34] *The Times*, 1 Oct. 1998.

[35] Ibid. See also Roy Calne, *The Ultimate Gift: The Story of Britain's Premier Transplant Surgeon* (London: Headline, 1998), 8 (on Milstein).

[36] Interview with Harold Ellis, 19 June 1998; *JC* 2 Feb. 1962, p. 6.

[37] Calne, *The Ultimate Gift*, 1, 8, 37.   [38] Ibid. 37, 38, 41, 47–9.

His sponsor, Harold Ellis, encouraged Calne to start a kidney transplant programme there. Partly because the patients were too ill at the time of the transplants, partly because some of the kidneys were too damaged before they were
removed, Calne's results were poor to begin with, but there were a few successes,
even when using kidneys removed from patients whose hearts had stopped
beating. In 1965 Calne was appointed professor of surgery at Cambridge and
consulting surgeon at Addenbrookes Hospital, where in 1968 he carried out the
first human liver transplant operation in the United Kingdom.[39]

Lipmann Kessel (1914–86) was one of a growing stream of South African-
born Jewish doctors, including also Woolf Herschell, Solly Morris Cohen, and
Arthur Jacob Jelfet (1907–89), who were trained as surgeons in England in the
1930s or just after the Second World War. Once demobilized Kessel returned
to St Mary's Hospital, where he became senior orthopaedic registrar to Valen-
tine Ellis, whose work greatly influenced him. Notwithstanding the bottleneck
which developed in the 1950s as a plethora of registrars sought positions as
consultants, Kessel, both a Jew and a Marxist, ended up as a consultant in
orthopaedic surgery at the small Fulham and St Mary Abbots hospitals. Here
Kessel, because of his undoubted talent, flourished, albeit with most distinction
in the academic rather than the practitioner world, eventually becoming director of studies and then professor at the Institute of Orthopaedics attached to
London University. He took a prominent part in the discussions which led to
the building of the new Charing Cross Hospital, where he became an honorary
consultant. During his years at the institute he wrote several important books
on orthopaedics, particularly on the surgery of the shoulder joint, and for many
years he was a world leader in the field, establishing an international organization for its study.[40]

The contrast between the career of Kessel and that of Alan Graham Apley
(1914–96) is illuminating. Apley was the son of Jewish immigrants from Poland
and went to a primary school in Battersea, where he came top of all London in
the London County Council scholarship examination for admission to a grammar school. But, according to the *Times* obituary, 'He was prevented from reap-
ing the full rewards of his achievement because of his background. This episode
coloured his attitude to religion and he later abandoned his faith.' Qualifying at
University College Hospital before the war, Apley was appointed a consultant
to the Rowley Bristow Orthopaedic Hospital, Pyrford, in 1947. Here he was
influenced by the innovating orthopaedic surgeon George Perkins and, an inspir-
ing teacher, established a scintillating course for training orthopaedic surgeons
which was always oversubscribed. The textbook which he wrote based on his

[39] Ibid. 73, 74, 84–108.
[40] *Lives of the Fellows of the Royal College of Surgeons 1983–1990*, 155 (on Helfet), 189 (on Lipmann
Kessel); *The Times*, 17 June 1986, *Lancet*, 12 July 1986 (obituary of Kessel).

lectures for this course, *Apley's System of Orthopaedics and Fractures* (1959), became a classic and went through seven editions. He also set up the first purpose-built accident and emergency centre in southern England, in Chertsey. The severing of his links to his Jewish faith may in some measure have smoothed the path for his promotion: Apley was appointed director of the orthopaedics department at St Thomas's Hospital in 1972, one of the first people from an east European Jewish background to achieve such a position in an older teaching hospital. On retirement, Apley became the editor of the *Journal of Bone and Joint Surgery*, which has gained an international reputation.[41]

Other Jewish surgeons also progressed through the medical schools and the network of advanced clinical institutes belonging to London University. Geoffrey Glazer, after serving as surgical registrar in Hillingdon, moved to St Mary's in the early 1970s, where he became senior surgical registrar and by 1976 honorary consultant and senior lecturer to St Mary's medical school. Eye surgery has always been an attractive career option for Jews—perhaps because of a propensity to short-sightedness which in the past was an advantage when fine work was required. Montague Ruben, having served as the ophthalmic registrar at Guy's and a lecturer at the Institute of Ophthalmology, was promoted to the rank of consultant at the Royal Northern Hospital. By 1962 he was consultant ophthalmic surgeon in the regional eye unit for Herts. and Essex Hospital, Harlow Hospital, and Hertford County Hospital; in 1969 he moved to become a consultant and director of the department of contact lenses and prosthetics at Moorfields Eye Hospital. Barrie Samuel Jay (b. 1929) was a senior registrar in the ophthalmic department of the London Hospital between 1962 and 1965, when he became a consulting surgeon to the London Hospital, remaining there until 1979. He then joined the Institute of Ophthalmology in 1980, first as sub-dean and then as dean, before in 1985 being promoted to professor of clinical ophthalmology at London University, a post he held until 1992. Since 1992 Jay has been a consulting surgeon to Moorfields Eye Hospital.

Alan Spencer Mushin is the son of Louis Mushin, an ophthalmic surgeon to hospitals in Tooting, Woodford, and St Albans; being a second-generation surgeon and entering the profession under more propitious conditions, he has had a more illustrious career than his father. Working as senior registrar in ophthalmology to University College Hospital and Moorfields Eye Hospital and lecturing at the Institute of Ophthalmology, Alan Mushin gained his FRCS in 1968 and was appointed consulting ophthalmic surgeon to the London Hospital in 1972. Irving Luke also chose to become an ophthalmic surgeon, perhaps influenced by the fact that his father was visually handicapped. Coincidentally, he followed Alan Mushin as senior registrar at University College Hospital. He was

---

[41] *The Times*, 28 Dec. 1996, *BMJ* 29 Mar. 1997 (obituary of Apley).

subsequently appointed a consultant ophthalmic surgeon in London—to St James's Hospital in 1976 and in 1981 to St George's Hospital, where he also held the post of honorary senior lecturer in ophthalmology.[42]

Gerald Westbury (b. 1927) was appointed consultant surgeon to the Westminster Hospital in 1960; he remained there until 1982, when he became honorary consultant to the Royal Marsden Hospital and also professor of surgery at the Institute of Cancer Research. Michael Baum (b. 1937), a leading breast cancer specialist with a sceptical view of the benefits of mass screening, served as professor of surgery at King's College Hospital between 1980 and 1990, after which he held similar positions at the Institute of Cancer Research and later at University College. In February 1993 Professor Irving Taylor took over as professor of surgery, head of the department, and chairman of the board of surgery of University College London.[43]

After the Second World War, the first Jews to become consultant gynaecologists in London teaching hospitals scaled perhaps the last bastion of resistance to their participation in medicine at this level. Gynaecologists could practise either as physicians or as surgeons, but most aiming at consultancy positions tended to take the examinations of the Royal College of Surgeons because of the Caesarean and other operative procedures they were required from time to time to undertake. Elliot Elias Philipp (b. 1915) was educated at Cambridge and the Middlesex Hospital but spent an interlude studying in Lausanne during the winter of 1937–8 as he was suffering from tuberculosis. At the Lausanne hospital there was a dynamic obstetrician and gynaecologist called Rochat, who on Elliot Philipp's first day in the lecture hall pointed to him to come down, calling him 'you American', but at first Philipp did not budge and Rochat made him the laughing stock of the class. In revenge Philipp took to following Rochat around, thereby developing an interest in the specialty which was enhanced by his family's friendship with the gynaecologist Elsie Landau. By 1947 Philipp was a registrar in the gynaecology and obstetrics department of the Middlesex Hospital, where his career was promoted by the senior consultant Carnac Rivett, who was, he said, 'a terribly nice man'. However, when Rivett unfortunately died of lung cancer, he was succeeded by an antisemite who pushed Philipp out of the department, forcing him to seek appointments at the same level at Cambridge in 1948 and then as senior registrar at the Royal Free Hospital. Afterwards Philipp became a consultant at the Oldchurch Hospital in

[42] *Medical Directory 1975*, i. 937, *Medical Directory 1976*, i. 945 (on Glazer); *Medical Directory 1960*, ii. 2003, *Medical Directory 1969*, ii. 1662 (on Ruben): *Who's Who 1996* (London: A. & C. Black, 1996), 1008 (on Jay); *Medical Directory 1970*, ii. 1899, *Medical Directory 1972*, ii. 1861 (on Mushin); *Medical Directory 1981*, i. 1666 (on Luke); interview with Irving Luke, 1 Dec. 1999.

[43] *Who's Who 1996* (London: A. & C. Black, 1999), 2040 (on Westbury); *Who's Who 1999* (London: A. & C. Black, 1999), 126 and *JC* 8 Sept. 1995 (on Baum); *JC* 5 Feb. 1993 (on Irving Taylor).

Essex; then, at the age of 50, he was made a consultant at the Royal Northern and City of London hospitals when the incumbent became blind.[44]

Meanwhile Albert Davis, who as noted in Chapter 3 moved from Manchester to London, joined the Prince of Wales, Dulwich, and St Giles's hospitals in London as a consultant gynaecologist. When Davis was appointed to the consultant staff of the combined King's College Hospital Group in 1966, 'this was only as a result of the London [County] Council's insistence as a condition of the merger. But it made me [Davis] the first acknowledged Jewish gynaecologist on the staff of a London Teaching Hospital.' He was followed by Frank Elias Loeffler, who by 1969 was serving as consultant obstetrician and gynaecologist to St Mary's Hospital, having held a similar position in the Central Middlesex and Willesden general hospitals; by 1970 Alan Gerald Amias held a similar position at St George's Hospital. Sir Stanley Simmons (b. 1927) was a registrar at St Mary's and then senior registrar at St Thomas's Hospital between 1960 and 1964, before becoming a consultant obstetrician and gynaecologist to the Windsor group of hospitals and later president of the Royal Society of Obstetricians and Gynaecologists from 1990 to 1993. In 1997 Professor Stuart Stanton was awarded a personal chair in pelvic reconstruction surgery and urogynaecology by London University, having lectured and operated in this specialty in a wide range of countries.[45]

Clearly, in the late 1940s and throughout the 1950s it was almost impossible for Jews to secure senior surgical posts in any field in the central London teaching hospitals and in Manchester and Leeds. Pre-war prejudices were slow to thaw, the restructuring of the appointments boards by the new NHS took time to implement, and the profession was overcrowded with able registrars jostling for promotion; all these factors delayed the selection of Jews to fill the top positions. During the 1960s and 1970s, however, the pace of change quickened and more Jews, including many from east European backgrounds, were appointed.

Having surveyed the various branches of surgery, I now turn to the growing acceptance of Jews as consultant physicians in the leading teaching hospitals in London and the provinces after the Second World War. Max Leonard Rosenheim (1908–72), after studying in Cambridge and at University College medical school, joined University College as medical registrar in 1936 and then succeeded Harold Himsworth as professor of medicine in 1950. As a clinician, he pioneered the use of mandelic acid to treat infections of the urinary tract; when this product was replaced by sulphonamides, he turned his attention to the

---

[44] Interview with Elliot Philipp, 18 July 1997, 16 Nov. 1998; *Medical Directory 1947*, i. 253, *Medical Directory 1948*, i. 258, *Medical Directory 1954*, ii. 1629 (on Philipp).

[45] Albert Davis to author, 18 Apr. 1997; *Medical Directory 1953*, i. 77, *Medical Directory 1967*, i. 562 (on Davis); *Medical Directory 1969*, i. 1126 (on Loeffler); *Medical Directory 1993*, i. 75 (on Amias). *Who's Who 1996* (London: A. & C. Black, 1996), 1765 (on Simmons); *JC* 18 Apr. 1997 (on Stanton).

treatment of high blood pressure with hexamethonium, a drug which had been developed by colleagues in his department. Rosenheim and other colleagues elucidated the nature of chronic pyelonephritis and devised the best treatment for this illness. Despite being shy and lacking small talk, Rosenheim was a brilliant administrator, incisive, yet with a friendly, humorous manner, and he was a notable networker. Like Lord Cohen, another outstanding medical administrator, he never married and was somewhat fixated on his mother. According to the *Jewish Chronicle*, 'he was proud of his Jewish origins and interested himself in Jewish educational activities, especially the Hebrew University, of which he was a governor'; yet one of his housemen, who knew him well socially, was amazed to learn that he was Jewish. As the first Jewish president of the Royal College of Physicians (between 1966 and 1972), Rosenheim transformed the venerable institution, democratizing the fellowship by including all medical disciplines and massively increasing the number of fellows who were elected, and establishing the faculty of community medicine. A life peerage was bestowed on him in 1970.[46] Subsequent Jewish presidents of the RCP included the eminent endocrinologist Sir Raymond Hoffenberg (b. 1923), who held the position between 1983 and 1989; and Lord Turnberg (b. 1934), professor of medicine at Manchester University from 1973 to 1997 and a leading authority on gastroenterology, who served as president from 1992 to 1997. During his term of office Turnberg tried to extend the spread of the college by setting up regional offices in Newcastle and Manchester, and to 'make the College more open to its fellowship'. The current president, who succeeded Lord Turnberg in 1997, is another Jew, Kurt George Matthew Mayer Alberti, professor of medicine in Newcastle, who devised simple methods of treating diabetic people in the rural populations of poorer countries.[47] The election of four Jews to this office since 1966 underscores the increased status of Jewish physicians within the medical profession as a whole.

Class was still an important element in the careers of Jewish physicians in the leading London hospitals after 1945. Rosenheim was accepted at University College Hospital because, as the son of a German Jewish merchant who had moved to England as a young man and as the product of an Oxbridge education, he was distinctly upper middle class—just like his predecessor, the pre-war assistant physician Philip Montagu D'Arcy Hart. By 1946 Rosenheim held an appointment as a consultant physician at University College Hospital, a position matched only by the Leeds-born Hugh Gainsborough at the smaller St George's Hospital. The only other Jewish physicians of consultant status in the

---

[46] *Dictionary of National Biography 1971–1980*, 735, 736; *JC* 8 Dec. 1972, p. 49; *Lancet*, 9 Dec. 1992; *BMJ* 16 Dec. 1972 (obituaries of Rosenheim).

[47] *Who's Who 1999* (London: A. & C. Black, 1999), 955 (on Hoffenberg), 2037 (on Turnberg); interview with Turnberg, 14 Mar. 2000; *Camden New Journal*, 6 Jan. 2000 (on Alberti).

London hospitals which possessed their own medical schools were (in 1960) David Pyke at King's College Hospital, who was partly of Jewish descent, and (in 1950) Kenneth Harry Tallerman and Bernard Schlesinger, paediatricians respectively at the London Hospital and University College. However, Samuel Leonard Simpson (1900–83), captain of boxing at Cambridge and later chairman of the family business Simpson's of Piccadilly, became a consultant endocrinologist at St Mary's Hospital in 1950. Married to Baroness de Podmaniczky, he was well established in the upper class, with a large farm in Sussex and a London residence at Hyde Park Gate. By contrast, Michael Kremer (1908–88), a neurologist of distinction at the Middlesex Hospital, where he was appointed physician to the neurological department in 1958, and a protégé of Samson Wright, appears to have been a self-made man who owed little to the standing of his family. His somewhat secular father was a tailor's baster in the East End, but Kremer was a brilliant scholarship winner; however, he had little time for Jewish causes and married outside the faith.[48]

A more significant change occurred in the 1960s, when the number of Jewish physicians at the teaching hospitals began to multiply, as can be seen by glancing at the returns for 1970. Abraham Guz was appointed by the Charing Cross Hospital, M. H. Lessof by Guy's, B. J. Freedman and P. H. Friedlander by King's College Hospital, R. D. Cohen by the London Hospital, and the partly Jewish John Nabarro by the Middlesex Hospital. In addition, Leon Julian Grant (the son of Cantor Grundstein of the Stepney Orthodox Synagogue) became a consultant chest physician at University College Hospital after a smaller hospital where he worked merged with that institution.[49] Three of these gentlemen, namely R. D. Cohen, Abraham Guz, and M. H. Lessof, became professors of medicine. Sir John Nabarro (1915–98), a general physician at the Middlesex Hospital, specialized in endocrinology and diabetes, raising the quality of care for diabetics throughout the country by his campaigning.[50]

Another important appointment indicative of social change was the selection of David Weitzman (1918–64) as consultant physician to the cardiological department at St Bartholomew's Hospital in 1961. He came from an east European Jewish background and was educated at Grocers' School. After qualifying as a doctor at St Bartholomew's, Weitzman received his cardiological training at the National Heart Hospital between 1952 and 1954. He then

[48] *Medical Directory 1950*, vol. ii, 2430–9; *Medical Directory 1960*, pt. 2, 2786–94; *Lives of the Fellows of the Royal College of Physicians of London*, viii. 538, 539 (obituary of Simpson); *Lancet*, 5 Nov. 1988, p. 1090 (obituary of Kremer); *Lancet*, 5 Nov. 1988, p. 1090; *Lives of the Fellows of the Royal College of Physicians of London*, viii. 265–7 (obituary of Kremer); Michael Kremer's birth certificate; interview with Jack Sakula, 10 Apr. 2000.

[49] *Medical Directory 1970*, pt. 2, 3141–50; *Lives of the Fellows of the Royal College of Physicians of London*, 223 (obituary of Grant).

[50] *Independent*, 14 May 1998; *The Times*, 21 May 1998 (obituary of Nabarro).

returned to Bart's as a tutor at the medical school and as a research assistant in the cardiological department, where he assisted in the establishment of a modern investigatory unit. When the head of the department retired, Weitzman succeeded him; but, stricken with heart disease himself, he died at the age of 45.[51] A year later Walter Graham Spector (1924–82) became professor of pathology at the same hospital, where formerly such appointments had been closed to Jews.[52]

When the background of the small number of Jewish consultant physicians in the London hospitals during the 1940s and 1950s is scrutinized, it becomes clear that the overwhelming majority were the scions of well-established Anglo-Jewish families. Educated at public schools, often as boarders, and Oxbridge, and retaining only tenuous links to their faith, they differed no more than marginally from their non-Jewish colleagues. David Pyke, the physician in charge of the diabetic department of King's College Hospital, was a grandson of the Victorian Jewish barrister Lionel Pyke. However, David Pyke admitted that, while his father was Jewish, 'he was never in any sense a practising Jew, having no religion at all . . . [and] I have never felt Jewish'.[53] Kenneth Harry Tallerman (1894–1981) was educated at Charterhouse School and Cambridge, completing his medical studies at St Thomas's Hospital. He joined the consultant staff of the London Hospital in 1931, becoming chief physician in the children's department after the war. Bernard Edward Schlesinger (1896–1984) went to another public school, Uppingham, and Cambridge, and then to University College medical school in London. After serving as a physician to the Great Ormond Street and Royal Northern hospitals before the war, he was appointed consultant paediatrician to University College Hospital in 1947, where he started an intensive care unit for premature babies which soon gained an international reputation.[54] It was not until 1967 that someone from a lower-class east European Jewish background, Simon Yudkin (1914–68), was appointed as a consultant paediatrician to a London teaching hospital.[55] Like Leonard Simpson, his fellow consultant endocrinologist Gerald Swyer not only attended public school but was Oxbridge-educated.

Abraham Guz (b. 1929), having been educated at Grocers' School in Hackney Downs, King's College London, and Charing Cross Hospital medical school, completed his clinical training at Charing Cross Hospital, where he qualified as a doctor in 1952. In 1948, at the time of the disturbances in Palestine, when Guz was still a medical student, he was subjected to an outburst from an older class-

[51] *BMJ* 22 Aug. 1964 (obituary of Weitzman).
[52] *Lancet*, 23 Jan. 1982, p. 233 (obituary of Spector); Hilton, 'St Bartholomew's Hospital', 33–4, 97.
[53] Medawar and Pyke, *Hitler's Gift*, p. xv.
[54] *Lives of the Fellows of the Royal College of Physicians of London*, vii. 567 (obituary of Tallerman); ibid. viii. 441, 442; *BMJ* 11 Feb. 1984, pp. 494, 495 (obituary of Schlesinger); *JC* 19 Apr. 1968, p. 47.
[55] *Lancet*, 27 Apr. 1968, pp. 928, 929 (obituary of Yudkin).

mate who said that 'We may need to take out guns here and shoot at Jews.' Guz became an assistant lecturer in pharmacology at the medical school and gained his membership of the Royal College of Physicians in 1954, after which he did his national military service with the British Army of the Rhine—which he found to be extremely beneficial for the advancement of his career. In 1956 he joined the postgraduate medical school at Hammersmith Hospital as a senior house officer, and in 1957 went to the United States, where he spent two years as a research fellow at the Harvard medical school under Professor Herman Blumgart and then held a similar position at the Cardiovascular Institute of the University of California under Professor Julius Comroe between 1959 and 1961. Guz returned as a lecturer to the Charing Cross Hospital medical school in 1961, rising through the ranks of senior lecturer and reader to become professor of medicine in 1973 and head of the department of the combined Charing Cross and Westminster medical school in 1982. This successful career was not achieved so easily as the mere facts might suggest. During the 1960s Guz was applying for various chairs of medicine when he was warned by a distinguished (non-Jewish) mentor that one of his referees, whom he had believed to be a friend, was a secret antisemite, who was submitting dismissive reports, and that he should select another referee. Again, when the two London medical schools were merged, a senior lecturer remarked to him, 'We have an ethnic problem here', referring to the preponderance of Jews on the staff of the Westminster Hospital, to which Guz retorted: 'You mean Jews.' Nevertheless, none of these skirmishes with antisemitism seriously blighted Guz's career, though the secret antipathy of one of his medical referees may have delayed his promotion to a chair of medicine. Among his hobbies in *Who's Who*, Guz proudly lists the study of Jewish culture.[56]

In Manchester and Leeds, the recruitment of doctors from east European immigrant backgrounds into the teaching hospitals occurred at a slower pace than in London. The pattern of progress, however, was similar. An able consultant physician, Norman Kletz (later Kletts), had gained entry into the Manchester Royal Infirmary before the Second World War, and though himself assimilated he retained sufficient Jewish feeling to inspire a number of bright Jewish students. Kletts may have encouraged two physicians who later became consultants, Moses Oelbaum at the Crumpsall Hospital in Manchester (1952) and Neville Roussak at the Withington Hospital in the same city (1954). Shortly after the Second World War, Hyman Lempert was the clinical pathologist at the Manchester Royal Infirmary. Samuel Oleesky (b. 1921) was the son of a Manchester kosher butcher and entered Manchester University in 1938 with a state scholarship, a university scholarship, and a Manchester city medical scholarship. Here he won many prizes, qualifying as a doctor in 1944 and pass-

---

[56] Interview with Professor Abraham Guz, 11 Dec. 2000.

ing his membership examination for the Royal College of Physicians in 1946. After a short period as lecturer in therapeutics in Sheffield, he was appointed consultant physician to the Crumpsall Hospital in 1953 and also to Ancoats Hospital in 1956. The greatest influence on Oleesky's postgraduate career was Robert Platt, who, he said, embodied every virtue as a 'clinician, teacher, researcher, and administrator'. In 1965 Oleesky relinquished his posts at the Crumpsall and Ancoats hospitals on appointment to the consultant staff of the Manchester Royal Infirmary, where he was a general physician with an interest in diabetes and hypertension; he was also part-time lecturer in medicine at the university. He was the first consultant physician at the infirmary to affirm his Orthodox Jewish identity freely and openly, having been president of the Manchester Jewish Students and serving on the council of the local B'nai B'rith and on his synagogue education committee.[57]

Leslie Turnberg (Lord Turnberg) came from a working-class family: his father was a machinist in a raincoat factory, although he later started his own small business. Turnberg attended the local grammar school before proceeding to Manchester University, where he qualified as a doctor in 1957. Enjoying hospital medicine, he was never tempted to become a general practitioner. Turnberg was senior house officer at the Ancoats Hospital, where he adopted Samuel Oleesky, then a junior consultant, as his role model. Turnberg became a registrar at the Royal Free Hospital specializing in gastroenterology, then held a similar position at the Manchester Royal Infirmary before returning to London for a short spell as lecturer at the Royal Free Hospital under the direction of Sheila Sherlock. Both Oleesky and Turnberg held registrar's positions at the Royal Infirmary, marking a clear break with the pre-war prejudice against east European Jews. In 1968 Turnberg spent a year in Dallas, Texas, working on a successful research project. 'My main research interest', he declared, 'was how the intestine works, how it absorbs fluid and salts, and how that all goes wrong with severe diarrhoeal diseases like cholera and childhood gastroenteritis, but I have a strong clinical interest in the treatment of Crohn's disease and colitis.' On the strength of his previous appointments and his outstanding research, Turnberg returned to the Manchester Royal Infirmary as a senior lecturer in 1968, remaining there until 1973. Next he moved to the Hope Hospital in Salford, where another teaching hospital was being established to cope with the expansion of Manchester's medical school, as professor of medicine. Dean of the medical school from 1986 to 1989, he progressed naturally from that position into national medical politics, becoming president of the Royal College of Physicians. While he was dean, Turnberg changed the curriculum of the medical school, presenting the students with clinical problems and forcing them to

[57] Letters from Samuel Oleesky to the author, 21 Mar., 26 Mar. 2000.

work out the answers by going back to first principles. Like Oleesky, Turnberg was a committed Jew and not fearful of displaying his identity; for example, he put a mezuzah (a small box containing a scroll bearing the profession of faith) on the entrance door of his official residence.[58] In Leeds, Jews were not permitted to hold senior posts in the General Infirmary until 1969, when a Jewish orthopaedic surgeon, who had an Anglicized name and did not look Jewish, was unwittingly appointed. In the same year the London-born Professor Monty Losowsky was placed in charge of the Leeds University department of medicine at St James's University Hospital.[59]

Just as there was an important group of Jewish Communist and radical lawyers in the 1930s and the post-war period (see Chapter 13), so there were also a number of equally radical Jewish doctors. Two we have already mentioned—Joshua Samuel Horn and Lipmann Kessel—but there were others, and one of these in particular, Dr Len Crome (Lazar Krom, 1909–2001), merits attention in some detail. He was born in Dvinsk in Latvia, then part of the Russian empire. Because his father had business connections in Scotland, he went to study commerce and medicine in Edinburgh and qualified as a doctor in 1932. A member of the Left Book Club, he was deeply affected by the events unfolding in Germany after Hitler's seizure of power, and on learning that volunteers were required for the Republican cause in Spain, he went there in the autumn of 1936 to join the Scottish Ambulance Unit; however, he left after discovering that they were also helping fascists who were in hiding. Instead, he served as an assistant in the field to the Chief Medical Officer of the 35th Division of the International Brigades, Domanski-Dubois. When the latter was wounded, Crome temporarily took his place, advancing rapidly in the medical hierarchy of the Republican army because of his skills at improvisation and his linguistic ability, and on Dubois' death at the later battle of Quinto he became permanent chief of the medical services of the division. When General Walter was recalled to the Soviet Union, Crome was made Chief Medical Officer of the 15th Army Corps. Len Crome, the highest-ranking Briton serving in Spain, was repatriated in the autumn of 1938, after the defeat of the Republicans, with other members of the International Brigades, about a quarter of whose members were Jewish. On his return to England, his attempt to join the British army was rejected because of his left-wing sympathies.

During the Second World War, Crome served as commanding officer of 152nd Field Ambulance and supervised medical services at certain prisoner-of-war camps and German military hospitals. At this time, he discovered that some members of his family had been killed by the Germans, while his father had perished in a Soviet labour camp. On demobilization, he trained as a pathologist

[58] Interview with Leslie (now Lord) Turnberg, 14 Mar. 2000.
[59] Letter from Murray Freedman to the author, 11 Sept. 1996; *Who's Who 1996*, 1185.

at St Mary's Hospital and later under Alfred Meyer at the Maudsley Hospital, where he specialized in the neuropathology of learning difficulty. In 1956 he was appointed pathologist at the Fountain Hospital in London, the leading centre for the treatment of learning disability. With the assistance of his colleagues, Crome produced the first comprehensive textbook of paediatric neuropathology, *Pathology of Mental Retardation* (1971). On returning from Spain, Crome had joined the British Communist Party; he remained a member until it was dissolved.[60]

When Martin Sarner qualified in 1959, the number of Jews who were consultants at London teaching hospitals could, in his words, 'be counted on the fingers of a mutilated hand'.[61] During the 1960s and 1970s this situation changed irrevocably as Jewish doctors spread into every nook and cranny of the medical world, instead of being squeezed into a few areas, such as psychiatry and pathology, as had been the case before the Second World War. As in surgery, the swiftest path for a Jewish physician from an immigrant background seeking promotion was to show academic excellence and to be appointed to a position in a medical school. The list of Jewish physicians is inexhaustible; rather than recite their names, here, it will be more informative to describe the careers of doctors from the various specialties who made significant contributions to medicine.

In two areas of medicine in particular there was a pronounced Jewish contribution: namely, psychiatry and the treatment of infertility. The attraction of psychiatry for Jews has been discussed in an earlier chapter; infertility was also a conscious choice for some, as Judaism attached great value to the scriptural injunction to 'Be fruitful and multiply.' In 1948 Bernard Sandler (1907–97) was appointed director of the infertility clinic at the Manchester Victoria Memorial Jewish Hospital, the first such specialist clinic to open outside London. Sandler developed his own method of unblocking fallopian tubes without anaesthesia and perfected the technique of artificial insemination by the donor; also, because (unusually at this time) he attached importance to male infertility, he examined both husband and wife at the beginning of each case. His high success rate in overcoming infertility attracted patients from all over northern England.[62] Gerald Isaac MacDonald Swyer (1917–95), after studying at Oxford, London, and California, became a consultant endocrinologist in 1951 at University College Hospital, where he established the endocrine and fertility clinics. 'His early work in the field of reproductive medicine was in the forefront of research, and many women who would otherwise have been childless owe their ability to have

---

[60] Letter from Professor Peter Crome to the author, 8 Mar. 2001; Len Crome, 'Autobiographical Notes' (MS); *The Times*, 8 May 2001 (obituary of Crome).

[61] Interview with Martin Sarner, 24 Nov. 1999.

[62] *Guardian*, 17 Oct. 1997; *JC* 31 Oct. 1997, p. 21 (obituaries of Sandler).

children to his work on fertility.' During the 1950s his research into the use of progestogenic hormones led to advances in the development of the contraceptive pill, while his later research concentrated on the detection and treatment of defective ovulation.[63] Dr Simon Fishel (b. 1954), formerly of Nottingham University, pioneered a technique known as SUZI for men with a low sperm count, in which sperm was injected 'into the space between the egg's outer surface and its outer coating', thus maximizing the chances of the woman becoming pregnant; the first baby conceived using this micro-injection technique was born in Italy in 1990. To promote successful pregnancies, Simon Fishel established the Rachel Foundation, arguing that the matriarch Rachel believed not only that life without children was worthless, but that unless a woman could conceive she would 'die' genetically, leaving nothing after her.[64]

Robert Maurice Lipson Winston was born in 1940, graduating from the London Hospital Medical School in 1964. During the 1970s Winston developed better sterilization techniques connected with microsurgery and 'carried out the first successful ovarian transplant and the first human tubal transplant'.[65] At the outset Winston was opposed to the technique of *in vitro* fertilization, in which the sperm and the egg are brought together in a dish, believing that fallopian tube transplants were a superior procedure. Despite the success of IVF with the birth of Louise Brown, the first child conceived in this way, in 1978, Winston continued to oppose this method of fostering pregnancy for another two years before a dramatic conversion, when he became an enthusiastic supporter.[66] In 1981 he started the first NHS *in vitro* fertilization programme at his Hammersmith Hospital unit, to which he later added a support group and counselling service. The Hammersmith fertility unit ranks only midway in the league tables for IVF because it is the only centre that treats people who have failed when using the technique elsewhere; and in any case only 15 per cent of such patients are able to conceive. By 1987 Winston had become professor of fertility studies at London University and then dean of the Institute of Obstetrics at the Royal Postgraduate Medical School, Hammersmith. During the 1980s Winston introduced a pioneering medical documentary series on television, following it up with series on IVF and on twins.[67] Made a life peer in 1995 by Prime Minister Tony Blair, he bravely initiated a national debate on the extent of government expenditure on the health service, which he claimed fell below the levels achieved elsewhere in Europe—probably wrecking his chances of appointment to ministerial office in the process.[68]

[63] *Guardian*, 13 Oct. 1995; *JC* 13 Oct. 1995, p. 21 (obituaries of Swyer).

[64] Jack Challoner, *The Baby Makers: The History of Artificial Conception* (London: Channel 4 Books, 1999), 9, 94–6; see also *JC* 30 July 1999; *The Times*, 26 Feb., 31 Mar. 2000 (on Fishel); *JC* 3 Mar. 2000, p. 11. [65] *Shalom*, 13 Dec. 1995, 1 May 1996. [66] Challoner, *The Baby Makers*, 37, 38.

[67] *Evening Standard*, 21 July 1999; *Sunday Times*, 11 Apr. 1999.

[68] *The Times*, 15 Jan., 25 Jan. 2000.

It could be argued that until the 1960s Jews often went into the least glamorous sectors of medicine, where hope for the patients had almost been abandoned—into care for the inmates of mental hospitals, into work with paraplegics, into combating unethical experiments on patients, into the rehabilitation of alcoholics, and into the treatment of geriatric patients. Max Glatt (1912–2002), a refugee from Germany and an 'eternal optimist who saw no evil in fellow human beings', was widely recognized as the 'father of the rehabilitation of alcoholics' in Britain.[69] Lionel Zelick Cosin (1910–94) was a pioneer of geriatric medicine, establishing a department at Oxford which has trained many of today's leading geriatricians. Intent on a career in surgery, he passed his exams for the fellowship of the Royal College of Surgeons and had been offered a post at the London Hospital when the war disrupted his plans. Shortly afterwards Cosin became the superintendent of a hospital at Orsett in Essex, where he had to look after war casualties; but by 1944 the numbers of these had fallen, and he had two empty wards where he could accommodate chronically sick patients transferred from other local hospitals. Among them were elderly people with broken hips earmarked for permanent care, as they were considered too fragile for surgery; but Cosin successfully operated on them, and sent them home. Cosin found that, by offering these elderly patients rapid treatment, the overwhelming majority could be rehabilitated and that after six months only one in five still needed hospital care. When he became a member of the Ministry of Health's Committee on the Chronic Sick in 1947, he helped to persuade the Chief Medical Officer to make this new approach national policy, by concentrating on geriatric units within general hospitals rather than expanding institutions for the chronically sick. Invited in 1950 to take charge of the Cowley Road Hospital in Oxford, he applied the policy developed at Orsett there and soon drastically reduced the number of patients needing permanent care. Cosin was clinical director of the geriatric unit of the United Oxford Hospitals from 1950 to 1976 and lecturer in geriatric medicine at Oxford University from 1976 to 1994. His most original idea was to set up the first purely geriatric day hospital in 1957; modelled on similar psychiatric ventures, the idea spread all over the country. A typical day centre had a treatment room, a therapy room for remedial work for patients with disabled limbs and muscles, a physiotherapy room, and a dining room. Cosin's advice was sought widely, particularly in the United States, where he advised on the establishment of a community health care programme in San Francisco and made representations to a Senate committee on ageing.[70] Another Jewish pioneer of geriatric medicine was Bernard Isaacs (1924–95) the first professor of geriatric medicine at Birming-

---

[69] *Guardian*, 25 May 2002; *The Times*, 7 June 2002 (obituaries of Glatt).

[70] *Independent*, 13 Apr. 1994; *BMJ* 16 July 1994, p. 189 (obituary of Cosin); Ivor Felstein, *Later Life: Geriatrics Today and Tomorrow* (Harmondsworth: Penguin, 1969), 66–8.

ham, who opened a gait laboratory which extended knowledge of balance in old age.[71]

It is appropriate at this point to mention the career of one of the outstanding mavericks in the world of medicine: Maurice Henry Pappworth (1910–94). Trained as a doctor in Liverpool, he served as registrar to the professor of medicine, Lord Cohen, but was too independent-minded as a diagnostician and soon fell out with his mentor. Having passed his examination for membership of the Royal College of Physicians in 1936, he was told when he applied three years later for a consultant's post that 'No Jew could ever be a gentleman.' Unable, despite a further stint as a registrar at the London Hospital, to secure a position as a consultant—no doubt hampered by his somewhat abrasive personality—Pappworth opened consulting rooms in Harley Street after the war; to supplement his income during the 1950s and 1960s he coached doctors hoping to pass the examination for membership of the Royal College of Physicians, and eventually trained 1,600 members of the college—stimulating it to improve its own training for physicians. During the post-war years Pappworth, a brilliant diagnostician, was offered jobs in less desirable parts of England, but held out in vain for a post in a major London hospital.[72]

Pappworth liked to quote Markus Herz, an eighteenth-century Jewish physician, who declared, 'May I never see in the patient anything but a fellow creature in pain.' The debate on medical ethics had been initiated by Professor Henry K. Beecher of Harvard University in his book *Experimentation on Man* (1959), but in a follow-up article in 1964 Beecher had avoided supplying the names of experimenters and the journal references identifying their work. Pappworth, too, was suspicious of risky surgery, the trial of drugs at a stage when their full effects were unknown, and the suffering caused by experiments on patients without their consent. Alerted by the post-war disclosures of the misdeeds of the Nazi doctors, Pappworth began to keep a record of unethical experiments and set about bombarding the medical press with letters expressing his disquiet.[73] In 1962 Pappworth wrote a trenchant essay in the journal *Twentieth Century*, later expanded into his seminal book, *Human Guinea Pigs* (1967), in which he described a large number of questionable experiments, seventy-eight of which had been carried out in NHS hospitals; he not only named the experimenters, but also gave the references to the journal papers relating to these experiments.[74] 'He was particularly harsh on the Hammer-

[71] *Independent*, 12 May 1995 (obituary of Bernard Isaacs).

[72] *BMJ* 10 Dec. 1994, p. 1577 (obituary of Pappworth).

[73] Neil Belton, *The Good Listener. Helen Bamber: A Life Against Cruelty* (London: Weidenfeld & Nicolson, 1998), 161–5, 188–91.

[74] Ibid. 202–8; M. H. Pappworth, 'Human Guinea Pigs: A Warning', *Twentieth Century* (Autumn 1962), 66–75; id., *Human Guinea Pigs: Experimentation on Man* (Harmondsworth: Penguin, 1969); *BMJ* 22 Dec. 1990, 1456–60.

smith Hospital, where the earliest cardiac catherisations and liver biopsies had been carried out in Britain', noted Christopher Booth.[75] As a result of Pappworth's plea, ethics committees were set up to regulate clinical research, and medical students were obliged to take ethics courses. Such was the opposition provoked by Pappworth's criticism of the profession that he was not elected a Fellow of the Royal College of Physicians until 1993, though he had passed their examination in 1936.[76]

Dame Albertine Louise Winner (1907–88) was trained at the University College medical school, where she qualified in 1933 and won the university gold medal. For a time Winner was an assistant physician to the Elizabeth Garrett Anderson Hospital for women, but after the war she joined the Ministry of Health, rising to the rank of Deputy Chief Medical Officer—the first woman to reach such a position. Max Rosenheim persuaded her to become an officer of the Royal College of Physicians; again, she was the first woman to serve in that capacity. She remained in post with the college as Linacre Fellow for eleven years, from 1967 to 1978, developing training posts all over the country: 'she did break ice, not as a feminist but simply as an extremely competent and reliable administrator who succeeded in getting to the top in what was at the time very much a man's world'.

Although the NHS provided excellent care for the acutely ill, it was at this time failing its terminally ill patients. When Dame Cicely Saunders was building up the hospice movement, she had drawn a favourable response from Winner in Whitehall; after she retired, Winner went on a clinical refresher course and became deputy medical director of St Christopher's, the first research and teaching hospice, working there part-time between 1967 and 1973 and helping to establish its clinical and administrative standards. Since not all the patients were cancer sufferers, Winner's special expertise in neurological medicine was of great value. She became chairman of St Christopher's in 1973 and its president in 1985; she also founded the North London Hospice, an institution with strong Jewish and inter-faith connections. What Rose Heilbron achieved in the legal profession, the formidable Dame Albertine Winner attained in the medical world, equally adept as she was at circumventing the obstacles that she encountered as a Jewish woman and a feminist.[77]

William Mushin (1910–93), though born in London, spent most of his professional career in Wales. He gained international recognition as an anaesthetist and played a major role in transforming the discipline from one 'practised by G.P.s, to a scientific speciality which is now the largest in the hospital service'. His father was the headmaster of the Great Garden Street Talmud Torah and a

[75] *BMJ* 10 Dec. 1994, p. 1577.   [76] *JC* 20 Jan. 1995 (obituary of Pappworth).
[77] *Lives of the Fellows of the Royal College of Physicians of London*, viii. 546–8; *The Times*, 17 May 1988 (obituary of Winner).

leading *shochet* (ritual slaughterer of animals).[78] At Oxford University, Mushin became first assistant to Sir Robert Macintosh, with whom he wrote *Physics for the Anaesthetist* (1946), now in its fourth edition, and *Local Analgesia: Brachial Plexus*. He was called to open a new department in Cardiff in 1947 because of concern at the excessive number of deaths caused by the anaesthesia of patients undergoing surgery. He stressed the importance to anaesthesia of the basic sciences, physics, pharmacology, and physiology, by appointing specialists in these fields to his team, thereby greatly reducing the number of fatalities during operations. While at Cardiff, Mushin wrote volumes on thoracic anaesthesia and *Automatic Ventilation of the Lungs* (1959), the latter 'for the first time classified ventilators as well as analysing their interaction with patients with varying lung function'.[79] He encouraged anaesthetists to play a more active role in intensive care units, contributing, according to Professor Michael Rosen, to the reduction of the mortality rate in these units 'over 20 years from 80 to 15 per cent. He also pioneered the application of acute pain relief for obstetrics and postoperative care, and chronic pain relief for cancerous patients.' His trainees later filled more than 100 consultant anaesthetist posts. As dean of the Faculty of Anaesthetists from 1961 to 1964, he was the leader of this specialty, and rejoiced at its enhanced status when a charter was bestowed on it as the Royal College of Anaesthetists in 1992.[80]

Harris Julian Gaster Bloom (1923–88), after training in radiotherapy in the Meyerstein Institute of the Middlesex Hospital, published a seminal study of breast cancer, suggesting a method of grading the degree of malignancy which was widely adopted. Joining the department of radiotherapy of the Royal Marsden Hospital in 1958, when high-energy linear accelerators were becoming available for use in clinical practice, he developed high-precision techniques. His dedication as consultant radiotherapist at the Royal Marsden, where he worked until 1987, was outstanding: his 'afternoon' clinics often ended at 9 p.m., sometimes at midnight. Afterwards he became an honorary visiting professor at the Institute of Cancer Research. He specialized in the treatment of urological and brain tumours, establishing a brain cancer unit at the Royal Marsden Hospital and devising new methods of treating advanced renal cancer with hormones, especially progesterone.[81]

His namesake Arthur Leslie Bloom (1930–92) was born in south Wales, the grandson of a rabbi and the son of a pharmacist. Joining a research team at

[78] *Lancet*, 6 Feb. 1993; *The Times*, 8 Feb. 1993; *JC* 12 Feb. 1993, p. 11 (obituaries of Mushin); interview with Bernard Mushin, 10 Mar. 2000.   [79] *Lancet*, 6 Feb. 1993; *The Times*, 8 Feb. 1993.

[80] *JC* 12 Feb. 1993, p. 11; Thomas G. Boulton, *The Association of Anaesthetists of Great Britain and Ireland 1932–1992 and the Development of the Speciality of Anaesthesia* (London: Association of Anaesthetists, 1999), 597.

[81] *Lives of the Fellows of the Royal College of Physicians of London*, viii. 32–4; *The Times*, 23 Dec. 1988 (obituary of Bloom).

Oxford in 1956, Arthur Bloom was at the forefront of a new field of scientific investigation when haematology separated itself from pathology as a separate discipline. 'He pioneered research on the molecular structure of blood-clotting proteins, especially Factor VIII, the substance defective in classical haemophilia, and he instigated early clinical trials in the UK on what were then unexplored therapeutic agents such as chemically purified Factor VIII from human and animal sources', declared a colleague. He was also interested in blood coagulation and thrombosis and wrote the authoritative text, *Haemostasis and Thrombosis* (1981). In acknowledgement of his work he was awarded a personal chair in Haematology by the University of Wales in 1976. As a physician he was a leading figure in the treatment of patients suffering from haemophilia, his advice being sought from all parts of the world.[82]

Jack (Jacob) Pepys (1914–96) was born in Johannesburg and entered the medical school at Witwatersrand University at the age of 15, graduating at 21. For fourteen years he worked in South Africa as a general practitioner with affiliated academic appointments before leaving for London in 1948. During the 1950s he set up an allergy clinic at the Brompton Hospital which soon achieved international renown, and from this base he developed a department of clinical immunology with a special interest in allergies—the first such academic department in Britain. In 1956 Pepys became head of the department of clinical immunology at the University of London Institute of Diseases of the Chest, and in 1967 was promoted to the professorship of clinical immunology; again, the first such chair. According to his obituary in *The Times*,

[Pepys'] talent was to unravel complex mechanisms in specific allergic processes. An association between farmer's lung [disease] and mouldy hay, for instance, had been known about since the 1930s, but the specific cause remained elusive . . . Pepys and his co-workers discovered the specific cause—allergy to moulds—and developed a blood test for farmer's lung which has remained routine in clinical practice ever since.

Pepys achieved worldwide fame for his research on allergic lung diseases caused by fungi. Equally important was his research into occupational asthma. Using simple inhalation tests, he showed a cause-and-effect relationship between a sensitivity to certain chemicals in the workplace and the onset of asthma; ultimately, asthma was recognized as an industrial disease, for which compensation could be claimed. In 1971 Jack Pepys founded and was the first editor of the journal *Clinical Allergy*.[83]

His son Professor Mark Pepys FRS (b. 1944) has had a career at least as distinguished as that of his father, who encouraged him to study medicine and to specialize in the field of immunology. After taking his first degree at

[82] *Independent*, 26 Nov. 1992 (obituary of Bloom).

[83] *The Times*, 26 Sept. 1996; *JC* 8 Nov. 1996, p. 25 (obituary of Pepys); Sheldon G. Cohen, 'Landmark Commentary: Pepys on Farmer's Lung', *Allergy Proceedings*, 11/2 (Mar.–Apr. 1990), 97–9.

Cambridge, Mark Pepys completed his training as a doctor at University College Hospital, where he came under the spell of Max Rosenheim, a 'fantastic clinician, [a] wonderful clinical teacher and a marvellous man'. The younger Pepys returned to Cambridge to work on a Ph.D. in the complement field.

It was to do with the mechanisms underlying antibody formation. I found that the complement system which is a system of proteins in the blood, about which [Professor] Peter Lachmann is a world authority . . . up to that point had been thought to become involved in the immune defences of the body only after the body had made antibodies, which are specific molecules that react with particular germs or other materials that the body encounters in the environment; and what I discovered was that in fact the complement system is involved in antibody formation before antibodies are formed.

For these findings, Pepys was not only awarded his Ph.D. but was elected to a fellowship at Trinity College, Cambridge. After gaining his doctorate, Pepys held various positions at the Hammersmith Hospital with a short interlude at the Royal Free as head of the immunology department, rising to become professor of immunological medicine and honorary consultant physician at the Royal Postgraduate medical school, later the Imperial College School of Medicine. In 1999 Pepys moved back to the Royal Free and University College medical schools as professor of medicine.

While Pepys was at the Hammersmith Hospital, Professor Christopher Booth advised him that the research he had undertaken at Cambridge was 'too fundamental . . . not clinical enough'; so Pepys changed direction and investigated 'C-reactive protein which is the classical acute phase protein . . . and in due course [he] became the world authority on that protein and related proteins, one of which is involved in a disease called amyloidosis'. Pepys explained that the protein 'is produced in greater quantities when you are sick for almost any reason, that is why it is called an acute phase protein because it goes up in the acute phase of illness . . . In 1988 we invented a new technique for diagnosing amyloidosis which . . . has revolutionised our understanding of this disease and its treatment.' In 1999 he took charge of the National Amyloidosis Centre, which is funded by the National Health Service. Other Jewish Fellows of the Royal Society in medicine were Professor Peter Lachmann of Cambridge and Professor Anthony Segal of University College.[84]

Arie Jeremy Zuckerman (b. 1932) trained at the Royal Free Hospital but for twenty-five years was attached to the London School of Hygiene and Tropical Medicine, where he conducted research into hepatitis. He served as professor of virology at London University between 1972 and 1975, after which he became professor of medical microbiology. Under his guidance his laboratory developed a vaccine against Hepatitis B, while a new Hepatitis A vaccine was

[84] Interview with Professor Mark Pepys, 12 Apr. 2000.

introduced later. In 1989 he returned to take charge of the Royal Free Hospital school of medicine as dean, at a time when its reputation was not high and its financial resources were somewhat straitened. Viscount Bearsted, chairman of the Council of the Royal Free, stated that 'Zuckerman had brought in outside investment, bringing new departments and specialties to the Royal Free, and brought the school from the brink of bankruptcy to triple the turnover to £30 m.' In his ten-year term of office as dean at the Royal Free, Zuckerman 'doubled the size of the medical school and created eight new university departments', in part by merging it with the University College Hospital medical school. The Royal Free, he claimed, had a renowned research department, noted 'as one of the principal centres for research into hepatitis, liver diseases, AIDS, bone marrow and liver and kidney transplantation'. When he retired in September 1999, the research rating of the medical school was joint second in the country.[85] Both the Royal Free and University College medical schools had a reputation for tolerance and openness, marked by the appointment of numerous Jewish consultants to their staff, equalled only by one of the smaller schools, that of Westminster Hospital.

Other distinguished Jewish doctors of the late twentieth century include Professor Michael Besser, head of the department of endocrinology and the medical professional unit at St Bartholomew's Hospital medical college and the Royal London School of Medicine; Dr Frank Clifford Rose, director of the London Neurological Centre and consultant neurologist at St Thomas's Hospital from 1963 to 1985; Dr Malcolm Godfrey, chairman of the Public Health Laboratory Service Board from 1989 to 1996; Sir Anthony Epstein, former professor of pathology at Bristol University and an authority on the Epstein–Barr virus; Sir David Goldberg, professor of psychiatry at the Institute of Psychiatry since 1992; Jeremy Morris, son of the great Jewish educationist Nathan Morris and professor of public health at London University 1967–78; Robert Souhami, a cancer specialist and professor of medicine at the Royal Free and University College London medical school; and the South African-born Lewis Spitz, professor of paediatric surgery at the Institute of Child Health, London. Professor David Baum (1940–99), the first president of the Royal College for Paediatrics and Child Health, was a leader in neonatal medicine, the inventor of the 'silver swaddler' for transporting sick premature babies, and a specialist in childhood diabetes. He refused a number of chairs in child health before accepting one at Bristol, stating that his family had to live in a suitably Jewish environment.[86] This list is far from complete; the point to be emphasized is how many of these doctors had remarkable careers in academic medicine.

[85] *Camden New Journal*, 5 Sept. 1996, 30 Sept. 1999, 7 Oct. 1999.
[86] *Who's Who 2000* (London: A. & C. Black, 2000), 165, 633, 777, 780, 1456, 1766, 1915, 1927. *JC* 24 Sept. 1999; *The Times*, 29 Sept. 1999 (obituaries of Baum).

I turn now to the influence of Jewish doctors on general practice in the post-war period. Within the British Medical Association, Dr Solomon Wand (1899–1984), having served on all the influential committees, became the first Jew to chair its council (1956–61). He was chairman of the BMA committee which negotiated the introduction of a comprehensive National Health Service, though at the time he was opposed to the service covering the whole population and to a full-time, salaried staff; he led a struggle with the minister of health to ensure adequate remuneration for doctors, culminating in the pay award by Mr Justice Danckwerts in 1952. This award, which Wand and the then secretary of the association achieved, decided that 'the "betterment" to be applied to the 1939 remuneration of general practitioners should be 100%—unequalled before or since'. Wand later led a deputation of the BMA which gave oral evidence to the Royal Commission on Doctors' and Dentists' Remuneration; the commission recommended the setting up of a review body to make pay awards, a system which favoured doctors. Thus Wand enabled doctors to remain independent and to secure high earnings in relation to other occupations, thereby in some measure restoring their prestige and halting the decline from their pre-war status. The next Jewish chairman of the BMA Council was Dr John Marks (b. 1925), who held that office between 1984 and 1990. The first Jew to hold the equivalent position in the Law Society was Sir David Napley in 1976/7, some two decades later; this gives an indication of the Jews' superior standing in the general ranks of the medical profession at an earlier date. Indeed, no other Jew has held the office of president of the Law Society, a position dominated by partners from the big City firms, where Jews gained a significant entrée only in and after the 1970s.[87]

'By the 1960s, the proliferation of specialists and the diminished proportion and prestige of general practitioners in most countries of the world had become a problem of acute contemporary general interest', noted John Burnham.[88] As a means of enhancing their status, general practitioners in England decided to organize and become a specialty. 'We were not second class hospital doctors, we were first class family practitioners', noted Dr Stuart Carne.[89] To reach this goal the College of General Practitioners was set up by Dr John Hunt in 1952; but a new theoretical framework for general practice was also required, and to this a number of Jewish doctors made important contributions. Foremost among them was Dr Michael Balint (1896–1970), who was born in Budapest and, after graduating as a doctor, trained as a psychoanalyst. Forced to flee to England in 1939 because of antisemitism in Hungary, he was appointed medical director of a child guidance clinic and later consultant psychiatrist to the Royal

---

[87] Josephs, *Birmingham Jewry*, 81, 82; *BMJ* 29 Sept. 1984, 841, 842 (obituary of Wand); Eckstein, *Pressure Group Politics*, 126–50.

[88] John C. Burnham, *How the Idea of Profession Changed the Writing of Medical History* (London: Wellcome Institute, 1998), 123.   [89] Interview with Stuart Carne, 10 Feb. 2000.

Northern Hospital in Manchester. Moving to London in 1945, he joined the staff of the Tavistock Clinic in 1948; retiring from here in 1961, he moved to University College Hospital. In 1952, while at the Tavistock Clinic, Balint started a seminar on general practice for doctors. He showed that 'the most frequently used drug in general practice was the doctor himself, i.e. it was not only the bottle or the box of pills that mattered, but the way the doctor gave them to his patient—in fact, the whole atmosphere in which the drug was given and taken'. Balint 'taught a whole generation of doctors that it was very important to listen to what patients were saying, and to listen without interpreting what they were saying, or telling them what they should be saying, or explaining to them better what to think', asserted Professor Marshall Marinker. According to Dr Philip Hopkins, another of his disciples, Balint 'concluded that there is a very important gap between the traditional [teaching] hospital-based training, and general practice medicine, which resulted in a continuous conflict between the disease-centred approach of hospital medicine, and the whole-patient-centred medicine which is required by so many more of the patients seen in general practice (probably more than 70%)'. Balint was a cultured man, with a forceful personality and an exceptional knowledge of literature, his conversation being peppered with quotations from Goethe, Rilke, and Talleyrand. However, his writings, notably *The Doctor, his Patient and the Illness* (1957), were criticized for being doctor-centred and ignoring the organic nature of illness.[90]

A number of Jewish doctors have been active in the leadership of the Royal College of General Practitioners, among them Dr John Fry FRCS (1922–94), one of the founder members of the college, who sat on its council for thirty years and inspired its study groups. Starting his own practice in Beckenham in 1947, Fry pioneered the description of common diseases in his own practice, charting their progression and outcome. He published over fifty books, the most popular of which were *The Catarrhal Child* (1961) and *Common Diseases* (1974), which went into a number of editions. In addition, he acted as editorial adviser to the *Journal of Postgraduate General Practice—Update*, which had been founded by Dr Abraham Marcus in 1968, and he was a visiting professor at the universities of Oxford and California.[91] Dr Stuart Carne (b. 1926) was the first Jewish president of the college from 1988 to 1991; the second was Dr Lotte Newman (b. 1929), who held the post in the years 1994–7 and was concerned with improving the position of women in the medical profession. Carne was treasurer of the college from 1964 for seventeen years, during which he saved it from bankruptcy

[90] *BMJ* 16 Jan. 1971, p. 179; *Lancet*, 16 Jan. 1971, p. 144 (obituary of Balint); Philip Hopkins, 'Who was Dr Michael Balint?', in John Salinsky (ed.), *Proceedings of the Eleventh International Balint Congress 1998* (Southport: Balint Society, 1999), 40–54; E. M. Tansey, D. A. Christie, and L. A. Reynolds (eds.), *Wellcome Witnesses to Twentieth Century Medicine* (London: Wellcome Trust, 1998), ii. 127.

[91] *Independent*, 3 May 1994 (obituary of Fry).

by doubling the annual subscription. By supporting special qualifying examinations for doctors who wished to become general practitioners, Carne hoped to make general practice respectable; to implement this scheme the college had to overcome the criticism of the consultant physicians. Carne also served from 1982 to 1986 as chairman of the Standing Medical Advisory Committee of the Ministry of Health, a post formerly held by Lord Cohen. He published *Paediatric Care* (1976), the first monograph on child health by a GP for his fellow general practitioners, and was the joint author of three editions of the government *Handbook on Contraceptive Practice*.[92]

Dr Harry Levitt, a South African Jewish chairman of the council of the college, approached an influential figure in the Privy Council to ascertain how to make the appropriate application to obtain the royal charter for the college that would enable it to become the Royal College of General Practitioners. He was successful in his endeavours, deftly sidestepping opposition from some of the other royal colleges, and in 1967 the charter was granted. By means of a joint approach with the chairman of the BMA, the leadership of the college helped overcome the misgivings of the Conservative minister of health and implement the rule by which, from February 1981, it became obligatory for doctors to participate in a three-year training scheme if they wished to qualify as general practitioners. Thus, by becoming a specialty, general practitioners consolidated the improvement in their status.

While many of the leading Jewish consultants, such as Sir Roy Calne and Sir Raymond Hoffenberg, had only minimal ties to the Jewish community, others, such as Professor Irving Taylor, Professor Mark Pepys, and Professor Stuart Stanton, have a strong attachment to Orthodoxy; in fact, Stanton's grandfather was Rabbi Dr Epstein, the Principal of Jews' College, the training centre for United Synagogue Ministers and part of London University. Many of the older generation of consultants, as we have seen, were sons of rabbis. An outstanding example was Professor Joseph Yoffey (1902–94), the eldest son of the rabbi of the Manchester Central Synagogue, who was professor of anatomy at Bristol University from 1940 to 1967. Well versed in the Talmud, 'he helped Israel's new medical schools and the rabbinical authorities to formulate policies on post-mortems and dissections'.[93] Among the first post-war generation of consultants at the teaching hospitals there was a tendency to conceal Jewish identity, as in the cases of Michael Kremer or Gerald Apley, or to assume a low Jewish profile, as in the case of Max Rosenheim. Even where individuals retained Jewish ties, there was a drift from Orthodoxy to the Reform movement because of the shock effect of Anglicization to those brought up in traditional Jewish households—a shock which was not so severely felt a generation later. For

[92] Interview with Stuart Carne, 10 Feb. 2000.   [93] *JC* 29 Apr. 1994 (obituary of Yoffey).

example, the father of Professor William Mushin was the headmaster of a Talmud Torah in the East End, but his son was a founder member of the Cardiff
Reform Synagogue.[94] If one wished to retain an unimpaired Jewish identity, the
London and Manchester Jewish hospitals remained a safe haven (until they
closed: the London Jewish Hospital in 1979, the Manchester Victoria in 1991);
or one could sometimes adopt the alternative messianic faith of Marxist ideology,
as a number of consultants did. However, a sure sign that Jews were feeling
more at ease in England was the fact that Dame Albertine Winner, who joined
the Christian foundation of St Christopher's as a 'sympathetic agnostic', was
later able to return to the faith of her fathers.[95] Moreover, whereas Professor
Jack Pepys was a member of the Upper Berkeley Street Reform Synagogue, his
son belongs to an Orthodox congregation.

During the 1950s the new system of meritocratic appointment was still being
implemented in the health service and vestiges of the old regime persisted in the
low-key stance adopted by consultants towards their Jewish identity, but by the
1960s and more clearly by the 1970s Jewish doctors were feeling sufficiently
self-confident to express their Jewishness openly, without the need to make any
compromises. In multiracial and multicultural British society, the espousal of
Judaism and the retention of Jewish values was no longer a burden.

[94] *The Times*, 8 Feb. 1993 (obituary of Mushin).
[95] *Lives of the Fellows of the Royal College of Physicians of London*, viii. 547 (on Winner).

TWELVE

Jewish Solicitors
1945–1990

A LTHOUGH the groundwork for the transformation of the position of Jews in the legal profession had been laid prior to the Second World War, the burgeoning careers of many solicitors were interrupted by service in the armed forces and were not resumed until the late 1940s. Practices left in the hands of managing clerks and neighbouring solicitors had run down, and it took a few years of sustained effort to restore many a practice to its former level. However, a group of enterprising Jewish solicitors did more than this: they seized the opportunities that existed in the 1950s and 1960s as a result of post-war rebuilding, the office and housing boom, and the consumer revolution, and sometimes hitched their fortunes to those of Jewish property entrepreneurs or entered the property market themselves. Others, too, through their financial and legal acumen, became directors of a wide range of companies. During the inter-war period the economic fortunes of British Jews, which had peaked in the Edwardian period, declined, and this was especially true of the old City of London merchant banking families of the Cousinhood. 'There can be little doubt that the post-war period has seen a considerable revival of the wealth of Britain's Jewish community, and it now seems probable that perhaps 15 per cent to 20 per cent of Britain's wealthiest men and women are Jews', declared W. D. Rubinstein in 1981; he suggested, moreover, that there was good reason to believe that this was an underestimate.[1]

Since the inter-war period the traditional Jewish trades of tailoring, furniture-making, and shoe-making had been in decline, with a corresponding diversification in the choice of occupation, leading to the creation of a broad-based Jewish middle class. These trends had accelerated in the 1940s and 1950s. Summing up the findings of research in 1962, Lionel Kochan stated that the end of the Second World War

inaugurated the era of higher mass consumption standards and it is on this basis that the great recent Anglo-Jewish fortunes have been founded—on hire purchase, foodstuffs,

---

[1] Rubinstein, *Men of Property*, 156, 241–2.

furniture, [electrical goods,] clothing, footwear, and their distribution through chain stores. As a notable by-product of the immensely enhanced importance of retail trade to the country's economy there has been a corresponding increase in property values, which has again proved of benefit to Jewish entrepreneurs and property developers. Higher housing standards have worked in the same direction. By the same token professions affiliated to property development, such as law, accountancy, and estate agency, have benefited. Similarly, medicine and dentistry have been other beneficiaries of the Welfare State, with its higher standards of medical care.[2]

A huge expansion of work for barristers and solicitors resulted from the introduction of the Legal Aid and Advice Act 1949, whose provisions were implemented slowly and started to take effect in about 1958. First legal aid was extended to civil litigants in the High Court, followed by the grant of similar assistance in the local county courts, for smaller claims. In 1903 the Poor Prisoners Defence Act had provided defendants charged with serious offences with representation in the higher criminal courts; in 1930 criminal legal aid was extended to trials or committal proceedings before magistrates. With the marked increase in crime following the Second World War and the more generous payments made under the scheme, there were more pickings to be had for the legal profession.[3]

During the post-war years of industrial expansion, property boom, and increased activity due to the vast extension of the legal aid scheme, the number of solicitors in England and Wales steadily climbed from 13,000 in 1945, the lowest number since 1882, to 18,000 in 1960.[4] The expansion continued through the following decades, with the number of solicitors holding practising certificates from the Law Society rising from 22,013 in 1973 to 32,957 in 1983—an increase of 50 per cent in ten years. Until 1965 the rate of admissions was static, with between 600 and 800 articled clerks entering the profession each year; but in that year the intake jumped to over 1,000, and it continued to increase until 1980, when it reached 3,500.[5] There is evidence that Jewish entry into the profession started to increase from the mid-1920s, accelerating in the post-war decades. Whereas in the early 1920s only three or four Jewish candidates were passing the Law Society finals at each of the three annual sittings, by 1926 the number had increased to six or eight and by 1929 had crept up to sixteen.[6] In a survey of Jewish students published in 1951, Raymond Baron found that 106 out of 817

---

[2] Lionel Kochan, 'The Present State of Anglo-Jewry', *AJR Information* (May 1962); Lipman, *A History of Jews in Britain*, 210–15.

[3] Abel-Smith and Stevens, *Lawyers*, 315–47; Napley, *Not Without Prejudice*, 30.

[4] Michael Birks, *Gentlemen of the Law* (London: Stevens & Sons, 1960), 285.

[5] Law Society, *A Statistical Summary of the Solicitors Profession 1984*, 1, 2.

[6] *JC* 21 Apr. 1922, p. 24, 27 July 1923, 23 Nov. 1923, p. 23, 28 Nov. 1924, p. 29, 9 Apr. 1926, p. 10, 23 July 1926, 26 Nov. 1926, 9 Dec. 1927, p. 32, 27 Dec. 1929, p. 12.

men (13 per cent) and 6 out of 258 women (2.3 per cent) intended to study law as a profession.[7]

In keeping with the huge expansion of the legal profession, particularly solicitors, between 1965 and 1980, the number of Jewish solicitors grew dramatically between 1970 and 1990. If we assume that this number had reached its pre-war level by 1950, with a few additions from the ranks of the refugee lawyers, then we would have around 310 Jewish solicitors in post-war London, a much smaller number than we would expect on the basis of current figures. We can check this calculation by once again employing Asher Tropp's method of extracting certain distinctive surnames from the professional directories and then multiplying the figure by 14.26 to obtain the overall number. In 1950 there were twenty-one solicitors with such distinctive surnames, which would give us a figure of 300 Jewish lawyers. In 1970 the records show forty-seven distinctive Jewish surnames, generating a total of 670 Jewish solicitors in London—slightly more than double the figure for 1950. When we inspect the directory for 1990, we find a great increase in the number of distinctive Jewish names to some 125, suggesting that there were approximately 1,782 Jewish solicitors in London. As in the case of Jewish doctors, this figure may be somewhat exaggerated, and a truer figure may be in the region of 1,300. While in the 1950s and 1960s there were hardly any Jewish women practising as solicitors in London, by 1990 there may have been between 150 and 170.[8]

*

Property values in England started to rise in 1944 before the Allied invasion of France and continued to soar until the devaluation of 1949; according to Oliver Marriott, 'Many of the great property fortunes were founded [on these rising values]. Often land was bought and sold again at a profit within a few months. Sometimes vacant buildings were bought and leased. Occasionally war-damaged offices were repaired.'[9] Lewis Silkin, a Jewish solicitor who had worked his way up through the London County Council to become a minister in the Attlee government, introduced the New Towns Act of 1946 and the Town and Country Planning Act of 1947 which imposed a 100 per cent tax on increased land values created by planning permission. This 'development charge', along with the concept of 'betterment' on which it was based—the rise in the value of land after planning permission had been granted—were scrapped in the new Town and Country Planning Act introduced in 1953 by the minister of housing and local government, Harold Macmillan; the following year Nigel Birch, the minister of

---

[7] *JC* 16 Feb. 1951, p. 13, 23 Feb. 1951, p. 9.

[8] Tropp, *Jews in the Professions*, 94–7; *Law List 1950*, 515–704; *Law List 1970*, 1047–93; *Solicitors and Barristers Directory 1990* (London: Waterlow, 1990), ii. 733–983.

[9] Oliver Marriott, *The Property Boom* (London: Hamilton, 1967), 1–6.

works, abolished building controls. Once these restrictions were removed, building development boomed. Whereas in 1952 the LCC granted planning permission for 2.4 million square feet of space, by 1955 this figure had climbed to 5.9 million square feet.

'The new legislation was predictably too complex to be effective, so almost anyone with a modicum of brain could get round it', declared Charles Gordon.

Its main restriction, plot ratio—the ratio of the size of a new building to the size of the plot—was a commercial joke and a commercial jackpot . . . Amidst all this, property development provided a money-making investment opportunity which was quite simply fantastic. Planning consents were oozing out from the planning committees of the local authorities for office buildings, shop developments and town centre schemes and a profusion of tenants with major covenants were eagerly looking for space and taking up leases. In particular, finance was freely available on fabulous terms to the borrower. Long-term rates were around 5% to 6%.[10]

In the early 1960s there was usually no provision for rent review in a fixed-term lease; however, during the decade they began to become more frequent: by 1965 the interval had been halved from fourteen to seven years.

The majority of the new breed of property developers were Jewish, from second-generation immigrant families. Most were estate agents who entered the property market because they appreciated the opportunities that existed for profit-taking better than anyone else. Of 108 property millionaires listed by Marriott, over 50 per cent started their careers as estate agents. Other Jewish developers emerged from the retail trades or manufacturing: for example, Joseph Littman (a furrier), Louis Mintz (a gown manufacturer), and Gerald Ronson (a furniture maker). Stephen Aris has pointed out that many Jewish boys from an immigrant background chose to go into estate agency as 'a compromise between a fully fledged commercial career and a full-blooded professional one'. Other reasons why young Jewish men chose this career were that self-employed estate agents did not have to work on the sabbath, and that it was a good way for someone without capital to make money—a quick route into becoming a property entrepreneur. Although Edward Erdman wanted to train for the law, his millionaire uncle, the timber merchant Reuben Gliksten, told his parents, 'You cannot afford to make your son a solicitor', and instead he took a job as office boy with a firm of estate agents.[11] He went on to become a leading West End property agent. Walter Flack was a failed solicitor, who graduated from being an estate agent into a millionaire developer at the head of Murrayfield Real Estate.[12] Max Rayne, later a prominent property developer, studied at evening

---

[10] Charles Gordon, *The Two Tycoons: A Personal Memoir of Jack Cotton and Charles Clore* (London: Hamilton, 1984), 16–20. [11] Erdman, *People and Property*, 1, 2.
[12] David Clutterbuck and Marion Devine, *Clore: The Man and his Millions* (London: Weidenfeld & Nicolson, 1987), 134.

classes to become a solicitor, but found the strain of combining his legal education and working in his father's tailoring business too much. 'Other boys in
much the same situation as Rayne faced similar pressures and it is for this reason
that so many of them, though they would perhaps have liked to be doctors,
lawyers or architects, turned to a slightly less rigorous profession, estate agency',
Aris suggested.[13] Despite these constraints, many other young Jews were able
to qualify as solicitors and, in the course of carrying out the conveyancing work
for property developer clients, came to see the hefty profits that they were
making, as a result of which they decided to undertake future developments
themselves.

In 1958 there were fifty quoted property companies on the Stock Exchange;
most were of pre-war origin and part of either a landed estate or an urban holding. By the early 1960s 150 new property companies had been floated by a new
type of entrepreneurial property developer. Charles Gordon has pointed out
'that the true groundswell of the property boom came from the explosive retail
expansion of the fifties [in which the new Anglo-Jewish middle class were the
front runners], not from the somewhat later boom in office building'.[14] Behind
the big names among the developers was an array of lesser but still important
Jewish figures, and the end result of this enterprise was a quantitative leap in the
wealth of the Anglo-Jewish community. Jews' participation in post-war urban
property development in the United States was equally significant, so much so
that there were probably similar underlying factors for their success in both
countries, notably a lack of sentimentality about land combined with a keen
appreciation of rising land values; entrepreneurial skill; willingness to take
risks; ability to mobilize capital; and exclusion from most of the banking and
insurance sectors.[15]

As noted above, a number of Jewish solicitors learned the property business
from their clients' ventures and drifted into property development themselves,
in the process becoming millionaires. Abraham Lazarus Dolland, the son of
immigrants from eastern Europe, is noteworthy because he was both a lawyer
and a pioneer among the post-war property developers. He qualified as a solicitor in 1934 and, after a complicated case involving two appeals, was suspended
from practising for two years in November 1944. Interestingly, he was charged
with acting in association with an unqualified individual or organization with
regard to pursuing an accident claim; it may be that he was a marginal figure in
the legal world, finding it difficult to obtain a sufficient caseload. A bachelor
who lived with his parents, an intellectual, a linguist, and a chess player, he

[13] Aris, *The Jews in Business*, 163–82.   [14] Gordon, *The Two Tycoons*, 21, 22, 30.
[15] Charles Silberman, *A Certain People: American Jews and their Lives Today* (New York: Summit,
1985), 133–6; Nathan Glazer and Daniel Patrick Moynihan, *Beyond the Melting Pot* (Cambridge,
Mass.: MIT Press, 1968), 151–5.

was perhaps an unlikely figure to embark on speculative property investment. Nevertheless, taking a risk, he bought the lease of a bombed site near Finsbury Square in the City. After an anxious time, he found a tenant in the South American export trade, thereby qualifying for a building licence, and a contractor who was prepared to raise the finances and carry out the building work. When the building was completed, it was worth over £250,000 more than it cost to construct. Dolland was so worried about putting similar development packages together that he sold adjoining sites to other developers. Next he put up two more buildings, again having the construction financed by the builder; he sold both of them in the early 1960s to the developer Bernard Sunley, making a profit of £2.11 million. 'I had such trouble letting my developments,' he told Oliver Marriott, 'it was such a nerve-racking experience that I thought the risk was too great to continue. I did not conceive of a boom.'[16]

Another bright intellectual, keen on chess and music, who became a property millionaire was Samuel Sebba, the son of a timber merchant: he studied law at London University and qualified as a solicitor in 1928. While carrying on his solicitor's practice in the City, 'he handled the legal formalities on behalf of property-investor clients', and decided to undertake some large-scale developments himself. For this purpose he formed Warnford Investments in 1960 and developed part of Portman Square in London's West End as well as buildings in some provincial towns; but his main focus remained the City, where he put up an office block with shops in London Wall, and Warnford Court facing the Stock Exchange. Around 1948 he purchased a site in Piccadilly with Maurice Wohl, an accountant and another well-known property developer, arranging the finances to construct the building known as Reed House. While Warnford Investments had a book value of £7.13 million in 1979, its directors believed that the properties owned by the company had a market value of £28 million.[17]

Moss Spiro (1915–96), who qualified as a solicitor in 1937, started his career as a divorce lawyer, but after marrying Jocelyn Shore, who had architectural skills, he switched to property development. Working in conjunction with legendary property developers such as Harry Hyams, Spiro developed various sites in the City and central London, sharing a profit of £530,000 with Hyams on the lease of a Grafton Street office block to Union Carbide, a gigantic American corporation. In the early 1960s the Spiros completed some developments themselves, including office buildings in west London and the redevelopment of existing structures at London Wall in the City. While his wife 'identified the locations, provided the design briefs and eventually managed the completed developments', Moss Spiro added the necessary legal and financial skills. 'With only a part-time secretary, they built over one million square feet of office

---

[16] Marriott, *Property Boom*, 51–3; *Law Society's Gazette*, Apr. 1945.
[17] Erdman, *People and Property*, 133, 134; *Estates Gazette*, 13 Oct. 1979.

accommodation, almost all of which was let straight off the drawing-board.' During the early 1970s Moss Spiro retired for a time from the property world, but returned later with a new idea, 'the construction of smaller buildings for single tenants'. Spiro was not only a member of St John's Wood Synagogue but also a strong supporter of Zionism; in 1971, while working on a residential complex at Watford, he encountered and exposed the building industry's compliance with the Arab boycott of any companies or individuals who had connections with Israel.[18]

Arnold Lee was a solicitor with conveyancing expertise who was articled to Malcolm Slowe, a West End lawyer, and was related to the well-known property developer Max Rayne, with whom he formed British Commercial Property to develop some sites. Having co-operated on half a dozen projects, their partnership came to an end when Rayne bought out Lee's share in the company in 1958. Arnold Lee formed another company, Imry Property, with a market value of £2 million in 1962; before selling it, he carried out a series of projects with financial backing from the Norwich Union Life Insurance Society to develop commercial properties in the West End of London and the suburbs. By 1982, when the major stakes in the company were owned by the Norwich Union and the Rothschild Trust, Imry Property had a market capitalization of £37.18 million but this was well after their takeover.[19]

Harold Wingate (1901–79), after taking a degree in chemistry, worked for Lever Brothers as an analytical chemist; later he qualified as a barrister, specializing (like a number of other Jewish practitioners) in patent law. For a short period he practised as a solicitor, but, finding this unsatisfying, he ventured into the property market, purchasing several cinemas and the Comedy Theatre. His company, Chesterfield Properties, was floated publicly in 1960, when it owned the Columbia Cinema building, the Curzon Cinema (which specialized in Continental films), and Chesterfield House. By 1974 Wingate was reporting net annual profits of £711,032 for his company and sales of properties in the City, Harrow, and Shrewsbury, as well as developments in Grosvenor Gardens near Buckingham Palace and smaller developments in Bristol and Leeds. He enjoyed becoming engrossed with architects in the design of a building and with solicitors in legal detail. In contrast to most other property entrepreneurs, Wingate decided that Chesterfield would retain the freeholds of the buildings which it owned, instead of following the practice of selling the freehold and buying back a long lease, the process known as sale and leaseback.[20]

Unlike the other Jewish solicitors and barristers who became property devel-

---

[18] *JC* 6 Dec. 1996, p. 15 (obituary of Spiro); Marriott, *Property Boom*, 6, 103.

[19] Marriott, *Property Boom*, 83, 84; *JC* 4 Oct. 1963, p. 29; *Estates Gazette*, 9 Jan. 1982.

[20] Erdman, *People and Property*, 131, 132; *JC* 5 Oct. 1979, p. 35 (obituary of Wingate); *Estates Gazette*, 3 Aug. 1974.

opers in the 1960s and 1970s, Louis Littman (1925–87) was the second generation of his family to work in this field. Littman was, as he put it, 'reluctantly' educated in America during the Second World War, and 'decided to return to England in 1944, working his passage across the Atlantic as a cabin boy aboard a small Polish ship carrying explosives'. His father, Joseph Littman, who migrated to Britain from Russia before the First World War, was one of the first Jewish property dealers from an east European immigrant background and is credited by Edward Erdman as 'perhaps being the originator of the leaseback method of finance which allowed him unlimited expansion without borrowing'. During the 1930s Joseph Littman bought shop properties on both sides of Kilburn High Road for the investment income; he then turned his attention to Oxford Street, acquiring a number of valuable sites.[21]

After reading law at Cambridge, Louis Littman practised as a solicitor in London between 1951 and 1967 before taking up farming in Dorset. He built up from scratch a huge estate of dairy farms, making prize-winning farmhouse cheese and becoming one of the largest producers of goats' milk in the country. At the same time, in London and elsewhere, he turned to property development, his Colette House in Piccadilly being commended by Westminster City Council as a building of architectural merit. In 1965 he established the Littman Library of Jewish Civilization as an act of charity in memory of his father Joseph, to publish scholarly works that explain and perpetuate the Jewish heritage; this, rather than any architectural masterpiece, has become his most enduring monument. A regular attender at the New London Synagogue, he was for a time vice-chairman of the Reform Synagogues of Great Britain and also served as chairman of the Library Committee of Leo Baeck College.[22]

Asher Lewis Shane (1911–91) was the grandson of rabbis on both sides of the family; his father was a clothing wholesaler and the owner of a small coal mine in Wales before the nationalization of the coal industry. After taking articles with a Cardiff firm of solicitors, he qualified in 1933 and came to London, where he acted for a number of property developer clients. In 1960 he formed the Equitable Debenture and Assets Corporation, successfully bidding in 1963 for the right to develop a four-acre shopping complex in Doncaster which was finished two years later. Because a number of factories in the Doncaster area made some of their employees redundant at this time, Shane had difficulties in finding tenants for the shopping centre, and matters improved only later. Despite this, he built up the Equitable Debenture and Assets Corporation into one of Britain's biggest privately owned property companies. Lewis Shane was described as 'a man of modest bearing and refined personality' who 'greatly enjoyed good conversation'. For a number of years he served as treasurer of the Jewish Historical

[21] *The Times*, 21 Dec. 1987 (obituary of Littman); Erdman, *People and Property*, 54–6.
[22] *JC* 11 Dec. 1987, p. 15; *The Times*, 21 Dec. 1987 (obituary of Littman); Probate Office records.

Society, and his library in his Hampstead home had 'perhaps the most important collection of Anglo-Judaica in private hands'. When it was sold in New York in 1998, his collection fetched £2.7 million.[23]

Among other solicitors who turned to property development were Ralph Yablon and Sidney Bloch. Legal and General Assurance supplied funds for a £1.5 million redevelopment in the centre of Paris to Yablon's Town and Commercial Properties in 1963. During the 1950s Sidney Bloch and Lewis Cohen formed a series of trusts to purchase housing estates, subsequently inducing the sitting tenants to buy their homes by means of mortgage advances from the Alliance Building Society. As Cohen's biographer comments, 'It was a licence to print money.' In 1959, however, after a dispute with Cohen, Bloch gained control of Hallmark Securities, the company they had founded together whose subsidiary built 830 houses in 1962–3. By 1970 Hallmark Securities was a finance, investment, and building company with a value of £37 million, and expected its profits to equal the previous year's figure of £1.4 million.[24]

David Ivor Young (b. 1932), later Lord Young, was a solicitor who combined property development with a political career; he rose to become Secretary of State for Trade and Industry from 1987 to 1989 in the Thatcher government. He was articled to his uncle Solomon Teff of the well-known firm Teff & Teff, who did a considerable amount of work for Jewish communal bodies, and qualified as a solicitor in 1955. Not staying long in the law, he joined Great Universal Stores in a junior capacity, where he was taken under the personal tutelage of Isaac Wolfson. 'At odd moments', Young recollected,

he would call me in and explain the inner workings and interpretations of balance sheets, often going through past triumphs and explaining what he first saw in the company and how it worked out in practice. At that time we were buying two companies a week. These were always by agreement but this gave me a marvellous grounding in commerce.

His father-in-law, a Mr Shaw, was a property developer concerned with erecting blocks of flats, and although David Young joined him for a short time, he soon left, as he was more interested in commercial property. Young obtained the option on a four-acre site at Stratford suitable for office development and raised half a million pounds by mortgaging the freehold. He then used these funds to create a trading estate near Bristol with over sixty factories, deliberately siting new warehouses near motorway intersections. He 'branched out into construction, plant hire, retail and manufacturing as well. Some did well, and some did not.' He sold his company to Town and City Properties, run by a

---

[23] Marriott, *Property Boom*, 252, 253; 'Asher Lewis Shane (1901–1991)' (obituary), *Jewish Historical Studies*, 32 (1990–2), pp. xvi, xvii; *JC* 10 July 1998, p. 27.

[24] *JC* 6 Sept. 1963, p. 37; *Estates Gazette*, 12 Oct. 1963, 14 Feb. 1970; David Winner, *They Called Him Mr Brighton: A Biography of the Socialist Peer Lewis Cohen* (Lewes: Book Guild, 1999), 46, 47, 49.

co-religionist, Barry East, and started some joint ventures with the Sterling Guarantee Trust, but as a result of the property market slide in the early 1970s Young's liabilities came to exceed his assets. He therefore established a new company, with an American bank, to lend money on property and this gradually prospered. After quitting politics, he served for a number of years as executive chairman of Cable and Wireless. Lord Young is a prominent communal figure and became president of Jewish Care in 1990; from 1989 to 1993 he was a governor of the Oxford Centre for Postgraduate Hebrew Studies, now the Oxford Centre for Hebrew and Jewish Studies.[25]

Overlapping with the property lawyers were a group of solicitors who became directors of leading companies and often extremely affluent. Norman Chinn (1909–97) was the youngest of six children from an impoverished Jewish family in a Welsh mining village. His father died after they moved to London, when he was 13; despite this, he qualified as a solicitor in 1932. With his brother Rosser he made a bid for a ramshackle garage in Soho in 1945, anticipating that there would be a great potential for motoring after the war; from these beginnings, Norman and Rosser Chinn developed the Lex chain of garages, now known as the Lex Service Group. As the group held large swaths of land, a subsidiary Rodwell–Lex Properties was set up to develop attractive sites; later, a new joint venture company was formed with Town and City Properties. Norman remained company chairman for thirty years until 1978, when he emigrated to the United States to become consultant for Lex's American holdings. From 1973 to 1978 he was chairman of the Ravenswood Foundation, a centre for mentally handicapped Jewish children, and also raised funds to send the British team to the Maccabi Games—the Jewish Olympics—in Israel in 1965.[26]

Another solicitor with wide business interests was a provincial lawyer, Hyman Stone, who died in 1961. Having gained a master's degree in law from Sheffield University, he was appointed lecturer in law there in 1929. In 1933 he came to London and practised as a solicitor. 'In the course of a highly successful legal practice, Mr Stone acquired many commercial interests and directorships. Among others, he was a Director of Poly Tours.' He too had a deep commitment to the Jewish community, serving as treasurer of the Jewish Historical Society, vice-president of the Anglo-Jewish Association, and honorary solicitor of the Residential School for Jewish Deaf Children.[27]

A little-known but greatly respected Jewish lawyer who went into business was David Lewis, who was admitted as a solicitor in 1936 and became a partner in B. A. Woolf & Co., a firm which had offices in Lombard Street in 1939 and

[25] Lord Young, *The Enterprise Years: A Businessman in the Cabinet* (London: Headline, 1990), 7–22; *Who's Who 1996* (London: A. & C. Black, 1996), 2134.

[26] *JC* 30 May 1997, p. 21 (obituary of Norman Chinn); *Estates Gazette*, 25 Dec. 1965, 10 Feb. 1968.

[27] *JC* 28 Apr. 1961, p. 27 (obituary of Stone), 8 Dec. 1995, p. 23.

which was later called Lewis, Lewis & Co. When the senior partner in his legal practice retired after the war, David Lewis started to act for Radio and Allied Industries, a company which manufactured radio and television sets. In 1961 GEC merged with Radio and Allied to secure the managerial services of Arnold Weinstock, and a couple of years later Lewis, with whom Weinstock had worked, was invited to join GEC as a director. Hitherto 'Lewis had been a professional director and . . . accepted invitations from all sorts of companies to become a director if it helped them.' Now, because of his knowledge of company tax legislation, Weinstock brought him into the board and inner circle of GEC. A group of three men, Weinstock, Kenneth Bond, and David Lewis, directed the expansion of GEC for thirty years into one of the major British technological companies. Among Lewis's specific contributions was his work as chairman of Osram, the electric light section, into which he was installed to shake up a somewhat underperforming division of the parent company.[28]

Two of the earliest solicitors with strong business links were Isidore Kerman and Ellis Birk, both of whom inherited some of their fathers' financial acumen. Isidore Kerman (1905–98) was the son of Hyman Kerman, an affluent moneylender who left an estate of £235,873. 14s. 1d. in 1926. Isidore was articled to a member of the firm of Strong & Co. and qualified as a solicitor in 1927, subsequently founding Forsyte Saunders Kerman, a medium-sized West End practice. (West End practices dealt with all kinds of property, including commercial property, whereas City practices dealt with banking and company work; later, West End practices also became involved in the corporate field.) The younger Kerman was involved in many business ventures: he was a director of City Centre Properties and a close friend of its co-founder Jack Cotton, who was also Jewish, from their schooldays together at Cheltenham; he was chairman of Scott's Restaurant in Mount Street; and he was also a director of the British subsidiary of Loew's hotel group of America, which owned the Churchill Hotel. Kerman had founded City Centre Properties with Cotton before the Second World War, travelling to Birmingham weekly to discuss property matters with him, and later he became trustee of Cotton's family trusts. After the war Cotton emerged as the biggest developer in the Midlands, and in 1954 Kerman advised him to purchase Central Commercial Properties from the Edgson family; it was this deal which enabled him to start outdistancing his rivals in the south and become a national figure. Cotton forged the links between developers and the insurance institutions, creating a new framework for the property market. In 1957 or thereabouts Cotton moved into a suite in the Dorchester, where he held nightly conferences with Kerman and his other advisers. He became

---

[28] *Law List 1939*, 607 and 737; Robert Jones and Oliver Marriott, *Anatomy of a Merger: A History of GEC, AEI and English Electric* (London: Cape, 1970), 216 and 221. Stephen Aris, *Arnold Weinstock and the Making of GEC* (London: Arum, 1998), 21, 24, 25, 28, 55, 171–3.

chairman of City Centre in 1958, initiating a series of spectacular deals and putting up the Pan-Am Building in New York. Later Kerman tried to dissuade Cotton from entering into a disastrous merger with Clore, and sadly had to persuade his friend to step down as chairman when the company encountered difficulties.[29]

Kerman, who had a country home in East Grinstead, Sussex, was a devoted racing enthusiast; he was chairman of Plumpton racecourse, purchased in part for its development potential, and also a director of the Fontwell Park Steeplechase Company. During the 1980s Kerman 'and a group of backers gained control of GRA, an ailing dog track operator which had just sold the White City stadium but still owned a number of sites with potential for development as superstores. Kerman's shareholding in the company multiplied 10 times in value when GRA was eventually sold to another property group.' Kerman also had a significant divorce practice, priding himself in being able to negotiate settlements between recalcitrant parties. Nevertheless, he remained primarily a business and property lawyer and investor.[30] In the 1960s he acted for Robert Maxwell, vouchsafing that 'Mr Maxwell is a man of undoubted integrity and Pergamon Press Ltd is well run', and attacked the *Sunday Times* for its 'shameful vendetta of slander'; but after the inquiries, conducted by the Board of Trade inspectors, into Pergamon, of which Kerman was a director, and his involvement as a witness, he could no longer act as Maxwell's solicitor. Having been criticized in the inspectors' report, Kerman tried to distance himself from Maxwell, praising him for his cleverness but suggesting that the publisher's 'megalomania' had ruined him.[31]

Like so many enterprising solicitors' firms with Jewish founders, Forsyte Saunders Kerman prided themselves on thinking in exactly the same way as their businessmen clients; in 1995 the company was 'particularly highly regarded for its top quality commercial property and corporate work; it has a substantial High Court litigation practice including a specialist property litigation team and an insurance claims team'.[32] A successful farmer, enthusiastic racehorse owner, winter sports enthusiast, and bridge player for considerable stakes, Kerman grew apart from his Jewish roots—he married out of the faith and his children were not brought up as Jews—but he did provide accommodation and funds for Jewish children fleeing from Nazi Germany. When he died in 1998 he left an estate of £14,126,988.[33]

---

[29] *Daily Telegraph*, 1 Aug. 1998 (obituary of Kerman); office copy of the grant of Letters of Administration to the estate of Hyman Kerman, 17 Nov. 1926; Erdman, *People and Property*, 95–6. Gordon, *The Two Tycoons*, 29–39, 90, 116, 204.   [30] *Daily Telegraph*, 1 Aug. 1998 (obituary of Kerman).

[31] Tom Bower, *Maxwell the Outsider* (London: Mandarin, 1992), 94, 192, 216, 225, 250, 258, 269, 285.

[32] *Chambers & Partners Directory of the Legal Profession 1995–1996* (London: Chambers & Partners, 1995), 647.   [33] *JC* 25 Dec. 1998, p. 17.

Ellis Birk was born in 1915 in Newcastle, the son of a prosperous banker who moved to Bishops Avenue in Hampstead Garden Suburb in 1932. Educated at Clifton College, in the Jewish House, and Jesus College, Cambridge, where he read classics and law, Birk was articled to David Jacobs of Nicholson, Graham & Jones, a small but lively firm of solicitors. Established in 1886, the firm had been built up by Willy Graham, described by Birk as 'a tiny little man with a very bad temper'. It numbered among its clients Sir John Ellerman, whose Ellerman Group was a gigantic conglomerate with substantial holdings in the Mirror Group (owner of the *Daily Mirror* and the *Sunday Pictorial*), Odhams Press and its subsidiary, the Amalgamated Press (the IPC Magazine Group), the Albert E. Reed Group (Reed International), a big newsprint manufacturer, a brewery, a considerable part of the Howard de Walden Estate of freehold properties in the West End of London, and a stake in Associated Television. Unusually for a non-Jewish City law firm, it had a Jewish partner, David Jacobs, who formed and nursed to success Wembley Stadium Ltd. Because of war service, Birk was not admitted as a solicitor until 1946, and then the sole surviving partner David Jacobs became seriously ill. One day Sir John Elvin, the chairman of Wembley Stadium, rang up Birk, saying, 'I can't have my company run by a firm of solicitors where the senior partner is ill and you're the only person who is left.' To this, Birk replied. 'Can't you? In which case bugger off now, at this moment.'[34]

With the help of 'extremely good managing clerks', Birk, who was a commercial lawyer with a growing interest in media law, reinvigorated the practice. On 24 March 1950 Ellis Birk joined the board of Sunday Pictorial Newspapers Ltd., the first of many company directorships which he held, including those of the *Jewish Chronicle*, of which he became chairman, and Reed International. Birk became a director of Associated Television, as a nominee of the Mirror Group, and was one of the 'backroom boys' in the nascent television industry, mainly concerned with the financial and commercial side of independent television.[35] Birk was invited to join the board of United City Merchants, an international trading group, and was a great friend of its founder Eric Charles Sosnow (1910–87).[36] *United City Merchants Investments Limited* v. *Royal Bank of Canada* (1982) determined that where on the face of it a letter of credit was genuine, the refusal of a bank to pay out on it 'did not extend to fraud to which the seller was not party'. When the property developer Maurice Wingate died suddenly, his son Stefan became managing director of Wingate Investments and Birk became chairman of the board of the company. By 1995, some ten

[34] Interview with Ellis Birk, 25 Sept. 1997; Silman, *Signifying Nothing*, 110.

[35] Interview with Ellis Birk, 25 Sept. 1997; biographical notes and list of companies of which Ellis Birk was director; David Pela, 'Tycoons and their Backroom Boys', *JC Supplement*, 24 Aug. 1962, p. v; Lew Grade, *Still Dancing: My Story* (London: Collins, 1987), 248.

[36] *Dictionary of National Biography 1986–1990*, 426, 427 (on Sosnow).

years after Birk had retired, Nicholson, Graham & Jones had thirty-four partners and a large number of assistant solicitors; its main strength lay in its company and commercial work, litigation and property departments.[37] Ellis Birk was also deeply involved in Jewish communal activities, being the joint treasurer of the Jewish Welfare Board and later its chairman, a member of the executive committee of the Hebrew University of Jerusalem, chairman of the finance and general purposes committee of the Institute of Jewish Affairs, and member of the executive of the Council of Christians and Jews.

In 1953 Julius Silman (1909–98), after a foray into building houses and acquiring property companies, joined Nicholson, Graham & Jones, developing a reputation as a shrewd commercial lawyer, brilliant at negotiating deals. Ellis Birk asked Silman to look after the affairs of Associated Television, which he did with great skill. He completed a multi-million-pound transaction for Lew Grade, covering the purchase of television and radio stations from an Australian company under great pressure of time, necessitating the deal's being concluded on a Sunday; on another occasion he negotiated the purchase of the Beatles' company which owned the copyright of their songs. Silman also acted for Joe Coral, assisting the latter in his building of a racing and casino empire. Another grateful client was Fred Stringer, a motor dealer, who formed one of the major distributors for the British Motor Corporation. Stringer decided to have Silman as his solicitor because he required 'someone with imagination', a business-orientated lawyer 'who can negotiate for me and resolve problems'. During the late 1960s Silman established Moorgate Mercantile, a finance house, which he steered through the fringe banking crisis of 1973–4 and sold for many millions in 1988.[38]

*

Although there were multifarious small Jewish law practices in the City of London, even in the decades after the Second World War Jews could not become partners in the large City firms, and if they were taken on at all by these giants, they were expected to become a fairly silent presence. When D. J. Freeman qualified in 1952, he was offered a position as an assistant solicitor with a large City firm. 'I'd prefer not to mention their name. I decided against them when I learned there were no prospects of partnership if you were Jewish.'[39] Similarly, Jeffrey Greenwood, later senior partner at Nabarro Nathanson, declared,

I was the first lawyer in my family, my father was in business . . . When I came down from Cambridge [in 1957], I wanted to get articles, and my father had a cousin, who was known as something in the City, in fact he was a manager with M. Samuel, the

[37] *Chambers & Partners Directory*, 790.
[38] Silman, *Signifying Nothing*, 112–27; *JC* 27 Feb. 1998, p. 25 (obituary of Silman).
[39] Michael Chambers, 'The Rainmaker', *Commercial Lawyer* (Mar. 1996).

merchant bank . . . and he said, 'Jeffrey, I will get you an interview with Slaughter & May . . . Jeffrey, I think that you should be low profile about your Jewishness,' and I said, 'What do you mean?' He said, 'Well, you will probably be able to get *Yom Kippur* [the Day of Atonement] off, but don't think about going home early on a Friday or getting the *Yomim Tovim* [festivals] off', and I said, 'You know, Harry, I couldn't work under those circumstances.'[40]

In another example, a solicitor who had since built up a large and successful practice told Stephen Aris,

I was not brought up as a Jew, but when I found I was going to be treated like one, I determined to act like one. I think I am an example of a chap who would never have built up his own practice . . . But when I realized I would never be president of the Law Society or a senior partner in one of the large firms, I said to myself: 'I'll show them that I am as good as the next man, if not better.'[41]

Michael Max was articled to Solomon Levy of S. A. Bailey & Co. between 1950 and 1955. Levy had grown up in the East End and had joined the firm as an office boy in 1913. He returned to the firm after serving in the trenches as a line signaller during the First World War—where the fact that 'he was knee high to a grasshopper' probably saved his life. After ten years Levy, by now a managing clerk, passed his solicitor's exams and qualified in 1930, after which he became a partner in S. A. Bailey. He later inherited a small but good general practice in Bloomsbury Way, WC1. Excellent at litigation, he acted for a non-Jewish builder from Bow as well as for a number of Jewish property developers.[42]

Michael Max had been thinking while doing National Service that only the larger firms, which could offer a range of specialized services, would succeed in the future; and, after the failure of negotiations to arrange a merger between S. A. Bailey and Paisner & Co., an expanding Jewish practice, he decided to move and attended a number of interviews. It soon became clear to him that none of the big non-Jewish firms would offer him a suitable position. One firm told him after an interview that went wonderfully well that he could certainly have a job, but he could never become a partner as their principal client had indicated that he would direct no further work to them if they took on a Jewish partner. At another firm, towards the end of the appointment, the interviewer remarked: 'Mr Max, I see you are partnered by Mr Lev-e-e. Are you Jewish?' To this, he replied: 'If the outcome of the interview depended on whether I was Jewish, you could have saved yourself from embarrassment by doing your homework before the interview.' Both were then medium-sized City firms; one is now very large.[43]

[40] Interview with Jeffrey Greenwood, 2 July 1998.
[42] Interview with Michael Max, 20 June 1997.
[41] Aris, *The Jews in Business*, 210–11.
[43] Ibid.

Behind the rapid progress of the large post-war Jewish solicitors' firms of Nabarro Nathanson, Brecher & Co., Titmuss Sainer & Webb, Paisner & Co., Berwin Leighton, and D. J. Freeman were the twin factors of the patronage of big Jewish property developers and businessmen, and the exclusion of able and ambitious Jewish solicitors from partnership opportunities in the City during the 1950s and early 1960s. But instead of being located in the City many of these new Jewish law firms sprouted up in the West End or other parts of central London. The removal of the statutory limit on the number of partners to twenty by the Companies Act 1967 both gave a fillip to the long-established City solicitors' firms and encouraged some of the new Jewish firms to mushroom in size.

As these new firms rose in importance in the post-war period, so the old elite Anglo-Jewish firms of Herbert Oppenheimer, Nathan & Vandyk, and Bartlett & Gluckstein declined, reflecting in some measure the waning power and influence of members of the Cousinhood within Anglo-Jewry. Whereas Bartlett & Gluckstein took a nosedive because of their dependency for work on J. Lyons, which succumbed to competition, Herbert Oppenheimer, Nathan & Vandyk had a flourishing and expanding practice, and imploded only because of feuding within the firm. After the first Lord Nathan's death, Fred Worms noted that 'Oppenheimers had a rapid succession of senior partners. . . . The revered old firm fell apart and sank without trace. Some partners joined Denton Hall . . . others went to Nabarro.'[44] According to the *Lawyer*,

Three factors played a major part in the collapse—disagreement about how profits should be divided up, about where the firm should locate itself and about the style in management . . . But the crunch came in the Spring [1988] when a number of junior partners demanded parity in equity with all profit sharers. 'From then, the firm was in a state of paralysis and trauma with nobody trusting anybody else,' says an ex-associate.

Until its demise in 1988 this firm had a wonderful clients' list, including Sainsbury's, Plessey, and Isaac Wolfson; it did much business with the United States during the 1950s, working closely in association with two leading American law firms; and as Leslie Cork, the brother of the accountant Kenneth Cork, was a partner, it also had a massive insolvency practice.[45]

Joseph Nunes Nabarro (1884–1948), a member of an old Sephardi family, qualified as a solicitor in 1909 and established Messrs J. N. Nabarro and Sons after being joined in practice by his sons, Alan in 1935 and Felix in 1937. During the inter-war years and into the 1950s it remained a small family firm with a largely small-business clientele, dealing chiefly with the Sephardi community. Joseph was an active communal worker, a *parnas* (president or warden) of the Spanish and Portuguese congregation, and a supporter of Zionism opposed to

[44] Worms, *A Life in Three Cities* (London: Halban, 1996), 323.
[45] *Lawyer*, 27 Sept., 4, 18, 25 Oct. 1988; Cork, *Cork on Cork*, 27–9.

the views of the diehards among the old Anglo-Jewish families. When Leslie Nathanson amalgamated his practice with the Nabarros to form Nabarro Nathanson, everything changed. Nathanson was the brother-in-law of the property developer Basil Samuel and with his partner Irvin Goldstein did the conveyancing work not only for him and his company, Great Portland Estates, but also for his cousin Harold Samuel, another, more famous, property tycoon who also happened to be a cousin of Nathanson. Harold Samuel, Baron Samuel of Wych Cross (1912–87), was an estate agent who became one of the most brilliant property developers and investors. Although Samuel came from an old Ashkenazi family, his branch did not belong to the Anglo-Jewish elite. Using the profits from a small company which he had acquired, Land Securities Investment Trust, Harold Samuel secured financial backing to acquire bomb sites and to rebuild the city centres of Plymouth, Exeter, Hull, Coventry, and Bristol. He took over not only the City of London Real Property Company but a number of other important property companies. Under his guidance Land Securities grew steadily and acquired assets worth £3 billion, becoming the biggest quoted property company in the world.[46]

Leslie Nathanson (1915–82) had a distinguished war record. Captured by the Germans in Italy, he escaped and was looked after by the partisans. After the war he set up charitable trusts for the education of poor Italian children as a mark of gratitude for the way in which he had been cared for by their compatriots. At the same time he established his own solicitor's firm, working exclusively for the Samuel cousins, and ably assisted by Irvin Goldstein until the latter's death in a motoring accident in Sicily in 1957. The loss of his partner compelled Leslie Nathanson to merge with another firm in order to keep on servicing the work of his important property clients. He was introduced to the Nabarros; the chemistry between Nathanson and the Nabarro brothers worked and Nabarro Nathanson was set up in 1958 with Leslie Nathanson as senior partner. The more the property companies associated with the Samuel cousins grew, the more Nabarro Nathanson expanded with them.

While it is true that Nabarro Nathanson was built up by members of old Anglo-Jewish families, albeit from branches outside the ranks of the elite in the 1960s and early 1970s, the renewed spurt in the growth of the property industry in the 1980s was handled by partners who had their origins in the east European immigrant community. When Jeffrey Greenwood joined the firm in 1961 there were five partners and the total staff did not exceed fifty; by the time he retired as senior partner in 1995 Nabarro Nathanson had 134 partners and a staff of over 1,000. So impressed were some non-Jewish property developers with the

---

[46] Interview with Jeffrey Greenwood, 2 July 1998; *JC* 25 June 1948, p. 15 (obituary of Joseph Nabarro), 22 Oct. 1971, p. 22 (obituary of Felix Nabarro); *Dictionary of National Biography 1986–1990*, 395 (on Samuel).

service offered by the firm to their Jewish business rivals that they decided to become clients. Moreover, Nabarro Nathanson was able to use its reputation to attract substantial business from American Jewish clients. Maintaining its commercial property division as the core of its business, Nabarro Nathanson also has expertise in mergers and acquisitions, corporate finance, banking, insolvency, European law and media and entertainment law.[47]

Another leading West End solicitors' firm which acted for developers and floated property companies in the early 1960s was Brecher & Co. It was started in December 1952 by David Brecher, who was joined a couple of years later by his brother Henry. Articled to Herbert Baron, Henry had an excellent training in conveyancing, and often acted for a Jewish developer of residential property. When selling properties from residential estates, Henry sent the purchaser's solicitors complete packages of all documents normally prepared by the purchaser's solicitors, as well as the vendor's contract and searches, long before this became fairly common practice. In the 1960s Brecher was the biggest firm acting for the property developers, dealers, and investors—bigger than Nabarro Nathanson. During the 1960s Brecher & Co. acted mainly for the developers of commercial sites and for insurance companies such as Eagle Star, Allied Dunbar, and Pearl, which invested funds in urban land development projects. However, it also took on as much residential work as it wanted, numbering among its clients the very active house-builder and commercial property developer Bernard Sunley. The firm invented many new ways of reducing the amounts of tax paid by its clients, particularly when its partners worked with Godfrey Bradman, an accountant and later property developer who worked out some complicated tax-saving schemes. During the 1970s and 1980s Brecher & Co. branched out into property banking and corporate work. 'We were known as the best firm of estate agents in the West End', David Brecher confessed, 'because we were either acting for the vendor, purchaser, mortgagee, or mortgagor and very often for more than one of them . . . we were trusted, we never charged anything but legal fees, we never charged commissions or anything like that, getting finance for clients or for putting clients together.'[48] The litigation department, headed by Sidney Prevezer (1929–97), 'grew on the back of [the] property practice'. Prevezer, later professor of law at Sussex University, 'was a great strategist and a formidable manager of large scale litigation who paid assiduous attention to detail. He soon had a strong following of clients.'[49]

The third outstanding West End firm of property lawyers was Berwin Leighton, founded in 1939 by Lionel Lazarus (1914–82). On leaving the air

[47] *Law Society's Gazette*, 15 Sept. 1982 (obituary of Nathanson); interviews with Michael Max, 20 June 1997, and Jeffrey Greenwood, 2 July 1998. *Chambers & Partners Directory*, 786, 787.
[48] Interviews with Henry Brecher, 24 Sept. 1998, 2 Dec. 1998; interview with David Brecher, 2 Dec. 1998.   [49] *The Times*, 16 May 1997 (obituary of Prevezer).

force after the war, Lazarus established a firm bearing his own name, but after changing his own name to Lionel Lazarus Leighton he also changed the name of his practice, to Lionel Leighton & Co. During the 1960s he worked for several West End property developers. 'A lot of his clients were pure market traders who had gone into the property business. They were risk takers who were interested in the deal, not the detail. They came to Leighton's because the firm was young and imaginative', declared Lawrance Heller.[50] Two of Leighton's brothers were surveyors and estate agents in the West End, so he had good contacts with the new generation of property tycoons; Instone Bloomfield of Oddenino's Property was a major client. Leighton was a close friend of the entrepreneur Louis Mintz (1909–87), who built his company Selincourt into one of the largest exporters of garments in the country and also had considerable property interests. Leighton served for a time as chairman of the Selincourt group of companies. When Stanley Berwin was invited to join the Rothschild merchant bank, he left S. J. Berwin in the hands of a junior partner, and Leighton & Co., which was then looking for City premises, felt that the merger of the two firms would work very well; so Berwin Leighton, a firm with a City orientation, emerged on 1 December 1970.[51] Leighton retired from work as a solicitor at the age of 58. Brought up in a traditional Jewish home in Stamford Hill and influenced by the example of his great-uncle Simha Becker, the founder of the first Jewish temporary shelter for homeless and jobless immigrants, Leighton was a dedicated chairman of the Jewish Welfare Board for the last ten years of his life.

Having gained experience in the flotation of property companies and takeovers at Titmuss Sainer, Lawrance Heller was recruited by Leighton & Co. and became one of the founders of Berwin Leighton. He explained that

Berwin Leighton brought West End, high quality conveyancing to the City, where nearly all the conveyancing was purely institutional in the 1960s. The underlying rationale and the actual property position were not understood by [City] solicitors; as far as they were concerned, they did mortgages, they bought a property, they sold a property, but they did not understand and they did not get involved in what the business aim was. The West End firms . . . really were a commercial complement to the actual developers, and property dealers and investors; and there was great understanding between them.

During the 1970s, however, attitudes in the City institutions were changing, and some of 'the young Turks at Hambros Bank used to like using us [for certain transactions] because we had that little extra understanding of business requirements', declared Heller. With a first-class degree in law from Cambridge, Heller, who later became senior partner of Berwin Leighton, was also editor of

---

[50] Interview with Lawrance Heller, 24 June 1999.
[51] Interview with Graham Drucker, 6 July 1999; *JC* 16 Apr. 1982, p. 24 (obituary of Leighton); *The Times*, 6 May 1987 (obituary of Mintz); *Commercial Lawyer* (Oct. 1998), 30.

Sweet & Maxwell's *Conveyancing Precedents.*[52] By 1995 Berwin Leighton was an important City player with fifty-seven partners and eighty-three assistant solicitors; property remained at the core of the practice, comprising 41 per cent of its workload, but company and commercial work, including corporate finance and banking, had grown to 28 per cent.[53]

Leonard Sainer (1909–91) was one of London's leading corporate lawyers for over forty years. The son of an East End tailor, he was educated at the Central Foundation School and London University, graduating in law in 1929. His father then paid a fee of 500 guineas for him to be articled to Messrs Bullcraig & Davis, a firm of solicitors situated near the Strand. In 1931 Sainer handled the purchase of the Prince of Wales Theatre for £700 on behalf of Charles Clore. Gradually Sainer took on an increasing amount of work for Clore, which enabled him to buy a partnership share in Titmuss Sainer & Webb. After the war Sainer was the sole remaining partner and moved into offices first in Carey Street and later in Serjeant's Inn. Sainer now dealt with all of Clore's business dealings and a vast quantity of work flowed into the firm. In 1953 Clore, with the assistance of Sainer and his accountant, made a successful hostile takeover bid for J. Sears & Co. (Trueform Boot Co.) Ltd., after studying the tactics used in similar operations in the United States. Although the 920 retail premises owned by the company had a book value of £6 million, their market value was £10 million, which greatly exceeded anything Clore would have to pay for the shares. Once he had won the battle for Sears, Clore, again with the assistance of Sainer, perfected a scheme originally invented by Joseph Littman and Isaac Wolfson for exploiting the value of retail property by selling the freehold and buying back a long lease, a device known as sale and leaseback.[54]

Contemporaries regarded Sainer as a workaholic; he would go out partying at night with Clore and then return home to pore over papers from 11 p.m. until 3 a.m. Very tall, he was always quietly spoken and immaculately dressed. Clore's entrepreneurial imagination gave Sainer an extraordinary amount of experience and a rare degree of exposure to City financial institutions. He was a brilliant lawyer with an amazingly quick grasp, but this was allied with a sound common sense.[55] Lawrance Heller, who worked for him, recollected that 'Sainer was no pure lawyer . . . but in terms of running transactions and understanding and negotiating in commercial terms he had no equal at that time.'[56] Sainer joined the board of Sears and spent much time helping Clore with a series of takeovers of other companies—including restraining his more rash schemes. Among the

---

[52] Interview with Lawrance Heller, 24 June 1999.   [53] *Chambers & Partners Directory*, 542.
[54] *The Times*, 2 Oct. 1991 (obituary of Sainer); Clutterbuck and Devine, *Clore*, 64–81; Erdman, *People and Property*, 55.
[55] *The Times*, 2 Oct. 1991; interview with Michael Max, 26 June 1997.
[56] Interview with Lawrance Heller, 24 June 1999.

companies absorbed by Sears were the bookmakers William Hill (both Clore and Sainer were fascinated by horse-racing) and the Lewis Investment Trust Ltd., which owned a number of provincial department stores and Selfridges. He became a member of the board of other companies, too, including Beautility the furniture maker and the First National Finance Corporation, and advised London and County Securities. On taking over as chairman of Sears in 1978, he resigned as a partner in Titmuss Sainer, although he continued to send clients to his old firm until 1988. When Sainer died, he left a fortune of £6,461,283.[57]

Having no children of his own, Sainer found it difficult to accept management of the firm being conducted on an innovative basis by younger partners. While he demanded a high standard of expertise and sound practice from his staff, he did not believe in them spending much time doing research, and advised them to send short instructions to counsel, whose chambers were in any case nearby, for the answers. His major concern was to serve existing clients, and if new clients were to be taken on he was happier with those he selected himself than those found by his younger partners. Certainly he had a knack of attracting clients and making them feel confident in his advice and with the work of his partners. Sainer's chance encounter with Paul McCartney's brother-in-law on a flight to America led to the Beatles becoming clients of the firm. Despite the fact that Titmuss Sainer acted for Sears and others in the purchase of huge New York office buildings, the American side of the work was handled by a small law firm, without any thought on Sainer's part of establishing a reciprocal relationship with a larger American law practice. Titmuss Sainer expanded throughout the 1950s and 1960s, and although, like Nabarro Nathanson, the bulk of its work continued to be in property, it was no longer a one-client firm. While the firm seemed to mark time in the 1970s, when the property boom was over, under new management in the 1980s it doubled in size between 1985 and 1989 to a total of over 300 partners and staff. In contrast to Sainer's somewhat cautious approach, under these new leaders it merged with a large American law firm Dechert Price & Rhoads, now known internationally as Dechert. The profile of the firm much resembles that of Nabarro Nathanson: it is strong not only in the property sector, particularly retail, commercial investment, and development, but also in mergers and acquisitions, flotations, financial services, construction, and planning.[58]

Leslie Paisner (1909–79) was articled in 1925 to Harris Chetham & Cohen of 25 Finsbury Square, London, at a premium of £260. He had attended Whitechapel Foundation School, his parents having established themselves as

---

[57] Probate Office records.

[58] Interview with Michael Max, 26 June 1997; Edward Fennell, *Titmuss, Sainer & Webb: 50th Anniversary Brochure* (London: 1997). *Chambers & Partners Directory*, 888, 889.

wholesale confectioners in London's East End after their arrival from Latvia in 1900. In 1932 he set up Paisner & Co., a firm based in Bedford Square for many years, and which grew into a medium-sized City practice. In the late 1960s he was joined by his two sons, Harold and Martin Paisner, who became his partners. Paisner & Co. had a very active property department, dealing with commercial property for investors, developers, and lenders; it also had an important private client department, dispensing advice on tax planning and the establishment of trusts to both Jewish businessmen and others. Paisner & Co. expanded in the area of charity law and now act for all the major Jewish charities, including the United Jewish Israel Appeal (UJIA) and Jewish Care.

Leslie Paisner's practice embraced a very broad spectrum, covering leaders of the business community such as Isaac Wolfson, Charles Forte, and Sir James Goldsmith, and figures in politics, the arts, and entertainment.[59] He had acted for many years for the brilliant Labour politician Richard Crossman, the publication of whose diaries after his death became the subject of widely publicized injunction proceedings brought by the government in 1974 in an attempt to suppress them. Paisner & Co. represented the executors of the estate. The judgment not only established a precedent in the laws of confidentiality but also achieved the hope, expressed by Crossman, of lighting up 'the secret places of British politics'. In early 1969 the firm successfully acted for the late Judy Garland and Talk of the Town in injunction proceedings seeking to restrain what proved to be her last London appearance.

Much of the firm's growth may also be attributed to Leslie Paisner's close association with Isaac Wolfson who, as we have seen, purchased other companies at a phenomenal rate during the 1950s and into the 1960s. Under Wolfson's leadership Great Universal Stores prospered, absorbing Burberry's, Waring and Gillow, Jays and Campbells, Hope Brothers, and Global Tours as well as many mail-order companies. When he died in 1991 GUS had a stock market valuation of £3 billion, ranking behind only Marks & Spencer and the three largest food supermarket groups.[60] As a trustee of the Edith and Isaac Wolfson Charitable Trust which was set up in 1958, Leslie Paisner guided the distribution of large charitable sums. He was not only vice chairman of the Oxford Centre for Postgraduate Hebrew Studies and the Hillel Foundation, which supports Hillel Houses for Jewish students at various universities, but also served on the boards of the Great and Central Synagogues in London.[61]

Unfortunately, in 1976, after a severe motoring accident in Spain and serious

[59] *London Jewish News*, 26 Mar. 1999; John Pritchard, *The Legal 500* (London: Legalease, 1991), 366; Richard Ingrams, *Goldenballs* (London: Deutsch, 1979), 62, 70; Richard Crossman, *The Diaries of a Cabinet Minister*, ed. Janet Morgan (London: Hamilton and Cape, 1976), ii. 518.

[60] *The Times*, 21 June 1991; *JC* 28 June 1991, p. 15 (obituaries of Wolfson).

[61] *JC* 6 Apr. 1979, p. 34 (obituary of Paisner).

illness, Leslie Paisner became involved in a sensational libel action, *Sir James Goldsmith v. Private Eye*, the consequences of which, coupled with his ill health, led to his retirement from practice.[62]

Stanley Berwin (1926–88) 'was one of the most distinguished solicitors to practise in the City of London in the post-War years'. Born and educated in Leeds, he was articled to a solicitor in Allen & Overy, a City law firm, who took him on despite the fact that he was Jewish because of his war service in the navy. After he qualified in 1954 Berwin stayed at Allen & Overy several years, but, not reaching partnership rank, eventually moved to Herbert Oppenheimer, Nathan & Vandyk, where his talents were recognized and he did become a partner. He was a company and trust expert rather than a property lawyer.[63] Lord Young, who became friendly with him at this time in the late 1950s, remembered that

Lord Nathan, the senior partner, would appear on occasion but all of the commercial work would fall to Stanley [Berwin]. He was a workaholic, an inveterate cigarette smoker, except in the company of Isaac Wolfson, and a solicitor of immense ability and energy. He would often come in for instructions on a new acquisition late one evening and then reappear at 7.30 a.m. the following morning with a thirty-page purchase and sale agreement.[64]

Berwin was described as having a nervous temperament, very much like that of a fine racehorse, and after dissension with some of his colleagues at Herbert Oppenheimer, Nathan & Vandyk left the firm, taking some of his clientele with him, including British Land, GUS, the Steinbergs, and the Gestetners. In 1966 he founded his own firm, Berwin & Co., which four years later—as discussed above—merged with the West End practice of Lionel Leighton to become Berwin Leighton.[65] Whereas the Leighton practice had a heavy emphasis on property transactions, only 30 per cent of the business Berwin's firm handled was connected with property matters, and the bulk of its fees came from company work. In 1970 Berwin was invited by Jacob Rothschild to serve as a senior director of N. M. Rothschild & Sons, the merchant bankers; he became chairman of the Rothschild Trust Company and also deputy chairman of the Gresham Life Assurance Society Ltd. In 1975 Lord Rothschild once again took over as head of the merchant bank and, there allegedly being a tense relationship with his son, Jacob Rothschild left. As a result of these changes, Berwin returned to the law full-time, first as a consultant at Berwin Leighton and later, in 1982, as the founder of S. J. Berwin & Co. 'To create two city [law] firms bearing his name must be a unique achievement, but even more impressive is the way in which,

---

[62] Ingrams, *Goldenballs*, 33–141; Ivan Fallon, *Billionaire* (London: Hutchinson, 1991), 284–99.

[63] *Law Society's Gazette*, 14 Sept. 1988 (obituary of Berwin); *Law List 1956*, 1041; *Law List 1957*, 1041; private information.   [64] Young, *The Enterprise Years*, 11.

[65] *Law List 1966*, 1049; *Law List 1967*, 1066.

under his leadership, S. J. Berwin & Co. has become in six years an established City firm of more than 30 partners for many of whose clients Stanley Berwin was a confidant as well as a lawyer.'[66] He was deputy chairman of the British Land Company as well as a director of Wickes. 'He had all the attributes of a businessman,' asserted the property tycoon John Ritblat, 'but he would never involve himself in a pecuniary way with his client's business . . . We were contemporaries but he had an almost avuncular reserve of advice.'[67] Again, it was said of him that 'While always acting as the lawyer he so obviously was, he nevertheless was able to think like the businessmen he represented. With Berwin a client was never left in doubt as to the legal niceties of the particular situation; he then had pointed out to him quite clearly the line of action he should take.'[68]

Since its founder's death S. J. Berwin has continued to prosper. 'Though it is almost halfway down the *Lawyer*'s size-based list of the Top 100 firms, S. J. Berwin appears regularly in the top 10 or 20 in league tables of City activity. But it has not been welcomed into this charmed circle of blue chip firms.'[69] In a league table compiled in 1997 of top legal advisers on the takeover of public companies in the United Kingdom, the firm emerged in fourth place, pushing Linklaters & Paines into fifth position.[70]

David Freeman started the firm of D. J. Freeman & Co. in March 1952. A free spirit even at the age of 24, when he realized that career opportunities in the older City firms were closed to him because he was Jewish he decided to set up on his own. He opened his first office in Cannon Street in the City, moving within a short time to the West End, where he gradually developed a flow of insolvency work from two firms of accountants and later, in 1958, from the insolvency specialists Cork Gully, whose senior partner, Kenneth Cork, he had impressed. Freeman first attracted public attention in 1959, when he represented the Jasper group of companies at the Board of Trade inquiry into its activities; he also acted for Harry Jasper at the trial at the Central Criminal Court in the following year, when he was acquitted on charges of fraud. During the property boom in the 1960s Freeman travelled around the country on planning appeals and acquired a growing clientele of property developers. He acted for Jarvis Astaire and Charles Burkeman, who respectively married the two daughters of A. L. Oppenheim, a leading property developer, and assisted them in the flota-tion of Perthpoint Investments Ltd., and he was instructed by Alec Coleman in the purchase of the Foundling Estate in Bloomsbury for £1,775,000. County and District also became a valued property client. During the collapse of the property market and the recession of 1973–4 Freeman reverted increasingly to insolvency work to rescue fringe banks and property companies, including the

[66] *Law Society's Gazette*, 14 Sept. 1988.
[67] *Lawyer*, 7 July 1988.
[68] Private information.
[69] *Lawyer*, 26 May 1992.
[70] *The Times*, 9 Jan. 1998.

Lyon Group, the Stern Group, Guardian Properties, and the Israel–British Bank. In 1977 he was appointed a Department of Trade inspector to inquire into the affairs of AEG Telefunken (UK) Ltd. and Credit Collections Ltd.— the first solicitor to hold a position usually reserved for QCs.[71]

Tony Leifer remarked that D. J. Freeman 'was still rather a sole practice when I joined in 1970'. The change came in 1976: in March of that year six salaried partners became equity partners alongside David, his wife Iris Freeman, and Arthur Brown. After studying psychology at London University, Iris Freeman (1927–97) was admitted as a solicitor in January 1970 and joined her husband as a partner, at the same time setting up an employment law department. 'She acted for many prominent businesses but her cases rarely made headlines—she liked to smooth out problems before the press took an interest.' Leifer claimed that

David [Freeman] was a great rainmaker. He would put deals to people, put people together, he was never shy. He'd ring Maxwell, Tiny Rowland—he knew them all whether in business or politics. If he met someone casually, he'd make a point of getting to know them . . . You couldn't approach people directly. You had to know their friends, as it were, or their auditors; you had to find ways of being introduced; and you had to be useful to them. You could always ring them up for a proper purpose, with a proposition for instance.

By the 1970s Freeman was acting for Prime Minister Harold Wilson, Barclays Bank, Pearsons, and Rush & Tomkins. Between 1975 and 1980 the turnover of the firm jumped from £846,000 to £2,386,000; by 1987 it had leaped to £7.5 million and by 1990 to £24 million, a remarkable expansion. Within the firm this rapid growth sparked a debate whether it should stay in the West End or move to the City, and in 1982 D. J. Freeman & Co. moved to Fetter Lane in Holborn—an attractive location, close to the courts and counsel.[72]

The firm restructured itself in 1987, adopting for the first time the corporate concept of a chief executive, a position held first by Colin Joseph and then by David Solomon, working alongside the senior partner. The collapse of the property sector in 1990 affected all legal firms with a significant property practice. D. J. Freeman & Co. commissioned a consultancy review which led to the firm identifying target business sectors of insurance, litigation, and property, and remodelling itself accordingly. David Freeman retired as senior partner in March 1992, being succeeded by David Solomon, but continued as a consultant.

During the 1960s the recruitment of suitable articled clerks was no problem

---

[71] Iris Freeman, *D. J. Freeman & Co.: The First Twenty Five Years* (privately published; n.d.), 1–17; Chambers, 'The Rainmaker'.

[72] Chambers, 'The Rainmaker'; interview with David Solomon, *Lawyer*, 31 Mar. 1992; Karen Dillon, 'D. J. Freeman, Chapters 1, 2, and 3 but not 11', *Legal Business* (Sept. 1991), 33–40.

for these vibrant and fast-growing firms. While these practices were thought of as Jewish, because they included a number of eminent Jewish partners, they also attracted a talented group of people who were not Jewish. Professor Raphael Powell of the law department of University College London was asked by Leslie Paisner to recommend bright Jewish graduates to him; and many other Jewish graduates knocked on the doors of these firms because they knew that their talent would be recognized and welcomed. While the big City firms had their pick of the recruits, the large Jewish firms could also trawl in a pool of very able non-Jewish youngsters who had not found places in the City.[73]

Why was there a change in the attitude of the big City firms to the recruitment of Jews in the 1970s? As these firms expanded in size, and into finance-based work and markets overseas, they had to seek persons of the right intellectual calibre and with the necessary expertise whatever their origin or background. With the number of partners no longer limited to twenty since 1967 there were many more staff vacancies to fill, and it was difficult to find the requisite number of male recruits from traditional sources; thus recruitment had to be 'more competitive and more meritocratic'.[74] As yet there were relatively few women solicitors in the profession—Linklaters & Paines, for instance, did not admit a female partner until 1981. The Sex Discrimination Act 1975 and the Race Relations Act 1976 both helped to change and shape new public attitudes less sympathetic to discrimination on the basis of gender or ethnic origin.[75] During the Second World War large American law firms acting for corporate clients started hiring Jews as associates and by 1963 some of them had been made partners; so established did this trend become that by the end of the 1960s Erwin Smigel concluded that the discrimination against hiring Jews in the Wall Street law firms had 'essentially gone'.[76] An increasing amount of American work was being done in London, generated by Jewish interests or represented by Jewish lawyers from the United States, and when these Jewish clients or lawyers encountered solid phalanxes of solicitors with a WASP background in the City solicitors' offices, this began to cause raised eyebrows. There was thus a knock-on effect from the United States, where attitudes to the recruitment of Jews had changed a decade or two earlier.[77] Moreover, City firms began to understand that by keeping their doors closed to a generation of successful Anglo-Jewish businessmen they had lost an immense amount of profitable work and had also allowed a group of dynamic semi-Jewish firms to grow strong and in many cases seize the initiative from them.[78]

[73] Interview with Michael Max, 20 June 1997; Ingrams, *Goldenballs*, 62.

[74] Interview with Michael Max, 26 June 1997; Galanter and Paley, *Tournament of Lawyers*, 57.

[75] Judy Slinn, *Linklaters & Paines: The First One Hundred and Fifty Years* (London: Longman, 1987), 207.

[76] Smigel, *The Wall Street Lawyer*, 65, 66; Auerbach, *Unequal Justice*, 29, 184, 185; Galanter and Paley, *Tournament of Lawyers*, 25, 26.   [77] Interview with Michael Max, 20 June 1997.   [78] Ibid.

Until the 1970s most big City firms did not have Jewish partners, apart from the occasional member of an old upper-class Anglo-Jewish family; Herbert Montefiore Cohen (1877–1946), for example, who was educated at Rugby and Balliol College, Oxford, was a partner at Linklaters & Paines from 1911 to 1946. The next Jew to become a partner at Linklaters was from an entirely different background. Leonard Terry Berkowitz (b. 1936) was the son of a businessman who emigrated from Lithuania to South Africa. Leonard Berkowitz qualified as both an advocate and an attorney, becoming a partner in 1963 at Hayman Godfrey & Sanderson, a law firm with a corporate practice in Johannesburg. After emigrating to England in 1964, he joined Linklaters as an articled clerk in 1967, combining this with running a part-time London office for Hayman Godfrey & Sanderson. Admitted as a partner at Linklaters in 1972, Berkowitz did a wide range of corporate work, including privatizations. Twenty years later he was discussing the changed situation with a Jewish colleague, who remarked that they could probably form a *minyan* (a quorum of ten men for prayer) out of the number of Jewish partners at Linklaters & Paines.[79]

Slaughter & May, another City giant, admitted its first ever Jewish partner, N. N. Jacobs, in 1973. It was alleged that his fee-earning capacity was such that he was bringing in more money than some of the existing partners and that he was propelled into a partnership position despite his initial reluctance.[80] Michael Sayers was made a partner at Norton Rose even earlier, in 1965, taking over the leadership of the corporate finance section in the firm ten years later, while by 1998 Norton Rose had given five Jews partnership status.[81]

Exceptionally, there were certain large City firms, such as Herbert Smith and Clifford-Turner, which welcomed Jews as partners. The remarkable Francis Mann became a partner at Herbert Smith in the late 1950s and in 1991 was one of the first two solicitors to be made honorary Queen's Counsel.[82] His protégé Dr (now Sir) Lawrence Collins, a leading authority on international law and general editor of *Dicey and Morris: The Conflict of Laws*, was made a partner in 1971 and went on to head the litigation department. Dr Mann and Collins were the only practising solicitors to be elected Fellows of the British Academy. Among Collins's landmark cases were those in which he acted for certain American banks in London during the Iranian and Libyan crises, when the Americans froze these countries' funds on a worldwide basis, but under English law the banks were obliged to repay their customers; he also acted for British Caledonian in the Laker conspiracy case against British Airways and other

---

[79] Interview with Leonard Berkowitz, 2 Feb. 1997; Slinn, *Linklaters*, 231, 239.

[80] Laurie Dennett, *Slaughter and May: A Century in the City* (Cambridge: Granta, 1989), 267, private information.

[81] Andrew St George, *A History of Norton Rose* (Cambridge: Granta, 1995), 204, private information.   [82] *Daily Telegraph*, 2 Oct. 1991.

transatlantic carriers.[83] In 1997 Dr Collins became the second solicitor to be appointed Queen's Counsel, enabling him to represent the government of Chile in Augusto Pinochet's appeal against extradition in the House of Lords. He has now been elevated to the High Court bench, 'the first solicitor to come direct from practice in a law firm'.[84] Clifford Chance, Britain's largest law firm with 272 partners in 1999, was created by the merger of Coward Chance and Clifford-Turner in 1987.[85] David Gottlieb (1941–81) worked as an assistant solicitor at Slaughter & May, without much hope of promotion, despite obtaining distinctions in four papers of his solicitor's finals, until he joined Clifford-Turner in 1967. Here he was made a partner in 1971 and, with another solicitor, was asked to create a taxation department, which at the time of his death consisted of six partners assisted by a large staff.[86] Sir Victor Blank, a specialist in the law of company takeovers and the son of a Stockport tailor, became a partner in Clifford-Turner in 1969, going on to become chairman of the Charterhouse Bank, deputy chairman of Great Universal Stores, and chairman of the Mirror Group. At a partnership meeting of the law firm when his promotion was under discussion, someone asked, 'Was it relevant that Blank was Jewish?'[87] While at Charterhouse, Blank arranged the acquisition of F. W. Woolworth, allegedly making a substantial sum from the deal which gave him the wherewithal to buy an Elizabethan country house near Oxford.[88] Like most of the property lawyers, both Blank and Collins had strong Jewish affiliations. Collins is a regular worshipper at an Orthodox synagogue; Blank is on the board of the UJIA and was chairman of a major review of the work undertaken by communal organizations for Jewish students in 1998.

By the 1970s some of the large City firms, in particular Linklaters & Paines, were beginning to set up their own powerful property departments to compete with the Jewish firms; Ashurst Morris Crisp tempted two property specialists, Laurence Rutman and Barry Walker, away from Paisners. At the same time, some of the fast-growing Jewish firms began to receive instructions from major banks as well as insurance companies. According to Jeffrey Greenwood, a former senior partner at Nabarro Nathanson,

the City solicitors very jealously guarded their patch, and as you know, the merchant banks, the accepting houses, were not allowed to be outside the Square Mile; and this meant that in order to work for the banks, and that was really where the most lucrative

[83] *Libyan Arab Foreign Bank* v. *Manufacturers Hanover Trust Co.* (No. 1) (1988); *British Airways Board* v. *Laker Airways* (1984).
[84] *JC* 4 Apr. 1997, 25 Feb. 2000; interview with Lawrence Collins, 16 July 1999.
[85] Slinn, *Clifford Chance*, 163, 179.
[86] *Law Society's Gazette*, 26 Aug. 1981 (obituary of David Gottlieb).
[87] Sir Victor Blank, speaking at the Clifford Chance Hanukah party, 11 Dec. 2001.
[88] *JC* 3 July 1998, *Sunday Times*, 24 Jan. 1999.

work came from on the corporate side, you had to be within the City, within the Square Mile. I think the Jewish firms came to prominence because they generally acted for the companies which were then floated by the banks, so that if you look at some of the flotations of the 1960s and the 1970s you will tend to see that the Jewish firms acted for the companies, the entrepreneurs, and the non-Jewish firms acted for the institutions that floated them . . . Paisner's acted for Isaac Wolfson's companies and we acted for many of the major property companies, when they floated, but we never normally acted for the banks and other institutions. When London was opened up to international competition beginning in the 1970s, when the American banks came over in force, the Americans did not distinguish between a City firm and a West End firm, they just wanted a good firm; and that is when, of course, the distinction between a City firm and a non-City firm went.[89]

The 1990s saw a number of well-known law firms such as Olswang and Pritchard Englefield, move from the West End to the City, and two of the premier property practices which had failed to adapt in the manner of Nabarro Nathanson and Berwin Leighton disappeared. Brechers, which was geared to property development, was hit hard by the recession of 1992–3 and possibly had an unwieldy structure; ultimately this may have contributed to the break-up of the practice and its merger with Nicholson, Graham & Jones in 1995. It was estimated that Brechers would be able to provide 25 per cent of the income of the new venture. Nicholson, Graham & Jones was now a medium-sized City practice whose corporate clients included East Midlands Electricity, Blue Circle Industries, Bass, Inchcape, and the bankers Singer & Friedlander; as noted earlier in this chapter, it was built up by Ellis Birk, and later by Philip Morgenstern, one of a group of solicitors who advised Robert Maxwell. So too, in 1998 Forsyte Saunders Kerman merged with corporate lawyers Lawrence Graham, a sixty-seven-partner firm based in the Strand, in order to reduce its reliance on income generated from property work.[90]

Not all the West End law firms prospered so mightily as some of the firms I have described; a good example of the successful smaller practices is provided by the career of Margaret Spector (Mrs Ellis, 1905–79), one of the few Jewish women practising as solicitors after the Second World War. When she was admitted as a solicitor in 1931, she was the youngest female graduate of the Aberystwyth University Law School, having grown up in Dowlais, Glamorgan. When her brother died after the Second World War she continued to run her law practice on her own in Bournemouth and also took over and rejuvenated his practice in the West End. She developed a close working relationship with a

---

[89] Interviews with Lawrance Heller, 24 June 1999, Jeffrey Greenwood, 2 July 1998.

[90] Michael Chambers, 'City versus West End: A Case Study', *Commercial Lawyer* (Sept. 1996), 20–4; *Lawyer*, 1 Aug., 12 Sept. 1995, 24 Feb. 1998; *Commercial Lawyer* (Dec. 1997), 39, 40; Bower, *Maxwell*, 79, 214, 338–9.

couple of Greek insurance brokers, and had a large clientele for whom she did conveyancing work and arranged mortgages and loans. In addition, she dabbled in the property market, acquiring a valuable Victorian apartment building at 48–50 Whitfield Street W1. At her death in 1979 she left an estate of £263,744.[91]

*

Three dynamic Jewish solicitors of the post-war period—Arnold Goodman, David Napley, and Victor Mishcon—deserve special attention as having gained a national standing unequalled since Sir George Lewis. The oldest and perhaps the most intellectually brilliant of them was Arnold—at first Aby, corrected to Abraham in 1931, and later Anglicized—Goodman (1913–95). While still articled to a solicitor at Rubinstein Nash & Co., Goodman graduated with a second-class degree in law from University College London, to which he added an LLM with first-class honours. He supplemented these academic achievements by also obtaining first-class degrees in Roman and Roman–Dutch law from Cambridge. Goodman was articled to Harold Rubinstein, who as we have seen acted for the literary establishment of the country in the 1930s and 1940s, and from 1946 to 1950 worked for Royalton Kisch. When Ronald Rubinstein, who ran Rubinstein Nash & Co.'s litigation department, died prematurely a few years after the war, Goodman rejoined the firm to take charge of this department. Once again Goodman was plunged into libel and copyright actions connected with the world of publishing and gave legal advice to, among others, leading novelists of the day including J. B. Priestley, Graham Greene, and Evelyn Waugh. Goodman's memoirs, written when he was ill, are not always accurate; he claims that he advised Waugh that an interview published by Nancy Spain, a journalist on the *Daily Express*, was probably libellous but that a novelist of his distinction should ignore it, evoking contempt from the celebrated author. In fact, after court proceedings Rubinstein Nash obtained damages of £2,000 plus costs against the newspaper for libel. Not content with this, Waugh, with his solicitor's assistance, compelled the *Daily Express* to pay him £3,000 for another hostile article verging on the libellous which was written by Nancy Spain, when the other action had not been concluded and was still *sub judice*.[92]

In 1953 Goodman left Rubinstein Nash to set up his own firm, Goodman Derrick & Co. According to his memoir his departure 'was a friendly one'; in fact, he took with him many clients from the literary world and elsewhere, causing much resentment among his former colleagues.[93] Goodman built up

[91] *JC* 11 Jan. 1929, p. 29; *Law Society's Gazette*, 26 Sept. 1979; *Estates Gazette*, 11 May 1968; *Spector v. Applefield Properties Ltd and Another, Spector v. Ageda*, 3 All ER 1971, p. 417; Probate Office Records.

[92] Goodman, *Tell Them I'm On My Way*, 22–96; interview with Michael Rubinstein, 20 Jan. 1997; Christopher Sykes, *Evelyn Waugh* (London: Collins, 1975), 387–9.

[93] Goodman, *Tell Them I'm On My Way*, 97–103; interview with Michael Rubinstein, 20 Jan. 1997.

a practice orientated towards literature, the theatre and the arts generally. In the early 1960s the expanding world of commercial television beckoned him and the complex and remunerative law of copyright and libel sang its siren song to good effect. Solicitors and accountants were much in demand on the boards of companies. Goodman became chairman of the newly constituted board of British Lion Films.[94]

Through his contacts in the world of television, first with Associated Rediffusion and then with Television for Wales and the West (TWW) and Granada, Goodman established a substantial practice in media and entertainment law. TWW purchased a group of theatres and also Dollond & Aitchison, one of the largest chains of opticians in the world, for which his firm did all the legal work.[95] He also acted for one of the leading post-war property developers Harry Hyams, and proposed a deal with the London County Council under which Hyams would buy all the land in St Giles Circus, surrender a portion to the LCC for a road and in return be allowed to build a taller office block—the building which became known as Centre Point.[96] Goodman strengthened his links with the property sector when he reorganized the Portman estate in the mid-1950s by selling valuable sites in central London, and he drew up the will and settlements of the property magnate Lewis Hammerson, subsequently advising his widow.[97]

In many respects Goodman's career resembled that of Sir George Lewis, particularly as a libel lawyer and an associate of the theatrical and literary elite, and was even more remarkable because of the influence he was able to wield. Richard Davenport-Hines has asserted that he 'emerged in the 1960s as one of the most effective fixers and freelance political advisers in twentieth century Britain. His nearest counterpart was Lord Esher . . . Yet Goodman was less serpentine and mischievous than Esher, genuinely keen to be helpful and do good, though not without his own form of sly self-importance.'[98]

Through George Wigg MP Goodman was introduced to such leading Labour politicians as Hugh Gaitskell, Harold Wilson, Aneurin Bevan, and Bevan's wife Jennie Lee. He first came to public prominence in 1957, when he won a celebrated libel action against the *Spectator* which came out with a slur against Bevan and other Labour politicians, accusing them of being drunk while on a trip abroad. His reputation was further boosted when he settled a strike in the television industry in 1964 but was reluctant to be named or photographed and hence was dubbed 'Mr X' by Harold Wilson, the Labour party leader.[99] Within

[94] *The Times*, 15 May 1995 (obituary of Goodman); see also *Independent*, 15 May 1995.
[95] Goodman, *Tell Them I'm On My Way*, 97–103; Brian Brivati, *Lord Goodman* (London: Richard Cohen, 1999), 74, 75, 94, 220, 224.   [96] Brivati, *Lord Goodman*, 253–8.
[97] Ibid. 94, 254, 284.   [98] *Times Literary Supplement*, 27 Aug. 1993.
[99] Goodman, *Tell Them I'm On My Way*, 163–70, 183–218; Brivati, *Lord Goodman*, 45–63, 83–4, 126–7.

months of the new Labour administration taking office he was made a life peer by Wilson, although he chose to sit on the cross benches, and was used by both Wilson and his Conservative successor, Edward Heath, to try to negotiate a settlement with Ian Smith in Rhodesia.[100] Richard Crossman treated Goodman as an invaluable unofficial adviser in the framing of the 1964 Rent Act, praising him as a resourceful man, full of ideas not only for overcoming gaps in the legislation but also for devising an acceptable formula for fixing a fair rent. On Sunday evenings Jennie Lee, the minister for the arts, would have dinner with Goodman, and after looking through his papers 'Goodman would suggest suitable memos that she might care to write to him, and suitable replies that she might care to receive from him.' Between 1965 and 1972 he was chairman of the Arts Council, working closely with Jennie Lee on many projects and in six years trebling the government's funding of the arts as well as raising money from philanthropists to rescue the London Festival Ballet.[101] Together with Lee, he pushed through the scheme for a National Theatre. Goodman also helped settle an unseemly squabble between Barbara Castle, the minister of health, and the consultants about private beds in NHS hospitals. He acted for a number of powerful newspaper proprietors including David Astor (with whom he forged a close relationship), Sir Max Aitken, and Rupert Murdoch, and from 1970 to 1975 he was chairman of the Newspaper Publishers' Association, negotiating adroitly with the printing unions. From 1976 to 1986 he was master of University College, Oxford, raising funds for fellowships and obtaining money from a benefactor that secured the future of the Oxford Union, the university's premier student debating society. At the time of his appointment as master he held the chairmanships of no fewer than nineteen important public bodies, including the Housing Corporation.[102]

Goodman advised several members of the royal family, including Prince Charles; when the heir to the throne sought legal comment about his matrimonial problems, Goodman steered him in the direction of another solicitor of Jewish origin, Fiona Shackleton of Farrer & Co. Ms Shackleton was a member of the Charkham, Salmon and Gluckstein families, although she had married into the non-Jewish family of the renowned explorer Ernest Shackleton. After completing her articles at Herbert Smith she moved to Brecher & Co., where she became a divorce lawyer, gaining a partnership at 25, and in 1984 she was approached to join Farrer & Co. 'Fiona has been handling the matrimonial problems of HRH because Lord Goodman pointed her out to the prince', a

---

[100] Brivati, *Lord Goodman*, 192–206; Goodman, *Tell Them I'm On My Way*, 219–29.

[101] Crossman, *Diaries*, i. 30, 40, 63, 75, 77, 78, 90; Patricia Hollis, *Jennie Lee: A Life* (Oxford: Oxford University Press, 1997), 227, 250–95.

[102] Brivati, *Lord Goodman*, 215–37, 262–5; Goodman, *Tell Them I'm On My Way*, 243–4, 440–1; *JC* 19 May 1995 (obituary of Goodman).

friend of Shackleton's claimed in 1996. 'It has only just emerged that she is advising the heir to the throne over his divorce, but it has been the case for some time.'[103]

Like Sir George Lewis, Goodman was consulted not only by members of the aristocracy but by the great and the not so good when they wished to conceal certain dark episodes in their lives; and, again like Sir George, Goodman was not above bullying his opponents with legal threats in order to protect his clients, even when he sometimes had doubts about the latter's veracity. On 12 July 1964 the *Sunday Mirror* proclaimed that a peer, who was 'a household name', had formed a homosexual relationship with a West End gangster infamous for his protection rackets. Wilson called in Goodman to protect the peer in question— a Conservative, Robert Boothby—because he feared that too much newspaper coverage of this story (although Boothby was not named initially) would divert public attention and undermine Labour's chances of victory at the impending election. A letter from Boothby (drafted by Goodman) denying the story was published by *The Times*, and with Scotland Yard refusing to reveal privileged information, Goodman forced the *Mirror*'s publishers to climb down and pay Boothby damages of £40,000. Again, when Norman Scott claimed that he had participated in a homosexual relationship with Jeremy Thorpe, the Liberal party leader instructed Goodman as his solicitor to conceal the truth. If a newspaper hinted about this relationship, Goodman 'would telephone the editor and point out that his client was an honest man and that Scott was a proven liar. If they were stubborn he fired off letters threatening terrible consequences if his client, the Rt Hon. Jeremy Thorpe, MP, PC, was accused of anything.' Further,

Lord Goodman deftly rewrote history and said that he had barely known Wilson or Thorpe and had certainly not been involved in the events leading to the trial at the Old Bailey [in 1979]. The obituaries after his death . . . did not mention Thorpe which was a posthumous triumph for Goodman. He had fought hard to protect him when Penrose closed in for the kill and spent the rest of his life insisting that he had not been involved with Thorpe.

On the other hand, it could be argued that Goodman felt that it was in Thorpe's best interests to be represented by the most brilliant criminal lawyer in the country, David Napley.[104]

According to Jeffrey Maunsell, a younger partner in Goodman Derrick & Co., Goodman 'had a combination which a lot of the very best solicitors have: an

[103] *Lawyer*, 29 Sept. 1992.
[104] *Sunday Times*, 8 Aug. 1993; Brivati, *Lord Goodman*, 84–8; Simon Freeman and Barrie Penrose, *Rinkgate: The Rise and Fall of Jeremy Thorpe* (London: Bloomsbury, 1996), 120, 129, 204, 225, 238–40, 273, 276–8, 289, 389.

extremely agile brain, a great academic intelligence . . . He coupled this with a great practical pleasure in dealing with matters, getting to the bottom of a problem and then negotiating.' To Lord Hoffman, he had 'an extremely quick mind able to pick up very rapidly what the issue was' between parties in contention; and then a facility 'by the exercise of personal charm' of 'lowering the temperature of a dispute'. Edward Walker-Arnott suggested that Goodman 'approached things tangentially, joking' and making the parties feel at ease, and then extracting 'concessions from them by good humour'. Hoffman declared that Goodman had a talent for persuading 'people to accept a form of words to bridge their differences'. Goodman, with a brilliant academic record at Cambridge and in the Law Society examinations, where he ranked equal second out of 500 candidates, was more than a mere fixer: he was a superb lawyer, a master of the profession consulted by other solicitors.[105]

Since his death, Goodman's standing as an honest broker has been questioned and he has been accused of siphoning £1 million (a sum which would today be worth £10 million) from the estate of Viscount Portman, a Tory peer, which he had administered for thirty years. It was alleged that 40 per cent of the money went to assist prominent Labour figures, including Harold Wilson, the former prime minister, and to buy influence. A writ was served by Lord Portman against Goodman and Goodman Derrick shortly before Goodman died. To settle this dispute and to reassure their clients, his partners in Goodman Derrick paid £500,000 to the trustees of the Portman estate, although they scrupulously accounted for every item that had passed through the account and denied all charges of impropriety.[106] The newspaper proprietor David Astor, a friend of Goodman, stated that 'I have been given enough confidential information about Lord Portman's allegations from reliable sources to say that these allegations and the way they have been publicly presented have given a false impression. That impression will be effectively demolished in due course.'[107] Another friend, the barrister and former editor of the *Jewish Chronicle* William Frankel, rebutted the accusations of Goodman's recent biographer that his subject was 'self-important, falsely modest and snobbish', saying, 'Few who knew him saw him in that light.'[108] On the contrary, Goodman's friends assert that he performed many acts of kindness to obscure individuals and helped little-known charities to raise funds, with little thought of self-advancement. In fact, he paid so little attention to financial matters that towards the end of his life he

---

[105] Iris Freeman interviews with Jeffrey Maunsell, Edward Walker-Arnott, and Lord Hoffman; Goodman, *Tell Them I'm On My Way*, 29–30; interview with Ellis Birk, 25 Sept. 1997.

[106] *The Times*, 19 Jan. 1999, 21 Jan. 1999, 25 Jan. 1999, 5 May 1999 (obituary of Viscount Portman); *Independent*, 18 Jan. 1999; Brivati, *Lord Goodman*, 274–8.   [107] Brivati, *Lord Goodman*, 278.

[108] *JC* 22 Oct. 1999.

had to sell a small collection of paintings to buy his retirement bungalow outside Oxford. As David Astor noted,

He was in fact distinguished in public and private life by his strict fidelity to the truth, his total confidentiality and his scrupulous care in all his dealings. This was the basis of all his many influential relationships . . . No doubt like the rest of us, he made mistakes. But when the details of whatever muddle he may have become involved in in his last years are revealed, they seem highly unlikely to have any serious effect on his great and real reputation.[109]

David Naphtali (1915–94), who later Anglicized his surname to Napley, qualified as a solicitor in 1937. As an insurance broker, his father had some contact with lawyers through insurance claims, and David was articled to Philip Emanuel, who, as described in an earlier chapter, ran a busy solicitor's office in Great Russell Street in central London. Napley, despite efforts in his memoirs to play down his own intellectual gifts, was exceedingly bright—as witnessed by a fellow articled clerk who saw him walk out halfway through a Law Society exam, having successfully completed the paper. After the Second World War he resumed his former partnership with Sidney Kingsley (1913–92), forming the firm of Kingsley Napley with a main office in Lincoln's Inn. Kingsley was a very able lawyer in his own right, respected for his 'commercial skill and experience in the property world' and 'his stamina as a negotiator'. This was yet another Jewish law firm whose fortunes were tied to the entrepreneurial skills of the new breed of Jewish property developers.[110]

Napley was at first interested primarily in the law of auctions and estate agents, writing *Law on the Remuneration of Auctioneers and Estate Agents* (1947) and the 1954 edition of Bateman's *Law of Auctions*. However, increasingly he felt himself drawn towards advocacy, and in 1946 opened a branch office of his firm near the Clerkenwell magistrates' court in King's Cross, where he built up a formidable reputation in criminal and licensing work.[111] He acted in many high-profile cases and played a leading role in the establishment in 1958 of the British Academy of Forensic Sciences. In 1968 he represented Robert Lipman, a wealthy young American who was convicted of murdering Claudie Delbarre while on an LSD trip—a conviction Napley always doubted, taking the view that she could have fallen and caused injuries to herself. In 1988 he acted for the actress Maria Aitken when she posted a series of envelopes from Peru to her London address which contained cocaine, but not for her own use. She pleaded guilty and was fined, but the envelopes continued to arrive; Napley and George

[109] *The Times*, 25 Jan. 1999.

[110] Napley, *Not Without Prejudice*, 12, 15; interview with Barnett Saffron, 15 May 1997; *Independent*, 16 Sept. 1992; *JC* 9 Oct. 1992, p. 11 (obituary of Kingsley).

[111] Napley, *Not Without Prejudice*, 238–55; *The Times*, 27 Sept. 1994, *Guardian*, 27 Sept. 1994, *Daily Telegraph*, 27 Sept. 1994 (obituaries of Napley).

Carman QC were able to persuade the Customs and Excise not to prosecute, as this was still part of the original offence. He was the solicitor for the Calvi family after what appeared to be the rigged suicide of the Pope's banker, and he was retained by Guinness after the Department of Trade and Industry's investigation into the company's affairs.[112] Other notable clients were Princess Michael of Kent (who obtained an out-of-court settlement); the surgeon at the inquest in November 1982 into the death of Helen Smith, a nurse who died in strange circumstances in Jeddah, Saudi Arabia;[113] and Sarah Tisdall, accused of leaking Foreign Office secrets to the *Guardian*. Moreover, through his expertise in licensing law, Napley saved the Mario & Franco chain of restaurants, which grew into a flourishing group of which he became chairman.

David Napley is best remembered for his role in the trial of Jeremy Thorpe for conspiracy to murder Norman Scott. In his memoirs Napley recounted how Arnold Goodman approached him, 'saying that . . . the police might wish to interview Jeremy [Thorpe], and as this impinged on a field more in my line than his he had suggested after discussion with Jeremy that I might take over the task of representing him'. The Crown's case against Thorpe rested on the evidence of Andrew Newton, a convicted man and perjurer, and Peter Bessell, a former Liberal MP who had been granted immunity from prosecution. For the first few weeks of taking instructions from Thorpe, Napley worked closely with John Montgomery, a partner in Goodman Derrick, 'with occasional meetings with Arnold Goodman at his London flat'. The nub of the prosecution case was based on the enquiries of two journalists, Barry Penrose and Roger Courtier, who had published a book called *The Pencourt File* (1978), and Thorpe was carefully questioned by Napley as regards the contents of the book.[114]

Napley, as was his custom, decided to conduct the committal proceedings, at the Minehead magistrates' court in November 1978, himself, instead of employing a barrister, and sought the concurrence of Arnold Goodman and George Carman, who had been instructed as counsel, on this point. Bessell praised Napley's decision to use old-style committal proceedings to cross-examine prosecution witnesses. 'The dress rehearsal', Bessell later declared, 'was used by the defence, and in particular by Napley himself, to probe and explore the weaknesses in an extremely complex case, in which the prosecution relied far too heavily on witnesses, including me, whose reputations and credibility were well open to attack.'[115]

The trial of Thrope and several other co-defendants opened at the Old Bailey on 8 May 1979. Napley invented a defence for Thorpe that Bessell and

---

[112] *Lawyer*, 4 Sept. 1990; *Guardian*, 24 June 1997.
[113] Paul Foot, *The Helen Smith Story* (London: Fontana, 1983), 296–8, 312–13, 359–60.
[114] Napley, *Not Without Prejudice*, 392–6.
[115] Ibid. 402–16; Freeman and Penrose, *Rinkgate*, 337–45.

Pencourt had 'orchestrated' the whole story—about Thorpe inciting others to murder Scott after he threatened to reveal their homosexual relationship—in order to make money by publishing their own sensational account. Peter Taylor, the prosecution counsel and later Lord Chief Justice, was aghast at the provision in Bessell's contract with the *Sunday Telegraph* by which his remuneration would be doubled if Thorpe were convicted, for he knew that when this came out in court it would destroy his credibility with the jury; and this is what happened. Taylor was scrupulous, some thought over-cautious, in not trying to introduce evidence about Thorpe's alleged homosexuality to the jury. Carman mercilessly cross-examined Scott, forcing him to admit that he had persistently lied and destroying his credibility as a witness. Fortunately for Thorpe, out of a sense of loyalty his co–defendants David Holmes and John Le Mesurier did not go into the witness box, for their evidence might well have undermined Thorpe's case and forced him to give evidence, something which he wished at all costs to avoid. In addition, the prosecution had been supplied with a letter from Thorpe to a friend in the United States which contained explicit allusions, but which they could not use unless Thorpe himself gave evidence. Holmes's solicitor David Freeman told friends that Thorpe was an 'unpleasant windbag with superficial charm', who had tricked his client into participating in the plot against Scott. In the event all the defendants, including Thorpe, were acquitted.[116]

Sir David Napley was knighted after serving as the president of the Law Society in 1976/7, the first Jew to head the solicitors' professional body. In a tribute to him in the *Law Society's Gazette* after his death, Sir Richard Gaskell wrote that 'From time to time, a practitioner of extraordinary stature emerges, standing head and shoulders above his peers. David Napley was such a man.' *The Times* remarked that 'Through his readiness . . . to give radio and television interviews and through his own prolific contributions to legal debate in the press, he achieved in his later years of practice the kind of status in the public mind that a few famous counsel had in the first half of this century.' Napley wore beautiful suits and drove around in a light brown Rolls-Royce which the press described as being gold-coloured. He was a flamboyant figure and a brilliant self-publicist, boasting that he had a supply of champagne in the boot of his car. He asserted that he was not only the best solicitor in the country but also the most expensive, a claim that appeared to be borne out in 1982 when it became known that in one case he was charging an hourly rate of £164, then a colossal sum. Yet he often represented solicitors who were appearing before the Law Society's disciplinary tribunal, sometimes free of charge; and if he believed that someone had been unjustly convicted, such as Michael Luvaglio, he would

116 Napley, *Not Without Prejudice*, 418–28; Freeman and Penrose, *Rinkgate*, 339, 347–66.

take his case to the Court of Appeal and the House of Lords, even though the legal aid fees paid in such cases were much lower than those he commanded in private practice. None the less, the more time that Napley devoted to enhancing the status of the profession, the less time he spent in the office; and it is noticeable that over the years his relations with his partner Sidney Kingsley cooled, so much so that he barely mentioned Kingsley in his memoirs.[117]

The third member of the triumvirate of charismatic post-war Jewish solicitors is Victor Mishcon (b. 1915), ennobled in 1978 as Lord Mishcon. His father, Arnold Mishcon, was the founder and rabbi of the Brixton United Synagogue and a *dayan* (judge in a rabbinical court); but he was also on friendly terms with all the local clergy, including the vicar, the Roman Catholic priest, and the Unitarian minister. Something of the same broadness of vision was inherited by his son.[118]

Victor Mishcon, having qualified as a solicitor at the age of 21 in 1937, opened a practice in the Brixton area, where he had many contacts in the local Jewish community. His father decided that Victor should become a solicitor because 'To be a barrister, in those days, one had to be wealthy.' After the war Mishcon retained his original Brixton office but opened additional south London offices in Wimbledon and Stockwell; his was very much a suburban and working-class practice, though he also had a central London office in Southampton Place. In the 1950s the Mishcon practice in Brixton throve under the guidance of Leon Simmons, its dedicated managing clerk. The clientele were mostly working-class, and it was so busy on Saturdays (when the work was handled by non-Jewish and non-Orthodox staff) that it had to close the doors of the office on the crowd of potential clients who had gathered outside. The practice mainly handled civil and matrimonial legal aid claims and did very little criminal legal aid work.[119]

In 1955 Ruth Ellis, the last woman to be executed in Britain for murder, instructed Mishcon to add a codicil to her will, and he went to see her in the condemned cell. Before her execution she made a full confession to Mishcon, stating that she was not the lone killer she had been portrayed as during her trial. Ellis told him that before the fatal shooting she had been drinking Pernod for many hours with her older 'sugar daddy', Desmond Cussen, who had handed her a loaded gun and driven her to David Blakely's home, where she killed her ex-lover, of whom Cussen was insanely jealous. Mishcon rushed to the Home Office to apply to the Home Secretary for a reprieve. But a prison officer present at the interview claimed that Ellis said that she had asked Cussen for the gun.

---

[117] *Law Society's Gazette*, 12 Oct. 1994; *The Times*, 27 Sept. 1994; Freeman and Penrose, *Rinkgate*, 338; *Guardian*, 27 Sept. 1994; Napley, *Not Without Prejudice*, 270–302.

[118] *JC* 18 Aug. 1995, p. 21.

[119] *JC* 18 Aug. 1995, p. 21; interview with Edward Toeman, 2 July 1998; *Law List 1957*, 1154, 1281, 1291.

Although the reprieve was not granted, the Home Office believed her account sufficiently some months later to consider having Cussen charged as an accessory to murder.[120]

During the 1940s and 1950s, following the example of Lewis Silkin, Mishcon plunged into local government politics and at the same time continued to be actively involved in the Jewish community, serving as president of the British Technion Committee, president of the Association for Jewish Youth, vice-president of the Board of Deputies, and chairman of the Institute for Jewish Studies. In the course of these activities he made many new contacts and clients. Shortly after the war he served as chairman of the finance committee of Lambeth Borough Council; he also became a member of the London County Council in 1946, rising through the ranks to hold various committee chairmanships, and in 1954 became the youngest twentieth-century leader of the council. However, despite four attempts in the 1950s to become an MP, Mishcon failed to be elected and thenceforth concentrated his energies elsewhere.[121]

During the 1960s and 1970s Mishcon had an interest in Blatchfords, a solicitors' practice based at Norwich House, Southampton Place, which undertook a considerable amount of litigation for trade unions, including the merchant seamen's and agricultural workers' unions. The office also dealt with an endless stream of industrial accident and motor insurance claims, sometimes almost being overwhelmed by the volume of work.[122]

By the late 1960s Mishcon had closed his Wimbledon office and the character of the practice was changing, with more and more commercial work being handled in his central London office; but it was still, as Anthony Julius remembered in 1981, a 'small, typical commercial practice with private client work', working for 'small companies, two or three public companies, a number of private clients, a lot of charities, [and] a lot of Jewish charities'.[123] Among Mishcon's business clients were Lord Palumbo, Robert Maxwell, and Gerald Ronson, whom he advised to pay back the 'success fee' of £5 million which he had received from Guinness to support their takeover bid for Distillers in 1986. Ronson has since been cleared by the European Court of Human Rights in Strasbourg for being denied his basic right to silence; with the implementation of the Human Rights Act, he is applying for a similar ruling in England, which could lead to the quashing of his conviction as opposed to a pardon.[124] Mishcon assisted Lord Archer in sorting out his finances to avoid bankruptcy, and acted

[120] *Guardian*, 19 Jan. 1999. The charge was never in fact brought.

[121] *Who's Who 1996*, 1346; *Sunday Times*, 28 Aug. 1994.

[122] Interview with Edward Toeman, 2 July 1998.

[123] *Law List 1966*, 1185 and 1249; *Law List 1968*, 1215; Dominic Egan, 'A Very Peculiar Practice', *Legal Business* (July–Aug. 1994), 22–31.

[124] *Sunday Times*, 28 Aug. 1994; Adam Raphael, *My Learned Friends* (London: Allen, 1989), 1–41; *The Times*, 4, 13 Jan. 2001.

for him in 1987 in a sensational libel suit against the *News of the World* and the *Star*, when it was alleged that Archer had offered a prostitute money to prevent her from talking about their relationship. The case went in Archer's favour, securing him damages of £500,000. But at a new trial in July 2001 Archer was convicted of lying and falsifying the evidence to secure victory in his libel action in 1987, for which he was given a four-year prison sentence.[125] Through Mishcon's friendship with Lord Palumbo, his services were recommended to the late Princess of Wales when she needed a lawyer to advise her on divorce proceedings, and the duchess of York also became a client.

Mishcon's eminence is said to have aroused jealousy in the legal profession. 'People just don't understand why a medium-sized, West End Jewish firm is acting for British royalty—to some in the Establishment, Diana's choice is inexplicable.'[126] In 1983 he became chief opposition spokesman on home affairs in the House of Lords; in 1990 he was appointed shadow Lord Chancellor and in 1992 was made an honorary QC. To one observer, in old age Mishcon's mind remained 'still as sharp as ever. He has great originality of thought and also kindness and stability. Though he will fight for his clients it is always done with good manners and an old-fashioned avoidance of personal acrimony. But never think he is a soft touch.'[127] For example, in the Archer libel action Mishcon telephoned the *Star*'s solicitors in January 1987, before the case came to court, suggesting a settlement whereby the newspaper would pay Archer a large sum of damages together with his costs, and print an apology on the front page. As the last point was unpalatable to the *Star* the offer was rejected—and at the end of the court proceedings the newspaper paid out much more than it need have done as a consequence.

By the time Lord Mishcon retired as senior partner in 1992 and became a consultant with Mishcon de Reya, his clientele resembled that of a pukka City firm rather than the Brixton-based office which he himself had started. Like Goodman Derrick, Mishcon de Reya had a particular expertise in commercial, property, and media work as well as some libel specialists on their staff. The resignation of so charismatic a figure as Mishcon left a power vacuum within the firm, and the individual best placed to fill it was Anthony Julius (b. 1956), Mishcon de Reya's young and dynamic litigation expert. Before Julius came along the litigation section was 'a service department', but by 1994 it had vastly expanded and was 'the engine room of the firm', accounting for 75 per cent of Mishcon de Reya's revenue in 1996.[128] Because of the success of his department, Julius became de facto head of the firm, causing, it is alleged, some

---

[125] *News of the World*, 21 Nov. 1999; *Evening Standard*, 2 Dec. 1999; *Evening Standard*, 19 July 2001; *The Times*, 20 July 2001.   [126] *Sunday Times*, 28 Aug. 1994.

[127] Raphael, *My Learned Friends*, 16–17.

[128] Egan, 'A Very Peculiar Practice', 25; *Legal Business* (Apr. 1998), 18; *JC* 4 Nov. 1994.

differences with colleagues. Between 1996 and 1998 about a third of Mishcon de Reya's partners left. Some cited clashes with Julius, but he denied that any partner had left because of him.[129]

In any event, Julius did much of the actual leg-work on Diana's behalf. When the *Mirror* published photographs of the leotarded princess exercising in a West London gym, she at first saw Lord Mishcon, but it was Julius who obtained an injunction against the newspaper and negotiated a settlement, with a payment being made to charity. A rapport was established between them, and it was natural that Julius would act for her in the divorce; in the process, while obtaining a £17 million divorce settlement for her, he ruffled the feathers of the royal family and their advisers, who allegedly found him 'far too abrasive'. On the other hand, his toughness attracted Gill Faldo when she divorced her golfer husband Nick, and Jerry Hall and Frank Bruno's wife also consulted him on domestic matters. Earlier in the 1980s, he was one of the lawyers who, according to the *Sunday Times*, by 'aggressive and largely successful' tactics prevented information about Robert Maxwell from being published. 'Maxwell never believed in subtlety or understatement,' Julius recalled, 'and was adamant about stopping bookshops from selling unauthorised biographies of him.'[130]

In revenge for Julius's victory against them in the affair of the gym photographs, the *Mirror* unleashed an outcry against Mishcon de Reya on 15 January 1998. Under a headline 'Shameful', they published the news that 'Diana's legal firm charges Memorial Fund £500,000 for 11 weeks' work.' The story was taken up by the rest of the national press, forcing the trustees of the fund to say that they would put all their future professional work out to tender; and Harbottle & Lewis eventually replaced Mishcon de Reya as legal advisers to the fund. Much of the criticism was in fact unfair, as Julius with his team of lawyers had gone to considerable trouble to establish unprecedented control over Princess Diana's image and name by registering them as trademarks in Britain, Europe, and the United States, in order to ensure that the profits from the sale of Diana memorabilia flowed into the trust fund; and a 20 per cent discount was allowed on Mishcon de Reya's fees, which was the equivalent of their normal profit margin. On 9 April 1998, however, after there had been a marked fall in the income generated by the litigation department, Julius left the partnership, continuing as a consultant for three days a week.[131] Despite this change of direction, Julius considerably enhanced his reputation by his successful defence of the historian Deborah Lipstadt in a libel action brought by David Irving against Ms Lipstadt and her publisher, Penguin Books, over the issue of Holocaust denial. Julius put

[129] *The Times*, 10 Jan. 1998.   [130] *Sunday Times*, 18 Jan. 1998; *Guardian*, 19 Jan. 1998.
[131] *Evening Standard*, 2 Dec. 1997, *Mirror*, 15, 16 Jan. 1998; *The Times*, 16 Jan., 21 Jan. 1998; *Sunday Times*, 6 Dec. 1998; *Legal Business* (Apr. 1998), 18.

the plaintiff on the defensive by persuading the court to grant wide-ranging discovery of Irving's papers, including his diaries.[132]

As far as the Jewish identity of these three lawyers was concerned, both Lord Mishcon and Lord Goodman had a strong Jewish identity, whereas Sir David Napley's ties with the Jewish community were tenuous. According to one informant, both Lord Goodman's parents were teachers at Hebrew and religion classes for children held at the Villareal School in the East End. His mother 'remained throughout her life a most devoted member of the Jewish community, an immense worker for Jewish causes and a passionate Zionist' and his father had a fine knowledge of classical Hebrew; neither, however, was particularly religious. William Frankel declared that Goodman's childhood home 'was kosher but not Orthodox, though permeated with Jewishness, imbuing Arnold with a profound sense of his Jewish identity which he always retained'. Lord Goodman regarded himself as 'not an Englishman, but a Jew born in England'. As for being Jewish, he was of the opinion that 'You should regard it as being a bonus. Because by and large, looking at it objectively, we are a sympathetic, kindly, charitable and morally responsible community.' Lord Goodman was a lifelong Zionist, a frequent speaker at events organized by the Jewish National Fund and the Joint Israel Appeal, and a supporter of the Jewish Welfare Board, ORT (an organization providing vocational training in Israel and elsewhere), and countless other organizations. In 1988 he accepted the presidency of the Union of Liberal and Progressive Synagogues—a shift from the Orthodox United Synagogue of his youth.[133]

Like Lord Goodman, Lord Mishcon is deeply involved in the Jewish community. His father, as noted above, was rabbi of Brixton Synagogue, while his mother Queenie, a teacher, was the daughter of the Revd Samuel Orler, who ministered in Falmouth and Stroud. Inheriting a sense of communal obligation from his parents, Lord Mishcon devoted considerable time and energy to various Jewish organizations as noted above, and he is still a member of the United Synagogue. Through his daughter Jane's schooldays friendship with the sister of the late King Hussein of Jordan, his country house was used several times during the 1980s as a venue for secret meetings between Shimon Peres, at that time the Israeli foreign minister, and the Jordanian king; Mishcon himself would shuttle between Israel and Jordan with notes to enable the two sides to clarify their ideas and, while keeping out of the actual negotiations, actively assisted in brokering the peace accord between the two countries.

---

[132] Charles Gray, *The Irving Judgment: David Irving* v. *Penguin Books and Professor Deborah Lipstadt* (Harmondsworth: Penguin, 2000).

[133] Interview with Ada Yudkin, 22 Feb. 1981; Goodman, *Tell Them I'm On My Way*, 2, 3; Selbourne, *Not an Englishman*, 1–15; *JC* 19 May 1995, p. 23, 22 Oct. 1999.

Anthony Julius is deeply interested in Jewish culture, sending his children to a Jewish school. While formerly an adherent of the (Conservative) Masorti Synagogue, since his second marriage Julius has become a member of the Orthodox Hendon United Synagogue.[134]

In contrast to Goodman, Mishcon, and his own partner Sidney Kingsley, the co-founder of the Hendon Reform Synagogue, Sir David Napley confessed to being 'probably the worst member' of the St John's Wood Liberal Synagogue and avoided membership of communal organizations; nevertheless, he had some deep-seated ethnic pride and relished his successful conduct of a case in a magistrates' court against a blatant antisemite.[135]

After the Second World War, the structure of Jewish law firms in London seemed to continue the pre-war pattern, with just a couple of such firms representing the old Anglo-Jewish elite and the bulk of the solicitors being concentrated in small offices. The property and consumer revolutions, by creating a boom in high street shopping centres and office building, changed all this. New firms founded in the West End by Jews in the 1950s and 1960s and linked to the property and business entrepreneurs grew rapidly and moved from the commercial property field into company and tax work, thereby challenging the dominance of the big City firms which had hitherto excluded Jews from their partnerships. Outside central London, the growth of legal aid encouraged the mushrooming of practices, both in the suburbs of the metropolis and in the provinces, specializing in criminal work and civil legal aid. By the 1970s, the lifting of the restrictions on the size of law firms and the meritocratic basis of recruitment in the City practices allowed women and Jews to become partners. As law firms move from the West End to the City or its fringes, the old distinctions among these firms, based on the ethnic origin of their founders, are in many cases beginning to disappear, and the meritocratic basis of recruitment has become even more marked. At the same time, Jewish members of the solicitors' profession have increased rapidly in numbers since the late 1940s; they are no longer merely of marginal importance, and in England at the end of the twentieth century there were probably more Jewish solicitors than Jewish doctors.

---

[134] *JC* 9 Feb. 2001, p. 37.

[135] *JC* 18 Aug. 1995, p. 21; *The Times*, 28 Oct. 1994; *JC* 28 Oct. 1994, p. 23; Napley, *Not Without Prejudice*, 77–9.

THIRTEEN

Jewish Communist, Socialist, and Maverick Lawyers

W HEREAS many Jewish solicitors viewed their profession primarily from a business perspective—and were extremely successful in both business and professional terms—another group of solicitors from the same east European background were driven by more altruistic motives, impelled by a zealous pursuit of justice on behalf of their clients or devoted to active campaigning for specific legal reform. Some of the sons and grandsons of immigrants were aroused by 'the [Jewish] values of protest and "justice hunger"' and were convinced of the importance of *tikun olam*, the 'repair or improvement of the world'. Some members of this latter group were communists; a larger number of the outstanding Jewish lawyers from the second generation of east European immigrants were associated with the Labour Party; still others were mavericks.[1]

Sydney Silverman (1895–1968) was born into a struggling Liverpool Jewish family. His father, who came to Britain from Romania, was a pedlar and credit draper; his mother's family had lived in England since the eighteenth century. By dint of scholarships to the Liverpool Institute, a prestigious grammar school, where he was nicknamed 'quicksilver', and Liverpool University, Silverman made his own way. Like Lewis Silkin (whose career is outlined below) he was awarded a scholarship to Oxford, but decided that he was too poor to take it up. During the First World War he registered as a conscientious objector and served some time in prison for his beliefs. As a CO he found himself unable to obtain employment as a teacher in Britain, so, after completing his degree, he became a lecturer in English in Helsinki. In 1925 he returned to Britain, obtaining a degree in law from Liverpool University with distinction and qualifying as a solicitor in 1927. Not having the fee to register as a solicitor, he borrowed the money from a bank and opened an office in Liverpool in 1928. He defended working-class clients who had fallen into debt or into arrears with their rent and were threatened with eviction; he represented sailors accused of fighting at the docks; and he acted for other clients charged with burglary or murder. 'Mr

---

[1] Interview with Aubrey Rose, 20 Jan. 1999; Lewis S. Feuer, *Einstein and the Generations of Science* (New York: Basic Books, 1974), 78; Gerald Sorin, *The Prophetic Minority: American Jewish Immigrant Radicals 1880–1920* (Bloomington, Ind.: Indiana University Press, 1985), 14.

Silverman spent a lot of time in Police Courts,' his secretary recalled, 'and . . . if he wanted to make a point nobody could stop him. He constantly made the headlines. On a number of occasions he walked out of Court. When he took a case his one concern was to win and he didn't care how much time he spent on it.' With his partner Harry Livermore (1908–89), who later served as Lord Mayor of Liverpool and was knighted, he rapidly built up one of the best criminal law practices in Liverpool; after becoming a Labour MP in 1935, Silverman also opened an office in London.[2]

One of Silverman's childhood ambitions had been to be a barrister, an ambition that had been frustrated by poverty, and his method of cross-examining in the magistrates' courts was devastating. In one case in Liverpool he questioned a police witness who claimed that the accused was wearing a fawn raincoat; the following exchange took place. 'Mr Silverman (holding up his client's raincoat): "Is this the coat?"— "It was a similar one to that." "Do you call that fawn colour?"—"Yes." "Would you be surprised if everyone else in the world called it grey?"—"Some might call it grey." Mr Silverman held aloft a very soiled raincoat and asked what colour it was.' As the witness would not answer, the magistrate interrupted, exclaiming that 'I think you have tied this witness up so much that he hardly knows how to answer you. I could not tell you the colour of the coat myself.' Selwyn Lloyd, later a senior Conservative politician but then a struggling young barrister in Liverpool, remembered how exciting it had been to be instructed by Silverman, 'the little figure bouncing up and down in front of one or beside one, pulling one's gown, passing notes in his illegible handwriting, pouring out ideas . . . convinced of his client's innocence and integrity'.[3]

Silverman sat as Labour MP for the Lancashire constituency of Nelson and Colne, from 1935 until his death in 1968. His experience as a criminal lawyer in Liverpool defending clients charged with murder led him to ponder on the finality of capital punishment, allowing no possibility of the rectification of an error or of a miscarriage of justice; as a result, innocent people were from time to time unjustly executed, and hence Silverman believed that the death penalty should be dropped. In 1948 he introduced an amendment to the Labour government's Criminal Justice Bill abolishing capital punishment, but the clause was rejected by the House of Lords—even when it was reintroduced with a number of exemptions for certain types of murder. In 1953 Silverman and his chief parliamentary ally, Reginald Paget MP, brought out a book, *Hanged—and Innocent?*, which outlined a number of cases in which men had been executed for murders which in all probability they had not committed. Outside Parliament, in July

---

[2] Emrys Hughes, *Sydney Silverman: Rebel in Parliament* (London: Skilton, 1969), 1–19; *Dictionary of National Biography, 1961–1970*, ed. E. T. Williams and C. S. Nicholls (1981) 941–4; *Law Society's Gazette*, 10 Jan. 1990 (obituary of Sir Harry Livermore).

[3] Hughes, *Sydney Silverman*, 22, 23, 34.

1955 Arthur Koestler and Victor Gollancz formed the Campaign for the Abolition of the Death Penalty as a pressure group to spearhead a national movement against capital punishment, but Silverman was not invited to join the organization because of the acrimonious relationship between him and Gollancz (though Koestler and Gollancz detested each other in equal measure). Nevertheless, it was above all Silverman's unflagging enthusiasm for the cause in the Commons which finally forced the abolition measure on to the statute book. In the Commons on 12 March 1956 Silverman secured a second reading of his Death Penalty (Abolition) Bill. The Lords rejected it. As a compromise, the Macmillan government passed the Homicide Act of 1957, which retained the death penalty for only certain categories of murder. With a Labour administration returned to power in 1964 Silverman tried once again, and in December of that year introduced the Murder (Abolition of the Death Penalty) Bill which, through his persistence and with government help, was passed in July 1965. The Lords, however, carried a Conservative amendment for the measure to lapse after a five-year period unless both houses passed motions for the permanent abolition of the death penalty; this they did in December 1969, a year after Silverman's death.[4]

In June 1946 Silverman secured the adjournment of the Commons in protest against British military action in Palestine and the imprisonment of Zionist leaders. He fought for the establishment of the State of Israel and wanted Jewish displaced persons to be settled in Palestine. Richard Crossman, a contemporary of Silverman's in the Commons, admired his colleague's courage as a passionate Zionist in standing up to the Foreign Secretary, Ernest Bevin, but was critical of him as a person. 'Nevertheless, he was vain, difficult and uncooperative. No one could get him to work in any kind of group. All his life he remained an individualist back-bencher.' This perhaps explains why Silverman, who was one of the best debaters in the House, was never offered a government position, in which his talent might have enabled him to accomplish far more.[5]

Another Labour MP of a similar social democratic mould to Silverman was Leo Abse (b. 1917), who qualified as a solicitor in 1949. 'Second sons have a notorious passion for justice', he claimed, 'and a constant suspicion of authority and sometimes it is best to accept, albeit wryly, the role determined by one's place within the family constellation. In my practice I did this with verve.' Throughout the 1950s Abse represented clients in the magistrates' courts in Cardiff, rapidly acquiring through the reports in the *South Wales Echo* a

---

[4] Hughes, *Sydney Silverman*, 144–92; R. T. Paget, S. S. Silverman, and Christopher Hollis, *Hanged—and Innocent?* (London: Gollancz, 1953); Elizabeth Orman Tuttle, *The Crusade against Capital Punishment in Great Britain* (London: Stevens, 1961), 59–143; Edwards, *Victor Gollancz*, 637–47.

[5] Crossman, *Diaries*, ii. 675.

considerable reputation as a criminal defence lawyer; but the practice also grew in the property and financial fields. One of his clients was the pools promoter and philanthropist Harry Sherman. Soon after he opened his office, he was joined in 1952 as a partner by Isaac Cohen, who took control of the financial affairs of the practice, thereby freeing Abse to pursue a parliamentary career. His success as an advocate when acting for workmen making industrial injury claims through the courts had brought Abse into close contact with the trades unions, and he was rewarded for his efforts with the nomination for a parliamentary seat.[6]

Leo Abse sat as Labour MP for Pontypool between 1958 and 1983 and, like Silverman, made a name for himself as a very effective backbencher. Indeed, Silverman's mantle seemed to fall on Abse, who led the final campaign in the Commons for the abolition of capital punishment in 1969. When Abse first made an attempt to implement some of the minor recommendations of the 1957 Wolfenden Report on homosexual law reform in a Tory-dominated Commons he was defeated, although the new Director of Public Prosecutions requested chief constables to consult him before prosecuting persons for homosexual acts committed in private. In 1966, under a Labour government, Abse reintroduced his ten-minute bill for full reform of the law on homosexual activity; and with the assistance of Roy Jenkins, the new Home Secretary, and John Silkin, the Chief Whip, who found time for the committee stages of the bill, it eventually passed into law as the Sexual Offences Act 1967. Henceforth homosexual acts between consenting adults in private were no longer illegal.[7]

In 1966 two groups issued reports advocating 'no fault' divorce: one was a body appointed by the archbishop of Canterbury, the other was the Law Commission. In 1969 Abse, who had considerable experience of matrimonial proceedings in the magistrates' courts, piloted the Divorce Reform Act through Parliament, thus enshrining the principle of no fault divorce in law. He had received help in drafting the bill from former colleagues and—in a clandestine fashion, for civil servants were not supposed to assist backbenchers—from members of the Law Commission.[8] Abse took the greatest pride, however, in sponsoring a bill in 1973 which he persuaded the government to adopt and which became the Children Act 1975. Under this measure, children could be adopted without the court first having to obtain the consent of their natural parents, and local authorities could give grants to facilitate adoption.

A few of these radical Jewish lawyers, imbued with the messianic urge to create a utopian society, joined the Communist Party, regarding their own work in acting for the unemployed, tenants, and demonstrators who clashed with the

---

[6] Interview with Leo Abse, 4 Dec. 1997; Leo Abse, *Private Member* (London: Macdonald, 1973), 25–32.   [7] Interview with Leo Abse, 4 Dec. 1997; Abse, *Private Member*, 28, 145–202.
[8] Lawrence Stone, *The Road to Divorce* (Oxford: Oxford University Press, 1995), 406–22; *The Times*, 28 Nov. 1997.

police as facilitating steps towards social revolution. Most, however, were on the left wing or in the mainstream of the Labour Party. As their practices grew, in many cases their early radicalism was tempered, and some of the firms changed character; Lewis Silkin & Co., for example, became a 'Westminster based high-profile commercial practice'.

Lewis Silkin (1889–1972) was the eldest of seven children whose parents had come to England from the Baltic region; he won an open scholarship to Worcester College, Oxford, but was too poor to take it up. Starting work as a clerk in the docks, he progressed to being the managing clerk of a solicitor's office and qualified as a solicitor in 1920. Elected to the London County Council in 1925, he helped secure the softening of the LCC's discriminatory scholarship policy, but when in 1934 he became chairman of the Housing and Public Health Committee, he did nothing to change a discriminatory housing policy under which 'aliens' were not eligible for assistance. Two years later he became the Labour MP for Peckham and served as minister of town and country planning in the post-war Attlee government.[9] Because of the expertise of Lewis Silkin and his sons in property development and planning, the practice naturally expanded in this field. One of Lewis's sons, John Silkin (1923–87), was minister of planning and local government (1974–6) and also, while practising as a solicitor, dabbled in various property deals—one of which involved his father and led to criticism in the national press. Jarvis Astaire, who encountered John Silkin when he was a member of a consortium which purchased Wembley Stadium in 1984, denounced him as 'an opportunist' and as 'someone prepared to bend rules to achieve what he wanted . . . Silkin lied because he pretended to have money and he didn't.' The other son of Lewis Silkin, Samuel Silkin (1918–88), having graduated with a first-class degree in law from Cambridge, became a barrister and Attorney-General in the Wilson government of 1974–6.[10] Lewis Silkin was raised to the peerage in 1950 and became a director of the City and Commercial Investment Trust, a far cry from his working-class origins.

A slightly younger contemporary of Silkin was Barnett Janner (1892–1982, later Lord Janner), who was born in South Wales, the son of immigrants from Lithuania. A gifted speaker, Janner wanted to be a barrister but was deterred by financial constraints; so, after being awarded a county scholarship to study law at university, decided on a career as a solicitor. For a while he practised as a solicitor in Cardiff, dealing with rent and lease problems, helping those struggling to pay off debts, and spending much time in court.[11] On moving to

---

[9] *The Times*, 12 May 1972 (obituary of Lewis Silkin); Geoffrey Alderman, *London Jewry and London Politics 1889–1986* (London: Routledge, 1989), 87–9.

[10] *Dictionary of National Biography 1986–1990*, 412–14 (on John Silkin and Samuel Silkin); Jarvis Astaire, *Encounters* (London: Robson, 1999), 182–91.

[11] Elsie Janner, *Barnett Janner: A Personal Portrait* (London: Robson, 1984), 12–14, 17–18; *JC* 7 May 1982, p. 34 (obituary of Barnett Janner).

London, he became secretary and solicitor to two companies run by his father-in-law, but then, in 1937, opened his own office in High Holborn with a nephew, Gerald Davis. This left him with time to pursue a parliamentary career as Labour MP for a Leicester constituency from 1945 to 1970 (he had previously sat for a brief period as Liberal MP for Whitechapel). Although a good speaker, he was a somewhat sloppy administrator and was not a high-calibre lawyer; nevertheless, he was successful in gaining admission to England for many refugees from Nazi persecution and took up the demand for compensation of Jews injured in riots in Aden in 1947, without asking for payment to his firm. In 1959 he guided the Restriction of Offensive Weapons Bill through the House of Commons; it became law, prohibiting flick-knives.[12] He was president of the Board of Deputies from 1955 until 1964 and also served as chairman of the Zionist Federation, acting as spokesman for Anglo-Jewry in the House of Commons.[13] In this he was succeeded by his son Greville Janner QC (b. 1928; now Lord Janner), a specialist in employment and industrial relations law, who followed him as MP for a Leicester constituency and as president of the Board of Deputies from 1979 until 1985. Greville Janner spearheaded the campaign for Nazi war criminals to be tried in British courts, which saw legislation enabling this passed in 1990, and in 1992 went on a secret mission to Yemen to secure the opportunity to emigrate for the remnants of the Jewish community there.[14]

A contemporary and ally of Silverman was Jack Gaster (b. 1907), whose father Rabbi Dr Moses Gaster (1856–1939) was the *ḥakham* (spiritual leader) of the British Sephardi community. Articled to Telfer Leviansky without payment of a fee, Jack Gaster was admitted to the roll of solicitors in 1931 and opened his own practice shortly afterwards. During the 1920s and 1930s he became an active public speaker for the Independent Labour Party, joining the Communist Party in 1935. Through his love of advocacy and his political associations, he frequently acted for the unemployed during the 1930s, and in 'very many cases of landlord and tenant disputes, and in collective rent strikes'. A friend of Wal Hannington of the National Unemployed Workers' Movement, Gaster often represented workers who had participated in the hunger marches and been arrested by the police. He also defended a large number of clients in the Thames Magistrates' Court who had been arrested after anti-fascist disturbances in the East End. When he heard the magistrate utter an antisemitic remark in a previous case, Gaster, on being called for his own case, protested, despite the hostility of the magistrate.

At the outbreak of the Second World War, the trade union leader Walter Citrine sued the *Daily Worker*, the Communist Party newspaper, for libel. Although Citrine was successful in his court action, Gaster had so split the

---

[12] Janner, *Barnett Janner*, 31, 69–71, 89, 119, 143–5; private information.
[13] *JC* 7 May 1982, p. 34.   [14] *JC* 21 July 1995 (profile of Greville Janner).

ownership of the assets of the newspaper among a company and penurious individuals, operating through a complex system of daily licences, that the victor was not able to recover one penny in damages. In 1946 there was a dockers' strike, 'when some Liverpool dockers and London dockers, were charged with conspiracy to break the emergency regulations which were then still in force'. Sydney Silverman acted for the Liverpool dockers and Gaster represented the London men; by conducting a filibustering defence at the Bow Street Magistrates' Court, Gaster so spun out the proceedings that the strike was able to continue despite the emergency regulations. A few years later in the Thames Magistrates' Court he defended some Canadian seamen caught up in a strike at the London docks, who were prosecuted under the Merchant Shipping Act, and 'by a miracle got them off'. After Gaster visited Korea during the middle of the war there, in 1950–1, on his return to Britain there was a clamour for him to be prosecuted for consorting with the enemy, but Sydney Silverman intervened successfully in the Commons on his behalf.[15]

Another well-known firm of Jewish left-wing lawyers which was established in London during the 1930s was Seifert Sedley. William Sedley (1909–84), one of six children of an East End tailor from an east European family, remembered scraping the scales off fish before doing his homework when his father later opened a fish and chip shop in Hoxton. After winning a scholarship to study economics at the LSE, he graduated in 1929 to find the employment situation in the commercial field so unpropitious that he decided to become a solicitor, qualifying in 1935. For a time he ran a 'poor man's lawyer' service in Bow; then he took a single room at 24 Holborn, London EC1, to open an office where he was afterwards joined by his brother-in-law Sigmund Seifert (admitted in 1936). Sedley developed an expertise in landlord and tenant matters and a complete mastery of the Rent Acts, which often enabled him to win cases for tenants by vindicating their rights in incisive correspondence. He also tried to protect clients who had fallen foul of moneylenders. By the time he established himself in Holborn, Sedley's radical sympathies had led him to join the Communist Party; however, although the Party had a materialist, secular orientation and was hostile to Judaism, this did not alienate him from his ethnic roots and he always retained a love of Yiddish literature.

Before the Second World War working-class families started buying houses in ribbon developments around London's North Circular Road. Building society surveyors allegedly colluded with the builders of jerry-built properties to pass them as structurally sound enough for mortgages to be granted on their security. In protest at this practice mortgage strikes were organized among the home-owners in London and Birmingham (where the practice was also

---

[15] Interview with Jack Gaster, 11 Nov. 1997; *Camden New Journal*, 9 Oct. 1997.

widespread) by Communist Party supporters, in a similar fashion to the rent strikes against landlords mentioned above; and Sedley was chosen to act for the mortgage strikers in a test case brought against them in the late 1930s by the Bradford Third Building Society, winning in the Chancery Division of the High Court only to see the decision overturned in favour of the building society on appeal.[16] Apart from Thompsons, the leading law firm connected with the trade union movement, which handled claims for workers injured in industrial accidents,[17] Seifert Sedley probably had the largest number of trade union clients of any firm after the war, when they absorbed the practice of John L. Williams and vastly increased their own union clientele. The firm continued to take on controversial cases, such as that arising from the death of Blair Peach during a peaceful demonstration, but during the 1970s and 1980s it expanded too rapidly, particularly in personal injury work, with catastrophic results leading ultimately to the closure of the firm in the early 1990s.[18]

An outstanding younger lawyer in the civil rights field was Benedict Birnberg, who was related to the Bentwich family. His first important case after qualifying as a solicitor in 1958 was *R. v. Clark*. George Clark, the field secretary of the Campaign for Nuclear Disarmament, was charged in 1963 with inciting persons to commit a public nuisance by obstructing the highway in and around Whitehall during a visit by the king and queen of Greece, for which he was duly convicted at the London Sessions. On appeal Birnberg instructed Elwyn Jones, who convinced the court that at the original trial there had been a misdirection to the jury because for the offence of public nuisance to have been committed the jury had to consider whether, granted the obstruction, there was unreasonable use of the highway, bearing in mind that the procession was lawful. As this had not been put to the jury, the conviction was quashed.[19] This success was followed by another in *Sweet v. Parsley*. On 14 September 1967 Miss Sweet, a teacher, was convicted at the Woodstock Petty Sessions under section 5(b) of the Dangerous Drugs Act 1965 of the management of premises which were used for smoking cannabis. Miss Sweet had sublet a farmhouse to a group of young people who, without her knowledge, were smoking cannabis there. Rose Heilbron QC, instructed by Birnberg for the hearing before the Court of Appeal, succeeded in her contention that absolute liability under the act should be kept within clearly defined limits, thus ensuring that Miss Sweet's conviction was quashed.[20] Further success on appeal was achieved for Dennis Brutus, who in July 1971

---

[16] *Borders v. Bradford Third Equitable Building Society* (1940). See Andrew McCulloch, 'The Mortgage Strikes', *History Today* (June 2001), 21–2.

[17] Harry Thompson was an uncle of A. J. P. Taylor, who was articled to him for a short time; see Adam Sisman, *A. J. P. Taylor: A Biography* (London: Sinclair-Stevenson, 1994), 68–9.

[18] Interview with Stephen Sedley, 29 Mar. 2000; Brook, *The Club*, 315.

[19] *Regina v. Clark (2)* (1963) 3 WLR, pp. 1067–71.

[20] *Sweet v. Parsley* (1970) AC, pp. 132–66; *Estates Gazette*, 29 June 1968.

demonstrated against apartheid at the Wimbledon tennis championships by stepping on to the court and distributing leaflets during a match, and later by staging a sit-down demonstration on the court. Brutus was charged with using insulting behaviour, whereby a breach of peace was likely to be occasioned under section 5 of the Public Order Act 1936. On appeal to the House of Lords in the landmark case of *Brutus and Cozens*, it was held that this conduct did not constitute insulting behaviour under the act in question.[21]

Shortly after opening his practice in 1962, Birnberg took on the Derek Bentley appeal on behalf of members of the family. Bentley, a 19-year-old with the mental age of 11, had been executed in 1953 for the murder of a policeman during a warehouse-breaking expedition, even though the fatal shot had been fired by his companion, Christopher Craig. Because Craig was only 16 at the time, he escaped hanging. Over the following decades successive Home Secretaries refused Birnberg's call for an inquiry; he was particularly upset by the response of Kenneth Clarke, who despite his opposition to capital punishment rejected an application to grant Bentley a free posthumous pardon. In 1993, however, his successor Michael Howard did recommend the grant of such a pardon; but Iris Bentley, Derek Bentley's sister, was dissatisfied with this and 'continued the campaign . . . to establish that her brother had been wrongly convicted of murder'.[22] Only when the Home Office's role in investigating miscarriages of justice had been transferred to the independent Criminal Cases Review Commission was the necessary action taken. On 30 July 1999 the Court of Criminal Appeal decided that the conviction was unsafe because of a flawed summing-up at the original trial by Lord Goddard, the Lord Chief Justice. Birnberg has also acted as the legal adviser in the campaign to secure the release from prison of Mordechai Vanunu, the Israeli nuclear spy.[23]

Edward Iwi (1904–66) was admitted as a solicitor in 1927. Imbued with a passion for justice, he wrote frequently to *The Times* and the *Jewish Chronicle*, pointing out procedural and other lapses which often were subsequently corrected. His book *Laws and Flaws* was published in 1956. 'Edward Iwi', declared John Shaftesley in a tribute, 'was in the line of English grand eccentrics . . . concealing with a transparent cloak of brusqueness the innate compassion which informed his countless good deeds . . . on numerous occasions he enjoyed "taking a rise" in a legitimate way out of other legal pundits or what he considered too stubborn authorities.' As a solicitor he dealt with a number of headline-grabbing Jewish cases, including 'the dispute between the Jewish Secondary Schools Movement and the headmaster, Mr J. D. Crystal and the Schtraks case [discussed in Chapter 14 below]'. He also became a remarkable constitutional expert whose views commanded respect. It has recently been revealed that the

---

[21] *Brutus and Cozens* (1973) AC, pp. 854–67.
[22] Francis Selwyn, *Nothing but Revenge: The Case of Bentley and Craig* (Harmondsworth: Penguin, 1988); *The Times*, 11 Feb. 1997, 31 July 1998, 31 Dec. 1998.   [23] *JC* 7 Aug. 1998, p. 7.

royal family changed its surname from Windsor to Mountbatten–Windsor in 1960 because of an intervention by Iwi—one that was not well received at the time: the Lord Chancellor wrote to Harold Macmillan, the prime minister, 'This is in very bad taste. Iwi must, must be silenced, he must go quietly.' To understand the legal nicety, it is necessary to know that Winston Churchill had prevented the queen from taking on her husband's surname of Mountbatten. Shortly before Prince Andrew was born, Iwi raised a point that no one seems to have noticed in respect of the elder siblings: namely, that if the future royal child bore the surname of Windsor, his mother's surname at birth, it would imply that he was born out of wedlock.[24]

A communal solicitor with a similar combative style to Iwi, though with different interests, was Lionel Bloch (1928–98). Born in Romania to a family of jewellers with stores scattered across Europe, Bloch had the cosmopolitan upbringing of the pre-war Jewish *haute bourgeoisie* and was multilingual. Having witnessed the pogroms perpetrated by the fascist Iron Guard and the communists' post-war expropriations at first hand, he was an enemy of all totalitarian regimes. According to his obituarist in the *Telegraph*,

For many years he served as legal adviser to the Israeli embassy; he represented countless Soviet bloc emigres in asylum hearings, thinking nothing of being woken in the middle of the night to help a Romanian sailor who had jumped ship; and he provided counsel to the journals *Encounter* and *Survey*, respectively edited by two of his closest friends . . . Bloch, who was a man of the utmost kindness in his private dealings, offered many of these services *pro bono*. In his public utterances, however, Bloch was a fierce controversialist.

He felt 'entitled to comment adversely on countries with different traditions and laws. Nobody complains', he wrote, 'when we describe cannibalism, or the mutilation of African women through circumcision, as barbarous.' Like Iwi, Bloch was an incessant writer of letters to newspapers, but his barbs were aimed at the excesses of the Russians and the Arab states.[25]

Aubrey Rose (b. 1926) qualified as a solicitor in 1951 and started as a sole practitioner. As a child of east European immigrants he was sympathetic to the wave of West Indians who migrated to Britain after the Second World War, and employed a Trinidadian as a clerk. Because of this connection he built up a considerable West Indian clientele. During the 1960s he acted in a notable case when the police arrested two West Indians, George Hislop, a teacher, and Desmond Allum, a barrister, falsely accusing them of trying to drive and take away cars in Finchley Road.[26] They were awarded record damages in the High

---

[24] *JC* 18 June 1966, p. 18 (obituary of Iwi); *Evening Standard*, 18 Feb. 1999.

[25] *Daily Telegraph*, 7 Nov. 1998; *JC* 20 Nov. 1998 (obituary of Lionel Bloch).

[26] Interview with Aubrey Rose, 20 Jan. 1999; Aubrey Rose, *Brief Encounters of a Legal Kind* (Harpenden: Lennard, 1998), 13, 20–3.

Court. In another significant case, a detective claimed that by looking out of a grille above a single toilet door he could see what was happening in the general lavatory area; as a result of his statement a number of men were arrested. When an expert witness inspected the grille and took photographs, it was clear that the policeman had been lying because he could only have had a restricted view of the area.[27] Rose belonged to a new generation of solicitors, who sometimes treated certain police evidence with a heightened degree of scepticism. 'What followed in the next three hours', Rose recalled, 'was the deadliest cross-examination [by Sebag Shaw QC and Michael Sherrard] I have ever heard. Lie after lie emerged from the officer, contradiction after contradiction, one untruth conceded, and explained away by another untruth . . . The prosecution, the judge nodding his assent, hastily asked to withdraw the charges.'[28]

In 1971 Rose entered into partnership with three other solicitors to form Osmond Gaunt & Rose. Here he was busy with commercial work, forming companies and transferring businesses, drafting commercial leases, and registering trade marks and trade names. But he also practised as an agent in the Judicial Committee of the Privy Council, and handled appeals in both murder and commercial cases for Commonwealth countries. He acted for a new Caribbean state which purchased the sugar industry located in its island; he participated in the Scarman inquiry into the Brixton riots of 1981; in 1990 he was invited to join the Commission for Racial Equality, of which he became the deputy chairman; and he acted as legal adviser to the campaign to establish a national lottery. He was also actively involved in communal affairs, serving as senior vice-president of the Board of Deputies in 1991 and 1994.[29]

Ben Hooberman was also from an east European background (his grandfather, Ben Ami Aaron Hooberman, was cantor in the Newcastle synagogue). He was admitted as a solicitor in 1950 and started his own firm, Lawford & Co., in 1954. Soon he was acting for a great number of trade unions, mainly in 'sectional fights between the Communists and Trotskyites and the moderates'. He recalled that the 1960s and 1970s were an exciting time, when he assisted in the legal moves which led to the eviction of the communists from the leadership of the Electricians' Union and then of the Engineering Union.[30]

Geoffrey Bindman (b. 1933) was the son of a doctor in Newcastle upon Tyne and the grandson of a minister to the local Jewish community. After studying law at Oxford he was articled to a partner in the firm of Rowleys Ashworth, which acted for trade unions, in particular the Electricians' Union and the General and Municipal Workers' Union. Here he gained experience of trade union law and personal injury claims, and qualified as a solicitor in 1959. He then spent a year

[27] Rose, *Brief Encounters*, 47.   [28] Ibid. 48.
[29] Interview with Aubrey Rose, 20 Jan. 1999; Rose, *Brief Encounters*, 80, 81, 88, 93.
[30] Iris Freeman, interview with Ben Hooberman, 9 July 1996.

as a teaching fellow at Northwestern University, Illinois, where he assisted Willard Wirtz, a labour law teacher, in the preparation of a celebrated lawsuit touching on racial discrimination, the *Deerfield* case. This was a class action against a local authority which excluded black people from buying houses. On his return to London, Bindman established a small law practice in Kentish Town which was one of the first firms to concentrate on legal aid work; later, in 1965, he became a partner in Lawford & Co., remaining with the firm until 1974. Here he handled among other matters a heavy caseload of personal injury claims for members of the Electricians' Union. In 1961 he participated in the inauguration of Amnesty International; he also joined the executive committee of Justice, whose secretary Tom Sargant recommended Bindman when a former conservative Attorney-General, John Foster, was consulted by the Race Relations Board when it wanted to find a legal adviser who was respected but not too radical. He was a member of the Street Committee, which reported in 1967, recommending changes in the law to prevent racial discrimination in housing and employment which were implemented in the 1968 Race Relations Act. (The committee was a private initiative set up by Roy Jenkins, Mark Bonham-Carter and Anthony Lester; Marks & Spencer paid the costs of producing the report.) Among the actions he fought for the Race Relations Board was *Mandla* v. *Dowell-Lee* (1983), which went to the House of Lords and established the right of Sikhs to be recognized as an ethnic group and of the particular Sikh schoolboy involved in the case to be permitted to wear his turban at school. Earlier, when this case had been considered by the Court of Appeal, Lord Denning had ruled that the Sikhs, unlike the Jews, were a religion and not an ethnic group, so that its members were not entitled to any relief under the Race Relations Act, a ruling that so irritated Bindman that he walked out of the court in disgust. He also branched out into libel law, acting for *Private Eye* for some fifteen years during the editorship of Richard Ingrams.[31]

In 1974 Geoffrey Bindman founded the firm of Bindman and Partners, which became known as a specialist in civil liberties and human rights issues, though this was not apparent at its inception. In fact, Bindman himself has remained an all-rounder, ready to try his hand in many different aspects of the law. Throughout the last quarter of the twentieth century Bindman continued to be associated with such organizations as Amnesty International and the Medical Foundation for the Care of Victims of Torture, an involvement culminating in his success against General Pinochet in 1999. Viviana Diaz, of the organization representing victims' families in Chile, claimed that, under the ruling by the law lords, the principle was affirmed that 'no head of state can torture or kill without being held accountable'; but this was not strictly accurate, as the judgment referred to a *former* head of state.[32] By frequently invoking the European

---

[31] Interview with Geoffrey Bindman, 4 Apr. 2000.   [32] *The Times*, 25 Mar., 30 Mar. 1999.

Convention on Human Rights on behalf of its clients, Bindmans established itself as the leading English law firm to appear at the European Court in Strasbourg.

In the A6 murder case, Bindman, as the Hanratty family solicitor, worked for twenty-five years to clear the name of James Hanratty, who was executed for the crime in 1962; finally, in March 1999, the Criminal Cases Review Commission announced that it was sending the case back to the Court of Appeal because the police had withheld vital evidence from the defence.[33] Meanwhile a partner in Bindmans, Brian Raymond (1948–93), the son of Jewish immigrants from Europe, represented the civil servant Clive Ponting, who was prosecuted under the Official Secrets Act for leaking the truth about the sinking of the cruiser the *General Belgrano* during the Falklands War, and secured his sensational acquittal in 1985. From the experience gained in acting in this case as head of the firm's criminal law department, Raymond learned how to mobilize the press and television to fight an injustice.[34] By the 1980s, especially after the Ponting acquittal, Bindmans had an increasingly high public profile, and outspoken professional people, such as Wendy Savage, Helen Zeitlin, and Graham Pink, flocked to consult Raymond. Wendy Savage, a consultant obstetrician, used controversial techniques when delivering babies, with the result that she was suspended on grounds that she was 'a danger to her patients'; but after an inquiry in which Bindmans presented her case she was completely vindicated. Many press and television companies seeking to protect their freedom from government constraints consulted Raymond. Another organization for which Bindmans acted was the World Development Movement, on whose behalf Stephen Grosz, a public law expert in Bindmans, secured a judicial review challenging the British government's right to allocate aid for Malaysia's Pergau Dam project, with the result that the court decided in 1994 that the Foreign Secretary's decision to grant such assistance was not within the law.[35] This caseload, with its emphasis on constitutional issues and questions of international law, was reminiscent of Iwi and in some contrast to the work handled by the other radical lawyers discussed here.

Since the disintegration of the Soviet Union in the early 1990s it has become apparent that the recruitment of Jewish lawyers into the Communist Party was a passing phase born out of the frustrations of the 1930s, and the misplaced idealism of the early 1950s. Towards the end of the century Jewish radicalism continued in new forms. Stephen Jakobi, after securing the release of two girls charged with smuggling drugs into Thailand, founded an advisory service

[33] Bob Woffinden, *Hanratty: The Final Verdict* (London: Macmillan, 1997), 391, 400, 401, 447–51; *The Times*, 30 Mar. 1999.

[34] *Independent*, 1 June, 3 June 1993; *The Times*, 10 June 1993 (obituary of Raymond); Clive Ponting, *The Right to Know: The Inside Story of the Belgrano Affair* (London: Sphere, 1985), 158–97.

[35] Audrey Poppy, 'Dam Shame', *Legal Business* (Jan.–Feb. 1995), 52–8.

called Fair Trials Abroad in 1994; and Daniel Machover, the son of anti-Zionist Israelis and the founder of Lawyers for Palestinian Human Rights, has rapidly become a leading civil liberties lawyer, instigating the prosecution of a number of warders at Wormwood Scrubs prison on a charge of assaulting prisoners.[36]

On the whole, the left-wing lawyers tended to have a more tenuous affiliation to the Jewish community than those associated with the property entrepreneurs or the world of business in general, though Sydney Silverman spoke out strongly on Zionist issues.

Apart from the commercial and radical lawyers, there were a large number of Jewish solicitors who built up their practices in the post-war period by advocacy in the magistrates' courts, and from their ranks emerged some distinguished Jewish criminal lawyers. The most prominent of these, Sir David Napley, has already been discussed in Chapter 12. According to John Platt-Mills QC, Ellis Lincoln 'appeared to have the London underworld as his client and the effect on my practice was that I moved into the Old Bailey for five years as Defence Counsel'. Bernard Perkoff was admitted as a solicitor in 1938 and founded the firm of Peters & Peters, becoming a formidable advocate in magistrates' courts and an expert in white-collar crime. So too, Jeffrey Bayes (1939–98) 'was regularly instructed in high-profile fraud and extradition cases'. Victor Lissak (1930–81) was one of the country's leading defence lawyers and among the first solicitors to be appointed a recorder.[37]

Jews not only continued to serve the world of the arts and the theatre, as in the past, but acted for many of the new commercial television companies. Sir Anthony Lousada (1907–94) 'specialised in private client work, particularly in the settlement of artists' estates', and was chairman of the trustees of the Tate Gallery (1967–9). Isador Caplan (1912–95), a partner in Forsyte Kerman, was Benjamin Britten's principal legal adviser and helped to set up the Aldeburgh Festival in 1948. In contrast, David Jacobs (1912–68) acted for many of the top stars in variety entertainment. Another solicitor who represented numerous showbusiness performers was Solomon Kaufman (1908–98); but he was better known for acting for Dr Soblen in extradition proceedings and for his successful defence of the author Leon Uris in a libel action, in which he persuaded the Polish authorities to release the Auschwitz hospital operations register for the trial.[38]

---

[36] *JC* 3 Nov. 1995, p. 10; *The Times*, 29 Mar. 2000 (on Jakobi); *Independent*, 4 Nov. 1999 (on Daniel Machover).

[37] *Law Society's Gazette*, 1 Feb. 1995 (obituary of Perkoff); *JC* 26 Feb. 1999 (obituary of Bayes); *Law Society's Gazette*, 10 Feb. 1982 (obituary of Lissack).

[38] *Independent*, 29 June 1994 (obituary of Lousada), 23 Jan. 1995 (obituary of Caplan); *JC* 20 Dec. 1968, p. 39 (obituary of Jacobs), 22 Jan. 1999, p. 23 (obituary of Kaufman). Dr Soblen was convicted in the USA of giving defence information to the Soviet Union. While on bail he fled to England and the Home Secretary issued a deportation order, under the Aliens Order, which was upheld by the Court of Appeal.

Probably the majority of Jewish solicitors in the 1970s were still working outside the City and the West End of London or were members of the smaller
provincial law firms. Usually these practices had a partner who specialized in
conveyancing and another lawyer who attended to the probate work and litigation. My own experience as a suburban lawyer took me on regular forays to the
local county court for landlord and tenant disputes and small monetary claims,
frequent trips to the divorce registry at Somerset House, and occasional outings
to the High Court for interlocutory proceedings and applications for summary
judgment. In addition, I attended hearings for petty crime at the local magistrates' court and instructed counsel for trials in the Crown Court, when the
charges were more serious. Occasionally there would be more exciting matters
to deal with, such as a tussle with solicitors acting for an insurance company to
secure the award of damages of £47,250 in 1978 for a passenger who was totally
incapacitated by injuries sustained in an accident when his friend's car went out
of control.[39] More memorable was the experience of acting for the plaintiffs in a
successful claim against Selico Ltd., a property company owned by the Bergers,
and their agents Select Managements Ltd. in 1984. Mr Justice Goulding, after
hearing the devastating cross-examination by counsel for the plaintiffs, found
that the managing agent's builder had attempted to conceal dry rot in a flat which
was sold to my clients. The turning point in the case was the evidence of the
lessee of a neighbouring flat, a timber expert, who said that he had discovered
dry rot in his own flat in 1977 and later in the plaintiffs' flat. From the appearance of the wood and its characteristic smell, the witness knew that the problem
was dry rot, whereas the managing agent's builder claimed that dry rot did not
smell. The judge declared that 'the dishonest act was done by . . . [the builder]
in the course of work ordered by Select within the scope of Select's authority as
the lessor's agent'.[40] It would seem that partly as a result of losing their appeal in
February 1986, and partly as a result of repeated allegations of neglect by councils and tenants, the Berger family, which owned over 100,000 homes, may have
started to move into the commercial property sector.

One of my last legal victories was to produce evidence from a metallurgist
to show that internal pipes in a flat had been deliberately tampered with and
fractured by a tenant, causing flooding and extensive damage to the flats in the
block; and that his claim for damages for lack of repairs by the landlord was
fraudulent.

[39] *Daily Express*, 6 Oct. 1978.
[40] *Gordon and Teixeira* v. *Selico Limited and Select Management Limited* (1984) 2 Estates Gazette Law
Reports pp. 79–85. *JC* 9, 23 May 1986.

FOURTEEN

Jewish Barristers
1945–1990

I HAVE already noted that few young men from humble east European family backgrounds succeeded at the Bar before the late 1950s, citing the examples of Eli Cashdan, Salmond Levin, and Sefton Temkin as able men who tried but failed to establish themselves through lack of connections and lack of work. Another example of such a failure was Hyman Diamond (1914–77). Brought up in Liverpool, where he qualified for the Bar, he reached the rank of major during the Second World War and was subsequently sent to Germany as a prosecuting officer with the British War Crimes Commission. Although he spoke with clarity, cogency, and wit, he was unable to find enough work; so he left the Bar and suffered a period of financial hardship until joining the Freshwater group of companies (owned by the Freshwaters, a Jewish family), one of Britain's leading landlords for rented accommodation.[1]

In the immediate post-war period, even if one had been successful as a junior member of the Bar there was no guarantee of continued success as a silk. Constantine Gallop (1893–1967) studied law at University College London, qualifying as a barrister at 21; after service in the First World War he undertook postgraduate study at Balliol College, Oxford, where he was elected president of the Union in 1919. 'His ability as a lawyer and advocate was such that all his friends expected that he would make a highly distinguished career. Joining the Midland Circuit, he quickly won a big practice, mainly in common law, especially in London.' But in spite of his fine career as a junior, after he took silk Gallop's career just petered out. He was appointed a special commissioner in divorce in 1953, conscientiously carrying out his duties in the divorce courts.[2]

On the other hand, certain exceptional individuals from a second-generation east European immigrant background managed to build up flourishing practices in the 1940s and 1950s. William Frankel (b. 1914) studied law at London University, being called to the Bar in 1944. He was a pupil in Herbert Garland's chambers, where he stayed after his pupillage doing work in the magistrates'

---

[1] *JC* 26 July 1991, p. 13 (obituary of Diamond); private information.
[2] *The Times*, 20, 21 Apr. 1967 (obituary of Gallop).

and county courts. During his first year at the Bar he earned 600 guineas, a sizeable sum in those days; in the normal run of things it was reckoned that a beginner at the Bar would have to work for three years before he could begin to recover his expenses. Frankel was one of the few lucky ones who achieved success at the Bar without connections. His chance came when he was visiting a friend in Constantine Gallop's chambers late one day and a clerk called asking for a junior counsel to do two cases in the Kingston Court the following day. There was no other junior counsel available at that hour, and Gallop's clerk suggested that Frankel be given a chance. When he appeared in court, the instructing solicitor from Feltham was impressed by the way in which he conducted the cases, and continued to send him work from then onwards. In 1952 Frankel joined the chambers of Leonard Caplan QC, specializing in commercial and divorce work until he left in 1955 to join the *Jewish Chronicle*; he became editor in 1958 and held the post until 1977.[3]

Partly because the provisions of the Legal Aid and Advice Act 1949 were starting to take effect, and partly because of the post-war upsurge in crime, there was a marked expansion in work for barristers in the late 1950s at much higher rates of pay than in the pre-war period. 'When I came to the Bar,' claimed Henry Cecil in 1975,

if a barrister volunteered to do what was called 'poor persons' work in civil cases or undertook dock briefs or had doled out to him easy briefs for the prosecution at Sessions or Assizes (known as 'soup'), he was either not paid at all or received a trifling amount. Under the Legal Aid scheme he is very handsomely paid . . . [A new recruit's income after six months' pupillage] may amount to anything from £1500 to £3000 for the first year and substantially more thereafter . . . Even as late as 1953 the prospects of success were poor. In a survey . . . published in *The Times* in 1953 it was stated that the writer had made a survey in seven or eight leading sets of chambers of all available juniors in these chambers. He found that the earnings of barristers of three years' standing averaged under £250 per annum, that those of from five to nineteen years' standing were under £800 and those of twenty years' standing or more were £2700.[4]

Much of the credit for this increase in the remuneration of barristers was due to a campaign launched in 1956 by two lawyers, Sir Milner Holland and Gerald Gardiner, which along with the growing volume or work helped triple barristers' incomes by 1964.[5]

During the late 1950s the Bar was still regarded as overcrowded, and graduates only slowly became aware of the better conditions of pay and employment prevailing there. The total number of barristers in practice sank from 2,010 in 1954 to 1,919 in 1960, climbing thereafter only gradually to 2,164 in 1965. None

---

[3] Interview with William Frankel, 23 July 1998.
[4] Cecil, *Memories*, 23, 24.
[5] Abel-Smith and Stevens, *Lawyers*, 417–26.

the less, by 1991 the consequence of the vastly improved rates of pay was that the number of practising barristers had quintupled, soaring to 10,000.[6] Here there were new opportunities for the children and grandchildren of Jewish immigrants from eastern Europe. Asher Tropp estimated that the number of practising Jewish barristers in 1991 was about 500, likewise a fivefold increase since the early 1930s.[7]

The expansion of legal aid and the subsequent growth of Jewish solicitors' practices specializing in criminal law boosted the opportunities for Jewish barristers; they were also helped by the multiplication of retail chains of shops in the clothing and electrical goods sectors, together with the establishment of large property companies, which in turn fostered a number of influential Jewish commercial law practices. Whereas the emergence of Jewish solicitors specializing in criminal law assisted the careers of some of those practising at the criminal Bar, the West End and City Jewish law practices with large numbers of business clients permitted the entry of barristers from families of east European immigrants into the commercial Bar and generated an appreciable volume of civil litigation. Accordingly, the increase in the number of Jewish solicitors' practices after the Second World War levelled the playing field for barristers from similar backgrounds, although these firms continued to instruct counsel from every creed and every ethnic group. Again, prominent Jewish solicitors sometimes assisted the careers of high-flying barristers who happened to be co-religionists. For example, Sir David Napley sponsored Sir Sebag Shaw; but he also talent-spotted George Carman, who was not Jewish. David Freeman helped to promote the careers of Sir Morris Finer and Michael Sherrard QC, while Lord Goodman discovered the forensic skills of Lord Hoffman.[8]

A small number of the Jewish barristers practising in the first three decades after the Second World War distinguished themselves in the divorce courts, but the overwhelming majority acted in criminal cases or with a mixed caseload of civil and criminal matters. Some, such as Dame Rose Heilbron and Sir Sebag Shaw, rose to prominence during the Second World War, when competitors were few; others, such as Ashe Lincoln QC and Bernard Gillis QC, rebuilt their pre-war careers in the criminal courts; others still, who were younger, such as Michael Sherrard QC and Sir Allan Green, began their careers after the war.

Rose Heilbron (b. 1914) was the daughter of Mr and Mrs Max Heilbron, owners of a boarding house for Jewish immigrants in Liverpool who subsequently went into the hotel business. She was educated locally and at Liverpool University, where she was awarded the LL B degree with first-class honours in 1935, becoming only the second woman in England to receive the degree. At 21

[6] Abel-Smith and Stevens, *Lawyers*, 420, 427, 428.   [7] Tropp, *Jews in the Professions*, 97.
[8] Napley, *Not Without Prejudice*, 13, 136, 340, 342, 343; Goodman, *Tell Them I'm On My Way*, 112, 113.

she won an entrance scholarship of £300 to Gray's Inn, the first woman to do so, and was called to the Bar in 1939. Rose Heilbron was from an Orthodox Jewish background, teaching a Bible class at the Princess Road Synagogue. As a student, she was treasurer of both her local student society and the Inter-University Jewish Federation. Her family, second-generation Jewish immigrants, were concerned with educational achievement and encouraged her to win a gold medal for elocution at 7 and an examination award for her skill at speaking at 16. Her mother, endowed with a feminist streak unusual in a Jewish mother, supported Rose in the ambition to read for the Bar which naturally flowed from her aptitude for speaking with eloquence, but sadly died a year before her daughter qualified.[9] Yet Rose Heilbron was 'anything but a blue-stocking. She . . . [was] attractive, charming, and vivacious and very feminine, particularly when it comes to discussing fur coats.'[10]

During the Second World War, when many men were serving at the front, Rose Heilbron's ability and willingness to confront judges on behalf of her clients quickly won her a reputation at the Bar as a criminal lawyer. She was frequently instructed by Silverman, Livermore & Co., who were rapidly emerging as Liverpool's leading firm of solicitors specializing in criminal law. Thus she was a protégée of both Sydney Silverman MP and Sir Harry Livermore. By 1946 she had already appeared in ten murder trials. 'Legal history was made last week', reported the *Jewish Chronicle* on 22 April 1949, 'when . . . Miss Heilbron of Liverpool, became one of the first two women barristers in England to be appointed King's Counsel.'[11] Her appointment as a silk at the age of 34 had been equalled only by Sir David Maxwell Fyfe MP. In a tribute to Rose Heilbron, Sydney Silverman noted that

Hers had been a career of great achievement. Nobody succeeded at the Bar on sentiment or chivalrous loyalty. Any success in law must be obtained on merit as a lawyer and an advocate, irrespective of sex. There had probably been some resistance to Miss Heilbron's appointment as a K.C., but she had overcome two handicaps—her sex, and the fact that she was Jewish. She had to prove that she was not only the equal of a man, but a little better.[12]

It was a remarkable feat for a young woman to crash both ethnic and gender barriers in the 1940s.

Such were Rose Heilbron's virtuoso performances in court that she became a significant figure on the national scene. During her defence of George Kelly in the Cameo murder trial in January 1950, she became the first woman KC to lead for the defence at a murder trial, just as earlier she had been the first woman to appear in the House of Lords without a leader. Rose Heilbron was instructed

[9] *JC* 6 Dec. 1935, p. 35, 22 Apr. 1949, p. 6.   [10] *JC* 9 July 1954, p. 26.
[11] *JC* 22 Apr. 1949, p. 6.   [12] *JC* 8 July 1949, p. 8.

by Harry Livermore on behalf of George Kelly, who at the first trial was jointly charged with Charles Connolly of murdering the manager of the Cameo Cinema. Rose Heilbron claimed that the cases of the two men were distinct and that 'Witnesses would say that Kelly on the night of the murder was nowhere near the Beehive public house and had nothing whatever to do with the murder.' She ridiculed the prosecution case, saying that it

had been most remarkable, bewildering, and fantastic. It was suggested that, in the public part of a public house, on the busiest night of the week, a plot was hatched to rob at the point of a gun the manager of the Cameo Cinema, that a gun was produced and loaded, and that a handkerchief was tied round a man's face to make a mask. Northam and Dickson, the two principal prosecution witnesses, she suggested, were quite unworthy of belief, and the evidence of Robert Graham (a prisoner at Walton gaol) was even more incredible . . . Miss Heilbron reminded the jury that no item in connexion with the murder had been traced to Kelly—no overcoat or mask which were alleged by the prosecution to have been worn, no gun, no bullet, and not a speck of blood, even on the underneath of his shoes.[13]

Kelly in his evidence denied shooting the manager and assistant manager of the Cameo Cinema and claimed to have an alibi. As Heilbron had sown sufficient doubt in the minds of the jury, they could not agree on a verdict, and the judge ordered a retrial; but not before Connolly had made specious and lurid allegations against Livermore, Kelly's solicitor, claiming that he had offered him £150 to change his evidence.[14]

At the second trial of Kelly in February 1950, when he was tried separately from Connolly, Miss Heilbron repeated her previous arguments in favour of the defendant, but this time was unable to save him: the jury took an hour to reach a verdict of guilty. She appealed on Kelly's behalf to the Court of Criminal Appeal, on the grounds that one of the jurymen had been convicted of a felony and was not entitled to sit on a jury. It was contended by her that the juryman, having been 'attainted' of a felony, was disqualified by virtue of section 10 of the Juries Act 1870; and that 'attainted' was equivalent to 'convicted'. If the court decided that the trial was a nullity, they should quash Kelly's conviction because there had already been two trials. The Chief Justice Lord Goddard delivered the court's verdict, dismissing the appeal.

The Juries Act 1870 dealt with three classes of person: those attainted of treason or a crime, those convicted of a crime that was infamous (buggery), and those who were under outlawry. Outlawry had been abolished in 1938, while the juryman in question had not been convicted of an infamous crime. The remaining point to be decided was whether or not the juryman was a person

[13] *The Times*, 13 Apr. 1949.
[14] *The Times*, 13, 14, 17, 18, 19, 20, 21, 24, 25, 26, 27, 28, 30 Jan. 1950.

attainted of felony. Once section 1 of the Forfeiture Act 1870 had abolished attainder, except in the case of outlawry, it was impossible that 'a person attainted of felony' could mean 'a person convicted of felony', capital or non-capital; the juryman in this case had been convicted of the non-capital felony of receiving and was not therefore attainted, so that no objection could be made to him.[15]

Rose Heilbron also went to the Court of Criminal Appeal on behalf of E. F. Devlin, who, with a companion, had been tried for the murder of a woman in Manchester in December 1951. A 15-year-old girl claimed that Julie Oldham, Devlin's ex-girlfriend, admitted that she had lied when she asserted that Devlin and Burns had plotted the robbery and asked her to participate in it. Lord Goddard refused to allow Miss Heilbron to submit new evidence, but told her to contact the Home Secretary, who appointed a senior barrister in April 1952 to review all the evidence. He concluded that Julie Oldham had not committed perjury. The solicitors acting for Oldham and Burns with the assistance of Miss Heilbron drafted a memorandum to the Home Secretary asking for a reprieve; it was rejected, and the men were executed. As a result of this episode, Lord Goddard put forward a motion in the House of Lords urging that the Court of Criminal Appeal should be granted fresh powers to order a retrial when fresh evidence came to light.[16]

Overlapping with these events, Miss Heilbron in February 1952 defended Louis Arnold Bloom, a Jewish solicitor from West Hartlepool, who was accused of murdering his mistress, Patricia Mary Hessler. Bloom had qualified as a solicitor in 1948 and had been consulted by Mrs Hessler in 1950; a close association had developed between them and there was talk of marriage. On 14 November 1951 Bloom told Mrs Hessler that his practice was beginning to deteriorate because certain clients objected to his association with her, but she pleaded with him that they should spend one last night together. Bloom in his evidence declared that he was in love with Mrs Hessler up to the time of the 'happening'. At 7 a.m., Bloom asked Mrs Hessler to leave his office, as the staff would be coming; and she exclaimed, ' "You can't palm me off so easily", and began to scream.' Moreover,

On a . . . [previous] occasion when they were staying at a hotel she would not stop shouting and screaming, and he got hold of her throat with both his hands. He pressed on her throat and she went on making a little bit of a noise. He pressed again and she stopped shouting and screaming. Afterwards there was a slight bruise but nothing serious.

In November 1951 they had spent the night in question love-making and she had been drinking. When he told her to leave, she became excited and he asked her to stop screaming many times.

[15] *The Times*, 3, 7, 8, 9, 18 Feb. 1950, and 7, 11, 16 Mar. 1950; *R.* v. *Kelly* I All ER 1951, pp. 806–11.
[16] Bresler, *Lord Goddard*, 214–18.

He then put his hands round her neck with his thumbs to the front. He applied a very slight pressure with his thumbs. Then he took his thumbs away and she was still making a noise. He pressed again with his thumbs, and when he took his thumbs away there was no noise. He noticed that her face looked lifeless . . . He had no reasons or motives to kill Mrs Hessler.

He had put his hands on her neck to quieten her and not to make him look a fool to the people in the shop below. In cross-examination Bloom denied using more pressure on Mrs Hessler's neck than on previous occasions.[17]

A pathologist called by the defence stated that chronic alcoholics, such as Mrs Hessler, tended to bruise more easily. He disagreed with the doctor called on behalf of the prosecution that considerable violence would have to have ensued to cause the injuries to Mrs Hessler's throat. A fractured cricoid (the cartilage which forms the lower and back part of the larynx), as sustained by the victim, did not always cause death. Mrs Hessler was under the influence of drink when Bloom put his hands around her neck and would not have paid attention to pain.[18]

Miss Heilbron submitted that it was not a case of

murder or manslaughter. Manslaughter was the unlawful killing of another without malice or an unlawful act where a man might unintentionally kill another by accident. If the act was not unlawful then the killing was not manslaughter but misadventure, and of course a verdict of Not Guilty would follow. There was no question of an unlawful act. On two or three occasions Bloom had got hold of Mrs Hessler's throat and not only had she never complained but she had told him to stop her if she ever behaved similarly again. If Bloom wanted to get rid of Mrs Hessler could the jury think of a more ridiculous place . . . than in his office? . . . What was more natural [than] for him [Bloom] to press on her neck and tell her to be quiet? But if one made a mistake and the pressure was a little too hard the damage was done. That did not mean to say that he did it deliberately.

In his summing up the judge told the jury that if the prosecution had satisfied them that Mrs Hessler was killed by an unlawful act, then it was manslaughter. They could not find Bloom guilty of murder, unless the prosecution had proved in addition that the killing was intentional. Bloom was found guilty of manslaughter by the jury and sentenced to three years in prison.[19]

Sir Sebag Shaw (1907–82) was born in the East End, where his father ran a successful photography business, and he attended the Central Foundation School, the *alma mater* also of Selig Brodetsky and Lewis Silkin. He then won a scholarship to University College London, where he took his LL B. After being called to the Bar in 1931, he decided to become a law teacher rather than a practitioner

---

[17] *The Times*, 19 Dec. 1951, 5, 6, 7 Feb. 1952.
[18] *The Times*, 7 Feb. 1952.
[19] *The Times*, 7, 8 Feb. 1952.

because of the limited opportunities for barristers then existing; he worked as a teacher for more than ten years. As a boy he had suffered from a severe attack of poliomyelitis which had left him lame, so that he was not called up for military service. During the war he abandoned his career as a lecturer and entered chambers, quickly gaining a considerable reputation as a criminal lawyer. Like Rose Heilbron he made his mark as a barrister in the war years, standing out in the depleted ranks of advocates. According to Bernard Gillis, 'At home, alike in criminal courts as in civil courts, he was much sought after as a junior, appearing from time to time for the Board of Trade, the Commissioners of Excise and Customs and for many local authorities and public bodies in important cases.'[20] 'A short man, with a pronounced limp and a mass of crinkly white hair, he did not have an obviously commanding presence, but when he rose and addressed a jury it was pure music to his listeners. I am satisfied that there is no one today at the Bar who could match his command of simple descriptive language, or his flow of eloquence and charm', wrote David Napley, who briefed him frequently, in 1982. When he took silk in 1962, 'He would like to have developed a practice on the civil side, but his clients, by continuing to instruct him in heavy criminal cases made this difficult.' In 1966, during the trial of the notorious Richardson gang, Sebag Shaw showed himself to be their master: 'Without any outward display of emotion, he proved himself to be lucid in exposition, powerful in argument, and deadly in cross-examination; the gang was smashed, and its leaders received well-deserved . . . punishment.'[21] As a silk, he was an outstanding leader and soon in the front rank. He headed a set of chambers with so many Jews in it that it was known as 'the Jewish chambers'.

Jack Messoud di Victor Nahum (1907–59) was the twin brother of the society photographer Baron and the son of a Sephardi Jewish communal leader in Manchester. He was educated in the Jewish House at Clifton College and Oxford; called to the Bar in 1929, he practised on the northern assize court circuit, where he made a name for himself as defending counsel in criminal cases, the most famous being the Merrifield murder trial. He took silk in 1953. Despite his family connections he had little interest in Jewish matters and was more concerned with sport; having played rugby for his Oxford college before the war, he went on to play for Manchester. His career may be contrasted with that of the distinguished paediatrician George Marcus Komrower (1911–89), who represented his county in rugby football and played an active role in Manchester social life, yet was proud of his ancestry.[22]

Among the next generation of those who sometimes practised in the criminal

[20] *The Times*, 4 Jan. 1983; *JC* 7 Jan. 1983, p. 22 (obituary of Shaw).

[21] Napley, *Not Without Prejudice*, 222.

[22] *JC* 3 Apr. 1959 (obituary of Nahum). *Lives of the Fellows of the Royal College of Physicians of London*, ix. 297–300 (on Komrower).

courts, Michael Sherrard (b. 1928) was awarded his LL B by London University and was called to the Bar in 1949.[23] As a junior, he was led by F. H. Lawton QC in 1960 on behalf of Dandy Kim (Michael Carbon-Waterfield), successfully arguing that the extradition warrant of the latter for theft of money from Jack Warner in France was invalid.[24] At the age of 33 Sherrard leapt to public prominence as James Hanratty's defence counsel in the A6 murder trial in 1962. Originally Victor Durand QC had been instructed to lead Sherrard on behalf of Hanratty, but he was suspended from practising at the Bar for a year and Sherrard, who had acted robustly for Hanratty in the committal proceedings, was at his client's insistence appointed to act in his place, though as yet he had not taken silk. His vigorous conduct of Hanratty's defence at the trial established Sherrard's reputation as a criminal lawyer and he acted for several other individuals accused of murder.[25] In 1963 his standing was further enhanced when he secured the dismissal of the charge brought against Donald Rooum (a well-known political cartoonist) at Marlborough Street Magistrates' Court of possessing offensive weapons, namely pieces of brick, at a protest meeting against the queen of Greece. This was one of the events which ultimately led to CID Detective-Sergeant Challenor's committal to a mental hospital; he had planted bricks on his victims. The affair received much publicity in the national press and a judicial inquiry was ordered.[26]

When Sherrard was a junior counsel, about 60 per cent of his work related to civil matters and 40 per cent to criminal cases, mainly commercial crime. He worked closely with the solicitor David Freeman and other counsel, particularly Morris Finer, Sherrard's pupil-master, on a number of high-profile cases concerning the financier Harry Jasper and John Bloom, who established Rolls Razor Ltd., a firm that sold washing machines.

Sherrard's first case after he became a QC in 1968 involved Bloom, and following its successful outcome he was asked to undertake more and more heavy fraud cases. In *Barclays Bank Ltd. and Quistclose Investments Ltd*. Sherrard and Arthur Bagnall QC successfully appeared in the House of Lords, when it was held that where a bank receives money knowing that the money is held in trust for shareholders it does not become the depositor's money if the depositor becomes insolvent.

During the last quarter of the century Sherrard also undertook a variety of civil and criminal cases in the Far East, mainly with a commercial slant. In addition, he sat as a recorder of the Crown Court at the Old Bailey from 1974 to 1993. Unfortunately, in the early 1980s when he was being considered for

---

[23] Interview with Michael Sherrard, 12 July 1999.

[24] *Regina v. Governor of Brixton Prison and Others. Ex parte Carbon-Waterfield* 2 QB 1960, pp. 498–512.

[25] Woffinden, *Hanratty*, 151, 152, 168, 169, 443.

[26] Mary Grigg, *The Challenor Case* (Harmondsworth: Penguin, 1965), 49–56.

appointment as a judge he declined because he was then in poor health. In 1996 he was elected treasurer of Middle Temple and became its first director of advocacy. For some years he did communal work for the Jewish Friendly Circle for the Blind, which met in Stepney, and he is a member of the West London Reform Synagogue.[27]

Allan Green (b. 1935), educated at Charterhouse and Cambridge, was called to the Bar in 1959. His father Lionel Green was formerly president and chief executive of the leading fashion company Windsmoor. Having excelled as a criminal prosecutor, securing convictions against the mass murderer Dennis Nilsen and the East German agents Rheinhard and Sonja Schulze, Green was appointed Director of Public Prosecutions in 1987; but he was forced to resign in October 1991 when he was caught by the police with a prostitute in King's Cross. He was, however, welcomed back as a defence counsel in his old chambers. Although Green was the first Jew to hold the office of DPP, his Jewish associations were minimal, confined to membership of the British Friends of Tel Aviv University.[28]

Among the younger generation, the outstanding divorce lawyer was Joseph Jackson (1924–87). One of eight children from a Jewish family of east European origin, his father was a tailor. He won scholarships to Cambridge to study history and then law, and undertook a postgraduate course at London University, where he received his LLM. He was called to the Bar in 1947. Jackson was chairman of the World Union of Jewish Students and 'In the immediate post-War period he did . . . relief work among Jewish students in Europe who had survived the Holocaust, and travelled widely to make himself familiar with the position and needs of the remnant.' In the early 1950s he disappeared from the Jewish communal scene, resigning from thirteen committees to concentrate on earning a living. Within a few years of qualifying for the Bar, he published the highly regarded *Formation and Annulment of Marriage*. He became the acclaimed editor of the fifth to fourteenth editions of *Rayden on Divorce*, the divorce practitioner's bible, and was torn between pursuing a career as an academic lawyer and practising in the courts. In 1959, in the case of *Gillon* v. *Gillon*, Jackson secured a declaration recognizing an Israeli certificate of divorce or *get* as valid, where both parties were Jewish and the husband was domiciled in Israel.[29]

When Seymour Karminski, a divorce judge from a patrician family, wrote a warm letter of congratulation to Jackson on his appointment as a QC in 1967, he commented that his 'only regret is that it has taken you so surprisingly long to

---

[27] Interview with Michael Sherrard, 12 July 1999; *Barclays Bank Ltd and Quistclose Investments Ltd AC* 1970, pp. 567–82; *JC* 23 Feb. 1962.   [28] *JC* 11 Oct. 1991, p. 6; *Sunday Times*, 7 Feb. 1993.
[29] *JC* 7 July 1961, p. 8, 22 May 1987, p. 13 (obituary of Jackson); interview with Madeleine Gottlieb (daughter of Joseph Jackson), 31 Aug. 1998.

get there'.[30] Perhaps, as a member of the Anglo-Jewish elite, he did not fully appreciate the difficulties facing those of his co-religionists setting out to make their way from modest immigrant backgrounds. Jackson became 'one of the country's most eminent authorities on divorce and . . . appeared in the cases of many well-known personalities', including Peter Sellers, Cynthia Lennon, and Rex Harrison. Jackson was instructed not only by the leading Jewish solicitors' firms such as Nabarro Nathanson, Victor Mishcon, and Paisner & Co., but by many others too, and 'was involved in virtually every leading matrimonial case of the day'. Besides acting for the rich and powerful, men such as Prince Radziwill and Adnan Khashoggi, he was still ready to accept a brief from a legally aided client.[31]

From the innumerable cases in which Joseph Jackson appeared, it is possible to select a sample to convey an inkling of his persuasiveness in court. In 1980 he represented a divorced mother, winning an appeal to the House of Lords which ruled that the Law Society had the power to postpone the enforcement of a charge for costs on the former matrimonial home and to transfer it to another property.[32] A year later, in the Court of Appeal, Jackson again acted for the mother, when in wardship proceedings the court decided that all three children should stay with her in England rather than being returned to their father, despite a pre-existing order of a rabbinical court in Israel.[33] On 29 January 1982 the Court of Appeal held that a judge had jurisdiction to set aside part of a consent order in matrimonial proceedings because the wife had no intention of carrying out the agreement on which the order was based.[34] Again, in the same year the Court of Appeal accepted Jackson's submission in *Hussain (Aliya)* v. *Hussain (Shahid)* that 'a marriage could only be potentially polygamous if at least one of the spouses had the capacity to marry a second spouse'.[35] In 1983 Jackson represented a legally aided husband when the House of Lords held that the needs of any relevant children formed only one consideration, and not the paramount one, in proceedings for the ouster of a spouse from the matrimonial home.[36] Finally, in *Barder* v. *Barder (Caluori intervening)* in 1986 Jackson was successful in the Court of Appeal, but in the following year the ruling was overturned by the House of Lords, which decided that where there was a 'clean break' order in matrimonial proceedings, if there was an unforeseen change in circumstances the husband could appeal out of time.[37]

[30] Seymour Karminski to Joseph Jackson, 24 Mar. 1967, Joseph Jackson Papers, in the possession of Madeleine Gottlieb.

[31] *JC* 22 May 1987, p. 13; interview with Madeleine Gottlieb, 31 Aug. 1998.

[32] *Hanlon* v. *Law Society, The Times*, 2 May 1980, *Daily Telegraph*, 2 May 1980.

[33] *Re: R, R, and R (minors), The Times*, 9 July 1981.

[34] *Thwaite* v. *Thwaite, The Times*, 5 Feb. 1982.

[35] *Hussain (Aliya)* v. *Hussain (Shahid)*, 24 June 1982; appeal from Manchester County Court, *Solicitors' Journal*, 24 Sept. 1982.   [36] *Richards* v. *Richards, The Times*, 1 July 1983.

[37] *Barder* v. *Barder (Caluori intervening), The Times*, 22 Apr. 1986 and 2 All ER 1987, pp. 440–54.

Blessed with a first-rate mind, Jackson was short and inclined to be somewhat pugnacious. When he sat as a commissioner of assizes in south Wales to see how he would fare as a judge there was an appeal from one of his decisions, and the Court of Appeal heavily criticized Jackson for interfering too much in his conduct of the case, utterly scotching his chances of becoming a High Court judge. As *The Times* remarked, 'It is a surprising feature of his career that he was not appointed to the High Court Bench but the authorities clearly thought that his tough forensic qualities did not suit him for judicial office.' Although Jackson still spoke to Jewish groups occasionally in the latter part of his life, in general his ties to the community became looser, and his second wife, Dame Margaret Booth, a former pupil and latterly a judge in the Family Division, was not Jewish.[38]

Jews from the patrician class, such as Lionel Cohen, Cyril Salmon, and Alan Mocatta, all dealt with a higher class of company and commercial work. Apart from Harold Lightman QC, few Jews from recent east European immigrant families made much headway in handling this type of work until the advent of Ingram Linder and Henry Burton.

Ingram Joseph Linder (1913–59) was being groomed for high office in the Jewish community as a successor to Lord Cohen as president of the Jewish Board of Guardians, and also looked set for promotion to high judicial office, when he died prematurely at the height of his powers, aged 46. Born in Stepney, the son of Polish immigrants, he was educated at the Northwold Road School in Stoke Newington, the North Hackney Central School, and Clifton College. His schooling indicates that he belonged to an upwardly mobile family; his father, a property dealer, was keen to see his son progress to higher things. Linder won a scholarship to Cambridge and was called to the Bar in 1935, taking silk in 1953. 'He was regarded as a leading advocate in the Chancery Division, dealing mainly with union and company matters.' Before the Second World War he was a regular speaker in north London in the campaign to combat antisemitism and took a great interest in the Jewish Friendly Society movement. After the end of the war Linder 'became identified with many of the community's charitable and political organisations'. Besides sitting on the Board of Deputies for the West London Synagogue, he was also active in the legal group of the Friends of the Hebrew University and on the Board of the United Restitution Organization. He became a member of various Jewish Board of Guardians committees, and as chairman of the Infirm Aged Committee in 1953 he played a notable role in the establishment of Tudor House in Grayshott for the elderly and infirm. He acted as a transitional figure between the old generation of patricians, who still ran many of the key institutions of Anglo-Jewry, and a new, highly urbane generation,

---

[38] *The Times*, 16 May 1987; private information.

populated by the sons of east European immigrants, that over time replaced most of them.[39]

Another such bridge-builder was Henry Burton (1907–52), who also died young, killed in a rail disaster at Harrow aged 45. He too was the child of east European immigrants, and was educated at Manchester Grammar School and Oxford. Called to the Bar in 1930 and taking silk in 1951, he became one of the best-known counsel on the Northern Circuit and specialized in common law and commercial law, frequently appearing in the Court of Appeal. Lord Justice Singleton praised him as someone who 'never missed a good point and never persisted in a bad one'. Neville Laski remarked that Burton 'was a most able attractive advocate, and a doughty fighter. He was possessed of great charm of manner.'[40] Like Linder, had his career not been cut short he would almost certainly have been promoted to the High Court, a position attained by his son Michael Burton QC.[41] Nevertheless, at the outset of Henry Burton's career, he found it difficult to find a place in chambers for his pupillage; and to assist other young Jews who encountered similar obstacles, he later formed his own set of chambers in Manchester. 'For four years—' noted Nathaniel Jacobs of the Council of Manchester Jews, 'from 1944 to 1948—he gave up his Sunday mornings to coach a group of raw recruits in the technique of public speaking to non-Jewish audiences in the cause of Jewish defence.'[42] He was on the board of governors of the Manchester Victoria Memorial Jewish Hospital and was a popular speaker at Jewish gatherings.

A barrister born in Merthyr Tydfil, who had a general practice with an emphasis on commercial work, was Leonard Caplan (1909–2001). His father, who came from Bialystok in Poland, was a dentist at a time when such a qualification could be acquired by watching more experienced practitioners at work; his mother was from the Austro-Hungarian province of Galicia. Like so many east European Jewish immigrants, his parents were ambitious for him, inculcating the idea in him as a child that he should become a barrister—which he understood as meaning 'bannister'. By the age of 20 Caplan was earning his living as a travelling propagandist for the Conservative Party, while simultaneously studying law; he was called to the Bar in 1935. He joined R. F. Levy's London chambers and developed a big general practice very quickly, so that when war broke out in 1939 he was well on his way to equalling F. E. Smith's record earnings of £5,000 in his fifth year at the Bar. Before the war Caplan was frequently instructed by Joseph Goldman, and was involved in many important bankruptcy cases. During the war he joined the army in the ranks but gained rapid promo-

---

[39] *JC* 29 May, 13, 5 June 1959, p. 13 (obituary of Linder); interviews with Judge Finestein, 6 Apr. 1998, Leonard Caplan, 22 Dec. 1998.

[40] *JC* 10 Oct. 1952, p. 8, 17 Oct. 1952, p. 9 (obituary of Burton).

[41] *JC* 26 Jan. 1996, *Solicitor's Supplement*, p. 2.   [42] *The Times*, 4, 10 Oct. 1952.

tion, and at the end of hostilities was Assistant Adjutant-General to Allied Forces in South-East Asia. Thereafter, R. F. Levy's chambers having been disbanded, Caplan set up his own set of chambers at 2 Harcourt Buildings in the Temple, of which the future Lord Justice Farquharson was an early member.[43]

Leonard Caplan became a QC in 1954, though it was not until 1961 that he became known to a wider public when he appeared in the Schtraks case. Yossele Schumacher, a boy aged 7, was kidnapped in Israel by his grandfather and uncle and removed from the custody of his parents because they feared that he would not be brought up as an Orthodox Jew. The uncle, Shalom Schtraks, fled to England, while the boy was spirited away to New York, where he was eventually found and reunited with his parents. When Schtraks was arrested in England, he appealed all the way up to the House of Lords, his lawyers raising the issues of whether the government of Israel had the right to extradite him for an act of perjury committed in Jerusalem, where the United Kingdom recognized the government of Israel as having only *de facto* authority; and whether his crimes were of a 'political character' within the meaning of the relevant section of the Extradition Act 1870. Caplan argued at the magistrates' court hearing that if the matter had now become a political issue in Israel this was irrelevant to the question of whether a crime had been committed, unless it could be shown that the crime had been committed in connection with a political measure. He submitted that the British government 'had granted *de facto* recognition to Israel's sovereignty over the Israeli-administered part of Jerusalem and that the courts of this country draw no distinction between *de facto* and *de jure* recognition arising from territory'. At the hearing before the House of Lords Caplan concentrated on showing that 'If parents have a right to possession of a child, and some person with intent to defeat that right places the child somewhere under a false name, it cannot be said that that intent was not to deprive the parents of possession to which they had a right and which in the ordinary way would have ripened into actual possession.' As to the appellant, and the reasons why he failed to surrender the boy, Caplan declared, 'Whether they are religious grounds, or reasons of filial piety, or whatever reasons they are, they are certainly not shown to be political reasons.' The law lords dismissed Schtraks's appeal, after which he was extradited to Israel, where he received a prison sentence of three years.[44]

Ten years later Leonard Caplan appeared in another sensational case, acting for Mrs Patricia Wolfson, the former wife of Sir Isaac Wolfson's nephew David. Having broken off her engagement to Ralph Stolkin, an American multi-millionaire, she refused to return jewellery and property worth £250,000. Caplan clashed with Stolkin's counsel, Joseph Jackson, in court and subjected

---

[43] Interview with Leonard Caplan, 22 Dec. 1998.
[44] *JC* 1 Sept., 6 Oct., 17 Nov., 15 Dec. 1961, p. 8, 5 Jan. 1962, p. 10, 19 Jan. 1962, p. 9; *H. L. E. Schtraks and Government of Israel and Others* AC 1964, pp. 575–7.

Stolkin to a bruising cross-examination before the case was settled.[45] Increasingly, however, Caplan acted in commercial matters; but he ordered his clerk to put up his fees for insolvency cases to a prohibitive level, as he did not wish to become known as 'Caplan the bankruptcy man'. In *Prudential Assurance Co. Ltd.* v. *Newman Industries Ltd. and Others* (1980) Caplan acted for the Prudential, successfully claiming that it was entitled as a minority shareholder in Newman Industries to sue for compensation on behalf of the company. 'In the same action Prudential was also held to be entitled to pursue a claim for damages for conspiracy in a direct personal capacity and in a representative capacity on behalf of other shareholders of Newman as at the date of the resolution.'[46] Caplan also acted in a three-month arbitration in London for the City of Nairobi, when French contractors tried to rescind a contract to build an earthen dam; his client's expert showed that despite the high moisture level of the area the soil would not turn into slurry as the contractors had alleged. Although he sat as a deputy High Court judge on numerous occasions, Caplan made it clear to the Lord Chancellor's Department that he had no desire to be elevated to such a position permanently, as he did not wish to be sent on circuit.[47]

The success of the careers of Linder and Burton, and perhaps also of Caplan (who handled a wider range of work) made it easier for other barristers from similar east European backgrounds, such as Morris Finer and Samuel Stamler, to achieve recognition at the commercial Bar. Morris Finer (1917–74) 'was born in the East End where his father was a tailor and he retained throughout his life a strong consciousness of his working-class origins . . . He was a thoroughly unpompous man renowned for his caustic wit.' When his family moved to Kilburn he was educated locally and at the London School of Economics, from where he graduated in 1939, being called to the Bar at Gray's Inn some four years later. Finer was a pupil of Arthian Davies, later Lord Justice Davies, in chambers which were predominantly Welsh in composition; after completion of his pupillage he had to take up a chambers residency elsewhere. In his early years at the Bar Finer augmented his income by writing articles for the *Evening Standard*, particularly humorous leading articles for the Saturday edition. Sometimes, though, he wrote serious leaders, taking up instances where an individual had been harshly treated by the operation of the law.[48] 'The interesting thing about the way he worked', Michael Sherrard recalled, was that 'he was one of the very few barristers who was a first rate typist. So he typed all his own work. For solicitors to get their paperwork typed almost by return was an enormous asset, but after research he also had the skill of being able to type the

---

[45] *The Times*, 29 Oct., p. 2, and 5, 6 Nov. 1971; *Daily Telegraph*, 5 Nov. 1971 (on the Wolfson case).

[46] *Prudential Assurance Co Ltd* v. *Newman Industries Ltd and Others*, *The Times*, 29 Feb. 1980.

[47] Interview with Leonard Caplan, 22 Dec. 1998.

[48] *JC* 20 Dec. 1974, p. 38 (obituary of Finer).

opinions and the advice straight off.'[49] Finer was predominantly a civil practitioner, but also knew his criminal law. 'He was very effective, very down to earth in his style [of oratory], very unpompous, and [had] a great gift of speaking plain English, short sentences, good timing'—a role model, indeed, for pupil barristers today.[50]

Although Finer came to wider public attention in 1960 in the State Building Society case, when acting with the assistance of Sherrard for one of the defendants, Harry Jasper, he was by then already responsible as a junior for a heavy caseload of commercial work, including landlord–tenant litigation and banking and insolvency work which received little, if any, publicity. On behalf of Jasper, Finer made a series of submissions which led to his client's being acquitted of making reckless and false statements to shareholders, whereas the other defendants were sent to prison for fraud.[51] Neville Faulks QC claimed in his memoirs that he recommended charging Jasper 'with obtaining money by false pretences' and that Finer told him 'that he would have advised him to plead "guilty" to such a charge'—a remark which seems out of character for Finer and not altogether credible.[52]

In spite of his application for silk being turned down three or four times, even though he was supported by judges at the Appeal Court level, Finer was at last made a QC in 1963, and, according to Iris Freeman, he 'was generally recognised to be the ablest commercial lawyer of his generation'.[53] Known for his great energy, he was capable of working a sixteen- or seventeen-hour day. Among his early victories as a silk were *Grangeside Properties Ltd.* v. *Collingwoods Securities Ltd. and Others*, where the mortgagees were held to be entitled to relief from forfeiture, and *Pick* v. *Josaron Investments Ltd.*, where the tenant's claim for compensation for giving her landlords vacant possession of property was allowed. Moreover, 'As an acknowledged expert on company law . . . and industrial affairs, he was in constant demand by private individuals (like the Beatles and Robert Maxwell), of the corporate bodies (like the Pilots' Union in the involved Trident disaster inquiry) and of the State (as in the Rolls Razor inquiry).'[54] In 1970, in *Re Pergamon Press Ltd.*, Finer argued on behalf of Robert Maxwell that the Board of Trade inspectors had to abide by the rules of natural justice and that the directors of Pergamon were entitled not only 'to see the transcripts of evidence of witnesses who speak adversely of them', but to cross-examine such witnesses. While rejecting the latter point, Lord Denning held that a director should be given 'a fair opportunity for correcting or contradicting what is said

---

[49] Interview with Michael Sherrard, 12 July 1999.   [50] *JC* 20 Dec. 1974, p. 38.
[51] *R.* v. *Grunwald and Others* 3 All ER 1960, pp. 380–90.
[52] Neville Faulks, *A Law Unto Myself* (London: Kimber, 1978), 23.
[53] Interview with Michael Sherrard, 12 July 1999; Freeman, *D. J. Freeman & Co.*, p. 9.
[54] *Estates Gazette*, 16 Nov., 21 Dec. 1963; *JC* 20 Dec. 1974, p. 38.

against him . . . An outline of the charge will usually suffice.'[55] As noted in Chapter 13, in *Brutus and Cozens* Finer showed that a demonstration involving a sit-in did not constitute insulting behaviour under section 5 of the Public Order Act 1936.

In 1972 Finer was appointed to the High Court bench; his judicial career, and other posts he held in the latter years of his life, are discussed in Chapter 15 below.

Stanley Burnton and Anthony Grabiner pointed out that 'When . . . Morris Finer took silk in 1963, Stamler was regarded by many as his natural successor, although they were not members of the same chambers.' Samuel Aaron Stamler (1925–94) was born to Jewish immigrant parents in Stoke Newington, where his father was a fur merchant of modest means, and was educated—like so many East End Jewish boys—at Central Foundation School. He later went on to Berkhampsted School before going to Cambridge in 1943. For a few years after graduating he stayed at Cambridge as a law tutor, before being called to the Bar in 1949. In 1966, with three colleagues, Stamler founded what has now become the largest commercial chambers in London at 1 Essex Court, Temple, with fifteen QCs and thirty-two junior barristers, of which he was head for twenty years.

Stamler's practice was entirely self-made . . . Despite its growth [1 Essex Court] . . . has retained an informality unusual in the profession. He was regarded as a father–figure by his colleagues; and his door was always open to the most junior tenant. He would strut around chambers and Essex Court in shirtsleeves, tie removed, accosting barristers, judges and clients with the latest of his enormous fund of jokes.[56]

Even as a junior Stamler appeared in weighty cases, and after previously having his application turned down for inexplicable reasons he took silk in 1971. His first important case was *W. J. Alan & Co. Ltd.* v. *El Nasr Export and Import Co.* (1972), which helped to clarify the concept of waiver in contract law. Although the seller had contracted to be paid for the supply of coffee in Kenyan shillings, he had none the less accepted payment in pounds sterling from the buyer, for whom Stamler was acting; then for a further shipment of coffee he had insisted on payment in the equivalent amount of Kenyan currency after the pound was devalued. As Lord Denning noted,

The principle of waiver is simply this: if one party by his conduct, leads another to believe that the strict rights arising under a contract will not be insisted upon, intending that the other should act on that belief, and he does act on it, then the first party will not afterwards be allowed to insist on the strict legal rights when it would be inequitable for him to do so.[57]

[55] Lord Denning, *The Discipline of Law* (London: Butterworths, 1979), 94–6; Bower, *Maxwell*, 270, 272, 282.   [56] *Independent*, 19 Nov. 1994; *JC* 25 Nov. 1994 (obituary of Stamler).
[57] *W J Alan & Co Ltd* v. *El Nasr Export and Import Co* 2 All ER 1927, pp. 127–47; Denning, *The Discipline of Law*, 214.

In *Town Investments* v. *Department of Environment* Stamler challenged the application of the Counter-Inflation (Business Rents) Orders on the grounds that the tenancies of the premises in question were held by the Secretary of State for the Environment and not the Crown; and that the premises were not occupied for the purpose of a 'business'.[58] His next major case was *Air Canada* v. *Secretary of State for Air (No. 2)*, dealing with airport landing charges and the disclosure of ministerial documents. It was held that a party desiring disclosure must show that the documents sought are likely to support him on an issue and that without such a document he would be deprived of proper representation.[59] Both these last two actions were ultimately lost by Stamler in the House of Lords, but he nevertheless ventilated fundamental issues of constitutional and public law. *Kleinwort Benson* v. *Malaysia Mining Corporation Bhd* (1989), which Stamler won for his client, was the leading case on the contractual obligations contained in 'letters of comfort' given by a parent company to a lender on behalf of a subsidiary. Lord Justice Gibson concluded that 'The defendants made a statement as to what their policy was, and did not in para 3 of the comfort letter expressly promise that such a policy would be continued in future.'[60]

Legal Business commented in respect of what was to be Stamler's last major court appearance that 'There is an old saying that 90 per cent of cases win or lose themselves, seven are lost by counsel and three are won by counsel. In the 3 per cent category is the result of the judicial review of the *Radio Authority*. Sam Stamler QC is said to have played a blinder for EMAP, the media group, in its support of the Authority.' EMAP wanted to take over TransWorld Communications, but by doing so it would have owned more local radio licences than permitted. By transferring a 50 per cent stake in one of its subsidiary companies to its merchant bankers, EMAP was able to convince the Radio Authority that it did not control the two licences held by its subsidiary. When the Guardian Media Group contested the decision of the Radio Authority, it was unable to satisfy the court that its interpretation of the statute was the correct one.[61]

Stamler's 'was a mind of the first rank and of great subtlety. No legal problem was so knotty, no set of facts was so complex, that he could not master it. The law reports contain numerous examples of judgements that reflect his arguments; and as Lord Lowry observed on an appeal to the House of Lords in 1990, Stamler's ability meant that a case presented by him "lacked nothing in thoroughness, ingenuity or force".'[62] The leading City solicitors in London, such as Freshfields, Slaughter & May, Ashurst Morris Crisp, and Herbert Smith,

---

[58] *Town Investments* v. *Department of Environment* AC 1978, pp. 359–403.

[59] *Air Canada* v. *Secretary of State for Air (No. 2)* 1 All ER 1983, pp. 161–89, 1 All ER 1983, pp. 910–27.

[60] *Kleinwort Benson* v. *Malaysia Mining Corporation Bhd* 1 All ER 1989, pp. 785–8; private information.   [61] *Legal Business* (Oct. 1994), 40; *The Times*, 11 Nov. 1994.

[62] *Independent*, 19 Nov. 1994.

brought a never-ending procession of bankers and businessmen to his chambers, which in the late 1970s and throughout the 1980s saw a marked increase in both the number of its members and its prestige. Richard Ireland recalled that he first instructed Stamler on behalf of Slaughter & May, the case being 'a trust problem and I knew from a friend of mine that Stamler was just ace at that kind of thing'. Despite the hubbub at the Chancery hearing, Stamler was 'so brilliant and eloquent and witty that everybody started listening and you could hear a pin drop'.[63] Burnton and Grabiner claimed that Stamler's 'analysis of facts and his powers of legal analysis were unique: he could see where none else could and problems for his opponents which they could not predict'. Michael Grade, who was a director of London Weekend Television in 1979, recalled that

We had a long day's consultation with . . . Stamler—and at five o'clock he took from his drawer a bottle, poured us all a huge whisky and proceeded to dictate a 15 page memo summarising all the options, recommending courses of action, referring back and forth, off the top of his head, and never drew a breath. I thought: that's a superior intelligence.[64]

Stamler's services were often sought in contested takeovers, including the Lonrho boardroom battle involving Tiny Rowland. His conduct of Heron International's 1982 attempt to thwart Robert Holmes à Court from acquiring Associated Communications was regarded as masterly; and if Holmes à Court could not be stopped, it would be compelled to pay a much higher price for its acquisition.[65]

Although he was made a Crown Court recorder in 1974, Stamler told a friend that he was reluctant to seek elevation to the High Court bench, as it would be a few years before he could move to the Appeal Court and in the interim the cases he would hear would be humdrum compared with the exciting proceedings in which he was accustomed to be engaged. He further believed that his inclination to intervene during court hearings because his quickness of mind made him grasp any side of an argument made him unsuitable for higher judicial office.[66]

Stamler was a learned Orthodox Jew, conducting a daily session of Talmud study during his undergraduate days at King's College, Cambridge. He became the national Jewish student leader, like Joseph Jackson assisting in the rebuilding of Jewish student life in Europe. He was friendly with Rabbi Kopul Rosen, founder of the prestigious Jewish boarding school Carmel College, which he served as a governor; and he became even more involved with the school when his younger brother David Stamler was appointed as its head. He was a firm

[63] *The Times*, 22 Nov. 1994 (obituary of Stamler).

[64] *Legal Business* (Jan.–Feb. 1995), 27.

[65] *Heron International Ltd and Others* v. *Lord Grade, Associated Communications Corporation plc and Others*, Butterworth's Company Law Cases 1983, pp. 244–72.

[66] Interview with Judge Henry Lachs, 22 Sept. 1999; private information.

supporter of Israel, organizing a number of fundraising functions for the Bar in aid of charities there.[67]

Once Morris Finer was appointed a Board of Trade inspector to inquire into the affairs of John Bloom's company in 1964, he increasingly received instructions from City firms, who often used him as an arbitrator to resolve disputes without recourse to the courts.[68] Samuel Stamler continued this trend and inaugurated a new era for the mass of Jewish barristers by winning the confidence of the leading City firms during the 1970s. The reputation he established resulted in an increased willingness on the part of City firms to hire Jewish barristers in important commercial cases, and his chambers at 1 Essex Court rapidly rose to prominence, enabling anyone with the necessary talents to break into the field of commercial law. Among the top silks who were Jewish and earning more than £1 million in 1998 or 1999 were Lord Grabiner, a pupil of Stamler, and Graham Aaronson QC, also from these chambers, while David Goldberg QC, Michael Flesch QC, Michael Crystal QC, and Jules Sher QC were based elsewhere; and Michael Burton, as already noted, moved on to become a High Court judge. All these individuals were from the tax, commercial, or Chancery Bar. Graham Aaronson, Michael Flesch, and David Goldberg were all specialists in the tax implications of company takeovers and were reputed to be among the highest earners at the Bar with an income of £1.5 million.[69] David Goldberg started to receive instructions from Linklaters in 1971 or 1972, when by chance a young Jewish solicitor with whom he had grown up in Plymouth happened to be working in the firm's revenue department.[70] Mark Littman QC (b. 1920), whose father had allegedly owned a textile business in Petticoat Lane, acted in some of the biggest commercial cases and was much in demand for international arbitration, but he held himself somewhat aloof from the Jewish community;[71] thus, according to the criteria adopted in this book, his not belonging to Jewish organizations meant that he was not a trend-setter.

There is a story that, after Israel won the Six Day War in 1967, the whole Bar mess stood up and applauded when a well-known Jewish counsel walked in; this is perhaps an indicator of the changing attitudes to Jewish barristers within the Bar, their acceptance as equals, which became more pronounced in the 1970s.

One other sector to which Jewish barristers made a notable contribution was in the area of human rights, starting with the French legal specialist Professor René Cassin, who played a key role in the drafting of the Universal Declaration of Human Rights in 1948. Sydney Kentridge (b. 1922), who grew up in Johannesburg and was called to the South African Bar in 1948, was a member of the defence team in the trials of black and white anti-apartheid activists on political

[67] *JC* 25 Nov. 1994. [68] Interview with Michael Sherrard, 7 Oct. 1999.
[69] *The Times*, 7 Sept. 1998, 27 Sept. 1999; *Evening Standard*, 14 Sept. 2000.
[70] Interview with David Goldberg, 25 Nov. 2000.
[71] Interview with William Frankel, 23 July 1998.

and treason charges. As a silk, he demonstrated to the world that Steve Biko, the founder of the Black Consciousness Movement, did not die accidentally but was murdered while in police custody. Tired of repeated clashes with unsympathetic judges on behalf of his black clients in South Africa, Kentridge transferred his practice to England, where he was called to the Bar in Lincoln's Inn in 1977. His progress, like that of Judah Benjamin, was rapid, and by 1984 he had become a QC. Lord Alexander described him as being 'softly spoken and sometimes understated. He lets the facts speak for themselves but presents them so skilfully that they are inevitably in favour of his own client.' Among his leading cases have been 'the defence of the P&O directors over the sinking of the *Herald of Free Enterprise*; for Dr Nigel Cox charged with murder by euthanasia . . . for the Serious Fraud Office in the claim by Ernest Saunders in Strasbourg that his trial was unfair; and in the International Tin Council bankruptcy saga'.[72] In *Regina* v. *Lord Saville of Newdigate and Others, Ex parte A and Others* (1999) he appeared for some of the soldier applicants when a Queen's Bench divisional court allowed an application by them to give evidence before the tribunal appointed to inquire into the events leading to 'Bloody Sunday' without revealing their names.[73] After the Bar sued Lord Hailsham, the then Lord Chancellor, in 1984 for his failure to raise legal aid fees for several years, Sydney Kentridge was chosen to present the barristers' case, which he did in so devastating a fashion that after his opening speech the government conceded defeat. If Kentridge had joined the English Bar earlier, there is little doubt that he would have become a law lord like some of his compatriots.

Another lawyer in a similar mould, who acted for prisoners on death row in the Caribbean, was Sir Louis Blom-Cooper (b. 1926). Called to the Bar in 1952 and taking silk in 1970, he was chairman of both the panel of inquiry into circumstances surrounding the death of James Beckford in 1985 and, from 1991 to 1992, the committee of inquiry into complaints about Ashworth high-security hospital. Between 1987 and 1994 he was chairman of the Mental Health Act Commission. According to Marcel Berlins,

As an advocate he was constantly arguing cases on behalf of the vulnerable and oppressed, when it was not fashionable or career-enhancing to do so. There are many who believe . . . that he never became a High Court Judge (which would have led to higher things) because at the time he should have gone on the bench on merit, he'd clashed with too many establishment judges at odds with his robustly expressed liberal views.[74]

Anthony Lester (b. 1936), now Lord Lester of Herne Hill, educated at Cambridge and Harvard universities, was called to the Bar in 1963. His father was Harry Lester (1907–84), the head of chambers at 12 King's Bench Walk, who

---

[72] *The Times*, 22 June 1999.　　　　[73] *The Times*, 5 Oct. 1999, Law Section, p. 5.
[74] *Guardian*, 29 June 1999.

had a civil law practice and fought a noteworthy case, *Bonsor* v. *Musicians' Union* (1955), up to the House of Lords; the judgment allowed members to be reinstated and to recover damages against their union for wrongful expulsion.[75] While serving as a special adviser to Roy Jenkins, when the latter was Home Secretary, Anthony Lester drafted a White Paper, *Equality for Women*, which was the basis of the Sex Discrimination Act 1975; a central feature was the establishment of the Equal Opportunities Commission with wide-ranging enforcement powers.[76] Lester, also played a key role in the framing of the Race Relations Act 1976, by setting up the Commission for Racial Equality which was itself modelled on the Equal Opportunities Commission. Lester admitted that, as far as racial discrimination was concerned, he 'was mainly inspired by ideas from across the Atlantic', though he refused to rely on conciliation committees for enforcement.[77] After taking silk in 1975, Lester conducted a number of cases in the European Court of Justice in the area of sex discrimination, and while at first the decisions of the court were unhelpful, from the mid-1980s it began to display a more positive attitude. For instance, *Johnston* v. *Chief Constable of the Royal Ulster Constabulary* decided that there was to be proper access to justice in discrimination cases.

When the European Convention on Human Rights was adopted in 1950, Britain long resisted making it enforceable; eventually, two years after its election in 1964, the Labour government of Harold Wilson accepted the right of individual petition and the compulsory jurisdiction of the European Court of Human Rights. From the 1960s Lester worked on some of the earliest British cases to go before this European court, including *Ireland* v. *United Kingdom* (1976) concerning torture perpetrated by the British army, *Times Newspapers Ltd.* v. *The United Kingdom* (1976) about the ban on a proposed article dealing with children suffering from the effects of thalidomide, and *Silver and Others* v. *The United Kingdom* (1980).[78] In the last case prisoners, including Silver, who wrote letters to the *Jewish Chronicle* and Rabbi Goren, complained that the prison authorities had stopped various letters which they had sent. As a result of the court's judgment, new regulations governing prisoners' correspondence were introduced in 1981.

With the publication of a pamphlet, *Democracy and Individual Rights*, in 1968, Lester started a thirty-year campaign for adoption of appropriate human rights legislation in Britain, culminating in the foundation of a pressure group,

[75] Harry Street, *Freedom: The Individual and the Law* (Harmondsworth: Penguin, 1977), 253; *JC* 11 Nov. 1955, p. 6.

[76] Roy Jenkins, *A Life at the Centre* (London: Macmillan, 1991), 375, 376.

[77] Lord Lester, 'Discrimination: What Can Lawyers Learn from History?', *Public Law* (1994), 224–37.

[78] Vincent Berger, *Case Law in the European Court of Human Rights 1960–1987* (Dublin: Round Hall, 1991), i. 86–91, 108–13, 213–17.

Charter 88; Lord Wade and Lord Lester, as he became, introduced human rights bills in the House of Lords in 1995 and 1997.[79] Meanwhile the judges, too, were changing in their attitudes to such a bill, because their decisions were being challenged in the European courts and they sought a British remedy for this impasse. The Labour leader John Smith, after the party's defeat in the election of 1992, made such a measure part of his programme, and Lord Lester claimed that he 'sought to persuade Derry Irvine [the Lord Chancellor] and I am glad to say that I succeeded'. Lord Lester's original bill favoured the Canadian model, which allowed courts to strike down statutes except where Parliament stated that this was not permissible. But because of the opposition of many leading judges, in his later bill Lester shifted to the New Zealand model, which would require judges to interpret law in accordance with the convention.[80] Under the Human Rights Act 1998, which followed this approach, David Pannick noted, 'legislation must be read and given effect in a manner compatible with rights guaranteed under the European Convention on Human Rights. Public authorities, including courts and tribunals, will have to act consistently with those rights.'

Lord Lester has also been involved in many important cases in the area of public law. In *Derbyshire County Council* v. *Times Newspapers Ltd* (1992), Lester almost persuaded Lord Justice Balcombe in the Court of Appeal to incorporate Article 10 of the European Convention on Human Rights into British law. Balcombe declared that since the article stated 'the right to freedom of expression and the qualifications to that right in precise terms', it could be utilized 'to help resolve some uncertainty or ambiguity in [British] municipal law'; and the Court of Appeal held that a municipal corporation was not entitled at common law to sue for libel to protect its reputation. When the council appealed to the House of Lords, Lord Keith would not go as far as that, but claimed 'that in the field of freedom of speech there was no difference in principle between English law on the subject and article 10 of the Convention . . . the common law of England is consistent with the obligations assumed by the Crown under the Treaty in this particular field'.[81] In *Pepper (Inspector of Taxes) and Hart*, Lord Browne-Wilkinson accepted Lester's submissions, stating that 'Subject to questions of the privileges of the House of Commons, reference to Parliamentary material should be permitted as an aid to the construction of legislation which is ambiguous or obscure or the literal meaning of which leads to an absurdity.'[82]

[79] *Silver and Others* v. *United Kingdom* 3 EHRR 1980, pp. 475–81, 486, 487, 523–30.

[80] *The Times*, 29 Oct. 1996, 5 July 1997, 18 May 1999; *Independent*, 15 June 1999; James Young, 'The Politics of the Human Rights Act', *Journal of Law and Society*, 26/1 (1999), 27–37; Lord Lester, 'UK Acceptance of the Strasbourg Jurisdiction: What Really Went On in Whitehall in 1965', *Public Law* (1998), 237–53.

[81] *Derbyshire County Council* v. *Times Newspapers Ltd* 1 QB 1992, pp. 770–818, AC 1993, pp. 534–51.   [82] *Pepper (Inspector of Taxes) and Hart* AC 1993, pp. 593–5, 630–5.

As Lord Irvine noted, here

the long established convention that the courts do not look at *Hansard* to discover the parliamentary intention behind legislation was reversed. It is strongly arguable that this was a consequence of the influence of Community law, where it is common to look for the purpose of a law in order to interpret that law and to look for that purpose in the legislative history.[83]

A landmark case in which Lord Lester acted which attracted widespread media attention was *Regina* v. *Human Fertilisation and Embryology Authority, Ex parte Blood* (1996). Mrs Diane Blood applied for a judicial review of the decision by the authority that her deceased husband's sperm could not be released so that she might have treatment for an artificially assisted pregnancy, on grounds that her husband's written consent was not obtained before the sample was taken. The couple had been trying to start a family when he was struck down by illness. Sperm which Mrs Blood had ordered his doctors to take from him, while he was unconscious and mortally ill, was kept in storage pending the decision of the court. Sir Stephen Brown, the president of the Family Division, ruled that Mrs Blood could not be inseminated artificially with the sperm taken from her husband because his prior written consent had not been obtained, nor could his sperm be exported to a country such as Belgium where written consent was not a prerequisite of treatment. When Lord Lester addressed the Appeal Court, he declared that 'The refusal of the authority to allow the export [of her dead husband's frozen sperm] is a restriction of Mrs Blood's right to obtain medical services in another European state as she is entitled to do under European law.' Giving judgment in the court, Lord Woolf ruled that

Under articles 59 and 60 of the EC Treaty, Mrs Blood had a right to receive medical treatment in another member state. The right was directly enforceable and therefore part of English law . . . the authority had not taken into account . . . that there should be no more cases after the instant case in which sperm was preserved without consent. Had the fact been appreciated, it could well have influenced the authority's decision.

A Belgian clinic carried out the artificial insemination and Diane Blood gave birth to a son in December 1998.[84]

It was rumoured that Lord Lester was offered a High Court appointment when he was 57, but declined the offer because he did not want to try criminal cases on circuit. Like Sydney Kentridge and Sir Louis Blom-Cooper, Lord Lester was not closely involved with Jewish communal affairs. Whereas his father, Harry Lester, was once deeply involved in communal organizations,

---

[83] Lord Irvine, 'The Development of Human Rights in Britain under an Incorporated Convention on Human Rights', *Public Law* (1998), 230, 231.

[84] *The Times*, 18 Oct. 1996, 15 Jan. 1997, 7 Feb. 1997, 28 Feb. 1997; *Sunday Times*, 13 Dec. 1998.

Lord Lester had little contact with them and it was only in middle age that he re-established some ties. Allan Levy QC, the leading specialist in cases concerning children who won a landmark decision in the European Court of Human Rights against corporal punishment for children, described himself as an 'assimilated Jew', though 'he supported a number of communal charities'.[85] On the other hand, David Pannick QC, another human rights and commercial lawyer, belongs to many Jewish organizations and is a member of the Radlett Synagogue. Whereas in the past Jewish barristers had to deal with institutionalized antisemitism, today they have to cope with long hours and career pressures which leave little time for communal involvement and encourage an increasingly secular lifestyle. Only the most dedicated, such as Eldred Tabachnik QC, former president of the Board of Deputies, and Romy Tager QC of the Jewish Book Council, care to spend their leisure hours on Jewish concerns.

[85] *JC* 11 Nov. 1955, p. 6, 16 Apr. 1999, p. 25 (obituary of Denise Pannick); Joshua Rozenberg, *The Search for Justice: An Anatomy of the Law* (London: Sceptre, 1995), 367; *JC* 2 Oct. 1998.

FIFTEEN

Jews in the Judiciary, 1945–1990

UNTIL the 1950s and 1960s it was uncommon for Jews to reach the higher levels of the English judiciary. True, there were outstanding individuals from the older Anglo-Jewish families, such as George Jessel and Rufus Isaacs, who graced the benches of the High Court; but none had ever been joined by a Jewish colleague. At first it seemed that this pattern was to be repeated when Lionel Leonard Cohen (1888–1973) was appointed as a judge in the Chancery Division of the High Court in 1943—another solitary Jew on the High Court benches. Descended from Levi Barent Cohen (1747–1808), the ancestor of the Anglo-Jewish 'Cousinhood', and a member of one of Anglo-Jewry's most illustrious families, with ties to the Rothschilds and Montefiores, Lionel Cohen was educated at Eton and New College, Oxford, where he obtained a first-class degree in history in 1909 and in law in the following year, and was called to the Bar in 1913. After service in the army during the First World War he joined the chambers of Alfred Topham, a leading specialist in company law, and soon acquired a considerable practice of his own; he was elevated to the rank of King's Counsel in 1929.[1] 'He was the first Jew to be appointed as a puisne judge, then the first Jew to become a Lord Justice of Appeal [in 1946] and finally the first to be made a Lord of Appeal in Ordinary [in 1951].'[2] On this last promotion to the House of Lords, the highest court in the land, he was made a life peer. Although Cohen retired as a Lord of Appeal in Ordinary in 1960, he still sat in the House of Lords from time to time, hearing cases, until 1967. According to Sir Raymond Evershed, Cohen was ' "the greatest living exponent of English law on corporations", possessing all the qualities required in his most eminent position: integrity of mind, accuracy of thought and expression, and distrust of the catchword'.[3]

Cohen was precluded from making a greater contribution to English law as a judge by his extensive role in public life and his involvement in the affairs of the Jewish community. He was chairman of the Company Law Amendment

---

[1] *Dictionary of National Biography 1971–1980*, 163, 164; *JC* 1 Mar. 1963, p. 16.

[2] *JC* 16 Nov. 1951, p. 1, 28 Dec. 1951, p. 11, 2 May 1952, p. 5.

[3] *JC* 1 Mar. 1963, p. 16; *Dictionary of National Biography 1971–1980*, 163, 164.

Committee, a post which enabled him to shape the Companies Act of 1948, the first major reconstruction of the law in this field since the beginning of the century; he also served as chairman of a number of royal commissions, as well as being one of the 'three wise men' entrusted by Harold Macmillan between 1957 and 1959 with devising an incomes policy.[4] 'Thus to write of Cohen as a law lord [with all these outside commitments] is to write of an almost hypothetical figure', argued Robert Stevens. 'His relatively rare appearances meant that he never achieved, judicially, the dominance one would have expected even in company and tax matters.'[5] Although 'outwardly a country gentleman, a devotee of golf and a keen shot', Cohen sometimes evinced liberal sympathies and was a convert to the abolition of capital punishment.

Cohen played a significant role in Anglo-Jewish life, serving as president of the Jewish Board of Guardians for seven years and for a time as vice-president of the Board of Deputies; he was also president of the Jewish Historical Society, and sat on the council of the Anglo-Jewish Association. A frequent visitor to Israel, despite never being 'a Zionist in any narrow sense'—as befitted a member of an old Anglo-Jewish family—he was chairman of the Friends of the Hebrew University, where the Lionel Cohen lectureship was established in his honour.[6] As a young man, he was a member of the Orthodox Central Synagogue, but later joined a Reform congregation.

When Seymour Karminski (1902–74) was appointed a High Court judge in 1951, the *Jewish Chronicle* proudly announced that 'two members of the Anglo-Jewish community, for the first time in its long history, sit on the Bench of the High Court—the other Judge, of course, is Lord Justice Cohen'.[7] Like Cohen, Karminski had the right Anglo-Jewish family connections and education for the position. His father was a distinguished banker, and Karminski was educated at Rugby School and Oxford University; after gaining a first-class degree in history, he was called to the Bar in 1925. Two years later he married the granddaughter of the eminent Jewish solicitor Sir George Lewis; and, as he specialized in divorce law, no doubt his practice was boosted by instructions from the family firm of Lewis and Lewis. He took silk in 1945. Having been appointed a judge of the Probate, Divorce, and Admiralty Division in 1951, he relinquished this position in 1969 when he was made a Lord Justice of Appeal. As a judge, 'He was courteous and patient. He was never ruffled or lost his temper. He was at his best at dealing with family matters . . . [but] He was a good judge, too, in Admiralty matters, where his [wartime] experience in the Navy proved invaluable.'

[4] *Dictionary of National Biography 1971–1980*, 163, 164.
[5] Robert Stevens, *Law and Politics: The House of Lords as a Judicial Body, 1800–1976* (London: Weidenfeld & Nicolson, 1979), 372, 373.
[6] *JC* 28 Dec. 1951, p. 11.   [7] *JC* 12 Jan. 1951, p. 1, 19 Jan. 1951, p. 6.

Like Lord Cohen and the wealthy individuals from old Anglo-Jewish families who controlled the communal institutions in the nineteenth century, Sir Seymour Karminski was very active in Anglo-Jewish affairs. He followed Lord Cohen by becoming president of the Jewish Board of Guardians; he presided regularly over meetings and addressed public gatherings, and he and Lady Karminski were frequent visitors to old people's homes, convalescent homes and youth clubs. He succeeded Lord Cohen as president of the Friends of the Hebrew University, delivering the Lionel Cohen lecture in 1962. He was vice-president of the Jewish Ex-Servicemen's Association, having served as a lieutenant-commander in the Royal Navy Volunteer Reserve during the Second World War. And as if all this were not sufficient, he was also president of the Trades Advisory Council, a council member of the Anglo-Jewish Association, and president of the Westminster Synagogue.[8]

Cyril Barnet Salmon (1902–91), whose father was a cousin of Sir Samuel Salmon, the managing director of J. Lyons, was another member of an affluent Anglo-Jewish family. Educated at Mill Hill School and Cambridge, he was called to the Bar in 1925 and became a pupil of Walter Monckton. Having built up a reputation in commercial law he took silk in 1945, becoming a leader with a busy and varied practice. As noted in an earlier chapter, when William Frankel applied to join his chambers as a young barrister, Salmon told him 'that he had heard good things about' him 'but he did not want to make his set into a Jewish set of Chambers'. Like Rufus Isaacs, Salmon had a wonderfully retentive memory, and his cases were conducted with the scantiest of notes, as he had the gift of retaining dates and page references without difficulty; they were also conducted in a fluid style, varying with the occasion. He had a tart wit, and once when interrupted by a judge in the Court of Appeal, exclaimed: 'My Lord, I apologize. I must take comfort from the fact that your Lordship's learned brethren grasped it [the point he was making] twenty minutes ago.' After a stint as recorder of Gravesend, he was appointed as a High Court judge in 1957, and first attracted press and public attention the following year, when he presided over a trial at the Central Criminal Court of a gang of white youths accused of beating up blacks during the Notting Hill disturbances. He gave the defendants stiff prison sentences, declaring that 'Everyone, irrespective of the colour of their skin, is entitled to walk through our streets in peace, with their heads erect and free from fear.' He seized this opportunity to denounce racialism, as he was 'conscious of his Jewish origin as a possible source of discrimination'.[9]

In 1964 Salmon was promoted to the Court of Appeal, where he continued to express his liberal views in a forthright manner. Here in 1968 he dismissed the

[8] *JC* 1 Nov. 1974, p. 42; *The Times*, 31 Oct., 1 Nov., 12 Nov. 1974 (obituary of Karminski).

[9] *The Times*, 9 Nov. 1991; Deborah Andrews (ed.), *The Annual Obituary* (Detroit and London: St James Press, 1992), 709, 710 (obituary of Salmon); interview with William Frankel, 23 July 1998.

appeal by the financier Savundra against conviction for insurance fraud, at the same time castigating the media for trial by television in having broadcast an ill-considered interview with Savundra a short while before his arrest. Among his other memorable judgments were his decision to quash the conviction for obscenity of the publishers of *Last Exit to Brooklyn*, his support for women's rights in declaring that a woman was entitled to be a racehorse trainer, and his refusal in the Privy Council to accept that the law required the execution of any prisoner for crimes committed when he was a minor. In 1972 he became a lord of appeal in ordinary, but thereafter was hampered by ill health until his retirement in 1980.[10]

Stevens has shown that in sitting as a law lord Salmon was rather less liberal in his decisions than during his time as a member of the Appeal Court, where he tended to side with Lord Denning. In the Lords he did not find with his colleagues for the Race Relations Board, and he was hostile to picketing. During his judicial career he presided over two royal commissions, one in 1966 into the working of tribunals of inquiry, the other in 1974 into standards of conduct in public life after the Poulson scandal.[11] Unlike Cohen and Karminski, he did not participate very actively in Jewish communal life, apart from being chairman of the legal group of Friends of the Hebrew University and a member of the Maccabeans; both his two wives were non-Jewish, and he lacked any ambition to become a communal insider.

In 1961 Alan Mocatta (1907–90) was elevated to the High Court bench and the *Jewish Chronicle* proudly announced that 'This is the first time that there have been three Jewish Judges in the High Court in the same period.'[12] The Mocattas, a Sephardi family from Spain, settled in England in 1671, establishing the banking house of Mocatta and Goldsmid. (Asher Goldsmid was an Ashkenazi Jew whose family had arrived from the Netherlands in the early eighteenth century.) Educated in the Jewish house at Clifton College and at Oxford, Alan Mocatta was called to the Bar in 1930. After being made a silk in 1951, he specialized in arguing points of law in commercial litigation; he would make his juniors stay up until the early hours of the morning, studying all the possible arguments which could be derived from the relevant authorities, and dismiss them at 2 a.m., saying he wanted to prepare an urgent opinion for one of his instructing solicitors. He enhanced his reputation by his report for a government committee on cheque endorsement in 1956. From 1936 until 1984 he was editor of six editions of *Scrutton on Charter Parties*. After being made a High Court judge in 1961, Mocatta sat in a variety of courts throughout the 1960s and 1970s, including the Restrictive Practices Court, and tried criminal

---

[10] *The Times*, 9 Nov. 1991; Andrews (ed.), *The Annual Obituary*, 709, 710 (obituary of Salmon); *JC* 15 Nov. 1991, p. 14 (obituary of Salmon).

[11] Stevens, *Law and Politics*, 578–83.　　　　　　　　　　[12] *JC* 6 Oct. 1961, p. 8.

cases on circuit, but it was in the Commercial Court that his judgments made the greatest contribution to the development of the law. He was not raised to the Court of Appeal and retired in 1981.[13]

Mocatta was a deeply committed Jew, an urbane chairman of the Council of Jews' College from 1945 to 1961, president for fifteen years of the board of elders of the Spanish and Portuguese Synagogue, and president of the Jewish Historical Society in 1969. For almost forty years, he assisted in the administration of the Beth Holim, the home for the aged of his congregation. He also enjoyed publicly chanting the *haftarah* (an extract from the Prophets or other sacred writings) in the synagogue on the sabbath.[14]

All these four post-war High Court judges came from well-established families belonging to the Anglo-Jewish elite. Three of them were educated in well-known boarding schools, while one attended a public day school; all of them went on to university at either Oxford or Cambridge. In 1969 Henry Cecil found that out of 'a random group of 36 judges of the Court of Appeal and the High Court . . . 31 had been to public schools (86 per cent) and 33 to Oxford or Cambridge (92 per cent)'. Two other judges in this period were born into Jewish families, though they did not practise the faith as adults: Sir Eric Sachs (1898–1979), who sat in the Court of Appeal, and Lord Simon of Glaisdale (b. 1911), who sat in the Lords. Both had been to public schools and Oxbridge.[15] Thus the first post-war Jewish judges had a class and educational profile similar to that of most other High Court judges. Much of the work of Cohen, Salmon, and Mocatta as barristers came from dealing with lucrative commercial disputes, while Karminski acted in many society divorce suits. Three participated in running some of the chief Anglo-Jewish communal institutions, while the fourth, Salmon, supported the legal section of the Friends of the Hebrew University and was always willing to speak at the functions of other Anglo-Jewish societies.

One outstanding Jewish advocate, of east European stock, who never quite made it to the top during the 1940s and 1950s was Richard Francis Levy QC (1892–1968). Among his notable cases he defended the Revd Harold Davidson, the rector of Stiffkey, Norfolk, on charges of immoral conduct in a sensational trial in 1932, and in 1950 he defended Donald Hume at the Old Bailey in his trial for the murder of Donald Setty, a car dealer whose dismembered body was thrown out of an aeroplane. He also clashed angrily with Gilbert Beyfus in a breach of promise action brought by Mrs Helen Dunhill, the wife of a tobacco magnate. Levy was educated at Hackney Downs School and London University, not quite matching the educational antecedents of other High Court judges. His reputation was somewhat unfairly sullied by his acting for money-

---

[13] *The Times*, 12 Nov. 1990 (obituary of Mocatta).   [14] *JC* 6 Oct. 1961, pp. 8, 11.

[15] J. A. G. Griffith, *The Politics of the Judiciary* (London: Fontana, 1985), 25–9; *Dictionary of National Biography, 1971–1980*, 751, 752 (on Sachs); *JC* 16 Feb. 1962, p. 6 (on Simon).

lenders as part of his pre-war practice. He never became a High Court judge, despite his undoubted abilities; instead he served as chairman of the Monopolies Commission between 1956 and 1965, but, rather shabbily, a knighthood was not conferred on him, though the honour went to both his predecessor and his successor in that office.[16]

In contrast with the earlier post-war appointments, the next batch of Jewish High Court judges in the late 1960s and early 1970s were mainly from east European immigrant families. The first, Sebag Shaw (1907–83), was placed on the High Court bench at the age of 61 in 1968 by Gerald Gardiner, the reforming Lord Chancellor in Harold Wilson's Labour government. Seven years later Sebag Shaw was promoted to become a lord justice of appeal. Here was a clear break with the past: promotion for a man who had grown up and been educated in the East End, and who headed a set of chambers known as the 'Jewish chambers'. 'People who knew him', said *The Times* in a tribute,

were sure that he would be a good . . . [judge], and they were right. While he was well able to carry out the full and varied range of work with which the Queen's Bench Division has to deal, successive Lord Chief Justices (Parker and Widgery) often relied on him as a sort of trouble-shooter in difficult criminal cases where a combination of strength and discretion were particularly required in the presiding judge.

When he sat as a judge, declared Bernard Gillis, 'the Bar and litigants always knew that they would be heard with patience: when they left his court, whatever the outcome, none could complain of having been subject to unfairness'. On criminological and penological issues, Sebag Shaw was a moderate liberal, opposing the removal of some of the provisions safeguarding the interests of accused persons and supporting the abolition of capital punishment; but the longer he spent on the bench, the more his sentencing policy hardened. Although he had an Orthodox upbringing and had as a child attended the Hambro Synagogue (now defunct), he later in life joined the Liberal Synagogue; nevertheless, he remained loyal to the ethical and cultural traditions of his Orthodox upbringing. He was a vice-president of the Magen David Adom (the Israeli equivalent of the Red Cross) and a prominent supporter of the Friends of the Hebrew University.[17]

Another Jewish judge appointed to the High Court bench by Lord Chancellor Gardiner was Sir George Bean (1925–73), a member of the Bonn family (the matza manufacturers). He was educated at the Liverpool Institute and Liverpool University, where he studied law, was president of the students' law club, and was actively engaged in student politics, becoming vice-president of

[16] *The Times*, 18 Dec. 1968; *JC* 20 Dec. 1968, p. 39 (obituary of Levy); private information; Adamson, *The Old Fox*, 198–204.

[17] *The Times*, 4 Jan. 1983; *JC* 7 Jan. 1983, p. 22 (obituaries of Shaw).

the National Union of Students. After being called to the Bar, he served in the army during the Second World War, rising to the rank of colonel. At the age of 45 he was made assistant presiding judge of the Liverpool Court of Passage and in 1965 recorder of Carlisle, in the meantime taking silk in 1963. He was appointed a High Court judge in 1969, 'and was an immediate success as a judge. He had the happy judicial knack of preventing the heat and smoke of forensic battle from obscuring the calm review that justice required.' Proud of his Jewish heritage, he was the leader of the Liverpool Jewish community, presiding over the Merseyside Representative Council. He founded the local Merseyside branch of the Association of Jewish Ex-Servicemen and Women, becoming national chairman of the whole organization in due course. 'In his early days in Liverpool Sir George took a keen interest in Jewish activities—notably the Jewish Lads' Brigade and youth club work.' On top of his judicial work and communal activities, he was asked by the Lord Chancellor to preside over a series of seminars on sentencing policy; it was at one of these that he suffered a heart attack, subsequently dying at the age of 58.[18]

The next Jewish High Court judge, Sir Phillip Wien (1913–81) was appointed in September 1970 by a Conservative Lord Chancellor, but his appointment may already have been in the pipeline when the new administration took over. Wien was born in Cardiff and educated at Canton High School, University College, Cardiff, and University College London, where he took his LL M. He qualified as a solicitor and briefly practised in Cardiff before the outbreak of the Second World War. During the war he commanded a squadron of armoured cars and rose to the rank of major. After the end of hostilities he participated in war crimes trials in Germany, where his ability was so noticed by members of the tribunals that he was encouraged to apply to the Bar on his return to civilian life. Wien was called to the Bar in 1946 and took silk in 1961. 'Thereafter, his qualities both as a lawyer and as an advocate were quickly recognized and he built up a large civil and criminal practice on the Wales and Chester Circuit', eventually becoming leader of the circuit. 'The many firms of solicitors who instructed him realized that in Phillip Wien they were able to call upon a skilled, articulate and powerful advocate . . . formidable and thorough . . . as a practitioner.' He was the leading counsel for the Coal Board in the inquiry into the Aberfan disaster, when the waste mound from a mine engulfed an elementary school, and the report in 1967 paid tribute to his 'great skill and persuasiveness'. From 1965 to 1969 Wien was recorder of Birkenhead and then briefly recorder of Swansea, where he displayed considerable judicial skill, so that it did not cause surprise when he was elevated to the High Court bench: 'In civil jurisdiction he was quick to see the point and in the criminal field, although outwardly

---

[18] *The Times*, 23 Nov. 1973; *JC* 23 Nov. 1973, p. 22 (obituaries of Bean).

he presented a stern figure, he was in reality a most compassionable and understanding man.'[19] Among other cases, Wien tried Robert Maxwell's claim in 1971 that the DTI inspectors' report breached the rules of natural justice, but was unsympathetic to the publisher's rambling interjections and concluded that the inspectors had acted 'eminently fairly'.[20]

In 1972 Sir Morris Finer (1917–74), one of the outstanding members of the post-war Bar (see the discussion in Chapter 14 above), was promoted to the High Court bench, again by a Conservative Lord Chancellor. It was a remarkable appointment. William Frankel commented that 'Morris Finer was known as the stereotypical Jewish barrister. He was aggressive, he was not very popular among his colleagues, but when he was appointed a High Court Judge that was symptomatic of a fundamental change . . . Sebag Shaw was also of East End antecedents . . . [but he] was altogether a more cultivated kind of person.'[21] Other contemporaries, however, viewed Finer differently and in a much less harsh light. He was also extremely busy off the bench: he was vice-chairman of the governors of the LSE, and in 1972 the government called on him to chair the committee on one-parent families, which reported in 1974 and turned him into a national figure. From his experience while serving on this committee, he tried to refashion 'the relationship between the private law of family maintenance and the public law of social security. From this stemmed wide-ranging proposals for the reconstruction of the respective roles of the courts and the social security authorities in dealing with family breakdown.' He also found time to participate in the Cinematograph Films Council and the National Book League. He sat as a judge in the Family Division of the High Court, but was able to sit only occasionally because of his committee work and his appointment in 1974 as chairman of the Royal Commission on the Press. This appointment, noted Charles Wintour, 'changed the outlook entirely . . . he not only knew what it was like to work in a newspaper; he had a vast commercial experience, an enquiring intelligence, an unslakeable appetite for mastering indigestible documentation, and, above all, that passionate belief in the value of open argument which is at the heart of the case for free speech'. Finer had a mastery of revenue law and in his judgments in the Family Division he tried to make the tax system mesh more closely with the provisions for relief under the social security system.[22] According to Lord Elwyn-Jones, the Lord Chancellor, Finer 'thought of the law as a purposive instrument of social betterment'.[23]

In 1956 Rose Heilbron QC (whose career at the Bar is discussed in Chapter 14 above) was made recorder of Burnley, succeeding Neville Laski, who had

---

[19] *The Times*, 13 June 1981; *JC* 19 June 1981, p. 14 (obituaries of Wien).
[20] Bower, *Maxwell*, 291–4. [21] Interview with William Frankel, 23 July 1998.
[22] *The Times*, 16 Dec. 1974 (obituary of Finer).
[23] Transcript of memorial meeting to Finer, 13 Jan. 1975, copy in the possession of Michael Sherrard.

been promoted to be a judge of the Crown Court in Liverpool. This was the first time that a woman had occupied this position. Despite Heilbron's national reputation, she was beaten in the promotion race by Elizabeth Lane, who leapfrogged over her to become the first woman county court judge in 1962 and later the first High Court judge. On the return of a Labour government in 1974, however, Dame Rose Heilbron was elevated to the Family Division of the High Court, where she sat until retiring in 1988. 'She was not, I think, an outstanding Judge', declared a colleague, 'but she was competent, easy to appear before, not a great lawyer but she wouldn't have appreciated that as being a compliment anyway.'[24]

When the first group of Jewish judges appointed after the Second World War are compared with their successors, a number of distinctions become apparent. The first batch of judges were from old Anglo-Jewish families and were educated at public schools and Oxbridge, whereas the later judges were the children of immigrants and attended local grammar schools and redbrick universities or London University. While three members of the first group were Anglo-Jewish communal leaders, the later judges tended to have looser communal ties, though Sir George Bean was a provincial Jewish leader. There was one notable exception to this finding, namely Sir John Alfred Balcombe (1925–2000), who belonged to a socially mobile east European Jewish family and was educated at Winchester and Oxford. He became a judge in the Family Division of the High Court in 1977, and in 1985 was promoted to the Court of Appeal, where he stayed for ten years. He was deeply involved with Jewish communal bodies, serving as president of the Maccabeans and (for ten years) as chairman of the Friends of the Hebrew University, for which he organized fund-raising activities. He was also a trustee of the Wimbledon Reform Synagogue and gave strong support to Norwood Child Care, a charity for Jewish children, and Nightingale House, a home for the Jewish elderly.[25]

As to the Jewish affiliation of some of the other judges, Finer was 'very proud of being Jewish', asserted his former pupil Michael Sherrard; 'he gave a lot to being Jewish; it gave a lot to him; but he could not bear the religious trappings. And it was for this reason that he did not wish a religious funeral.'[26] His attendance at a dinner in 1969 in support of the Joint Israel Appeal was a rare event. As for Dame Rose Heilbron, although she came from an Orthodox background and had been treasurer of the national Jewish students' federation (IUJF), she had little time once she was a barrister to participate in Jewish organizations; and Sir Phillip Wien had no connections with Jewish communal organizations.[27] Nearly

---

[24] Private information.
[25] *JC* 14 July 2000, p. 23 (obituary of Balcombe).
[26] Transcript of memorial meeting to Finer, 13 Jan. 1975.
[27] *JC* 22 Apr. 1949, p. 6, 19 June 1981, p. 14.

all the first group of judges specialized in commercial law, but apart from Finer none of the latter had a commercial law practice and most were more at home in the criminal or divorce courts.

Despite his brilliance and the speed with which he dispatched business, so that two judges were required to replace him, Neville Laski (1891–1969) remained a judge of the Liverpool Crown Court until he was 72, reluctantly retiring only in 1963. His regime of tough sentences, preceded by whiplash remarks to the criminals concerned, reduced crime in the city of Liverpool; but he also attracted adverse criticism in the national press and was more or less forced to retire.[28] Equally harsh when sentencing was Ewen Montagu (1901–85), who 'was one of the last of the old-fashioned bullying chairmen of [the Middlesex] Quarter Sessions. Outside court a man of great charm and wit, inside, whenever a mother entered the witness box to give evidence in mitigation, he would write GBAH to stand for good boy at home as she took the oath. It rarely did the child much good.' Both men held senior communal positions, Laski as president of the Board of Deputies and of the Sephardi elders, Montagu as president of the United Synagogue.[29]

Quite a few slightly younger Jewish judges sat for the first time in the Central Criminal Court, the Old Bailey. Myer Alan Barry King-Hamilton (b. 1904) came from an old Anglo-Jewish family of Dutch origin which had settled in England in the late seventeenth century; his great-grandmother on his mother's side was a Quaker, a member of the famous Fox family. Educated at grammar school and Cambridge, he was called to the Bar in 1929 and took silk in 1954. He did a mixture of civil and criminal work while he continued to deal with traffic licensing, in which he had specialized since his early days at the Bar. He held the recorderships of Hereford, Gloucester, and Wolverhampton in succession, but for family reasons he declined an offer by the Lord Chancellor, then Kilmuir, to sit as recorder of Liverpool, which was a full-time post. When the City of London (Courts) Act 1964 provided for the appointment of additional judges at the Old Bailey, King-Hamilton was one of the first two judges selected to fill this role (with Bernard Gillis). As an Old Bailey judge between 1964 and 1979 he tried a number of notable cases, including those of the fraudulent insurance promoter Emil Savundra; Janie Jones, who was charged not only with running a call-girl racket but also with blackmail and deception; and Peter Hain, who was falsely charged with theft because of a plot by the South African security

[28] *JC* 16 Dec. 1960, p. 12, 4 May 1962, p. 6, 28 Mar. 1969, p. 53 (obituary of Laski); Doreen Tanner, 'He gave Liverpool the Severity it Needed' [*c.* Aug. 1963], Neville Laski Papers, Southampton University, Parkes Library, MS 134, AJ 33/204; transcript of farewell to Laski on his retirement, 1 Aug. 1963, AJ33/201.

[29] *JC* 30 Jan. 1953, 13 July 1985, 26 July 1985, p. 15 (obituary of Montagu); James Morton, *Bent Coppers: A Survey of Police Corruption* (London: Little, Brown, 1993), 111.

service. King–Hamilton was a committed Jew who served as president of the West London Reform Synagogue from 1967 to 1975.[30]

Bernard Gillis (1905–96), the son of Rabbi Julius Kyanski of Newcastle, was a close friend of King–Hamilton and the two men's careers ran remarkably parallel. Both were educated at Cambridge, although Gillis was called to the Bar in 1927, two years before King–Hamilton. Both served in the Royal Air Force during the Second World War and both rose to the rank of squadron leader. On demobilization, Gillis built up a reputation at the Bar by sifting through the detail of fraud cases. Gillis and King–Hamilton took silk at the same time in 1954, while on the same day ten years later they were appointed additional judges at the Old Bailey. When sitting as a judge at the Central Criminal Court it was Gillis's task to try the many involved cases of fraud.

Movements of valuable cargoes, great advances in international financial business and the increase in the number of banks and finance houses, exchange controls, new customs and excise regulations, the avoidance and evasion of tax, the rise of newly independent countries without adequate financial experience, all these factors have attracted clever but dishonest men who with false documents and by other fraudulent means, have created a world wide machinery to rob banks and insurance companies and those engaged in international trade; dishonest interference in companies accounts for millions stolen each year. This largely new area of very serious crime is in addition to the familiar cases of fraud arising within these shores.[31]

In 1980 King–Hamilton and Gillis shared a retirement party at the Old Bailey together.

Until he joined the bench Gillis played a prominent role in British Jewry, becoming chairman of the Association of Jewish Ex-Servicemen and Women, serving as a governor of Carmel College, and participating in the work of the Board of Deputies; but he was never 'able to accept some of the ritualistic or restrictive standards and practices of strictly Orthodox Judaism', though he was inspired by the prophets and the Old Testament, 'with its codes of social and economic justice'. In consequence he broke with his Orthodox upbringing and became a member of a Reform synagogue.[32]

Another judge who sat in the Old Bailey was Alexander Karmel (1904–98). Educated at Newcastle Royal Grammar School and Trinity College, Dublin, he spent several years in his father's tailoring business before being called to the Bar in 1932. As a barrister on the Northern Circuit, he built up a thriving personal injuries practice and also appeared in some criminal cases. A cousin of David Karmel, the recorder of Wigan, he was himself made recorder of Bolton in 1962 and an additional judge at the Old Bailey in 1968. 'Barristers were

---

[30] King-Hamilton, *And Nothing but the Truth*, 1–125.   [31] Gillis, 'Once Round Only', 5, 113.
[32] *JC* 24 May 1996; *The Times*, 27 May 1996 (obituary of Gillis).

invariably charmed by Karmel's good manners, instinctive sense of fairness and rather relaxed approach to time-keeping', eulogized the *Daily Telegraph*. 'Violent criminals, on the other hand, found him frighteningly firm. Karmel was the first English judge to refer to "mugging", in a 1972 case involving a gang of youths who had attempted to rob a detective on a train at Stockwell station.' Another obituary recorded that he was a member of the West London Reform Synagogue, but added that he 'admits to no communal activities'. He was chairman of the croquet committee of the Hurlingham Club.[33]

Sir John Hazan (1927–88) attended King's College, Taunton and then London University, gaining an outstanding reputation as a prosecutor for the Inland Revenue 'in a number of sensational trials involving protection rackets, murder, drugs and spying', but he died after completing less than eight months' service as a High Court judge. Although not communally active, he supported several Jewish charities.[34]

Lord Taylor asserted that most people thought that judges were 'white, male, public school, Oxbridge and Establishment minded'; a survey carried out in 1997 by the Labour Research Department, backed by the trade unions, confirmed this impression, showing that 82 per cent of High Court judges had indeed attended public schools and that 88 per cent were Oxbridge-educated.[35] How closely did Jewish judges follow these trends after the era of Sebag Shaw and Finer? Eight Jewish High Court judges were born during the 1930s, namely Lord Taylor, Lord Woolf, Lord Millett (b. 1932), Lord Hoffman (b. 1934), Sir Harry Henry Ognall (b. 1934), Sir Simon Denis Brown (b. 1937), Sir Stephen John Sedley (b. 1939), and Sir Gavin Anthony Lightman (b. 1939). Of these eight, five went to public school and three went to state schools, while six attended one of the Oxbridge colleges. Six Jewish High Court judges were born during the 1940s, namely Sir Robert Robin Raphael Hayim Jacob (b. 1941), Sir John Anthony Dyson (b. 1943), Sir Bernard Anthony Rix (b. 1944), Sir Alan George Moses (b. 1945), Sir Hugh Ian Lang Laddie (b. 1946), and Sir David Edmond Neuberger (b. 1948). Of these, one went to both public and state schools, another to Leeds Grammar School, and the other four to public school; all six of them were educated at an Oxbridge college.[36] Thus, whereas the Jewish judges born during the 1930s diverged a little from the general trends, those born in the next decade were identical with the overall trends, showing the rapid upward social mobility of a select group of Jewish parents.

When Peter Taylor, Lord Taylor of Gosforth (1930–97), was appointed the second Jewish Lord Chief Justice in 1992, he followed the footsteps marked out nearly eighty years earlier by Rufus Isaacs. Peter Taylor's father, Dr Herman

[33] *JC* 19 Jan. 1968, p. 9; *Daily Telegraph*, 10 Oct. 1998 (obituaries of Karmel).
[34] *The Times*, 22 Aug. 1988; *JC* 26 Aug. 1988, p. 13 (obituaries of Hazan).
[35] *Financial Times*, 7 July 1997.   [36] Rozenberg, *The Search for Justice*, 5.

Louis Taylor, was one of the first Jewish scholarship winners to qualify as a doctor in Leeds; moving to Newcastle, he married the sister of his partner, Dr Harry Shokett, another Leeds graduate. Peter Taylor's grandfather was a tailor from Vilna called Teiger, a surname which an immigration officer decided to alter, renaming him Taylor. His family were steeped in Zionism, 'with no fewer than 33 Rabbis among their ancestors'.[37]

Taylor was educated at the Royal Grammar School, Newcastle upon Tyne, and Cambridge, where he read history, before being called to the Bar in 1954. He joined the chambers of John Harvey Robson as a pupil and later practised mainly on the North-Eastern Circuit, apart from a few cases of national significance in his later years as an advocate. Both his uncle and his brother were distinguished solicitors in Newcastle, no doubt assisting the launching of his career. 'Over a period of twenty years he did every sort of work. Crime, divorce, Civil Litigation of all types, Planning, Licensing—the lot', noted Mr Justice Potts.[38] In 1974 he prosecuted Poulson, the corrupt property developer: 'Aficionados of that art rate his interrogation of George Pottinger, the brilliant but bent head of the Scottish Office, as one of the most devastating cross-examinations of the century . . . the clever and sophisticated mandarin fell to an opponent who outmatched him, even in Latin epigrams.'[39] In the trial of Jeremy Thorpe in 1979, the Liberal leader avoided going into the witness box to face Taylor; his acquittal was assured when the *Sunday Telegraph*, by coming to an arrangement with Peter Bessel, Taylor's chief witness, to double a payment for his story on a conviction, undermined Bessel's credibility with the jury. Like Rufus Isaacs, Taylor was possessed of a prodigious energy and an eloquent command of English, even as a schoolboy. He took silk when he was 36 and by 1980 had reached the top of his profession, becoming the leader of the North-Eastern Circuit and then chairman of the Bar Council. He also sat as recorder of Huddersfield from 1969 to 1970 and of Teeside from 1970 to 1971, being made a recorder of the Crown Court in 1972.[40]

Having been made a High Court judge in 1980, Taylor was elevated to the Court of Appeal in 1988. A keen sports enthusiast and captain of Northumberland at rugby, he was chosen to head the inquiry into the Hillsborough football stadium disaster. His sensitive report of 1989, which laid blame for the tragedy on the police and the owners of the ground, led to the introduction of all-seater stadiums in football grounds, though he rejected a proposal mooted by the government for a football identity card system. Among his recommendations was that racist chanting should be banned at football matches, and the Home

---

[37] *JC* 9 May 1997, p. 21 (obituary of Lord Taylor).
[38] Transcript of address given by Mr Justice Potts at the memorial service for Lord Taylor, 15 July 1997. [39] *Guardian*, 30 Apr. 1997.
[40] *Independent*, 30 Apr. 1997 (obituary of Lord Taylor).

Secretary, David Waddington, brought in a new, tougher law to deal with this problem.[41] His membership of a religious minority may have fostered his humane outlook, professionally and personally. For example, he sprang to the defence of one court clerk, who had retired as a barrister through ill health and used to go into the barristers' robing room for a chat until an older barrister told him he had no right to be there. Peter Taylor gave his colleague a dressing-down, indignantly telling him: 'Leo is a practising barrister and is not only entitled to come in but is welcomed by all of us.'[42] As a judge, he granted bail to the Bradford Twelve, a group of Pakistani youths wrongly treated as terrorists when they stockpiled and abandoned petrol bombs which had been made to protect their community from attack by the National Front; and in 1984 he made MI5 justify their behaviour for the first time, when they tapped the telephones of the Campaign for Nuclear Disarmament.[43]

In 1992 Sir Peter Taylor was made Lord Chief Justice and became Lord Taylor. He took over at a time when public confidence in the country's criminal justice system had been shaken by the quashing of the convictions of the Guildford Four, the Birmingham Six, and the Tottenham Three. He shared these misgivings, remarking when one man whom he had successfully prosecuted for rape was shown by DNA tests to be innocent, 'I think judges will be a great deal more cautious in the way in which they direct juries on the facts, and I hope the police will be a great deal more cautious in how they go about their investigations.'[44] He developed a judicial agnosticism, believing that the Court of Appeal should develop rules to protect the possibly innocent. 'If trial judges made mistakes, appeals must be upheld even if the probably guilty went free (although sensibly he made more use of the power to order re-trials in such cases)', noted Geoffrey Robertson QC. 'It has been a most difficult era, requiring a delicate balance between the demands for a fair trial and the need for the state to protect valuable criminal informants and to use in evidence fruits of electronic surveillance. His judgments have struck this balance, not always successfully but by genuine attempts to be fair.'[45] As part of this balance, Taylor decided in a 1993 appeal that the prosecution could apply *ex parte* to a judge as to why certain evidence should be withheld from the defence to protect police witnesses, and that, exceptionally, they did not have to inform the defence of such an application. He understood that the law was inherently biased against blacks and women. He tried to do something about the mandatory life sentence for murder given to women, and in the case of Kiranjit Aluwhalia, who had killed her husband after suffering years of violent abuse at his hands, he tried to use the principles of diminished responsibility and provocation to avoid such harsh

[41] *The Times*, 30 Apr. 1999.   [42] Letter from Leo Blair, *The Times*, 7 May 1997.
[43] *Guardian*, 30 Apr. 1997.   [44] *The Times*, 30 Apr. 1997.   [45] *Guardian*, 30 Apr. 1997.

sentencing. When he retired in 1996, public confidence in the judicial process had in good measure been restored.[46]

Taylor tried unsuccessfully to have wigs and possibly gowns abolished to give courts a more modern air, and permitted women barristers to wear trousers in court. He believed that 'As time goes on more women and members of ethnic minorities would be appointed [to judicial posts]. But it would be wrong artificially to achieve proportionate representation of women and ethnic minorities on the Bench.'[47] Taylor clashed with Lord Mackay, the Lord Chancellor, over legal aid funding, condemning the 1993 cutbacks as 'an abdication of responsibility to a large section of those for whom the legal aid system was devised'.[48] Michael Howard, as Home Secretary, wanted to introduce automatic life sentences for those convicted for a second time of violent and sexual offences, and stiffer sentences for burglars and drug dealers. Taylor delivered a swingeing attack on these proposals, telling the Lords that 'Quite simply, minimum sentences must involve a denial of justice.'[49] One of his last judgments was to reject the appeal of the murderer and sexual molester Rosemary West on commonsense grounds: 'The concept of all these murders and burials taking place at the applicant's home and concurrently grave sexual abuse of other young women being committed by both husband and wife together without the latter being party to the killings is clearly one the jury were entitled to reject.'[50]

Like his predecessor Rufus Isaacs, Peter Taylor had an equivocal attitude to his Jewish roots. His father was a member of the Jewish congregation in Newcastle but held somewhat aloof, mixing mainly with the local consultants. Taylor claimed that his Jewish background would make him 'more sympathetic and responsive to the needs of minorities', but he also stressed that 'I am a judge who is Jewish, not a Jewish judge.'[51] On the other hand, his brother was not only a solicitor for his Newcastle synagogue, but a member of Ajex (the Association of Jewish Ex-Servicemen). Taylor was, he admitted, 'out on a long leash from Judaism . . . [and] just that much further away from it than he is, and my wife the same'; but, he continued, 'we do get involved in Jewish organizations'. He was a member of both the Friends of the Hebrew University and the Friends of Tel Aviv University; he was also a member of the Maccabeans, the annual subscription to the society being paid by his mother until she died. 'She thought it was a way of trying to keep me within the fold', he wryly confessed.[52] He had no sympathy for isolationism, as he told the Zionist charity Emunah:

I remember when my children went to *cheder* [Hebrew classes], and they were told by the rabbi not to go to parties given by non-Jews. That seems to me to be quite

---

[46] David Rose, *In the Name of the Law: The Collapse of Criminal Justice* (London: Cape, 1996), 189.
[47] *The Times*, 30 Apr. 1997.   [48] *Independent*, 30 Apr. 1997.
[49] *Law Society's Gazette*, 26 Feb. 1992.   [50] Rozenberg, *The Search for Justice*, 229.
[51] *JC* 28 Feb. 1992, p. 1.   [52] *JC* 1 May 1992, back page.

deplorable. It creates tension and fosters anti-Semitism . . . It upsets me to hear Jews who should know better talk about *schwartze[r]s* [blacks] and *goyim* [non-Jews] . . . Let us have respect for our Jewish traditions—combined with an understanding for the world outside.[53]

According to his close friend Lord Woolf, who spoke at the memorial service for Lord Taylor at St Paul's Cathedral, Peter Taylor would not have attached more importance to being Jewish than to being a Geordie. Although Taylor retained his own identification as a Jew, the ambiguities in his thinking meant that he was unable to pass on the idea of communal involvement so clearly to his children, most of whom married out of the faith.

Harry Kenneth Woolf, Lord Woolf of Barnes (b. 1933), came from a prosperous Jewish family of Lithuanian origin; his father was a successful builder and developer of housing estates. He was educated at Whittingehame, a Zionist-orientated school, and the exclusive Fettes College, Edinburgh, during the war years, and thereafter at University College London, where he was awarded his LL B, but was not an academic high achiever. Woolf was called to the Bar in 1954, shortly thereafter being diverted into national service, which he served in the Royal Hussars and the army legal services. Returning to civilian practice, he often appeared in a variety of cases against Patrick Medd, who sometimes sat as recorder of Abingdon; in Woolf's words, 'He out of the blue recommended me for the job of revenue junior, and I had never done a tax case in my life . . . They wanted a good advocate, a person with common sense.'[54] From 1973 to 1974 he was junior counsel to the Inland Revenue, and he so impressed those instructing him that when a more senior post quickly fell vacant he was appointed first Treasury junior counsel, a position which he held from 1974 to 1979 and in which he established his reputation as an expert in public law. 'Well, I can fairly say that the cases I lost as Treasury junior', admitted Woolf, 'are really the landmark cases of the early stages of the development of public law in this country [the Gouriet case, Congreve, and Laker Airways]. So I was appearing regularly before . . . Denning and regularly losing . . . I always used to say to my team [of Treasury lawyers], don't worry about the result of a particular case; what you are worried about is to make sure that the courts get it right.'[55]

Woolf rose rapidly through the judicial hierarchy, being appointed a recorder in 1972, a High Court judge in 1979, a lord justice of the Appeal Court in 1986, and a law lord in 1992. In the same year he was passed over when the office of Master of the Rolls fell vacant; some considered that this was because it was felt to be inappropriate for two Jews to occupy the two most senior positions in the judiciary at the same time.[56] Woolf became nationally known for his inquiry

[53] *JC* 29 Jan. 1993, p. 1.   [54] *Sunday Times*, 17 Oct. 1993.

[55] Interview with Lord Woolf, 17 Feb. 2000.

[56] Joshua Rozenberg, *Trial of Strength: The Battle between Ministers and Judges over who Makes the Laws* (London: Richard Cohen, 1999), 215 n. 18.

into the riots in the Strangeways prison in Manchester in 1990, when he recommended better food and hygiene, better educational facilities, and an end to 'slopping out' and overcrowding.[57] A judicial liberal, he upset right-wingers when in 1985 he dismissed an action brought by Victoria Gillick to ban contraceptives being given to persons under 16. He ruled that a group of Asians charged with assaulting some members of the National Front should be tried in an area with Asian residents.[58] In 1993 he caused a furore when he stated that those who failed to look after their property carefully should be fined, but claimed that he was merely referring to car theft.[59]

Woolf was regarded as 'soft' on sentencing and as favouring a wider ambit for the judicial review. Indeed, John Griffiths asserted that the whole process of reviewing the administrative decisions of the government was extended by Woolf in the early 1990s.[60] It was Woolf's belief that judges could decide whether or not powers conferred by a parliamentary statute were being exercised fairly and reasonably. In *M* v. *Home Office* (1994), Woolf delivered the leading judgment as the authority on judicial review, concluding that government ministers could be guilty of contempt for not complying with court orders. In *Mallinson* v. *Secretary of State for Social Security* Woolf upheld the right of Mr Mallison, who was blind, to claim an attendance allowance under section 35(1) of the Social Security Act 1975.[61] David Robertson pointed out that 'Instead of arguing that he [Mallison] cannot be helped in seeing because he is blind, Woolf asserts that "the only help that can be given to a person in connection with a sight handicap is to provide the assistance to enable that person to do what he could do physically for himself if he had sight." '[62] 'Concern has been expressed', Woolf remarked, 'that to allow attention [by a carer for a blind person claiming the allowance] to qualify which relates to walking in unfamiliar surroundings would lead to a situation which is difficult to administer or enforce', but he did not accept that this would be the result. In May 1996, on Sir Thomas Bingham's appointment as the new Lord Chief Justice, Woolf was finally promoted to Master of the Rolls. A few months later, sitting in the Court of Appeal, he ruled that the decision of Michael Howard, the Home Secretary, that the boys who had killed the toddler James Bulger should serve a minimum fifteen-year term, was illegal. In respect of an application by the Al Fayed brothers for British citizenship, Woolf suggested that if the Home Secretary rejected the application he should be guided by the principle of fairness, telling the Al Fayeds

[57] *Law Society's Gazette*, 16 Sept. 1992.
[58] *Sunday Times*, 17 Oct. 1993.   [59] *The Times*, 25 May 1996.
[60] Griffith quoted in Kate Malleson, *The New Judiciary: The Effects of Expansion and Activism* (Aldershot: Dartmouth, 1999), 19; Rozenberg, *Trial of Strength*, 9, 133; id., *The Search for Justice*, 30–3.
[61] *Mallison* v. *Secretary of State for Social Security* 2 All ER 1994, pp. 298–307.
[62] David Robertson, *Judicial Discretion in the House of Lords* (Oxford: Clarendon Press, 1998), 92–7.

of his reservations so that the brothers should be able to address the areas of concern in Mr Howard's mind before he reached his final decision. In February 1997, sitting in the Court of Appeal, he upheld the decision of a lower court and decided that those seeking political asylum who are denied state benefits must be given food and shelter by local authorities.[63]

Woolf has been hailed as a master of judicial creativity. 'It is extraordinary', one Queen's Counsel exclaimed of his judgment in the Diane Blood case (see Chapter 14 above): 'a judgment of Solomon—a creative use of adjudicatory powers which recognises the force of law but also the need to take a compassionate view in exceptional circumstances.' In *Grovit* v. *Doctor* Woolf enunciated the principle that delay could amount to an abuse of the legal process and supply the grounds for striking out, if the plaintiff had no intention of bringing the action to trial. In *Attorney-General* v. *Blake* Woolf resolved that in cases where there is skimped performance or the defendant does the opposite of what he promised to do, compensatory damages would be inadequate and that restitutionary damages should be awarded instead. Thus George Blake had promised not to disclose information obtained from his activities as a spy, but in breach of this undertaking published his memoirs. Although the Attorney-General neglected to claim the profits secured by Blake, the court nevertheless set out the circumstances in which such restitutionary damages could be claimed.[64]

The 1980s were a period, Woolf believed, when if public law was going to develop properly it needed its own identity.

In particular . . . it was all about duties and what the Courts were doing were really ensuring that public bodies do their duty. Now public law has come of age and . . . what we want to do is to reintegrate public law into the law generally; and the principles which have been developed now very extensively in public law could well be in the new situation developed in what was previously . . . called private law . . . [Since 1979] a lot of areas which used to be public as a result of privatization are now private. I think that is a phenomenon of society which we have got to accommodate. It is also more in keeping with the sea change in our constitutional approach which will result from the Human Rights Convention.

Although it was rumoured that Woolf wanted to become the senior law lord to oversee the implementation of the convention, this position was filled by Lord Bingham and instead Woolf was promoted in June 2000 to the vacant position of Lord Chief Justice, becoming the third Jew to occupy this august office.[65]

---

[63] *Independent*, 31 July 1996; *The Times*, 18 Feb. 1997.

[64] *The Times*, 7 Feb. 1997; Craig Rose, 'The Reformer: An Interview with Lord Woolf', and the 'Opinion of Christopher Style', *Commercial Lawyer* (Mar. 1998), 32, 33, 70, 72.

[65] Interview with Lord Woolf, 17 Feb. 2000; *The Times*, 7 June 2000.

George Jessel, Woolf's Victorian Jewish predecessor as Master of the Rolls, had chaired a committee which devised the procedure to be followed in the reformed High Court.[66] Other notable contributions towards revising the rules regulating civil procedure were made by Master Arthur Sigismund Diamond (1897–1978) and Sir Jack Jacob (1908–2000), editors of the 'White Book', the High Court annual practice volume. During a slack period at the Bar in the mid-1950s, Jacob successfully applied for the post of a High Court Queen's Bench master, and helped to transform the importance of the position. 'At the time it was considered a low-grade job for failed barristers, who presided over a round of short procedural hearings often attended by inexperienced court clerks.'[67] So too, in 1996 Lord Woolf made a series of recommendations to improve civil litigation, including dividing claims into fast-track, for those involving sums under £3,000, and multi-track, for those concerning amounts over £10,000. His promotion to the office of Master of the Rolls was made partly to enable him to oversee the implementation of these reforms.[68] He has encouraged more judicial management of cases and the exchange of witness statements by parties to try to facilitate the settlement of disputes before they come to trial. So far it is possible to give only an interim report on these reforms, to the effect that while promoting a fall in litigation, the new procedure makes small claims often too expensive to pursue.

A slightly older colleague of Lord Woolf who followed a similar route to judicial promotion through government service was Peter Millett (b. 1932), Lord Millett of St Marylebone. His father's family arrived in Britain from the Austro-Hungarian province of Galicia in the 1880s, while his mother's family, which was of rabbinical descent, came in the mid-nineteenth century from Frankfurt in Germany. Peter Millett won an exhibition from his preparatory school to Harrow, proceeding on a major scholarship to Cambridge, where he read classics and law and obtained a first-class degree in both parts of his tripos. Doubting whether his oratorical talents would be sufficient to bring him success at the criminal bar, he toyed briefly with becoming a tax specialist before taking up Chancery practice, drafting wills, conveyances, and leases. He was called to the Bar in 1955 and admitted that 'In those days . . . it took you five years to get on your feet at all, you didn't make any money.' His first real break came in 1965, when he was junior counsel in *Re: B*, the 'tie-of-blood' case which took hold of the public imagination. An older married man had an affair with a younger woman, resulting in the birth of a child, who was given away for adoption. Unwilling to see the child brought up by adoptive parents, the father patched up his marriage and was able to offer the little boy a loving home. The

---

[66] Finestein, 'Sir George Jessel', 267.

[67] *JC* 21 Dec. 1962, p. 20, 10 Mar. 1978, p. 26 (obituary of Diamond); *Guardian*, 1 Jan. 2001 (obituary of Jacob). [68] *The Times*, 6 Aug. 1996, 26 Oct. 1999, Law Section, pp. 10, 11.

judge ruled that a child, if at all possible, should be brought up by his natural parent, and the Appeal Court upheld his decision. Two years later Millett fought the Enfield Comprehensive School case with a leader, Hugh Francis QC. The case arose when the Labour council in the London Borough of Enfield, realizing that the party was going to be defeated in the next election, rushed through an ill-thought-out scheme to turn the schools under its control into comprehensives. The scheme was opposed by a group of parents whose children attended a local grammar school; Millett and Francis won the case for the parents in the High Court, but lost when the council went to the Court of Appeal. Also in 1967 Millett was appointed one of the panel of junior counsel to the Board of Trade, often appearing in the Companies Court to wind up insurance companies without the requisite paid-up share capital. In 1971 he was junior counsel for the Department of Trade and Industry before a tribunal of inquiry which was investigating its conduct in relation to the Vehicle and General Insurance Company, then the country's second biggest motor insurer. In 1972 he led for the department in relation to a successful application to wind up Koskot Interplanetary UK Ltd., a pyramid selling company. Taking silk shortly afterwards he was then appointed an inspector by the Department of Trade and Industry to investigate the affairs of J. H. Willment & Sons, a building company, and when that assignment was completed he inquired into the affairs of a larger, fraudulent company.[69]

As a QC Millett was both incisive and, in his own words, 'just lucky', appearing for the Inland Revenue 'in a series of cases dealing with artificial tax avoidance, all of which went to the House of Lords and all of which we[re] won'. The cases were *Floor and Davis*, *W. T. Ramsay Ltd. and the Inland Revenue Commissioners*, and *Eilbeck (Inspector of Taxes) and Rawling*.

They established the principle that the Court will . . . disregard artificial steps in a . . . tax avoidance scheme; they were circular schemes; they were relatively easy, followed by *Furniss (Inspector of Taxes) and Dawson* which wasn't a circular scheme. Now those cases were heard in the early 1980s in the House of Lords . . . I was involved in them from about 1977 onwards.

He had also made a name for himself by appearing in some leading cases on estoppel, a bar to a person's right of action arising out of their own act, notably *E. R. Ives Investments Ltd.* v. *High* (1966) and *Crabb* v. *Arun District Council* (1975). In 1986 Millett was appointed to the bench as a judge in the Chancery Division of the High Court, where he dealt with insolvency cases but also decided a number of important actions on restitution. In 1994 Millett was elevated to the Court of Appeal, where he gave judgments in *Mougheu* and *Thackerar*, both of

[69] Interview with Lord Millett, 23 Apr. 1999.

which arose out of mortgage frauds and were concerned with the fiduciary duties of solicitors.[70]

In 1998 Millett was promoted to the highest court of the land and became a law lord. When the Pinochet case went to the House of Lords for the second time, Millett sat on the panel of judges and delivered a judgment concurring with the majority of his colleagues that Senator Pinochet should be extradited to Spain on a limited number of charges. But he also went further, allowing the appeal in respect of the charges 'to torture and conspiracy to torture wherever and whenever carried out'. He held that the International Law Commission

rejected the principle that international responsibility for crimes against humanity should be limited to crimes committed in connection with war crimes or crimes against peace . . . the Commission proposed that acts would constitute international crimes only if they were committed at the instigation or the toleration of state authorities. This is the distinction which was later adopted in the Convention against Torture (1984).

Further, Millet averred that the landmark decision of the Israeli Supreme Court in *Attorney-General of Israel* v. *Eichmann* (1962) established three propositions. First, 'There is no rule of international law which prohibits a state from exercising extraterrorial criminal jurisdiction in respect of crimes committed by foreign nationals abroad.' Second, 'War crimes, and atrocities of the scale and international character of the Holocaust are crimes of universal jurisdiction under customary international law.' Finally, 'The fact that the accused committed the crimes in question in the course of his official duties as a responsible officer of the state and in exercise of his authority as an organ of the state is no bar to the exercise of the jurisdiction of a national court.' It is no coincidence that a Jewish judge growing to adulthood in the aftermath of the Holocaust should have very strong views on human rights issues.[71]

Born in South Africa in 1934 and the son of a prominent lawyer, Leonard Hoffman was partly educated there and partly at Oxford, where he was a Rhodes scholar. Returning to South Africa in 1957, he married and practised law there for two years before migrating to Britain in June 1960. Because the industrialist Maurice Mauerberger happened to be one of his father's most important clients and also the uncle of Arnold Goodman, Hoffman came to work in Goodman's office as a law clerk, but went back to Oxford University in 1961 to teach law. He then decided to become a barrister, taking a sabbatical for six months to do his pupillage with Jeremiah Harman (later Mr Justice Harman), and was called to the Bar in 1964. It was not until 1966 that Hoffman started to practise law, regularly commuting from Oxford University, where he

[70] Ibid.
[71] *R.* v. *Bartle and the Commissioner of Police for the Metropolis and Others ex parte Pinochet,* House of Lords Session 1998–9, Opinions of the Lords of Appeal, pp. 93–106.

continued to teach.[72] A member of Chancery Chambers at 9 Old Square, Lincoln's Inn, he at first handled mostly property work and in particular landlord and tenant cases. This led to his first appearance before the Court of Appeal in 1969 in *Luganda* v. *Service Hotels Ltd*, where he successfully argued that a licensee occupying a furnished room in premises described as a 'hotel' which were plainly a house was protected from unlawful eviction by the Rent Acts.[73] Gradually Hoffman's practice expanded to include a full range of commercial work, including the takeover of companies. He took silk in 1977 and by the mid-1980s, with a yearly income of £500,000, was reputed to be one of the highest earners at the Bar. According to Goodman, the success of the British Steel Corporation in an action against Granada Television over a journalist's leaking of confidential information, a case which went to the House of Lords, 'was in large part attributable to . . . [Hoffman's] skill in argument'.[74]

Hoffman was elevated to the High Court bench in 1985, promoted to the Court of Appeal in 1992, and made a law lord in 1995. His judgment in the Court of Appeal in *Airedale NHS Trust and Bland*, concerning the withdrawal of feeding from Anthony Bland, a teenager who had been in a persistent vegetative state since the accident at the Hillsborough football ground, was mainly concerned with the moral aspects of the matter and is often cited in academic and philosophical works. At the outset of his judgment, Hoffman acknowledged the help of conversations with Professor Ronald Dworkin, who held the chair of jurisprudence at Oxford, and the philosopher Professor Bernard Williams. 'The mere fact that he [Bland] is still a living organism means that there remains an epilogue of the tragedy which is being played out', declared Hoffman.

This is because we have a strong feeling that there is an intrinsic value in human life, irrespective of whether it is valuable to the person concerned . . . Those who adhere to religious faiths which believe in the sanctity of all God's creation and in particular that human life was created in the image of God himself will have no difficulty with the concept of the intrinsic value of human life. But even those without any religious belief think in the same way.

To my mind this is a distinctively Jewish concept which has been incorporated into the Western value-system. It was also important, Hoffman asserted, for 'the individual human being' to have the 'right to choose how he should live his own life. We call this individual autonomy or the right of self-determination'; but the principles of the sanctity of life and the right to self-determination 'are not always compatible with each other [quoting from Isaiah Berlin's *Two Concepts of Liberty* on this issue]'.[75]

---

[72] Interview with Lord Hoffman, 16 Jan. 2001; *Guardian*, 8 Dec. 1998; *Sunday Times*, 20 Dec. 1998; *The Times*, 18 Dec. 1998; Iris Freeman interview with Lord Hoffman.

[73] *Luganda* v. *Service Hotels Limited* 2 Ch. 1969, pp. 209–20.

[74] Goodman, *Tell Them I'm On My Way*, 108–16.

[75] *Airedale NHS Trust* v. *Bland* AC 1993, pp. 824–34.

'Similarly', Hoffman asserted, 'it is possible to qualify the meaning of the sanctity of life by including, as some cultures do, concepts of dignity and fulfilment as part of the essence of life.' He thought that it was fallacious to assume

that we have no interests except in those things of which we have conscious experience ... At least a part of the reason why we honour the wishes of the dead about the distribution of their property is that we think it would wrong them not to do so. Most people would like an honourable and dignified death and we think it wrong to dishonour their deaths, even when they are unconscious that this is happening. We pay respect to their dead bodies and to their memory because we think it an offence against the dead themselves if we do not.

It was, therefore, an incomplete picture of Anthony Bland's interests to confine 'them to animal feelings of pain or pleasure ... we think it more likely that he would choose to put an end to the humiliation of his being and the distress of his family'.[76]

Legal Business described Hoffman as 'the most dominant personality in the Lords today by a mile, significantly outscoring the others in the number of leading judgments he has given' with a tendency to 'carry the rest of the court with him'. For example, in *Meridian Global Funds Management Asia Limited and Securities Commission* (1995) Hoffman decided that

In fast-moving markets [the act in question compelled] the immediate disclosure of the identity of the persons who become substantial security holders in public issuers. Notice must be given as soon as that person knows that he has become a substantial security holder. In the case of a corporate security holder, what rule should be implied as to the person whose knowledge for this purpose is to count as the knowledge of the company? ... the person who, with the authority of the company, acquired the relevant interest.[77]

A year later, in *South Australian Asset Management Corporation and York Montague Limited and Others*, Hoffman gave a judgment on the scope of the duty and care owed by surveyors to clients. He found

that a person under a duty to take reasonable care to provide information on which someone else will decide upon a course of action is, if negligent, not generally regarded as responsible for all the consequences of that course of action. He is responsible only for the consequences of the information being wrong ... The principle thus stated distinguishes between a duty to *provide information* for the purpose of enabling someone else to decide upon a course of action and a duty to *advise* someone as to what course of action he should take. If the duty is to advise whether or not a course of action should be taken, the adviser must take reasonable care to consider all the potential consequences

76 Ibid.
77 *Legal Business* (Oct. 1998), 53; *Meridian Global Funds Management Asia Limited and Securities Commission* 2 AC 1995, pp. 503–12.

of that course of action. If he is negligent he will therefore be responsible for all the foreseeable loss which is a consequence of action having been taken.[78]

Despite the setback to his career when his failure to disclose his connection with the charity Amnesty International led to the overturning of the judgment in the Pinochet case and a rehearing, Hoffman has outmanoeuvred his critics and re-established himself as a significant figure among the law lords. His judgment stripping barristers of their immunity from being sued for negligence during court proceedings was far-reaching. Describing himself as 'a Jew by race rather than religion', his principal interest outside the law has been in the arts, where he has served on the board of the English National Opera and on the Arts Council Advisory Committee on London orchestras.[79]

Easily the most distinguished Jewish woman judge currently practising is Dame Rosalyn Higgins (b. 1937), a former professor of international law at the London School of Economics, who has sat as a judge at the International Court of Justice at The Hague since 1995. As a silk she practised in international and petroleum law, appearing as counsel for Britain in the Lockerbie case, in which two Libyans were tried on charges relating to the blowing up of a Pan-Am airliner over Scotland in 1988, and for Portugal in the case concerning East Timor.[80] No other Jewish woman judge in Britain has reached her level of distinction, nor that of Dame Rose Heilbron. All those now sitting—Myrella Cohen, Valerie Pearlman, Dawn Freedman, Adrianne Uziell-Hamilton, and Ingeborg Bernstein—are circuit judges, although Myrella Cohen sits regularly as a judge in the High Court.[81]

When Myrella Cohen started training as a barrister, women found it difficult to obtain a place in chambers, and were rarely instructed in high-profile civil work which involved acting for big business or insurance companies, so they drifted into family and criminal law; even later, in the mid-1960s, Dawn Freedman remembered that 'Many chambers restricted their number [of female members], unofficially or otherwise.' Myrella Cohen, 'As a newlywed in 1953 . . . was the first woman barrister to have chambers in Newcastle' and the first to become a QC in the city. Appointed a circuit judge and deputy judge of the Family Division of the High Court in 1972, she was only the third English woman judge ever, and the youngest to reach this rank. After presiding over courts in the north-east for nineteen years before moving to London, she found commuting from Edgware to the Old Bailey too exhausting and transferred to the Harrow Crown Court, where she became the senior resident judge.[82]

---

[78] *South Australia Asset Management Corporation and York Montague Limited and Others* AC 1997, 210–24.   [79] *The Times*, 21 July 2000; *JC* 12 Feb. 1999, p. 11.

[80] *JC* 21 July 1995, p. 10; *The Times*, 29 Feb. 2000; Clare McGlynn, *The Woman Lawyer Making the Difference* (London: Butterworths, 1998), 189–91.

[81] *JC* 17 Nov. 1995, p. 16; *Legal Executive Journal*, June 1990.

[82] Interview with Judge Myrella Cohen, 7 Mar. 1997; *Independent*, 19 Feb. 1993 (on Freedman).

Deborah Rowland 'made legal history in 1971 when, on her appointment as a county court judge, she became the first Jewish woman judge [three years before Rose Heilbron and three months before Myrella Cohen]. She was subsequently appointed a circuit judge.' To men who she believed had maltreated their wives she could sometimes be shrill, but to the wives who had been victimized she could be compassionate, and she was admired by them.[83]

*

Until the late 1960s no Jew could become a High Court judge unless he— and it was 'he'—belonged to the Anglo-Jewish elite, which differed little in educational attainments and lifestyle from the rest of the English upper class, even if, like R. F. Levy, he was exceptionally able. Starting in 1968 during the last years of Harold Wilson's Labour administration, Lord Chancellor Gardiner began to appoint Jewish barristers from middle-class backgrounds and of east European family origin to the High Court bench; these men had for the most part been educated in local grammar schools and redbrick universities. This policy was continued both by the Conservative Heath government and by Labour administrations in the 1970s. Even so, Sir Rudolph Lyons (1912–91), who 'came from a Leeds Jewish family of modest means', was never elevated to the High Court bench, 'which he would have graced with distinction', and this despite the fact that he 'held in succession the two most senior judicial posts outside London'.[84] Before the 1990s a number of maverick personalities, who seemed eminently qualified in most respects, were excluded from the High Court bench. Gilbert Beyfus was considered too much of a ladies' man, although Hartley Shawcross recommended him for promotion, albeit somewhat half-heartedly, in 1950.[85] Both Joseph Jackson and Lewis Hawser were said to be too forceful in court. When Hawser agreed to an appointment as an Official Referee in 1978 to try building disputes, *The Times*' legal correspondent commented that 'Mr Hawser has for many years been considered by most of his colleagues to be of High Court quality at least, and it has been a source of puzzlement and concern that men considered to be less able have achieved that rank.'[86] Sir Louis Blom-Cooper was alleged to be too liberal for Conservative administrations to contemplate moving him on to the High Court bench, though his even more radical younger colleague at the Bar Sir Stephen Sedley (b. 1939) reached this rank in 1992. On the other hand, some high-flying Jewish QCs, such as Caplan and Stamler, excluded themselves from the bench for their own personal reasons.

[83] *JC* 2 Jan. 1987, p. 12 (obituary of Rowland); personal knowledge.

[84] *JC* 1 Feb. 1991, p. 24; *The Times*, 26 Feb. 1991 (obituary of Lyons).

[85] Robert Stevens, *The Independence of the Judiciary: The View from the Lord Chancellor's Office* (Oxford: Clarendon Press, 1993), 85.

[86] *The Times*, 13 Apr. 1978, 1 Aug. 1990 (obituary of Hawser).

There were also a number of High Court judges of Jewish origin who were brought up as Christians or who no longer wished to affiliate; these included Sir Eric Sachs, Lord Simon of Glaisdale, Sir Anthony Lincoln (1920–91), Sir Michael Kerr (b. 1921), and Sir Michael Sachs (b. 1932).[87] This illustrates the continuing, indeed arguably accelerating, process of radical assimilation in Anglo-Jewry.

For a time in the late 1960s and early 1970s, Jews born in quite modest middle-class homes or in more humble circumstances were elevated to the High Court bench, bearing witness to a new and remarkable flexibility and social open-mindedness in the appointments process. If these judges are contrasted with those Jews appointed to the higher levels of the judiciary in the 1990s, most of whom were educated at public schools and Oxbridge, it can at once be seen that by the end of the century the system had become somewhat ossified; but, on the other hand, it could be argued that this merely reflected the social mobility of their fathers and the bulk of Anglo-Jewry. Also, the selection process had both expanded and changed. Whereas in the mid-1970s there were 'still no more than 50 [judicial] appointments made each year',[88] by 1997 this number had risen to 600 such appointments, and the procedure for selecting judges followed guidelines under which the candidates were marked for communication skills, courtesy, and humanity. Under Lord Mackay, the Conservative Lord Chancellor in the early 1990s, the higher judiciary increasingly became a meritocracy, with suitable candidates being promoted whatever their ethnic origin, gender, political affiliation, or religion. Certain Jewish judges, such as Lord Woolf, Lord Hoffman, Sir Simon Brown, Sir Stephen Sedley, and Sir Gavin Lightman, boosted the liberal element in the judiciary, making radical pronouncements in various areas, particularly in public law.[89]

How Jewish were these High Court judges in their personal affiliation? Unlike the first post-Second World War generation of judges, who were deeply involved in the running of communal institutions, those appointed during the 1980s and 1990s had—with some notable exceptions—much looser ties to the Jewish community. Lord Millett was president of the West London Synagogue, while Sir Gavin Lightman was a vice-president of the Hillel Foundation, which fostered the welfare of Jewish students, and was associated with the Legal Friends of Haifa University. Sir Bernard Rix was vice-chairman of the Central Council for Jewish Community Services, a director of the Spiro Institute, and chairman of the Friends of Bar-Ilan University. Lord Woolf was much more closely connected with Jewish causes than his friend and colleague Lord Taylor. Woolf was a member of three Orthodox synagogues as well as being intimately

---

[87] *Dictionary of National Biography 1971–1980*, 751, 752 (on Sachs); *JC* 16 Feb. 1962, p. 6 (on Lord Simon); John Roskill KC, the father of Lord Roskill, was also reputed to be Jewish.
[88] Malleson, *New Judiciary*, 80, 81.   [89] Rozenberg, *The Search for Justice*, 84.

involved with multifarious Jewish institutions as president of the Central Council for Jewish Social Services, governor of the Oxford Centre for Hebrew and Jewish Studies, and chairman of the Bar and Bench Committee of the JPA (the Joint Palestine Appeal, predecessor of the UJIA) and the Jewish Chronicle Trust.

Jewish judges differed in their attitudes to the observance of the sabbath and Jewish festivals. Whereas Sir John Balcombe, who celebrated his bar mitzvah in the Hampstead Synagogue, believed that Jewish judges could take only the High Holidays off, his younger colleague Sir Gavin Lightman was of the opinion that all the Jewish festivals could be observed, provided that the time was made up on other occasions. Of the eight Jewish High Court judges who were born in the 1930s, at least five had Jewish wives and half of them attended functions connected with Jewish charities. Of the six Jewish High Court judges born during the 1940s, three had non-Jewish wives and avoided involvement with the Jewish community.

On the whole, the more communally active of the Jewish judges were to be found at circuit level. Israel Finestein QC, a circuit judge who often sat as an acting High Court judge, was very active in Anglo-Jewry, serving as president of the Board of Deputies and Norwood Child Care as well as being a noted historian of the Anglo-Jewish community. He was a founder member of the Hillel Foundation, later becoming its president.[90] Judge Alan Lipfriend (1916–96) was appointed a circuit judge in 1974 and 'sat regularly on crime, family and Queen's Bench cases, sometimes in the capacity of official referee'. He was chairman of Rabbi Louis Jacobs's New London Synagogue from 1982 to 1988, a position also held by Judge Leonard Krikler.[91] Judge Henry Lachs (1911–2000) was a circuit judge in Liverpool for twenty years as well as being president of the Liverpool Yeshiva.[92] Among the woman judges Myrella Cohen and Dawn Freedman were the most communally involved, particularly in work to enhance the rights of Jewish women who went through the divorce courts;[93] and Rosalind Wright, the director of the Serious Fraud Office from 1997, was a trustee of the Jewish Association for Business Ethics.

Overall there was in the post-war period a drift among the judges and QCs (again with some notable exceptions) out of Orthodoxy and into the Reform movement, and a further tendency to cut or loosen their remaining ties to the Anglo-Jewish community. Among others Lord Cohen, Sir Sebag Shaw, Sir John Balcombe, and Sigismund Diamond all relinquished the Orthodox synagogues of their youth and joined one or another Reform congregation. Pressure

[90] Interview with Judge Finestein, 16 Feb. 2000.
[91] *JC* 12 Apr. 1996, p. 17 (obituary of Lipfriend).
[92] *The Times*, 21 Feb. 2000 (obituary of Lachs).
[93] Lecture by Judge Myrella Cohen on 'Divorce Jewish Style', 25 Feb. 1997.

of work led Joseph Jackson QC to curtail his activities in Jewish organizations drastically. As a young man, Sir Jack Jacob chaired the University of London Jewish Students' Union; but after he lost his faith his membership of the Friends of the Hebrew University was almost his only connection with the community.[94] In fact, a large number of Jewish High Court judges have no community affiliations of any kind.

In sum, the ethos of the legal profession became much more important in the lives of many late twentieth-century Jewish judges than either Judaism or their ethnic background. This was marked in the case of benchers by the church services held in their memory, in which there was sometimes an uneasy juxtaposition of invocation of the Holy Spirit and recitation of the Kaddish, the Jewish prayer recited in memory of dead relatives. Explaining why both the Kaddish and the Lord's Prayer were recited at the memorial service to Lord Taylor in St Paul's Cathedral, his friend Lord Woolf remarked that 'Peter knew that church services are part of the life of the law. He would have appreciated the Dean and Chapter arranging such a beautiful service, sensitive to his background.' The combination of this relaxed ecumenicalism and a shared pattern of school and university education meant that there was often little to distinguish Jewish High Court judges from their non-Jewish colleagues.[95]

[94] *The Times*, 2 Jan. 2001, *JC* 12 Jan. 2001, p. 25 (obituary of Jacob).
[95] Personal knowledge and *JC* 18 July 1997.

Conclusion

URING the late Victorian age and the Edwardian era it was possible for a
few Jews from patrician or wealthy merchant families to rise to the top of
the Bar, or the front rank of the medical profession, while retaining a Jewish
identity. Examples include doctors such as Ernest Hart and, more emphatic-
ally, Gustave Schorstein and Bertram Abrahams, and lawyers such as George
Jessel, Arthur Cohen, and Rufus Isaacs in the earlier phases of his career. But
until 1914 the total number of Jewish professionals in England was small, with
no more than ninety or 100 doctors practising in London and perhaps a slightly
smaller number of Jewish barristers. At the same time there were prominent
members of these professions, such as the surgeon Sir Felix Semon or the international lawyer Judah Philip Benjamin, who were only marginally Jewish; others
again, such as the eminent solicitor the first Sir George Lewis, were Jewish, but
preferred mixing with non-Jewish artists and writers, neither emphasizing their
Jewishness nor denying it. As these Jewish doctors and lawyers were relatively
few in number and acculturated, they posed no threat to their non-Jewish
colleagues, and their progress in their chosen profession was accepted without
demur.

Between the two world wars English society was much less open than in the
late Victorian and Edwardian years. This was a time of heavy unemployment
and economic malaise, disfigured by sharpening antisemitism which did not abate
until a decade after the Second World War. The massive influx into the medical
profession of children of east European Jewish immigrants started during the
First World War, when, with so many young men absent on active service,
women and Jews were admitted into the medical schools in larger numbers than
hitherto. Nevertheless, despite Professor Kushner's caveats about the children
of the immigrants finding 'formal and informal barriers' being imposed during
the 1930s and 1940s to impede their entry into the professions because of
increasing antisemitism,[1] I could not find much evidence of this. On the contrary, during the inter-war period a rising number of Jewish students enrolled
in the London and provincial medical schools. Many of the earliest recruits to
the medical profession in England were the sons of rabbis or other officials of

[1] Kushner, 'The Impact of British Anti-Semitism', 201.

the Jewish community, the heirs of the educated minority, and they served as role models for their schoolfriends. In addition, the immigrant Jewish communities based in large urban areas, and with their tradition of valuing education, probably benefited disproportionately from the scholarship ladders which education authorities had in place in the 1920s and 1930s.

At the London Hospital during the 1920s Russian Jewish students whose parents had not been naturalized were sometimes discriminated against because of anti-alien and anti-Bolshevik scaremongering; but most of them found places in other medical schools in the capital, which were so numerous as to undermine the enforcement of any quota system. This prejudicial attitude on the part of the London Hospital was on a par with the discriminatory policy of the London County Council in refusing to award scholarships to the children of aliens; this policy was phased out after 1928, and it is likely that the hospital followed suit in its own admissions policy. Again, after 1933 certain English medical schools refused to admit or would accept only limited numbers of German Jewish students who had partially completed their medical training; but between fifty and seventy-five of these refugee students did qualify as doctors and an additional number of refugees, who had received some schooling in England, were also accepted. As for the trouble at the Leeds Medical School in 1945, described in Chapter 11 above, it was short-lived, caused by demobilized soldiers competing for university places with school-leavers.

In the years between the two world wars the number of Jewish doctors in London jumped from about 100 to 800, a rate of increase matched in Leeds, Liverpool, and Manchester. Most of the medical students from east European families who qualified in the 1920s and 1930s became general practitioners, buying panel practices, often in run-down neighbourhoods. Thus the movement of Jewish doctors into private practice at the lower level was governed by market forces, albeit distorted by some discrimination practised by local authorities in respect of public appointments, and was little affected by the antisemitism and fascism so prevalent during the 1930s.

It is equally true that no restrictions were placed on Jewish entry into English law schools in the 1920s and the 1930s. Any constraints inhibiting young Jews from becoming solicitors or barristers were economic: the cost of the legal training and the difficulty of setting up in practice as a solicitor or barrister. During the 1920s and 1930s a new and enterprising Jewish middle class began to emerge, but it was not sufficiently broad-based to support many Jewish professionals, so that the number of Jewish solicitors in London, for example, rose moderately, from about 100 in 1920 to 290 by 1939. There was considerable discrimination practised against Jews who applied for positions as assistant solicitors; as a consequence the number of Jewish sole practitioners mushroomed during the 1930s. Dubious practices among some Jewish lawyers—touting for work, ambulance-chasing, and undercutting conveyancing costs—seem to indicate that it was sometimes difficult to earn a satisfactory income, and there was probably a substantial underclass among these newly trained lawyers. The result of this discrimination in the employment market as far as Jewish solicitors were concerned was that they had to be more enterprising and more business-orientated than their non-Jewish colleagues.

Most of the hundred or so Jewish barristers practising during the 1920s and 1930s were recruited from the Anglo-Jewish elite; at this time, few entering the profession were of east European origin. Of those from immigrant families who did join the profession, many, such as A. S. Diamond or Bernard Gillis, were the sons of Anglo-Jewish ministers, coming from families unable to provide career openings in other fields and with a tradition of both academic distinction and public service. Others climbed to prominence at the Bar through their connection with the Labour Party: David Weitzman, Moss Turner-Samuels, Leslie Solley, and Julius Silverman all became MPs. Others still, such as Ashe Lincoln and Frederic Landau, were sons of solicitors and descendants of an earlier wave of immigrants from eastern Europe.

'Before the beginning of the nineteenth century, all Jews regarded Judaism as a privilege', proclaimed Mordecai Kaplan; 'since then, most Jews have come to regard it as a burden.'[2] This concept of Judaism as a burden was very much the viewpoint in the 1920s and 1930s of those assimilated Jews at the top of the professions, whose tenuous ties to their faith and lack of self-esteem made them particularly vulnerable to criticism; the self-lacerating comments of Rufus Isaacs and Sir Felix Semon will be recalled. During the inter-war period, in an atmosphere of anti-alien scares provoked by a fear of Russia and in the presence of a fascist threat at home and abroad, antisemitism in Britain reached a new level of intensity. In this environment Jewish doctors seeking to attain positions as consultant physicians and surgeons in the teaching hospitals needed to conceal their identity, by mixing with their non-Jewish colleagues, often by inter-marrying, and, above all, by not openly displaying any signs of their Jewish-ness. Almost all of them—Otto Leyton, Adolphe Abrahams, Edward Gustave Slesinger, Stanford Cade, Arnold Sorsby, Norman Kletts—married outside the faith, and at least two of them—Cade and Abrahams—seem to have converted to Christianity. No Jewish judges were appointed to front-rank (High Court) positions between the wars, with the sole exception of Sir Henry Slesser, who was a convert to the Church of Rome. When large numbers of Jews from east European backgrounds applied for positions as consultants in major hospitals, they were regarded as not being quite English, almost as members of a foreign nationality, and invariably their applications were rejected. In contrast, their

---

[2] Silberman, *A Certain People*, 28.

co-religionists from the Anglo-Jewish elite, armed with a public-school and Oxbridge education and a low Jewish profile, were deemed to be acceptable. Nevertheless despite widespread discrimination at the consultancy level Jewish doctors were able to find openings in the LCC hospitals, the new Jewish hospitals, and the smaller provincial hospitals.

The few eminent Jewish doctors and lawyers who cared about the fate of the community were overworked; often their professional careers suffered, and some, such as Maurice Sorsby and Cyril Picciotto, died prematurely. Neville Laski saw his practice at the Bar dwindle during the 1930s because of his communal workload; Professor Samson Wright was left with insufficient time for his scientific research.

Jewish barristers who were members of chambers and belonged to the Inns of Court, and consultants working in teaching hospitals and elected as fellows of the Royal Colleges, were enmeshed in a collegiate and institutional framework and could not escape from the pressure to conform if they wished to win acceptance and succeed in their chosen calling. So too, Jews in leading solicitors' firms, such as the Simmons brothers in the City, the second Sir George Lewis, and some members of the Rubinstein family who acted for celebrities in the world of the arts, also went down the path of radical assimilation. Self-hatred, arising from the combination of the negative image of Jews prevalent in the wider society and the need to conform to obtain professional advancement, resulted in the internalization of this negative image and a renewed wish to assimilate. In contrast, high street lawyers and the general practitioners among the doctors were more independent and were free of the constraints imposed by the wider society; they could adhere to Orthodoxy, or adopt a more secular Zionist orientation or a messianic belief in the triumph of socialism, and a few of them would follow the substitute faith of communism.

Although the old regime appeared to persist throughout the 1950s in both the legal and medical worlds, the establishment of the National Health Service by the post-war Labour government in 1948, the most radical measure of the Attlee administration, wrought fundamental changes. Among many innovations it set up new machinery for the selection of registrars and consultants, who were henceforth to be chosen on the basis of merit, thus allowing Jews who were the children or grandchildren of immigrants to gain appointments as consultants in the leading teaching hospitals in London and the provinces. Partly because of the return of large numbers of doctors from war service and partly because too many registrars were trained during the 1950s, the new regime did not start to operate effectively until the following decade. Since then, so ingrained have the new procedures become that some Jewish consultants have admitted that they have been appointed even by antisemitic heads of hospital departments because they were the best available candidates. Whereas in the past, apart from a successful group of assimilated consultants at the main teaching hospitals, Jews tended to be bunched up in a few less glamorous specialties, such as pathology, anatomy, physiology, and psychiatry, since the Second World War they have spread to every major department, including surgery. It is a myth that few Jews chose surgery as a career; there were many Jewish surgeons after the war, among them some respective innovators, such as Sir Roy Calne and Ralph Shackman. Moreover, the Nobel Prizes won by refugee medical scientists after the war—including Sir Hans Krebs and Sir Bernard Katz—enhanced the prestige of Jews in English medicine, making them more acceptable as colleagues at the highest levels.

Although there was a handful of prominent Jewish individuals in the legal profession in the Victorian and Edwardian periods, and between the two world wars, Jewish lawyers were relatively few in number compared with the degree of Jewish representation in the medical profession. After the Second World War, many factors stimulated the establishment of solicitors' firms by Jews: the consumer revolution and the growth of related retail outlets; the creation of huge national companies by Jewish entrepreneurs and property developers; the discrimination practised against Jews by the big City law firms until the 1970s; and the vast expansion of legal aid. In addition to the well-known names among the property developers there were many hundreds of smaller Jewish property investors, and among those who were spectacularly successful was a group of Jewish solicitors who decided to venture into the property market themselves. A cluster of law firms founded by Jews and connected with the big property companies—notably Nabarro Nathanson, Brechers, and Berwin Leighton—emerged in the West End, as did new firms on the fringes of the City, such as D. J. Freeman and Titmuss Sainer. The number of Jewish solicitors in London leapt from about 310 in 1950 to over 1,300 by 1990 and continued to rise with a large intake of bright Jewish graduates into City law firms, so that by the end of the century Jewish lawyers almost definitely outnumbered Jewish doctors practising in the capital; and the multiplicity of Jewish business enterprise enabled barristers from immigrant families to break into the area of commercial and tax law. After the Second World War a number of Jewish solicitors, through their involvement in local politics, became lord mayors of important towns, notable examples being Joshua Samuel Walsh in Leeds, Harry Sotnick in Portsmouth, and Arthur Goldberg in Plymouth, while others rendered outstanding service in public bodies at the national level.[3]

The shake-up in the legal world came a decade later than the upheavals in the health service, being in part a response to deep changes in social structure, in part a response to the ebbing of antisemitism, and in part a response to the

[3] *JC* 8 May 1970, p. 43 (obituary of Sotnick); *Law Society's Gazette*, 16 Mar. 1983 (obituary of Goldberg).

ripples flowing from the race relations legislation of the 1960s. It was not until 1968 that judges from east European family backgrounds were appointed to the High Court bench on a regular basis, and it was only in the 1970s that some of the biggest City law firms began to recruit women and Jews on a meritocratic basis and make Jews partners.

Throughout the 1930s a rigid hierarchical structure existed in the legal and medical professions in which Jews and women were allotted a subordinate place. Until the 1960s and 1970s it was on the whole necessary to conform to the public school and Oxbridge stereotype to be eligible for positions in the highest strata of the professions. Women, who had been admitted as medical students in large numbers during the First World War, found that most of the London medical schools were closed to them in the 1920s, while non-assimilated Jews were discriminated against in the City law firms and for appointments at senior hospital staff level. After the Second World War, and particularly in the 1960s and 1970s, Jews and women asserted their right to equality and challenged the 'nostalgic and antimodern vision of a smoothly functioning, non-egalitarian social order', demanding selection on the basis of merit.[4]

So far as the professions were concerned, the model espoused by Tony Kushner of pervasive antisemitism in the liberal society unless there was total conformity with its values is flawed, because exclusionary discrimination was practised against Jews in the higher levels of the professions specifically during the inter-war period rather than generally. On the other hand, William Rubinstein is also misguided in asserting that because Britain was a democratic and plural society antisemitism existed only at the margins. So far as Jewish general practitioners and young solicitors were concerned, there was antisemitism in the employment market before the Second World War. Nevertheless, the huge number of Jews graduating from the London and provincial medical schools between the wars, the ease with which panel practices were purchased by them in the open market, the admission of refugees into the British medical schools, and the ban on discriminatory advertising in the *British Medical Journal* all indicate that antisemitism, however fierce on occasions, had only a marginal effect on the entry of Jews into the medical profession.

Again, despite the discrimination in the job market for lawyers, the growth in the number of Jews in the legal profession was impeded more by structural factors, such as the modest degree of affluence enjoyed by the Anglo-Jewish community before 1939 and the restricted degree of legal aid available to potential clients, than by antisemitism, which was only of marginal importance as a direct barrier. Contrast this with the situation prevailing in Nazi Germany and Vichy France, where Jews were purged from the liberal professions by legislation;

[4] Paula E. Hyman, *Gender and Assimilation in Modern Jewish History: The Roles and Representation of Women* (Seattle, Wash.: University of Washington Press, 1995), 137.

'restrictions on "foreign influences" in law and medicine had been contemplated by France during the 1930s and the "invasion of the semites" specifically bemoaned'.[5] However, my research has shown that before the Second World War antisemitism was rife in the hospital system in England, and even after 1960 it influenced the selection of High Court judges and partners in City law firms. Thus until the 1960s and 1970s racial discrimination distorted the employment of Jews in the professions and hindered their advancement into the highest strata. Anesta Weekes QC echoed this finding when she claimed in 1999 that 'Some black professionals see two glass ceilings they have to get through: the Jewish level and then the white level.'[6]

Although the bulk of Anglo-Jewry has remained middle-class, a new, larger elite had emerged within the community by the 1990s. Its members, mostly of east European origin, were wealthy property developers and businessmen, top professionals in medicine and law firms, and High Court judges. Members of this elite may construct their own identity and are free to choose whether to lead a fully Jewish life or to assimilate, focusing solely on core professional values; within multiracial and multicultural Britain there is no longer any imperative to adhere to all the values of a liberal society with hidden agendas of its own, which were often corrosive of Jewish culture—as, for example, in the pressure on many top Jewish consultants of the 1930s to hide their identity, and in the Christian memorial services for Jewish benchers of the various Inns of Court. Antisemitism in Britain slowly declined once the State of Israel was established in 1948 and British troops were no longer in daily conflict with Jews. In addition, third-generation Jews were more comfortable in English society and more at ease with themselves. The social mobility of the east European immigrant Jews over three generations has been not only astonishing in itself but the most rapid of any ethnic group in Britain over this period. By dogged determination, hard work, and sheer ability, Jewish professionals broke through a succession of barriers in the 1960s and 1970s, so that the scandals involving Jews which erupted after that in the business world, such as the Guinness débâcle or the Robert Maxwell affair, did not interfere with their steady progress in the professions. Nevertheless, the conviction of the three Jewish defendants in the Guinness case caused much resentment in the community, the *Jewish Chronicle* remarking that 'there remains a considerable question mark over the imposition of prison sentences on

---

[5] Richard H. Weisberg, *Vichy Law and the Holocaust in France* (Amsterdam: Harwood Academic, 1996), 84, 85. 'It is difficult not to see the influence of the former Confédération des Syndicats Médicaux, as well as its other middle-class analogues, on Vichy's anti-Jewish program . . . the fact that these groups had put forth nearly all these demands in their prewar programs and had called for restrictions not only on foreigners but also on recently naturalized citizens, and even on citizens not born of French fathers, suggests a direct influence': Vicki Caron, *Uneasy Asylum: France and the Jewish Refugee Crisis, 1933–1942* (Stanford, Calif.: Stanford University Press, 1999), 326.

[6] *JC* 19 Nov. 1999, p. 19.

defendants found guilty of crimes in the takeover field at the time when this involved a very grey area of the law'.[7] These reservations were well justified; the European Court of Human Rights held that the trial was unfair and the defendants took their case to the Court of Appeal. Anger was also expressed by Jews at Clifford Longley's remark that they and Catholics 'feel slightly excluded from the dominant class and view the conventions of the country as being someone else's rather than being binding' on them.[8]

During the 1950s and 1960s there was a predominance of Jewish doctors over Jewish lawyers in England, but by the 1990s this situation had been reversed and Jewish lawyers were in a majority. Since the 1990s, there has been a decline generally in the number of applicants for medical schools in England, including Jewish school-leavers. The negative factors are the six-year training course for doctors and the tuition fees of £50,000, which can leave a trainee deeply in debt. Instead young Jews are going into banking, City law firms, accountancy, and management because they offer attractive starting salaries and good career prospects. A new wave of Asian recruits is entering the medical schools, re-enacting the involvement of Jews with the medical profession.[9]

Among these professionals today there is on the one hand an imperceptible drift by some out of the community, without pressure from the necessity for radical assimilation, and a switch by another group of professionals from the Orthodoxy of their fathers to Reform Judaism, which they find more compatible with the daily rhythm of their careers. It is quite possible that in post-war England, when there was a rapid expansion of Reform congregations in the suburbs and elsewhere, professionals may have spearheaded the flight of members out of Orthodox synagogues. On the other hand, despite the pressures on the leading professionals to conform with, for instance, memorial services in a Christian format for benchers of the Inns of Court, the close of the century witnessed a remarkable efflorescence of Jewish Orthodoxy, evident in the lunchtime *shiurim* (religious study sessions) in City law firms; top solicitors wearing a *kipah* (skullcap) on their heads, and not being afraid to leave early on Friday afternoons in the winter so as to be home before the sabbath; a Lord Chief Justice who is an adherent of an Orthodox synagogue; and a recent president of the Royal College of Physicians who is strongly identified as a Jew. Paradoxically, the coming of a multiracial and multicultural society in England, while giving some professionals the space to distance themselves from the Jewish community, gave others the sanction to be themselves and, like Samuel Stamler QC and David Goldberg QC among the lawyers and Professor Irving Taylor and Professor Stuart Stanton among the doctors, to adhere to Orthodoxy with a

---

[7] *JC* 31 Aug. 1990, p. 18.   [8] *JC* 7 Sept. 2001, p. 8.

[9] Mark Silvert, 'Is There a Doctor in the House? Maybe, but not a Jewish One', *London Jewish News*, 8 Mar. 2002.

new ease. And yet acceptance of Jews has been somewhat less than total, as indicated by the strange reluctance to clarify whether or not a Jew may occupy the position of Lord Chancellor, the highest law office in the land. As Anthony Julius has asserted, 'there is a certain resistance to them that is rarely expressed, and never legislated'.[10]

[10] 'England's Gifts to Jew Hatred', *Spectator*, 11 Nov. 2000.

Bibliography

Archives and Libraries

Board of Deputies Archive, London Metropolitan Archives (formerly Greater London Record Office)

Board of Deputies Defence Committee Archives, Board of Deputies Office, London

Bodleian Library, Oxford

British Library, National Sound Archive, London

British Medical Association Archive, London

Cambridge University Library

    Redcliffe Nathan Salaman papers, Cambridge University Library, Add. MS 8171, Box 1

Central Zionist Archives, Jerusalem, A255/881

    Norman Bentwich's diary

Committee of Vice-Chancellors and Principals Archive, London

David Cheyney Papers in the possession of the author

Education Aid Society, annual reports, London School of Jewish Studies

Home Office Medical Advisory Committee Records in the possession of Dr Philip D'Arcy Hart

Jewish Health Organisation of Great Britain, annual reports, University College Library, London

Jewish Museum, Finchley, London

London Jewish Hospital Medical Society Records in the possession of Dr Charles Daniels

London Metropolitan Archives (formerly Greater London Record Office)

Manchester Jewish Museum

Royal London Hospital Archive

    London Hospital Medical College Minute Book

    Redcliffe Salaman, 'The Helmsman Takes Charge' unpublished memoirs (n.d.)

Society for Jewish Jurisprudence, annual reports, London School of Jewish Studies

Southampton University, Parkes Library

    Education Aid Society, Minute Book, General Committee

    Neville Laski Papers

University of Leeds Archive

    University of Leeds Graduation List 1915–1922

    Faculty of Medicine Students' Record, vols. i and ii

Wellcome Library, London
　　Moran Papers
　　Plesch Papers
　　Charles Joseph Singer Papers

Parliamentary Papers

Report of the Joint Committee of the House of Lords and the House of Commons on the Moneylenders Bill PP 1924–25, vol. viii

Report of the House of Lords and House of Commons to Consider the Solicitors Bill 1939, PP 1938–9, vol. viii

Select Committee on the Conduct of a Member (Mr Boothby) PP 1940–41, vol. ii

Newspapers and Periodicals

AJR Information [AJR: Association of Jewish Refugees]
American Jewish Historical Quarterly
British Journal of Ophthalmology
British Medical Journal (BMJ)
Camden New Journal
Commercial Lawyer
Daily Express
Daily Mirror
Daily Telegraph
Estates Gazette
Evening Standard
Guardian
Ham & High
Independent
Jewish Academy
Jewish Chronicle (JC)
Jewish Historical Studies [formerly *Transactions of the Jewish Historical Society of England*]
Jewish Social Studies
Korot
Lancet
Law Society's Gazette
Lawyer
Legal Business
Legal Executive Journal
Leo Baeck Institute Year Book

London Jewish News
New York Law Journal
News of the World
Public Law
School Hygiene
Shalom
Solicitors' Journal
Sunday Times
The Times
Victorian Studies

Reference Books

The Annual Obituary, ed. Deborah Andrews (Detroit and London: St James's Press, 1992)

Chambers & Partners Directory of the Legal Profession 1995–1996 (London: Chambers & Partners, 1995)

Dictionary of Labour Biography, 10 vols.: vol. ix, ed. Joyce M. Bellamy and John Saville (Basingstoke: Macmillan, 1993)

Dictionary of National Biography

Sidney Lee (ed.), *Dictionary of National Biography* (London: Smith, Elder & Co., 1912), Second Supplement

J. R. H. Weaver (ed.), *Dictionary of National Biography* (London: Oxford University Press, 1937)

L. G. Wickham Legg (ed.), *Dictionary of National Biography 1931–1940* (London: Oxford University Press, 1949)

L. G. Wickham Legg and E. T. Williams (eds.), *Dictionary of National Biography 1941–1950* (Oxford: Oxford University Press, 1959)

E. T. Williams and C. S. Nicholls (eds.), *Dictionary of National Biography, 1961–1970* (Oxford: Oxford University Press, 1981)

Lord Blake and C. S. Nicholls (eds.), *Dictionary of National Biography 1971–1980* (Oxford: Oxford University Press, 1986)

Jewish Encyclopedia

Jewish Encyclopedia, vol. vii (New York: Funk & Wagnall's, 1916)

Jewish Encyclopedia (New York: Funk & Wagnall's, 1916), vol. xi

Jewish Year Book

Isidore Harris (ed.), *The Jewish Year Book 1909* (London: Greenberg & Co, 1909)

Isidore Harris (ed.), *The Jewish Year Book 1910* (London: Greenberg & Co, 1910)

Isidore Harris (ed.), *The Jewish Year Book 1922* (London: Jewish Chronicle, 1922)

S. Levy (ed.), *The Jewish Year Book 1933* (London: Jewish Chronicle, 1933)

The Jewish Year Book 1990 (London: Vallentine Mitchell, 1990)

The Law List (London: Stevens & Sons)

Volumes for 1919 (ed. Henry Birtles), 1929 (ed. Charles Connolly Gallagher), 1935 (ed. Frederick Greenwood), 1939 (ed. Percy Martin), 1949, 1950, 1955, 1956, 1957, 1966, 1967, 1968, 1970 (all ed. Leslie C. E. Turner)

Law Reports

The Times Law Reports, All England Law Reports, Appeal Cases, Bankruptcy and Companies Winding-up Cases, Butterworth's Company Law Cases, Chancery Division Reports, European Human Rights Reports, Weekly Law Reports

Lives of the Fellows of the Royal College of Obstetricians and Gynaecologists

John Peel (ed.), *Lives of the Fellows of the Royal College of Obstetricians and Gynaecologists* (London: Heinemann, 1976)

Lives of the Fellows of the Royal College of Physicians of London (Munk's Roll)

G. H. Brown (ed.), *Lives of the Fellows of the Royal College of Physicians of London 1826–1925*, vol. iv (London: Royal College of Physicians, 1955)

Richard Trail (ed.), *Lives of the Fellows of the Royal College of Physicians of London*, vol. v (1968)

Gordon Wolstenholme (ed.), *Lives of the Fellows of the Royal College of Physicians of London Continued to 1975*, vol. vi (Oxford: IRL, 1982)

Valerie Luniewska and Christopher Booth (eds.), *Lives of the Fellows of the Royal College of Physicians of London Continued to 1993*, vol. ix (London: Royal College of Physicians, 1994)

Lives of the Fellows of the Royal College of Surgeons of England

R. H. O. B. Robinson and W. R. Le Fanu (eds.), *Lives of the Fellows of the Royal College of Surgeons of England 1905–1956* (London: E. & S. Livingstone, 1970)

R. H. O. B. Robinson, W. R. Le Fanu, and Cecil Wakeley (eds.), *Lives of the Fellows of the Royal College of Surgeons of England 1952–1964* (Edinburgh and London: E. S. Livingstone, 1970)

Sir James Paterson Ross and W. R. Le Fanu (eds.), *Lives of the Fellows of the Royal College of Surgeons of England 1965–1973* (London: Pitman Medical, 1981)

E. H. Cornelius and S. F. Taylor (eds.), *Lives of the Fellows of the Royal College of Surgeons of England 1974–1982* (London: Royal College of Surgeons of England, 1988)

Ian Lyle and Selwyn Taylor (eds.), *Lives of the Fellows of the Royal College of Surgeons of England 1983–1990* (London: Royal College of Surgeons of England, 1995)

The Medical Directory (London: J. & A. Churchill)

Volumes for 1872, 1910, 1919, 1925, 1929, 1939, 1942, 1943, 1947, 1948, 1953, 1954, 1960, 1967, 1969, 1970, 1972, 1975, 1981, 1990, 1993

Solicitors and Barristers Directory 1990, ed. E. O'Connor (London: Waterlow, 1990)

Solicitors' Diary and Directory 1975, ed. William H. Edwards (London: Waterlow, 1975)

Transactions of the Jewish Historical Society of England 1924–1927, vol. 11 (1928)

The University of Leeds Calendar 1915–1916 (Leeds: Jowett & Sewry, 1915)

Who Was Who 1941–1950 (London: A. & C. Black, 1967)

Who's Who (London: A. & C. Black): volumes for 1996, 1999, 2000

General

ABEL-SMITH, BRIAN, and ROBERT STEVENS, *Lawyers and the Courts* (London: Heinemann, 1967).

ABINGER, EDWARD, *Forty Years at the Bar* (London: Hutchinson, 1930).

ABSE, LEO, *Private Member* (London: Macdonald, 1973).

ADAMSON, IAN, *The Old Fox* (London: Frederick Muller, 1963).

ALDERMAN, GEOFFREY, *London Jewry and London Politics 1889–1986* (London: Routledge, 1989).

—— *Modern British Jewry* (Oxford: Clarendon Press, 1998).

ALLFREY, ANTHONY, *Edward VII and his Jewish Court* (London: Weidenfeld & Nicolson, 1991).

ANDERSON, STUART, *Lawyers and the Making of English Law* (Oxford: Clarendon Press, 1992).

ANDREWS, JONATHAN, *et al.*, *The History of Bethlem* (London: Routledge, 1997).

ANNING, S. T., and W. K. J. WALLS, *A History of the Leeds School of Medicine: One and a Half Centuries 1831–1981* (Leeds: Leeds University Press, 1982).

ARIS, STEPHEN, *Arnold Weinstock and the Making of GEC* (London: Arum, 1998).

—— *The Jews in Business* (Harmondsworth: Penguin, 1973).

ASHBEL, RIVKA, *As Much As We Could Do* (Jerusalem: Magnes, 1989).

ASTAIRE, JARVIS, *Encounters* (London: Robson, 1999).

ASTOR, J. J., *et al.*, *Professor Samson Wright (1899–1956) in Memoriam* (London: Favil, 1956).

AUERBACH, JERROLD S., 'From Rags to Robes: The Legal Profession, Social Mobility and the American Jewish Experience', *American Jewish Historical Quarterly*, 66/2 (Dec. 1976), 249–84.

—— *Unequal Justice: Lawyers and Social Change in Modern America* (New York: Oxford University Press, 1972).

AYLETT, SYDNEY, *Under the Wigs* (London: Eyre Methuen, 1978).

BAKER, MICHAEL, *Our Three Selves: A Life of Radclyffe Hall* (London: Hamilton, 1985).

BARNETT, HENRIETTA, *Canon Barnett: His Life, Work and Friends* (London: Murray, 1921).

BARTRIP, P. W. J., *Mirror of Medicine: A History of the* British Medical Journal (Oxford: Clarendon Press, 1990).

BECKLEY, ELIZABETH, and DOROTHY USHER POTTER (eds.), *Ida and the Eye:*

A Woman in British Ophthalmology from the Autobiography of Ida Mann (Tunbridge Wells: Parapress, 1996).

BECKMAN, MORRIS, *The Hackney Crucible* (London: Vallentine Mitchell, 1996).

BEHLMER, GEORGE K., *Child Abuse and Moral Reform in England, 1870–1908* (Stanford, Calif.: Stanford University Press, 1982).

BELTON, NEIL, *The Good Listener. Helen Bamber: A Life Against Cruelty* (London: Weidenfeld & Nicolson, 1998).

BENTWICH, MARGERY, and NORMAN BENTWICH, *Herbert Bentwich: The Pilgrim Father* (Jerusalem: Hozaath Ivrith, 1940).

BENTWICH, NORMAN, *My Seventy Seven Years* (London: Routledge & Kegan Paul, 1962).

—— *They Found Refuge* (London: Cresset, 1956).

—— *The United Restitution Organisation 1948–1968* (London: Vallentine Mitchell, 1968).

BERGER, VINCENT, *Case Law in the European Court of Human Rights*, vol. i (Dublin: Round Hall, 1991).

BERGHAHN, MARION, *Continental Britons: German-Jewish Refugees from Nazi Germany* (Oxford: Berg, 1988).

BIRKS, MICHAEL, *Gentlemen of the Law* (London: Stevens & Sons, 1960).

BLACK, GERRY, 'Health and Medical Care of the Jewish Poor in the East End of London 1880–1914', Ph.D. diss. (Leicester University, 1987).

—— *Lender to the Lords, Giver to the Poor* (London: Vallentine Mitchell, 1992).

—— *Lord Rothschild and the Barber* (London: Tymsder, 2000).

BLAKENEY, MICHAEL, *Australia and the Jewish Refugees* (Sydney: Croom Helm, 1985).

BLOK, GEOFFREY D. M., 'Jewish Students at the Universities of Great Britain and Ireland Excluding London, 1936–1939: A Survey', *Sociological Review*, 34/3, 34/4 (1942), 183–97.

BOASE, FREDERIC (ed.), *Modern English Biography*, 6 vols.: vol. ii (London: Cass, 1965).

BOULTON, THOMAS G., *The Association of Anaesthetists of Great Britain and Ireland 1932–1992 and the Development of the Speciality of Anaesthesia* (London: Association of Anaesthetists, 1999).

BOWER, TOM, *Maxwell: The Final Verdict* (London: HarperCollins, 1996).

—— *Maxwell: The Outsider* (London: Mandarin, 1992).

BRESLER, FENTON, *Lord Goddard: A Biography of Rayner Goddard, Lord Chief Justice of England* (London: Harrap, 1977).

BRIVATI, BRIAN, *Lord Goodman* (London: Richard Cohen, 1999).

BROCKBANK, WILLIAM, *The Honorary Medical Staff of the Manchester Royal Infirmary 1830–1948* (Manchester: Manchester University Press, 1965).

BRODETSKY, SELIG, *Memories: From Ghetto to Israel* (London: Weidenfeld & Nicolson, 1960).

BROME, VINCENT, *Ernest Jones* (London: Caliban, 1982).

BROOK, STEPHEN, *The Club: The Jews of Modern Britain* (London: Pan, 1989).

BROOKS, MELVYN H., *Dr Hannah Billig 1901–1987. The Angel of Cable Street: Memories* (Karkur, Israel: privately printed, 1993).

BROWNE, DOUGLAS G., *Sir Travers Humphreys: A Biography* (London: Harrap, 1960).

BURNHAM, JOHN C., *How the Idea of Profession Changed the Writing of Medical History* (London: Wellcome Institute, 1998).

CALNE, ROY, *The Ultimate Gift: The Story of Britain's Premier Transplant Surgeon* (London: Headline, 1998).

CANTOR, NORMAN F., *The Sacred Chain: The History of the Jews* (New York: Harper-Perennial, 1995).

CARON, VICKI, *Uneasy Asylum: France and the Jewish Refugee Crisis, 1933–1942* (Stanford, Calif.: Stanford University Press, 1999).

CECIL (LEON), HENRY, *Memories and Reminiscences* (London: Hutchinson, 1975).

CESARANI, DAVID (ed.), *The Making of Anglo-Jewry* (Oxford: Blackwell, 1990).

CHALLONER, JACK, *The Baby Makers: The History of Artificial Conception* (London: Channel Four Books, 1999).

CHANCE, BURTON, *Ophthalmology* (New York: Hafner, 1962).

CLARK-KENNEDY, A. E., *The London. A Study of the Voluntary Hospital System: The Second Hundred Years* (London: Pitman Medical, 1963).

CLARKE, F. G., *Will-O-Wisp: Peter the Painter and the Anti-Tsarist Terrorists in Britain and Australia* (Melbourne: Oxford University Press, 1983).

CLINE, SALLY, *Radclyffe Hall: A Woman Called John* (London: Murray, 1997).

CLUTTERBUCK, DAVID, and MARION DEVINE, *Clore: The Man and his Millions* (London: Weidenfeld & Nicolson, 1987).

COHEN, LUCY, *Arthur Cohen* (London: Bickers & Son, 1919).

COHEN, SHELDON G., 'Landmark Commentary: Pepys on Farmer's Lung', *Allergy Proceedings*, 11/2 (Mar.–Apr. 1990), 97–9.

COLLINS, KENNETH, *Go and Learn: The International Story of Jews and Medicine in Scotland* (Aberdeen: Aberdeen University Press, 1988).

COLLINS, LAWRENCE, 'Dr F. A. Mann: His Work and Influence', *British Year Book of International Law*, 64 (1993), 55–111.

—— 'Francis Alexander Mann 1907–1991', *Proceedings of the British Academy*, 84 (1994), 393–407.

COOPER, JOHN, 'The Bloomstein and Isenberg Families', in Aubrey Newman (ed.), *The Jewish East End* (London: Jewish Historical Society of England, 1981).

—— *The Child in Jewish History* (Northvale, NJ: Aronson, 1996).

COOPER, R. M. (ed.), *Refugee Scholars: Conversations with Tess Simpson* (Leeds: Moorland, 1992).

CORK, KENNETH, *Cork on Cork* (London: Macmillan, 1988).

CROCKER, WILLIAM CHARLES, *Far from Humdrum: A Lawyer's Life* (London: Hutchinson, 1967).

CROSSMAN, RICHARD, *The Diaries of a Cabinet Minister*, ed. Janet Morgan, 2 vols. (London: Hamilton and Cape, 1975, 1976).

DAGLISH, N. D., 'Robert Morant's Hidden Agenda? The Origins of the Medical Treatment of Schoolchildren', *History of Education*, 19/2 (1990), 139–48.

DANBY, FRANK, *Dr Phillips: A Maida Vale Idyll* (London: Keynes, 1989).

DEARDEN, HAROLD, *The Fire Raisers: The Story of Leopold Harris and his Gang* (London: Heinemann, 1934).

DEESON, A. F. L., *Great Swindlers* (London: Foulsham, 1971).

DENNETT, LAURIE, *Slaughter and May: A Century in the City* (Cambridge: Granta, 1989).

DENNING, LORD, *The Discipline of Law* (London: Butterworths, 1979).

—— *The Due Process of Law* (London: Butterworths, 1980).

DICKENS, HENRY, *The Recollections of Sir Henry Dickens KC* (London: Heinemann, 1934).

DUNMAN, DANIEL, *The English and Colonial Bars in the Nineteenth Century* (London: Croom Helm, 1983).

DUNNAGE, JAMES ARTHUR, *The Modern Shylock* (London: E. J. Larby, 1926).

ECKSTEIN, HARRY, *Pressure Group Politics: The Case of the British Medical Association* (London: Allen & Unwin, 1960).

EDER, DAVID, *David Eder: Memoirs of a Pioneer*, ed. J. B. Hobman (London: Gollancz, 1945).

EDWARDS, RUTH DUDLEY, *Victor Gollancz: A Biography* (London: Gollancz, 1987).

EFRON, JOHN M. *Medicine and the German Jews* (New Haven: Yale University Press, 2001).

EMDEN, PAUL H., *Jews of Britain* (London: Sampson Low, Marston, 1943).

ENDELMAN, TODD M., *Radical Assimilation in English Jewish History, 1656–1945* (Bloomington, Ind.: Indiana University Press, 1990).

—— 'The Social and Political Context of Conversion in Germany and England 1870–1914', in id. (ed.), *Jewish Apostasy in the Modern World* (New York: Holmes & Meier, 1987).

ERDMAN, EDWARD L., *People and Property* (London: Batsford, 1982).

EVANS, ELI N., *Judah P. Benjamin: The Jewish Confederate* (New York: Free Press, 1988).

EYLER, JOHN M., *Sir Arthur Newsholme and State Medicine 1885–1935* (Cambridge: Cambridge University Press, 1997).

FALLON, IVAN, *Billionaire* (London: Hutchinson, 1991).

FAULKS, NEVILLE, *A Law Unto Myself* (London: Kimber, 1978).

FELDBERG, W., 'The Early History of Synaptic and Neuromuscular Transmission by Acetylcholine: Reminiscences of an Eye Witness', in A. L. Hodgkin *et al.* (eds.),

The Pursuit of Nature: Informal Essays on the History of Physiology (Cambridge: Cambridge University Press, 1977).

FELSTEIN, IVOR, *Later Life: Geriatrics Today and Tomorrow* (Harmondsworth: Penguin, 1969).

FENNELL, EDWARD, *Titmuss, Sainer & Webb: 50th Anniversary Brochure* (London: Titmuss, Sainer & Webb, 1997).

FEUER, LEWIS S., *Einstein and the Generations of Science* (New York: Basic Books, 1974).

FINESTEIN, ISRAEL, 'Arthur Cohen, Q.C. (1829–1914)', in John M. Shaftesley (ed.), *Remember the Days* (London: Jewish Historical Society of England, 1966).

FLEMING, G. H., *Lady Colin Campbell, Victorian Sex Goddess* (Milton-under-Wychwood, Glos.: Windrush Press, 1989).

FLETCHER, LORD [ARNOLD], *Random Reminiscences* (London: Bishopsgate, 1986).

FOOT, PAUL, *The Helen Smith Story* (London: Fontana, 1983).

FORMAN, DENIS, *To Reason Why* (London: Deutsch, 1991).

FRAENKEL, G. J., *Hugh Cairns: First Nuffield Professor of Surgery* (Oxford: Oxford University Press, 1991).

FREEMAN, IRIS, *Lord Denning: A Life* (London: Hutchinson, 1993).

FREEMAN, SIMON, and BARRIE PENROSE, *Rinkgate: The Rise and Fall of Jeremy Thorpe* (London: Bloomsbury, 1996).

FRIEDLANDER, SAUL, *Nazi Germany and the Jews: The Years of Persecution, 1933–1939* (London: Weidenfeld & Nicolson, 1997).

GALANTER, MARK, and THOMAS PALEY, *Tournament of Lawyers: The Transformation of the Big Law Firm* (Chicago: University of Chicago Press, 1991).

GARNER, JAMES STUART, 'The Great Experiment: The Admission of Women Students to St Mary's Hospital Medical School, 1916-1925', *Medical History*, 42 (1998), 68–88.

GAVRON, DANIEL, *Saul Adler: Pioneer of Tropical Medicine* (Rehovot: Balaban, 1997).

GIDNEY, R. D., and W. P. J. MILLAR, 'Medical Students at the University of Toronto 1910–1940: A Profile', *Canadian Bulletin of Medical History*, 13/1 (1996), 29–52.

GILBERT, BENTLEY B., *The Evolution of National Insurance in Great Britain* (London: Joseph, 1966).

GILLIS, BERNARD, 'Once Round Only' (unpublished memoirs).

GILMAN, SANDER, *The Jew's Body* (London: Routledge, 1991).

GLAZER, NATHAN, and DANIEL PATRICK MOYNIHAN, *Beyond the Melting Pot* (Cambridge, Mass.: MIT Press, 1968).

GOLDBERG, JACOB A., 'Jews in the Medical Profession: A National Survey', *Jewish Social Studies*, 1 (July 1939), 327–37.

GOLDSCHEIDER, CALVIN, and ALAN S. ZUCKERMAN, *The Transformation of the Jews* (Chicago: University of Chicago Press, 1984).

GOODHART, ARTHUR L., *Five Jewish Lawyers of the Common Law* (London: Oxford University Press, 1949).

GOODMAN, ARNOLD, *Tell Them I'm On My Way: Memoirs* (London: Chapman, 1993).

GOODMAN, RONALD A., *The Maccabeans: The Founding Fathers and the Early Years* (London: Maccabeans, 1979).

GOODMAN, SUSAN, *Spirit of Stoke Mandeville: The Story of Sir Ludwig Guttman* (London: Collins, 1986).

GORDON, CHARLES, *The Two Tycoons: A Personal Memoir of Jack Cotton and Charles Clore* (London: Hamilton, 1984).

GRADE, LEW, *Still Dancing: My Story* (London: Collins, 1987).

GRANSHAW, LINDSAY PATRICIA, 'St Thomas's Hospital, London, 1850–1900', Ph.D. diss. (Bryn Mawr College, 1981).

GRAY, CHARLES, *The Irving Judgment: David Irving v. Penguin Books and Professor Deborah Lipstadt* (Harmondsworth: Penguin, 2000).

GRIFFITH, J. A. G., *The Politics of the Judiciary* (London: Fontana, 1985)

GRIGG, MARY, *The Challenor Case* (Harmondsworth: Penguin, 1965).

GRUZENBERG, O. O., *Memoirs of a Russian-Jewish Lawyer*, ed. Don C. Rawson (Berkeley and Los Angeles: University of California Press, 1981).

HACKER, ROSE, *Abraham's Daughter: The Autobiography of Rose Hacker* (London: Deptford Forum, 1996).

HAMANN, BRIGITTE, *Hitler's Vienna: A Dictator's Apprenticeship* (New York: Oxford University Press, 1999).

HAVERS, MICHAEL, EDWARD GRAYSON, and PETER SHANKLAND, *The Royal Baccarat Scandal* (London: Kimber, 1977).

HAZARD, GEOFFREY C., and DEBORAH L. RHODE (eds.), *The Legal Profession: Responsibility and Regulation* (Westbury, NY: Foundation, 1988).

HENDRICK, HARRY, *Child Welfare in England 1872–1989* (London: Routledge, 1994).

HENRIQUES, H. S. Q., *The Jews and English Law* (Oxford: Oxford University Press, 1908).

HENRIQUES, ROBERT, *Sir Robert Waley Cohen 1877–1952* (London: Secker & Warburg, 1966).

HENRY, TERESA, *Partnership: The Story of Simmons & Simmons* (London: Granta, 1996).

HILTON, CLAIRE, 'St Bartholomew's Hospital London, and its Jewish Connections', *Jewish Historical Studies*, 30 (1987–8), 21–50.

HOLLIS, PATRICIA, *Jennie Lee: A Life* (Oxford: Oxford University Press, 1997).

HOMA, BERNARD, *Footprints in the Sands of Time* (Charfield, Glos.: Charfield, 1990).

HONIGSBAUM, FRANK, *The Division in British Medicine* (London: Kogan Page, 1979).

HOPKINS, PHILIP, 'Who was Dr Michael Balint?', in John Salinsky (ed.), *Proceedings of the Eleventh International Balint Congress 1998* (Southport: Balint Society, 1999).

HORN, JOSHUA S., *Away With All Pests: An English Surgeon in People's China* (London: Hamlyn, 1969).

HUGHES, A. G., 'Jews and Gentiles: Their Intellectual and Temperamental Differences', *Eugenics Review* (July 1928), 89–94.

HUGHES, EMRYS, *Sydney Silverman: Rebel in Parliament* (London: Skilton, 1969).

HURST, ARTHUR, *A Twentieth Century Physician* (London: Arnold, 1949).

HURST, GERALD, *Closed Chapters* (Manchester: Manchester University Press, 1942).

HYDE, H. MONTGOMERY, *Norman Birkett* (London: Reprint Society, 1965).

—— *Sir Patrick Hastings: His Life and Cases* (London: Heinemann, 1960).

—— *Strong for Service: The Life of Lord Nathan of Churt* (London: Allen, 1968).

HYMAN, LOUIS, *The Jews of Ireland* (London: Jewish Historical Society of England, 1972).

HYMAN, PAULA E., *Gender and Assimilation in Modern Jewish History: The Roles and Representation of Women* (Seattle, Wash.: University of Washington Press, 1995).

INGRAMS, RICHARD, *Goldenballs* (London: Deutsch, 1979).

ISAACS, GERALD RUFUS, *Rufus Isaacs, First Marquess of Reading*, 2 vols., i: *1860–1914*; ii: *1914–1935* (London: Hutchinson, 1942, 1945).

JACKSON, ALAN A., *Semi-Detached London* (London: Allen & Unwin, 1973).

JACKSON, ROBERT, *The Chief: The Biography of Gordon Hewart, Lord Chief Justice of England 1922-40* (London: Harrap, 1959).

JACOBS, ALETTA, *Memories: My Life as an International Leader in Health, Suffrage, and Peace* (New York: Feminist Press at the City University of New York, 1996).

JACOBS, JOSEPH, *Studies in Jewish Statistics: Social, Vital and Anthropometric* (London: D. Nutt, 1891).

JACOBY, N. M., *A Journey through Medicine* (Sussex: Book Guild, 1991).

JAMES, RICHARD RHODES, *Bob Boothby: A Portrait* (London: Hodder & Stoughton, 1991).

JANNER, ELSIE, *Barnett Janner: A Personal Portrait* (London: Robson, 1984).

JENKINS, ROY, *A Life at the Centre* (London: Macmillan, 1991).

JOHNSTONE, QUINTIN, and DAN HOPSON, *Lawyers and their Work: An Analysis of the Legal Profession in the United States and England* (New York: Bobbs-Merrill, 1967).

JOLOWICZ, J. A., and T. ELLIS LEWIS, *Winfield on Tort* (London: Sweet & Maxwell, 1963).

JONES, ROBERT, and OLIVER MARRIOTT, *Anatomy of a Merger: A History of G.E.C., A.E.I. and English Electric* (London: Cape, 1970).

JOSEPHS, ZOE (ed.), *Birmingham Jewry*, ii: *More Aspects, 1740–1930* (Birmingham: Birmingham Jewish History Research Group, 1984; vol. i 1980).

JUDSON, HORACE FREELAND, *The Eighth Day of Creation: Makers of the Revolution in Biology* (London: Penguin, 1995).

JUXON, JOHN, *Lewis and Lewis* (London: Collins, 1983).

KADISH, SHARMAN, *Bolsheviks and British Jews: The Anglo-Jewish Community, Britain and the Russian Revolution* (London: Cass, 1992).

KAPRALIK, C. I., *Reclaiming the Nazi Loot: The History of the Work of the Jewish Trust Corporation for Germany* (London: privately printed, 1962).

KELLY, THOMAS, *For the Advancement of Learning: The University of Liverpool 1881–1981* (Liverpool: Liverpool University Press, 1981).

KERSHEN, ANNE J., and JONATHAN ROMAIN, *Tradition and Change: A History of Reform Judaism in Britain 1840–1995* (London: Vallentine Mitchell, 1995).

KESSNER, THOMAS, *The Golden Door: Italian and Jewish Immigrant Mobility in New York City 1880–1915* (New York: Oxford University Press, 1977).

KING-HAMILTON, ALAN, *And Nothing but the Truth* (London: Weidenfeld & Nicolson, 1982).

KLEIN, EMMA, *Lost Jews* (Basingstoke: Macmillan Press, 1996).

KOKOSALAKIS, N., *Ethnic Identity and Religion: Tradition and Change in Liverpool Jewry* (Washington, DC: University Press of America, 1982).

KOVACS, MARIA M., *Liberal Professions and Illiberal Politics: Hungary from the Hapsburgs to the Holocaust* (New York: Oxford University Press, 1994).

KREBS, HANS, *Reminiscences and Reflections* (Oxford: Clarendon Press, 1981).

KUCHEROV, SAMUEL, *Courts, Lawyers and Trials under the Last Three Tsars* (New York: Praeger, 1953).

KUSHNER, TONY, 'The Impact of British Anti-Semitism 1918–1945', in David Cesarani (ed.), *The Making of Anglo-Jewry* (Oxford: Blackwell, 1990).

—— *The Persistence of Prejudice: Antisemitism in British Society during the Second World War* (Manchester: Manchester University Press, 1989).

LACHS, PHYLLIS S., 'A Study of a Professional Elite: Anglo-Jewish Barristers in the Nineteenth Century', *Jewish Social Studies*, 44 (1982), 125–34.

LESTER, ANTHONY, and GEOFFREY BINDMAN, *Race Law* (London: Longman, 1972).

LEVY, ARNOLD, *History of the Sunderland Jewish Community 1755–1955* (London: Macdonald, 1956).

LEWIS, AUBREY, 'Psychiatry and the Jewish Tradition', in *The Later Papers of Sir Aubrey Lewis* (Oxford: Oxford University Press, 1979).

LEWIS, J. R., *The Victorian Bar* (London: Hale, 1982).

LIPMAN, V. D., *Social History of the Jews in England 1850–1950* (London: Watts, 1954).

LIPMAN, VIVIAN, *A Century of Social Service 1859–1959: The History of the Jewish Board of Guardians* (London: Routledge & Kegan Paul, 1959).

—— *A History of Jews in Britain since 1858* (Leicester: Leicester University Press, 1990).

LIPSTEIN, KURT, 'The History of the Contribution to Law by German-Speaking Jewish Refugees in the United Kingdom', in Werner E. Mosse (ed.), *Second*

Chance: Two Centuries of German-Speaking Jews in the United Kingdom (Tübingen: Mohr, 1991).

LOVELL, RICHARD, 'Choosing People: An Aspect of the Life of Lord Moran (1882–1977)', *Medical History*, 36 (1992).

—— *Churchill's Doctor: A Biography of Lord Moran* (London: Royal Society of Medicine, 1992).

MCGLYNN, CLARE, *The Woman Lawyer Making the Difference* (London: Butterworths, 1998).

MCLEAVE, HUGH, *A Time to Heal: The Life of Ian Aird, the Surgeon* (London: Heinemann, 1964).

MALLESON, KATE, *The New Judiciary: The Effects of Expansion and Activism* (Aldershot: Dartmouth, 1999).

MANN, KALMAN JACOB, *Reflections on a Life in Health Care* (Jerusalem: Rubin Mass, 1994).

MARGOLIN, A. D., *The Jews of Eastern Europe* (New York: Seltzer, 1926).

MARKS, D. W., and A. LOWY, *Memoir of Sir Francis Goldsmid* (London: Kegan Paul, Trench & Co., 1882).

MARRIOTT, OLIVER, *The Property Boom* (London: Hamilton, 1967).

MATTHEWS, LESLIE G., 'The Aldersgate Dispensary and the Aldersgate Medical School', *Pharmaceutical Historian*, 13/3 (Sept. 1983), 7–10.

—— 'Will of Dr Jonathan Pereira', *Pharmaceutical Historian*, 14/1 (Mar. 1984), 5.

MEDAWAR, JEAN, and DAVID PYKE, *Hitler's Gift: Scientists who Fled Nazi Germany* (London: Richard Cohen, 2000).

MORTON, JAMES, *Bent Coppers: A Survey of Police Corruption* (London: Little, Brown, 1993).

NAPLEY, DAVID, *Not Without Prejudice: The Memoirs of Sir David Napley* (London: Harrap, 1982).

O'NEILL, JAMES E., 'Finding a Policy for the Sick Poor', *Victorian Studies*, 7/3 (Mar. 1964), 256–84.

ORCHARD, DOROTHY JOHNSON, and GEOFFREY MAY, *Moneylending in Great Britain* (New York: Russell Sage Foundation, 1933).

PAGET, R. T., S. S. SILVERMAN, and CHRISTOPHER HOLLIS, *Hanged—and Innocent?* (London: Gollancz, 1953).

PAPPWORTH, M. H., *Human Guinea Pigs: Experimentation in Man* (Harmondsworth: Penguin, 1969).

—— 'Human Guinea Pigs: A Warning', *Twentieth Century* (Autumn 1962), 66–75.

PATERSON, M. JEANNE, *The Medical Profession in Mid-Victorian London* (Berkeley and Los Angeles: University of California Press, 1978).

PERLMANN, JOEL, *Ethnic Differences: Schooling and Social Structure Among the Irish,*

Italians, Jews and Blacks in an American City 1880–1935 (Cambridge: Cambridge University Press, 1988).

PHILLIPS, LAURENCE, *London Jewish Hospital Medical Society* (London: n.p., 1964).

PLESCH, JOHN, *Janos: The Story of a Doctor* (London: Gollancz, 1947).

PODMORE, DAVID, *Solicitors and the Wider Community* (London: Heinemann, 1980).

PONTING, CLIVE, *The Right to Know: The Inside Story of the Belgrano Affair* (London: Sphere, 1985).

PORTER, ROY, *The Greatest Benefit to Mankind* (London: Fontana, 1999).

PRITCHARD, JOHN, *The Legal 500* (London: Legalease, 1991).

PROCTOR, ROBERT N., *Racial Hygiene: Medicine under the Nazis* (Cambridge, Mass.: Harvard University Press, 1988).

PRYWES, MOSHE, *Prisoner of Hope* (Hanover, NE: Brandeis University Press, 1996).

PYKE, DAVID A., 'The Great Insanity: Hitler and the Destruction of German Science', *Journal of the Royal College of Physicians of London* (May/June 1995).

RAPHAEL, ADAM, *My Learned Friends* (London: Allen, 1989).

READING, EVA, *For the Record: Memoirs of Eva, Marchioness of Reading* (London: Hutchinson, 1973).

RICE, ROBERT, *The Business of Crime* (London: Gollancz, 1956).

ROBERTS, GEOFFREY DORLING, *Law and Life* (London: Allen, 1964).

ROBERTS, JEFF, and MALCOLM PINES (eds.), *The Practice of Group Analysis* (London: Routledge, 1991).

ROBERTSON, DAVID, *Judicial Discretion in the House of Lords* (Oxford: Clarendon Press, 1998).

ROGERS, JOSEPH, *Reminiscences of a Workhouse Medical Officer* (London: Unwin, 1989).

ROSE, AUBREY, *Brief Encounters of a Legal Kind* (Harpenden, Herts.: Lennard, 1998).

ROSE, DAVID, *In the Name of the Law: The Collapse of Criminal Justice* (London: Cape, 1996).

ROSENFELD, LOUIS, *Thomas Hodgkin: Morbid Anatomist and Social Activist* (Lanham, Md.: Madison, 1993).

ROSS, ALEXANDER MICHAEL, 'The Care and Education of Pauper Children in England and Wales', Ph.D. diss. (London University), 1955.

ROTH, CECIL, *The Great Synagogue 1690–1940* (London: Edward Goldston, 1950).

ROZENBERG, JOSHUA, *The Search for Justice: An Anatomy of the Law* (London: Sceptre, 1995).

—— *Trial of Strength: The Battle between Ministers and Judges over Who Makes the Laws* (London: Richard Cohen, 1999).

ROZENBLIT, MARSHA L., *The Jews of Vienna 1867–1914: Assimilation and Identity* (Albany, NY: State University of New York, 1983).

RUBINSTEIN, STANLEY, *John Citizen and the Law* (Harmondsworth: Penguin, 1947).

RUBINSTEIN, W. D., *A History of the Jews in the English-Speaking World: Great Britain* (Basingstoke: Macmillan, 1996).

—— *Men of Property: The Very Wealthy in Britain since the Industrial Revolution* (London: Croom Helm, 1981).

RUPPIN, ARTHUR, *The Jews in the Modern World* (London: Macmillan, 1934).

SABELL, A. G., 'The History of Contact Lenses', in Anthony J. Phillips and Janet Stone (eds.), *Contact Lenses: A Textbook for Practitioner and Student* (London: Butterworths, 1985).

SACHER, HARRY, *Zionist Portraits and Other Essays* (London: Blond, 1959).

SACKS, OLIVER, *Uncle Tungsten: Memories of a Chemical Boyhood* (London: Picador, 2001).

ST GEORGE, ANDREW, *A History of Norton Rose* (Cambridge: Granta, 1995).

SAKULA, ALEC, 'Samson Wright (1899–1956), Physiologist Extraordinary', *Journal of the Royal Society of Medicine*, 92 (Sept. 1999), 484–6.

—— 'Sir Arthur Hurst (1879–1944), Master of Medicine', *Journal of Medical Biography*, 7 (1999), 125–9.

SALAMAN, REDCLIFFE, *The History and Social Influence of the Potato* (Cambridge: Cambridge University Press, 1985).

SAMUEL, EDGAR ROY, 'Anglo-Jewish Notaries and Scriveners', *Transactions of the Jewish Historical Society of England*, 17 (1953), 113–59.

SAMUEL, RAPHAEL, *East End Underworld: Chapters in the Life of Arthur Harding* (London: Routledge & Kegan Paul, 1981).

SARGANT, WILLIAM, *The Unquiet Mind* (London: Heinemann, 1967).

SAUNDERS, JAMES, *Nightmare: Ernest Saunders and the Guinness Affair* (London: Arrow, 1990).

SCHWAB, WALTER M., *B'nai B'rith. The First Lodge of England: A Record of Fifty Years* (London: Wolff, 1960).

SEFTON, W. VICTOR, 'Growing up Jewish in London 1920-1950: A Perspective from 1973', in Dov Noy and Issachar Ben-Ami (eds.), *Studies in the Cultural Life of the Jews in England* (Jerusalem: Magnes, 1975).

SEIDLER, FRITZ, *The Bloodless Pogrom* (London: Gollancz, 1934).

SELBOURNE, DAVID, *Not an Englishman: Conversations with Lord Goodman* (London: Sinclair-Stevenson, 1993).

SELWYN, FRANCIS, *Nothing but Revenge: The Case of Bentley and Craig* (Harmondsworth: Penguin, 1988).

SEMON, FELIX, *The Autobiography of Sir Felix Semon* (London: Jarrold, 1926).

SHERMAN, A. J., *Island Refuge: Britain and Refugees from the Third Reich 1933–1939* (London: Frank Cass, 1994).

SILBERMAN, CHARLES, *A Certain People: American Jews and their Lives Today* (New York: Summit, 1985).

SILMAN, JULIUS, *Signifying Nothing* (London: Minerva, 1997).

SILVERT, MARK, 'Is There a Doctor in the House? Maybe, but not a Jewish One', *London Jewish News*, 8 Mar. 2002.

SKIDELSKY, ROBERT, *John Maynard Keynes: Fighting for Britain 1937–1946* (London: Macmillan, 2000).

SLINN, JUDY, *Clifford Chance: Its Origins and Development* (Cambridge: Granta, 1993).

—— *Linklaters & Paines: The First One Hundred and Fifty Years* (London: Longman, 1987).

SMIGEL, ERWIN O., *The Wall Street Lawyer* (Bloomington, Ind.: Indiana University Press, 1969).

SOKOLOFF, LEON, 'The Rise and Decline of the Jewish Quota in Medical School Admissions', *Bulletin of the New York Academy of Medicine*, 68 (1992), 497–517.

SOLOMON, FLORA, and BARNETT LITVINOFF, *Baku to Baker Street: The Memoirs of Flora Solomon* (London: Collins, 1984).

SOLOMONS, BETHEL, *One Doctor in his Time* (London: Johnson, 1956).

SORIN, GERALD, *The Prophetic Minority: American Jewish Immigrant Radicals 1880–1920* (Bloomington, Ind.: Indiana University Press, 1985).

SORSBY, ARNOLD, 'John Zachariah Laurence: A Belated Tribute', *British Journal of Ophthalmology*, 16 (1932), 727–40.

STAR, LEONIE, *Julius Stone: An Intellectual Life* (Melbourne: Oxford University Press, 1992).

STARR, PAUL, *The Social Transformation of American Medicine* (New York: Basic Books, 1982).

STENGEL, ERWIN, *Suicide and Attempted Suicide* (Harmondsworth: Penguin, 1964).

STEVENS, ROBERT, *The Independence of the Judiciary: The View from the Lord Chancellor's Office* (Oxford: Clarendon Press, 1993).

—— *Law and Politics: The House of Lords as a Judicial Body 1800–1976* (London: Weidenfeld & Nicolson, 1979).

STONE, LAWRENCE, *The Road to Divorce* (Oxford: Oxford University Press, 1995).

STREET, HARRY, *Freedom: The Individual and the Law* (Harmondsworth: Penguin, 1977).

SULLIVAN, A. M., *The Last Serjeant: The Memoirs of Serjeant A. M. Sullivan QC* (London: Macdonald, 1952).

SYKES, CHRISTOPHER, *Evelyn Waugh* (London: Collins, 1975).

TANSEY, E. M., D. A. CHRISTIE, and L. A. REYNOLDS (eds.), *Wellcome Witnesses to Twentieth Century Medicine*, vol. ii (London: Wellcome Trust, 1998).

TEMKIN, SEFTON, *Bertram B. Benas: The Life and Times of a Jewish Victorian* (Albany, NY: State University Press of New York, 1978).

TEVETH, SHABTAI, *Ben-Gurion: The Burning Ground 1886–1948* (London: Hale, 1987).

THIRLWELL, ANGELA, *A Century of Practice: Isadore Goldman & Son 1885–1985* (London: Isadore Goldman & Son, 1985).

TOBIAS, J. J., *Prince of Fences: The Life and Crimes of Ikey Solomon* (London: Vallentine Mitchell, 1974).

TROPP, ASHER, *Jews in the Professions in Great Britain 1891–1991* (London: Maccabeans, 1991).

TUTTLE, ELIZABETH ORMAN, *The Crusade against Capital Punishment in Great Britain* (London: Stevens, 1961).

WAKOV, SEYMOUR, *Lawyers in the Making* (Chicago: Aldine, 1965).

WALKER-SMITH, DEREK, *Lord Reading and his Cases* (London: Chapman & Hall, 1934).

WASSERMAN, MANFRED, and SAMUEL KOTTEK (eds.), *Health and Disease in the Holy Land* (Lampeter: Mellen, 1996).

WAYDENFELD, STEFAN, *The Ice Road* (Edinburgh: Mainstream, 1999).

WEBSTER, CHARLES, *The Health Service since the War*, vol. i (London: HMSO, 1988).

—— *The National Health Service: A Political History* (Oxford: Oxford University Press, 1998).

—— (ed.), *General Practice under the National Health Service 1948–1997* (Oxford: Clarendon Press, 1998).

WEINDLING, PAUL, 'Austrian Medical Refugees in Great Britain: From Marginal Aliens to Established Professionals', *Wiener Klinische Wochenschrift*, 110/4–5 (27 Feb. 1998), 158–61.

—— 'The Contribution of Central European Jews to Medical Science and Practice in Britain: The 1930s-1950s', in Werner E. Mosse (ed.), *Second Chance: Two Centuries of German-Speaking Jews in the United Kingdom* (Tübingen: Mohr, 1991).

—— 'The Impact of German Medical Scientists on British Medicine: A Case Study of Oxford, 1933–45', in Mitchell G. Ash and Alfons Sollner (eds.), *Forced Migration and Scientific Change* (Cambridge: Cambridge University Press, 1996).

—— 'Jews in the Medical Profession in Britain and Germany: Problems of Comparison', in Michael Brenner, Rainer Liedke, and David Rechter (eds.), *Two Nations: British and German Jews in Comparative Perspective* (Tübingen: Mohr Siebeck, 1999).

WEISBERG, RICHARD H., *Vichy Law and the Holocaust in France* (Amsterdam: Harwood Academic, 1996).

WEIZMANN, CHAIM, *The Letters and Papers of Chaim Weizmann*, ser. A, 23 vols. (Jerusalem: Israel Universities Press, 1968–80): vol. xi, ed. Bernard Wasserstein (1974); vol. xiv, ed. Camillo Dresner (1977).

—— *Trial and Error* (London: Hamish Hamilton, 1949).

WEIZMANN, VERA, *The Impossible Takes Longer* (London: Hamilton, 1967).

WENGER, BETH S., *New York Jews and the Great Depression* (New Haven: Yale University Press, 1996).

WESTMAN, STEPHEN K., *A Surgeon's Story* (London: Kimber, 1962).

WILD, RONALD, and DEREK CURTIS-BENNETT, *'Curtis': The Life of Sir Henry Curtis-Bennett KC* (London: Cassell, 1937).

WILLIAMS, BILL, *The Making of Manchester Jewry 1740–1875* (Manchester: Manchester University Press, 1985).

WINNER, DAVID, *They Called Him Mr Brighton: A Biography of the Socialist Peer Lewis Cohen* (Lewes: Book Guild, 1999).

WOFFINDEN, BOB, *Hanratty: The Final Verdict* (London: Macmillan, 1997).

WOOLF, LEONARD, *Sowing an Autobiography of the Years 1880 to 1904* (London: Hogarth, 1960).

WOOLF, SIDNEY, *The Winding-up of Companies by the Court* (London: Reeves & Turner, 1891).

WORMS, FRED S., *A Life in Three Cities* (London: Halban, 1996).

YOUNG, LORD (DAVID), *The Enterprise Years: A Businessman in the Cabinet* (London: Headline, 1990).

YOUNG-BRUEHL, ELISABETH, *Anna Freud* (London: Macmillan, 1991).

Index of Personal Names

Index of Subjects

Printed and bound by CPI Group (UK) Ltd, Croydon, CR0 4YY

27/10/2024

14580406-0004